The History of
ORTHOPAEDICS

Multum egerunt, qui ante nos fuerunt.

Seneca

The History of ORTHOPAEDICS

An Account of the Study and Practice of
Orthopaedics from the Earliest Times to the Modern Era

David Le Vay

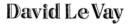

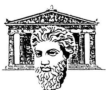

The Parthenon Publishing Group
International Publishers in Science, Technology & Education

Casterton Hall, Carnforth,
Lancs, LA6 2LA, UK

120 Mill Road, Park Ridge,
New Jersey, USA

Published in the UK by
The Parthenon Publishing Group Limited
Casterton Hall, Carnforth,
Lancs, LA6 2LA, England

Published in the USA by
The Parthenon Publishing Group Inc.
120 Mill Road,
Park Ridge,
New Jersey 07656, USA

British Library Cataloguing in Publication Data
Le Vay, David, *1915–*
  A history of orthopaedics.
  1. Medicine. Orthopaedics, history
  I. Title
  617′. 309

  ISBN 1-85070-145-8

Library of Congress Cataloging-in-Publication Data
Le Vay, David.
  A history of orthopaedics/by David Le Vay.
    p. cm.
  ISBN 0-940813-81-5 : $75.00 (est.)
  1. Orthopedics–History. I. Title
  [DNLM: 1. Orthopedics–history. WE 11.1 L656h]
RD725.L4 1989
617.3′009-dc20
DNLM/DLC   89-2548S
for Library of Congress   CIP

Phototypesetting by Lasertext Ltd., Manchester
Printed and bound in Great Britain by
Butler & Tanner Ltd., Frome and London

Contents

Section 3. Special Subjects

Section 4. The Turn of the Century

Section 5. The Effects of War on Orthopaedic Surgery

Preface

It is a quite remarkable fact that until now there has been no true history of orthopaedics, in any language, dealing with the subject in its entirety from antiquity to the present day. Why this should be so is perhaps not difficult to understand: to put it briefly, the clinicians have been too busy and the historians have lacked the practical knowledge. Of essays, articles and chapters in books there has been no dearth; even the busiest surgeon can find time to write about his special interests and such writings have been valuable in the compilation of this work. There are also a few books of great interest but essentially fragmentary: fascinating to read but not true histories methodologically considered. These include Keith's *Menders of the Maimed* (1919), Bick's *Source Book of Orthopaedics* (1948) and Mercer Rang's *Anthology of Orthopaedics* (1966).

The nearest approach to a true continuous history is Valentin's *Die Geschichte der Orthopädie* of 1961. It was possible for Valentin to produce this work of great scholarship only because, when he had reached the heights of clinical and academic orthopaedic achievement, he was expelled from Germany by the Nazis and courageously made use of the opportunity. When I came to translate this, my eyes were opened. I knew all about Hugh Owen Thomas, in Britain, for I had written his *Life*[1]. I did not know that among the fathers of orthopaedics we must also include Venel of Switzerland and Delpech of France, for no-one had ever brought them to general notice. Even now, their names are not exactly household words in our discipline. Nevertheless, Valentin's book, though required reading, had its defects. It did not extend beyond 1900, it was Central European in style and orientation, and it was virtually silent on many important topics. The author himself described it as 'only a torso' and used to discuss with me what more needed to be done.

It therefore seemed that an imperative imposed itself, though the task was a daunting one. My qualifications, such as they were, were that I had managed to combine a career as head of the orthopaedic department of a large London hospital with a parallel career as an author, editor and translator. A year's secondment to the World Health Organization as an editor and a long-lasting association with *Excerpta Medica* of Amsterdam and then with Springer-Verlag of Heidelberg had provided experience in the management of masses of technical material. Given the time, something might yet be done. This time was encroached on by the demands of work in the Third World, by an intrinsic inertia and by life-threatening illness; but, once I had committed myself, the problem was to know where to stop, a problem familiar to those engaged in such undertakings. I sometimes wondered whether such a book were not more properly work for a committee rather than an individual; but the only good book written by a committee is the Authorised Version of the Bible.

Once embarked, I received the greatest help and encouragement from the individuals and institutions listed below. The perennial problem was whether to organize the too-abundant material by topic or by epoch, by individual or by country; in the event, I have tried to combine these approaches, with what success it is for the reader to say. He will assuredly be able to point to this error and that omission, and to deplore some of my enthusiasms, but I hope to have at least touched on most of what is relevant. Ideally, I would like to absorb the criticisms and have a second innings, but that is not in my hands.

Any history of orthopaedics must deal with the history of orthopaedic disease; the history of orthopaedics as a discipline, i.e. the evolution of a natural history and of principles of management; and the history of orthopaedic surgery. Orthopaedic disease is simply something that happens to vertebrates and is to be found in Stone Age man and in the fossil record. The discipline began in ancient Egypt and Greece, India and China, thousands of years ago. But orthopaedic surgery, in anything like the form we know today, is a relative upstart, with its history a matter of a mere 200 years or so. Yet the pace of recent technical advance has been so rapid that the whole subject has become, as it were, foreshortened; we are in danger of forgetting our origins and the ineluctable rules of biologic process, so dazzling are the new techniques.

Although it is not quite true that there is nothing new under the sun, it is nevertheless chastening, and amusing, to discover how often procedures thought to be new had been practised long before, or thought of before the appropriate technology was available. The first hip replacement was attempted in the 1890s, at much the same time that Lister was experimenting with the penicillin mould in the wards of King's College Hospital in London. It can almost be laid down as an axiom that, if a surgeon claims loudly to be doing something for the first time, he is wrong. Conversely, whenever in the past the eminent have argued that a projected advance was impracticable, or arrogant, or against the will of God, they too were usually proved wrong very smartly – as if the coming event, whether of the magnitude of anaesthesia or of the prevention of poliomyelitis, had cast such a shadow before as to defeat rational consideration.

What is history? The current texts I read as a student are certainly historical by now. When I was presumptuous enough, many years ago, to write a *Synopsis of Orthopaedics*, the books I then relied on – the great *Textbook* of Jones and Lovett, the *Robert Jones Birthday Volume*, Brailsford's *Radiology of Bones and Joints* and others – have now been swept into the past, though still worth reading. The pace of advance is such that what was written even a few years ago is already out of date. If you read the journals systematically backwards, as you must in this endeavour, there is a very queer, even ghostly, moment when you realise that what you are holding is *of the past*: it has happened imperceptibly, the boundary cannot be defined, but one has stepped from the present into history. Sometimes the landmarks seem clear enough. Anaesthesia, asepsis, radiology, antibiotics and joint replacement seem to demarcate epochs as sharply as armistices. But this is probably illusory, for biologic process does not change and Nature, as Horace remarks, will return even if we expel her with a pitchfork.

I am not a professional historian, but I imagine that the essential problem in writing about any discipline is that no system can be defined in its own terms; we need an external stance, and do not have one. The past may look ordered enough when written down, but that is factitious; even if we can see where we have been we are in no position to judge the present; all we can predict about the future is that it is unpredictable.

I often think of Professor Henry Mankin's dictum: 'Future changes in orthopaedics will be based in biology and more specifically in our ability to understand and alter its basic unit, the cell'[2]. The most striking current technical advances may prove to be blind side-shoots of surgical evolution.

To leave the sententious, I hope that this book will serve to remind present-day orthopaedic surgeons of the immense antiquity of their discipline, of the strivings of their predecessors against the old familiar problems, above all of the importance of mastering new concepts without forgetting permanent truths. Our progress has not been the uniform movement of a wave but more that of an extended battle-line – advancing in little local rushes, retreating or hesitating here or there, often stagnant, sometimes marked by a great breakthrough. However, if we are to speak in military terms in what consists the victory? Anyone who thinks in terms of the mastery of Nature is as mistaken as it is possible to be. It is tragic that, because what orthopaedic surgeons do must so often be largely mechanical, we are tempted to regard our patients as mere mechanisms. One of my teachers, Philip Wiles, wrote in 1952: 'However important surgery may be now, it should be the aim of all doctors, including surgeons, to limit and ultimately abolish it'[3]. Our aim must be as all the great precursors recognized, to supplement and not supplant Nature, a truth to which too many of us pay lip-service and then turn our backs. To work with Nature, to aid natural methods of repair and recovery, to encourage function, to promote self-respect and independence: it is the same now as it has always been. To recapitulate these millennia, to offer the orthopaedic surgeon a sane perspective of his origins, that is the aim of this book. If I am reproached with borrowing rather freely, my defence is that of Ambroise Paré's: that he had no more compunction in so doing than in lighting his taper from another's candle. I find it difficult, at this point, to refrain from quoting some remarks of Boswell, in his *Advertisement* to the first edition of his *Life of Johnson*:

The labour and anxious attention with which I have collected and arranged the materials of which these volumes are composed will hardly be conceived by those who read them with careless facility...the nature of the work, as it consists of innumerable detached particulars...has occasioned a degree of trouble far beyond that of any other species of composition. Were I to detail the books which I have consulted, and the inquiries which I have found it necesary to make by various channels, I should probably be thought ridiculously ostentatious...And after all, perhaps, hard as it may be, I shall not be surprized if omissions or mistakes be pointed out with invidious severity.

To which one can only add that sad remark of the Great Cham himself. 'It is a most mortifying reflexion for any man to consider, *what he has done*, compared with *what he might have done*.' But then, Johnson was looking at himself. 'Every other author may aspire to praise; the lexicographer can only hope to escape reproach.' Bearing in mind that he defined the lexicographer in his great *Dictionary* as 'a harmless drudge', I am willing that a collector of the minutiae of orthopaedic history should be similarly categorized.

REFERENCES

1. Le Vay, D. (1956). *The Life of Hugh Owen Thomas*. Edinburgh and London, Livingstone
2. Mankin, H.J. (1983). Orthopaedics in 2013: A Prospection. *J. Bone Jt. Surg.*, **65A**, 1180
3. Wiles, P. (1952). Surgery and the surgeon. *Proc. Roy. Soc. Med.*, **45**, 493

Acknowledgements

These must begin and end with Bruno Valentin, whom I first came to know around 1962, when his publishers, Georg Thieme of Stuttgart, invited me to translate his *Die Geschichte der Orthopädie*. For commercial reasons the translation was never published but it led to a close collaboration with Valentin, who acknowledged the defects in his splendid book, urged me to take up the task anew, and bequeathed me his unpublished material.

Professor Valentin had been Chief Surgeon at the Annastift Orthopaedic Clinic in Hanover from 1924 to 1936, when, as a 'non-Aryan', he was compelled to abandon his appointment and practice. He had already had contacts with Brazilian colleagues and, he wrote, 'in 1938 I finally emigrated to Brazil, but not without first having been maltreated in the most evil manner by the Gestapo in Hanover'. His years in Brazil were far from easy, because of poverty and inability to practise; fortunately, the Swiss drug firm Ciba made him director of a newly created scientific division. He harboured no enmity and was active in German relief and the foundation of a Brazilian–German Cultural Institute in Rio de Janeiro after the war. He was also instrumental in the dissemination of German publications after 1950: 'I played a considerable part in restoring a proper place and its former respect to German medical literature.'

Valentin had written on aspects of orthopaedic history before his emigration. He was now, in the 1950s, to receive grants from various official bodies in Germany to pursue these studies in libraries and archives throughout the world, culminating in his *History* of 1960. He left his rich collection of books and memorabilia to the Orthopaedic Museum and Library of the University of Würzburg, now housed at the König-Ludwig-Haus, the famous orthopaedic centre in that city. His hopes of a second edition, or even a translation, of his book were not to materialize, but no-one who reads it can fail to be impressed by his immense erudition and his emphasis on personalities. He urged me to make the freest use of this and other material, and I have not hesitated to do so.

I have also resorted very freely to certain other publications, notably Edgar M Bick's *Source Book of Orthopaedics*, now out of print. The sheer volume of information this contains is staggering and without equal; but it is organized mainly by topic, a ground on which I could not have hoped to compete, so that I prudently concentrated on the chronology of developments in individual countries. I also obtained much useful information from Sir Arthur Keith's *Menders of the Maimed* of 1919, the *Robert Jones Birthday Volume* of 1928 (edited by Fairbank, Bristow and Platt) and Mercer Rang's fascinating *Anthology of Orthopaedics* of 1966. I also made use of material from my own *Life of Hugh Owen Thomas* of 1956.

A great deal of help was forthcoming from various libraries. There were the rich resources of the library of the Royal College of Surgeons of England in Lincoln's Inn Fields in London, where the former Librarian, Mr Eustace Cornelius, introduced me to the mysteries of the computer search. (I hasten to add that I have had no other dealings with computers, word-processors or even card-indexes). The present Librarian, Mr Ian Lyle, and his staff have been uniformly helpful. The library of the Wellcome Institute for the History of Medicine in London is world famous. In particular, I am grateful to Mr Eric J Freeman there for an introduction that led to a visit to the great library of orthopaedic history at Würzburg, mentioned above, by courtesy of the then Professor, Dr A Rütt. It was a matter for keen regret that my exploration of this treasure-house had to be so short: a year would not have sufficed.

This work was written after retirement from my London clinical post, i.e. during secondments of varying length in Australia, Southern Africa and many parts of the United Kingdom, and it was rare for any of these sojourns to be entirely unfruitful on matters of orthopaedic history. I am particularly grateful to Mrs Janice Mayhew at the fine library of the Lord Mayor Treloar Orthopaedic Hospital at Alton, Hampshire in England. More recently, a visit to the Biomedical Library of the University of California at San Diego unearthed many valuable items. Information on the history of the *Société Internationale de Chirurgie Orthopédique et de Traumatologie* was available in *SICOT: 50 years of achievement* by the late E Vander Elst, published by Springer-Verlag (1978), to whom thanks are due for permission to reproduce illustrations.

Naturally, the American and British Volumes of the *Journal of Bone and Joint Surgery* were a mine of information, and both have been very kind as regards the use of illustrations. The Royal Society of Medicine in London has kindly allowed me to reprint the bulk of a talk I gave there in 1973 on the history of the name 'rickets'.

A most useful and beautifully produced little brochure was *Zur Geschichte der Orthopädie* by Günter Döderlein, published by Aesculap Werke AG of Tuttlingen, West Germany. Another valuable source was the first (1939) one volume edition of Willis C Campbell's *Operative Orthopaedics* (Mosby Co), which I purchased in 1940 for three pounds sterling!

The greatest possible help was derived from the series of *Classics* published in *Clinical Orthopaedics and Related Research* (present Editor-in-Chief, Marshall R Urist). For many years each issue included a reprint in English of a historic publication collected and sometimes edited by Bick, a tradition now continued by Leonard F Peltier. A first collection of these appeared in book form as *Classics of Orthopaedics* by Bick, published by Lippincott of Philadelphia in 1976. The technical articles in the same journal also proved useful sources and again thanks are due for permission to use certain figures. In general, acknowledgements for permission to use illustrations accompany the legends to the figures from whatever source.

Certain individuals have been very helpful in supplying material or suggestions: Professor Maurice Hinsenkamp, of Brussels, for information on Belgian orthopaedics and on matters to do with SICOT; Dr Edgar R Matthies, Chief of Department, Central Institute of Traumatology and Orthopaedics, Moscow, on Russian topics; Mr C M Hooker, of Hamilton, New Zealand, on developments in that country; Dr Andrew Bassett of the College of Physicians and Surgeons of Columbia University, New York, on the history of electricity in osteogenesis; Dr Baumann, of Aachen, German Federal Republic, for information on his teacher, Pauwels. I hope that I have not omitted any names. In all these cases, any errors or omissions are mine and mine alone.

Sincere thanks are due to Georg Thiene Verlag of Stuttgart, for the use of many figures from Professor Valentin's book, most of which are of quite remote provenance.

A number of passages have been translated by me from the original French, German, Italian or Latin, and again I accept responsibility for any errors. It is matter for regret that my ignorance of the Slavic languages has led to a certain lack of coverage.

It is a pleasure to add that much of the actual work of writing this book was carried out during successive annual summer locums at the North-Western Regional Orthopaedic Centre in the General Hospital of delectable Sligo, in Ireland. I am grateful to my colleagues there, Brendan Healy and Fintan Shannon, for their understanding.

Finally, as the foundation of all else, I have at all times had the greatest possible help and encouragement of Mr David G T Bloomer, Managing Director of Parthenon Publications. It is impossible to construct and research a book of this kind over several years without full confidence and support from one's publishers; and this I have had.

Section 1

The Earliest Times

CHAPTER 1

The Earliest Times

THE FOSSIL RECORD

Since one definition of orthopaedic disease is that it is a condition that affects vertebrates, one might expect to find evidence of such lesions in fossil vertebrates and this is the case. The subject was well researched by Moodie[1], particularly in his *Palaeopathology* of 1923[2]. Moreover, some two per cent of the bones in the Cleveland-Lloyd Dinosaur Collection exhibit some form of pathology[3]: degeneration, necrosis, ossification of tendons or spinous ligaments, fractures and amputations, some with secondary osteomyelitis, ankylosing or osteophytic arthritis (mainly affecting the caudal vertebrae of the long and vulnerable tail). Definite evidence of true neoplasms is very rare. Some dinosaur long bones, 70 million years old, exhibit periosteal lesions once thought to be those of periosteal sarcoma; but these are now regarded as akin to contemporary avian osteopetrosis[4]. All this material relates to fossil reptiles. Little or nothing is known of pathology in the hosts of Cretaceous fishes.

PREHISTORY AND ANCIENT EGYPT

The earliest men suffered from familiar diseases. A skeleton from the New Stone Age shows healed tuberculous destruction of the 4th and 5th dorsal vertebrae with kyphosis[5]. Many skeletons the world over exhibit evidence of inflammation, arthritis and tumours, of fractures sustained and healed, as do fossil vertebrates before man. A Java man, *Pithecanthropus erectus*, had a large benign osteochondroma growing from the lower end of the femur and a similar tumour has been found in a 5th Dynasty femur from the Giza pyramids cemetery[6]. Degenerative lesions, ankylosis and injuries of the spinal column were particularly common. There is evidence of surgical procedures (with flint or obsidian knives) that included amputation of the fingers[7], even

3

limbs, and trephining of the skull – this last in both the Old and New Worlds. Models or statuettes showing kyphosis, dwarfism or other deformities from prehistoric times are scattered the world over.

Our firsthand studies of ancient Egyptian pathology are rather like those of palaeontology: we have almost only the skeleton to go on; the soft tissues were so changed by the process of mummification as to make disease processes largely unidentifiable unless they caused bony lesions. Much of our knowledge of the pathology of the period is derived from field-work in the Nubian desert carried out by a famous anatomist and anthropologist, originally Australian, who became professor of anatomy in Cairo and then at University College, London, Sir Grafton Elliot Smith (1871–1937)*, often in collaboration with Sir Marc Armand Ruffer (1859–1917), before the first world war. Once we depart from the skeletal findings, we are dependent on the sparse written material, the few surgical instruments that survive, the reliefs and inscriptions, wall paintings and the mummies.

Elliot Smith and Ruffer state that spinal arthrosis was so widespread as sometimes to be present in every adult skeleton in a burial ground, from predynastic times to the Persian Dynasties of the 6th–4th centuries BC[8]. They identified the traces of a psoas abscess originating from caries of the

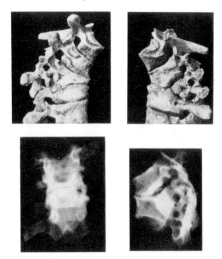

Figure 1 Tuberculosis of the dorsal spine in a New Stone Age skeleton: healing with angulation and bony fusion. (Bartels, P. [1907] *Arch. Anthrop.*, **34**, 243)

---

* The writer was one of Elliot Smith's students at University College and well recalls his silver-haired avuncular presence, like the best type of English butler. Lord Zuckerman has told us how, when walking home with Elliot Smith in 1932 from the Anatomy Department in Gower Street, the latter described some symptoms he had just begun to experience, correctly attributed them to an impending stroke, and located the affected vessel. He resumed lecturing after recovery, but with a hemiparesis and dribbling saliva, and died in the year that the author qualified at University College Hospital.

11th–12th dorsal and 1st lumbar vertebrae in the mummy of a hunchback from the 21st Dynasty (*c.*1000 BC)[9] and Ruffer described a number of other cases of Pott's disease in his *Studies in the Palaeopathology of Egypt* (Chicago University Press 1921). Smith and Jones, in a survey of Nubia in 1910[10], found ankyloses in skeletons that seemed to have been caused by rheumatoid arthritis, while Smith and Dawson concluded that osteoarthrosis was the preeminent disease of ancient Egypt and Nubia[11]. Ankylosis of the spine was as common then as now (Hamada and Rida 1972)[6] and, on the basis of findings showing hyperostosis, one wonders whether fluorosis was then endemic.

Fractures are common findings in ancient Egyptian skeletons, particularly of the left ulna, and this is attributable to self defence against a blow from a stick; the present writer has often seen this injury under contemporary conditions in African countries. Splints have been found applied to the forearms of mummies, some apparently for fractures sustained during post mortem handling. These splints were made of bamboo, reeds, wood or bark, padded with linen, and it is interesting that the splints used in France

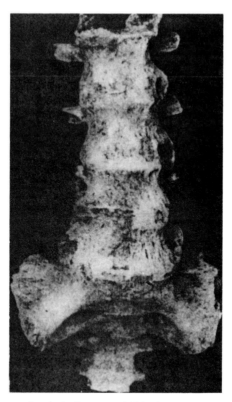

Figure 2 A specimen of ankylosing spondylitis from ancient Egyptian skeletons. (Hamada, G. and Rida, A. [1972] *Clinical Orthopaedics and Related Research,* **89**, 253)

thousands of years later were sometimes colloquially termed *joncs* (reeds). In some cases the splint has been applied over the interosseous space to spring the forearm bones apart, as in ancient and even modern China (see p. 470).

Elliott Smith also found a number of club and equinus feet in the royal mummies in 1912[12] and 1924[13]. There are also examples of hip and femoral fractures, and a well known temple relief shows *genu recurvatum* said to be due to a malunited fracture of the femur but more probably due to poliomyelitis[6]. Spinal fractures were common in building workers after falls.

In 1862, the robbers of a rock tomb at Thebes found a papyrus which they sold to an American egyptologist, Edwin Smith. Though the name of its author is not given, it is surmised to be the work of Imhotep, usually described as architect and chief minister to King Zoser of *c*.2800 BC. Imhotep devised the step pyramid at Sakkara which preceded the great pyramids and directed the scores of thousands of labourers engaged in their erection. Some say that he was deified by the Greeks, who identified him with Aesculapius, others that he was an illiterate peasant who was himself a labourer. However this may be, and whether or not Imhotep was the author, this papyrus is the oldest Afro-Asian surgical treatise and evidences a mass of careful clinical observation of injuries and their treatment, though we should bear in mind that the surviving papyrus is not in its original form but was copied and recopied over a thousand years and that the section on the lower limbs is missing. It is a collection of 48 specimen clinical records, beginning with injuries of the head and passing to the face, neck, clavicle, upper arm and sternum; in each group the more superficial injuries are described first. This detailed accurate record of the features and treatment of injuries of a host of workers engaged in a great project reminds one of the early experience of Robert Jones as the surgeon supervising the building of the Manchester Ship Canal, a much later accident service.

The author relates how the priest or physician (often one and the same) examined the pulse 'to discover the action of the heart, from which vessels

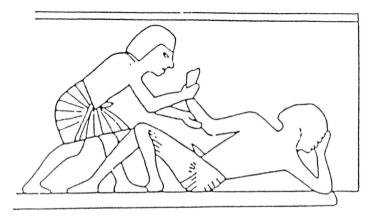

Figure 3   From a wall painting in the tomb of Ipuy, 1200 BC. Is this Kocher's manoeuvre? Metropolitan Museum of Art, New York

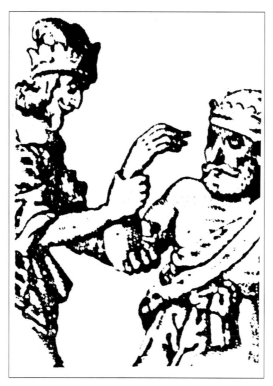

Figure 4   Reduction of an elbow dislocation: Scultetus, *Armamentarium Chirurgicum*, Ulm 1655

go to all the limbs, hands and feet', something unknown to Hippocrates. He classifies the injuries in relation to their prognosis in three categories: 'an ailment which I will treat' i.e. with a favourable prognosis; 'an ailment with which I will contend', which might go either way; and 'an ailment not to be treated', a hopeless case, what German army surgeons in World War II would have called a *Spritzfall*, fit for an injection of morphine and nothing else.

Case 3 is a compound fracture of the skull vault; digital probing of the wound is advised. Case 5, a depressed fracture, is not to be treated. Case 6 refers to 'a gaping wound of the head, penetrating to the bone, smashing the skull and rending open the brain', the gyri of which are compared to the corrugations of molten copper, 'throbbing and fluttering under the fingers'. This man had nose-bleeding and neck stiffness, because the wound had 'broken open the fluid within the skull'. The case was not to be treated. Case 8 is an excellent description of hemiplegia after head injury, for the eyes are askew in conjugate deviation, the gait shuffling and the hand cannot be closed. In Case 25, 'if you examine a man having a dislocated mandible, and the mouth is open and cannot be closed, you should place your thumbs on the ends of the rami within his mouth and your two hands under his chin and cause them to fall back and so restore them to their place.'

Case 31 is often quoted because of its appreciation of the morbid anatomy and prognosis of cervical spine injuries. 'If you examine a man having a dislocation of a vertebra in his neck, and find him insensible of both his arms and both legs as a result, while his penis is erect on account of it and urine drops from this member without his knowing... it is a dislocation of a vertebra of his neck extending to his backbone which causes him to be insensible of his arms and legs. If, however, the middle vertebra of his neck is dislocated, it is a seminal emission that befalls his phallus*. You should say of him: 'an ailment not to be treated'. Case 32 is that of a man 'having a displacement in a vertebra of his neck, whose face is fixed, whose neck cannot be turned, and if you say to him 'Look at your breast and both shoulders' and he cannot ... you should say of him: 'One having a displacement in a vertebra of his neck, an ailment that I will treat'. This sounds like an acute torticollis of benign nature without skeletal damage. Case 33 refers to 'a crushed vertebra in the neck' with insensibility of arms and legs and loss of speech, not to be treated.

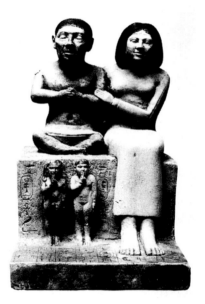

Figure 5   Model of achondroplastic court official Seneb, normal wife, one achondroplastic and one normal child (Fifth Dynasty) (Cairo Museum)

---

* As is sometimes seen in judicial hanging. In the Middle Ages, the mandrake was thought to spring from where the semen fell to the ground.

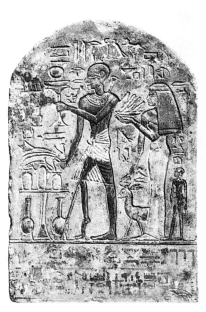

Figure 6 Stele from temple of Ishtar, goddess of healing, Memphis, Fifth Dynasty, c. 1550–1350 BC, showing Ruma the doorkeeper priest with wasted lower limb, shortening and equinus. Source: New Carlsberg Glyptothek, Copenhagen

In the treatment of a fracture of the clavicle (Case 35), 'you should lay him flat on his back with something folded between his shoulder-blades and spread out both his shoulders so as to stretch apart hs collar-bone until the break falls into place. You should apply two splints of linen, one on the inside and one on the underside of his arm' (presumably because, with a pad in the axilla, bringing the arm to the side applies leverage to the fracture. Short of operation, this is still the only method that approaches a perfect result in the treatment of such a fracture in a slender young woman and is also recommended in the ancient Indian literature.

Case 44 is that of a man with 'a sprain of a vertebra of his spinal column. You should say to him: "Straighten your legs and contract them again." When he straightens them, he contracts them both immediately because of the pain this causes in the vertebra of his spinal column. The diagnosis is "One having a sprain of a vertebra in his spinal column. An ailment that I will treat"'. The treatment, unfortunately never completed, was to lay him on his back and make him ... But make him do what? We shall never know. This may have been a 'sprung back' or a disc prolapse with restriction of straight leg raising (a sprain is defined elsewhere as 'a rending of two members though each is still in its place').

Thirty-three of these cases were simple or compound injuries of bones or joints, 12 were flesh wounds of the scalp, face, throat or chest. The papyrus several times refers to the discharge of *ryt*, presumably pus, from what must have been posttraumatic osteomyelitis; and then a sequestrum might be extruded or need to be removed. So here we have an acute clinical observer of nearly 5000 years ago whose knowledge of the pulse, inflammation, cerebral compression and cervical fractures and dislocations in some respects exceeded that of Hippocrates.

Hussein[14] tells of a sculptor to Rameses II in 1200 BC, one Ipuy, who made a mural painting for his own tomb, a detail of which appears to depict Kocher's method of reducing a shoulder dislocation. This may be so; but, as Beasley points out[15], it is also very like the reduction of a dislocated elbow as illustrated by Scultetus in his *Armamentarium Chirurgium*, published

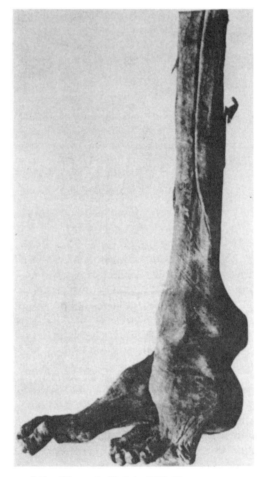

Figure 7   Mummy of the Pharaoh Siptah, 19th Dynasty; severe equinovarus and shortening in the left leg. (Hamada, G. and Rida, A. [1972] *Clinical Orthopaedics and Related Research*, **89**, 253)

at Ulm in Germany in 1655. The artistic evidence of orthopaedic disorders is indeed extensive. There are statuettes and wall-paintings of achondroplastic dwarfs, who were court favourites. Ptah, the god of death, was depicted as an achondroplastic, perhaps because the bodily proportions in this condition approximate those of the embryo and thus express a future life; but his descendants are similarly depicted, so that the condition was known to be inherited.

Did poliomyelitis exist in Ancient Egypt? There is a famous wall stele, or votive tablet, from the temple of Ishtar, goddess of healing, at Memphis from the 18th Dynasty, c.1550–1350 BC, which shows Ruma, the doorkeeper priest, with a totally wasted lower limb, shortening and equinus. He has a supporting staff and his wife and son are behind him. This stele, now in the New Carlsberg Glyptothek in Copenhagen, is often taken as a portrayal of the effects of poliomyelitis, to the extent that it has been adopted by the Danish National Association for Infantile Paralysis as its emblem, though some have regarded the lesion as due to spastic paralysis or even hip disease. The mummy of the Pharaoh Siptah, of the 19th century BC, shows total equinus of the left foot, balancing 4 cm of shortening, and this too has been attributed to poliomyelitis[16] and this attribution, too, has been disputed. The odd thing is that there is no relation of anything like an epidemic of poliomyelitis in the ancient and mediaeval literature, or even in the 17th and 18th centuries. Nor did Elliot Smith find any evidence of syphilis[17], and rickets, too, seems to have been totally absent in Egypt, probably because of climatic conditions.

In Babylonia, after 2000 BC, there was a strict medical code, that of King Hammurabi, the only notable orthopaedic element of which is the provision that, if a physician's treatment leads to the loss of a nobleman's life or sight, his hands shall be cut off, a provision recently revived for malefactors in the Moslem world.

In modern Egypt, specialized orthopaedics did not begin until around 1929, before when it was in the hands of general surgeons and bonesetters. The Egyptian Orthopaedic Association was also founded by Hussein, in 1948, and its *Journal* in 1966. Its emblem is an obelisk with the name of the journal in hieroglyphics. Hammada and Rida point out that Paget's disease is rare in Egypt, as is congenital dislocation of the hip unless there has been intermarriage with Europeans. Primary arthrosis of the hip is also rare; and, though this has been attributed to the use of the squatting position, it is more probably related to the rarity of congenital dysplasia.

ANCIENT INDIA

The Sanskrit sacred books, the *Vedas*, were written in the Vedic Period of 3500–1000 BC. The oldest of these, the *Rig Veda*, resembles the Greek legends in that the early physicians, the *Ashwani Kumaras*, were divinities, capable of curing paralyses and shattered limbs. We learn that Queen Vishpla had a leg amputated in a battle, and an iron leg fitted to enable her to fight on. Similar tales are told about the Silver Hand of Ireland and the wooden limbs of Norse heroes; others, less fortunate, had to continue on their stumps.

The last or *Altharva Veda* describes crutches, compression for haemostasis, and treatment aimed at securing healing by first intention, 'bone to bone, flesh to flesh, skin to skin'. Skeletal tuberculosis is also described, including gravitational abscesses and paraplegia, and there are references to lepromatous lesions of the skeleton.

The *Epic Era* (1000–600 BC) saw skilled surgeons at work in the Court and on the battlefield, dealing with arrow wounds and fractures. The subsequent development of the body of knowledge known as the *Ayurveda* relates mainly to traditional medication (600 BC–700 AD), but the rise of Yoga introduced valuable remedial and postural exercises called the Asanas.

The great surgical sage, who lived around 800 BC – the date is disputed – the Indian counterpart of Hippocrates, was Susruta, the father of Indian surgery. His corpus of writings is the *Susruta Samhita* and deals with the scope and methods of surgery, ignored in the other four great Ayurvedic texts. They describe the requisite instruments and were translated into Persian and Arabic by 800 AD. Susruta also resembles Hippocrates in his attention to detail: the surgeon must be clean, his nails short, well-mannered, the operating-room clean and fumigated. He must use inspection, palpation, percussion. The operation site is to be shaved. Instruments were many and various and fell into several main groups. The *yantras* were blunt; if they were forceps with handles, they were called *swastika yantra* for obvious reasons; there were also probes and hooks and *sastras* or sharp instruments, knives and scissors.

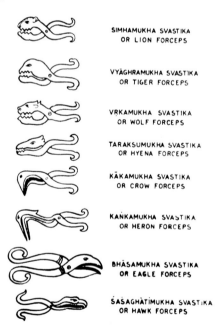

SIMHAMUKHA SVASTIKA
OR LION FORCEPS

VYĀGHRAMUKHA SVASTIKA
OR TIGER FORCEPS

VRKAMUKHA SVASTIKA
OR WOLF FORCEPS

TARAKSUMUKHA SVASTIKA
OR HYENA FORCEPS

KĀKAMUKHA SVASTIKA
OR CROW FORCEPS

KAṄKAMUKHA SVASTIKA
OR HERON FORCEPS

BHĀSAMUKHA SVASTIKA
OR EAGLE FORCEPS

ŚAŚAGHĀTĪMUKHA SVASTIKA
OR HAWK FORCEPS

Figure 8 Svastika, yantra or cruciform instruments. (Duraiswami, P. K. [1971]. *Clinical Orthopaedics and Related Research*, **75**, 269)

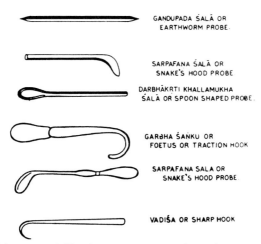

Figure 9 Salaka or rod-like instruments (Duraiswami, P. K. [1971]. *Clinical Orthopaedics and Related Research*, **75**, 269)

Duraiswami and Tuli[18] say that contemporary anatomy was inadequate for structures other than the skeleton, muscles and ligaments, because of the peculiar method of dissection by scraping away successive layers after burying the body under a river bed. Therefore, there was an esoteric system in which

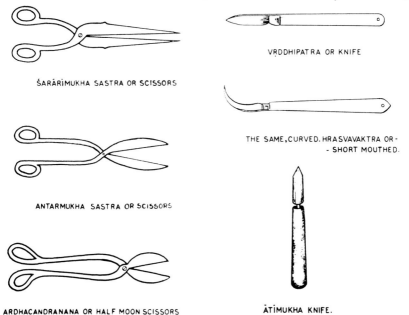

Figure 10 Sararimukha sastra or scissors (left) and vrddhipatra sastra or knives (right). (Duraiswami, P. K. [1971]. *Clinical Orthopaedics and Related Research*, **75**, 269)

initiates in the surgery of particular regions instructed each other. Structures, lesions, sutures, instruments, dressings and operations were all carefully listed and classified. Sutures were of cotton, leather, horsehair, animal tendons or vegetable fibres. Procedures included incision, excision, scraping, probing. There were 310 bones in the body, categorized as flat, cylindrical and others, and 210 joints: hinge, ball-and-socket, cuplike, coronoid (crow's-beak) and others. There were 500 muscles, 900 ligaments, 700 vessels, there was an account of the synovial membrane and synovial fluid. Fractures were classified as spiral, oblique, comminuted, transverse, greenstick, impacted, complicated, fissured and articular and their symptoms included pain, swelling, crepitus (its earliest historic mention) and loss of function. 'The cartilaginous bones bend, the tubular bones break, the flat bones become fissured and the small bones crack'. Reduction was much as now. Fractures of the femur and tibia required massage and traction. Splints were of bark (or bamboo or banyan), wrapped in ghee-soaked cloths and a bandage applied overall. Fractures became stable in a month in children, in two in the middleaged, in three in the elderly; refracture might be necessary for malunion. 'The fracture should be considered as having united well if the union is painless, without any shortening of the parts, without irregularity, and allowing free and easy movement. The surgeon should so endeavour that the fracture does not suppurate, as suppuration of muscles, vessels and ligaments renders cure difficult.' Subperiosteal haematoma was recognized, and subungual haematoma, to be treated by drilling the nail.

There were various types of dislocation, complete and incomplete. Shoulder dislocation was to be reduced with a 'club' in the armpit, the dislocated hip by traction via a pulley or 'the wise surgeon should reduce the dislocated thighbone by a circular motion' (*cf.* Bigelow in 1845!) For cervical fracture dislocation the patient was to be lifted with the surgeon's hands on the nape and round the sides of the jaw. There was a fracture table with movable pegs, to be arranged as required, a method often used in conjunction with the Hippocratic *scamnum*.

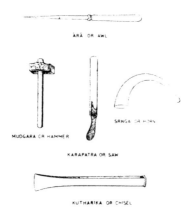

ÁRÁ OR AWL

MUDGARA OR HAMMER

SRNGA OR HORN

KARAPATRA OR SAW

KUTHARIKA OR CHISEL

Figure 11   Miscellaneous instruments. (Duraiswami, P. K. [1971]. *Clinical Ortho-paedics and Related Research*, **75**, 269)

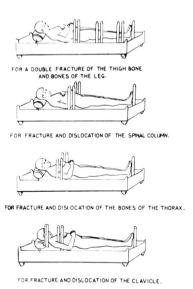

FOR A DOUBLE FRACTURE OF THE THIGH BONE
AND BONES OF THE LEG.

FOR FRACTURE AND DISLOCATION OF THE SPINAL COLUMN.

FOR FRACTURE AND DISLOCATION OF THE BONES OF THE THORAX.

FOR FRACTURE AND DISLOCATION OF THE CLAVICLE.

Figure 12   Kapata-Sayana or fracture bed of the Hindus. (Duraiswami, P. K. [1971].
Clinical Orthopaedics and Related Research, **75**, 269)

After the 6th century BC there was a large medical school at Taxila (now in Pakistan) and public hospitals in the major cities. Nevertheless, the cripple was often regarded as an incarnation of evil, just as he was often shunned in Europe at this period. The great authority of the 6th–7th centuries AD was Vagbhata, and there was another great teacher, Bhava Misra, in Banaras in the 16th century. However, dissection had declined after Susruta and with the spread of Buddhism; by 7–800 AD, surgery had been relegated to lower-class practitioners and stagnated after the first millennium, being largely taken over by charlatans.

The entire story is dominated by the figure of Susruta, who behaved like the author of the Edwin Smith papyrus in regarding some conditions as not to be treated. 'Fractures of the skull and waist as also their dislocations and subluxations, as also crushing of the hip-bones, should be excluded from treatment by the physician.' He also defined and rejected pathological fractures: 'Bones and joints which were abnormal even prior to injury, or were so from birth, or those fractures which, even though properly reduced, have become complicated due to improper immobilization or bandaging or due to movement, should be excluded from treatment'.

In modern times, British (and Portuguese and French) rule brought European methods. The communication was two-way. In 1857, Hugh Owen Thomas recorded the reduction of a ten-months-old dislocated shoulder in a seaman ('Aid at first trials, seven men; last trial, ten men'). 'At Singapore consulted the best surgical authorities, ten Man-of-War surgeons, but after ineffectual attempts they gave it up. Then some of the Indians tried, but failed also. I ought to relate that, before attempting reduction, they made him unconscious by repeated blows along the spine, ceasing only when he fell down exhausted, then the dislocation was manipulated.'[19] This was *not* in the canon of Susruta, who used wine and herbs (cannabis) pre- and postoperatively.

CHINA

Surgery is mentioned during the reign of the Emperor Huang Ti over 4000 years ago[20-22]. 'Yu Fuma, doctor of Huang Ti, employed manipulation, baking and radical excision. If necessary, he made incisions through the skin, loosened the muscles (? tenotomy), identified the blood-vessels, sutured divided tendons, exposed the spinal cord and cleaned various viscera.' One must be allowed a little scepticism: all the great civilizations refer to these early, superhuman figures. At around 1200 BC, Chou Kung wrote *The Medicine of Wounds*, one of whose four sections was on fractures.

During the Chou Dynasty (1121–249 BC) surgeons were classed as inferior to physicians and only lower-grade doctors were put in charge of surgical departments, for Confucian dogma held the body as sacred and not to be mutilated. The most famous surgeon of China was Hua T'o, often worshipped in temples as the god of surgery. Born in or around 190 AD, he is credited with miraculous diagnostic insight and surgical achievements under an anaesthetizing potion, including splenectomy. He stressed the role of movement and exercise, but Chinese surgery and anaesthesia seem to have halted with his death. There is a figure showing him operating on a general for necrosis of the arm. Surgery was recognized as a special branch of medicine in the Tang dynasty (619–901 AD) and this included the orthopaedic treatment of fractures and dislocations and the removal of sequestra. The Imperial Medical College was founded in 1076 AD and reestablished after an interregnum in 1191; it produced ten major texts, one on *Fractures and Wounds*. In 1573, Chou Yu-Fan published a book on paediatric massage therapy, widely used for both traumatic and systemic conditions. Such massage was well esteemed and included manipulation of the neck, spine and limbs. From the earliest times attention was paid to physical culture: breathing, boxing and gynmastics. Later, the Christian missionaries set up numerous mission hospitals. For modern developments, see p. 469.

JAPAN

Japan had sent envoys to China around 600–900 AD, much as the Scots had visited Ireland in the early days of the Christian Church, and these returned to diffuse Chinese teachings. The general medical influence of China on Japan was very much like that of Greece on Rome. The first known Japanese surgical monograph was a survey of Chinese surgery, the *Chi-so-ki* by Fukuyoshi, in the Showa Era of 834–847 AD, and deals with salves, bandaging, plasters, and chalk and powdered oyster-shells for wounds.

During the Muromachi Period (1334–1568), wounded soldiers and others unfitted for warfare took up the study of medicine and cared for the wounded, the *Kinso-i* or wound surgeons.

The Azuchi-Momoyama Period (1569–1615) and later was marked by the influence of Europeans, particularly the Dutch. These came from around 1570 on and brought the knowledge of their ships' surgeons with them. This was the origin of several schools named after individual Dutchmen, such as the Caster school of surgery, and it continued even after the expulsion of foreigners in general and the ban on foreign trade of 1603 and the banning of Christianity. A leading local figure of this time was Dosan Manase, who wrote the *Keiteki-Shu*, with chapters on diseases of the bones and wounds and a special section on diseases of the elderly[23].

The Dutch trading influence brought European books which stimulated the practice of dissection and Portuguese and other missionaries built a church in Kyoto in 1568, the *Nambanji* (church of the southern barbarians) where operations were done, and founded the *Namban-Ryu Geka*, the surgery of the southern barbarian school. In 1654, Gensho Mukai published the *Komorgu-Geka-Hiyo*, a translation of the surgical aspects of lectures by the Dutch physician, Mestruans Jonan. Nevertheless, surgery was not taught systematically until 1822 when the *Yoi Shinsho* (*A New Work on Surgery*) was published by Gempaku Sugita and Gentaku Otsuki. Extraordinarily enough, this was a translation of a work by the mediaeval Nuremberg surgeon, Lorenz Heister (1683–1758) (p. 54), which included sections on wounds, bandages, fractures and dislocations. During the 19th century, other European surgical texts were translated, including Stromeyer's *Textbook of Surgery* in 1865.

An indigenous publication of 1837 in 19 volumes, the *Yoka Hiroku* (*Theory and Practice of Surgery*) was a great stimulus to Japanese surgery and includes a fascinating line drawing of the surgical repair of club-foot, showing the excision of an oval of skin on the dorsolateral aspect of the foot exactly as practised by Robert Jones in England in the late 19th century. The *Seikotsu-Jutsu* was a system of surgical treatment confined to fractures and dislocations, begun in the second half of the 17th century and associated with a sect of specialists known as the *Seikotsukai*, very skilful manipulators, who published the *Seikotzu Han* in 1808. Two of their more famous figures were Ken Ninomiya and Bunken Koumu. For modern developments in Japan, see p. 473.

ANCIENT GREECE

The medicine of ancient Greece was influenced by that of Egypt, whose physicians were praised by Homer, and in its turn had a lasting influence on European thought although it was obscured for a time in the Dark Ages and owed its reintroduction, via the Byzantines, to the translations of the rising Arab civilization.

From the Minoan period on, diagnosis and treatment were matters for priests and the infirmaries were temples, even until after the Hippocratic period. The Minoan sanctuaries often contained many small models of human limbs, probably votive offerings. The Greek theology of therapeutics goes back to Apollo, son of Zeus. Apollo had many roles: that of importance to us is evoked in the first clause of the Hippocratic Oath, 'I swear by Apollo the Healer'. He grew up in Delphi, where he taught Cheiron the Centaur, who himself taught Achilles, Jason and Apollo's son, Asklepios. Achilles' medical skills are reported in the *Iliad* and figure in the famous chalice design by Sosias, where he is shown bandaging Patroclus.

Asklepios (later latinized to Aesculapius) may have been a real practical physician at the beginning of the first millennium BC. The legend has him slain by his grandfather, Zeus, because he was saving too many lives for Pluto's liking. At all events, he became the Graeco-Roman god of healing from the 7th century BC to the 6th century AD. He is classically portrayed with the potent serpent-rod symbol of the Minoans and of Aaron, the sign of medicine down the ages. Temple-infirmaries were found all over Greece, notably at Epidaurus, and in Cos, Pergamos and other Greek colonies in Asia Minor. Our interest is that temple inscriptions and votive offerings refer to victims of paralysis, muscle spasms and joint stiffness, who were treated

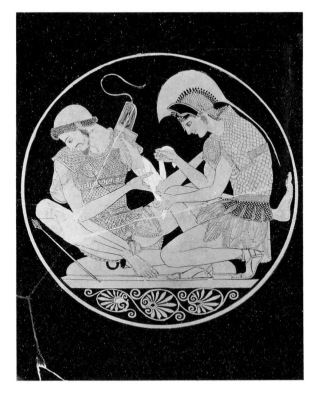

Figure 13   Achilles bandaging Patroclus: chalice design by Sosias. (Printed with permission from Bildarchiv Preussischer Kulturbesitz, Berlin)

as resident patients in hostels near the shrine. The priests' treatment was magico-religious, with fasting, bathing, suggestion, sleep and dream interpretation as its pillars, plus nocturnal visits from the sacred snakes. Sometimes healing took place during sleep. There is a definite association here between fervent belief and longing for cure, groves and caves and water, which we see again in the Lourdes of the 19th century AD.

The Trojan War, as narrated by Homer in the *Iliad*, was roughly contemporary with the origins of Asklepios; indeed, Homer tells us that the sons of Asklepios, Machaon and Podalirius (who figure in the arms of the Royal College of Surgeons of England) were the surgeons to the Greek forces on the plain before Troy. When Machaon was himself wounded, Idomeneus says: 'Quick, my lord Nestor ... pick up Machaon and drive with all speed to the ships. A surgeon who can cut out an arrow and heal the wound with his ointments is worth a regiment'. Yet Machaon was also a warrior by profession, and the heroes themselves performed surgical procedures; surgery had been laicized and was no longer the preserve of priests*.

Among other things, the Iliad is a textbook of traumatology and military surgery. Homer depicts some 147 types of wound and discloses a considerable knowledge of anatomy, especially in his accounts of transfixion wounds. The reader may amuse himself by searching these out. Let us just select the first forequarter amputation, when 'Diomedes ... struck the other with his great sword on the collar-bone by the shoulder, so that the shoulder was severed from the back and neck (V, 146); or there is a brachial plexus injury, when 'Hector ... struck his shoulder with the jagged stone on the weakest spot, where the clavicle leads over to the neck and breast ... his fingers and wrist were numbed, he sank to his knees, and the bow dropped from his hand' (VIII, 325). Evidently, this was an anatomic site that fascinated Homer, the best lethal approach to a mailed warrior, 'Hector's body was completely covered by armour ... except for an opening at the gullet where the clavicles lead over from the shoulders to the neck, the easiest place to kill a man' (XXII, 324). Again, 'Meriones struck him in the right buttock and the spearhead passed right through the bladder and came out under the bone' (XIII, 651). He describes injuries of the acetabulum; and Achilles performed a sort of tendon transplant on the corpse of Hector, when 'he slit the tendons at the back of both feet from heel to ankle, inserted leather traces and made

---

* Although Machaon was the first surgeon, his name also has a murderous connotation, meaning 'slaughterer', with the same root as the Greek word for battle. Other healer gods or heroes, sons of Machaon, also have warlike names, combining the attributes of warriors and physicians. But it is only man's wounds that can be healed, not man himself: Machaon wounds and heals, but in essence he is incurable. The warrior surgeon dies of his wounds: 'Wounding and being wounded are the dark premises of healing: it is they that make the medical profession possible, and indeed a necessity for human experience. For this existence may be conceived as that of a wounding and vulnerable being who can also heal.[48]' It is relevant that Machaon cured the wound in the heel of Philoctetes, abandoned for 10 years on Lemnos because of the stench of chronic osteomyelitis; he was wanted back on duty because of his skill in tipping arrows with deadly poison.

them fast to his chariot, leaving his head dragging' (XXII, 396).

Beasley[24], to whom we owe so much in this field, points out that the Iliad also contains references to deformities. The god Hephaestus, smith or artificer, is described as 'cavus-footed' and is addressed by his mother, Hera, (who had, in the manner of the period, tried to destroy him when he was born a cripple) as 'god of the crooked foot'; and yet, though of monstrous bulk and limping, he was nimble on his slender legs (XVIII, 410), evidently a case of bilateral equinovarus and reminiscent of the equally nimble ostler, Hippolyte, on whose club-foot Flaubert's Dr Bovary operated to such ill effect[25]. Then there is Thersites, characterized by Shakespeare in *Troilus and Cressida* as 'a deformed and scurrilous Greek', sometimes regarded as the archetypal muck-raking journalist, 'the ugliest man that came to Ilium; he had a game foot and was bandy-legged, his rounded shoulders almost met across his chest, and above them was an egg-shaped head' (II, 216). Beasley diagnoses him as a case of cranocleidodystosis.

There is less surgical information in the *Odyssey* because there is less fighting. However, we are told of Ulysses' thigh wound by a wild boar, how it was 'bound up wisely', and how the flow of black blood was staunched by preliminary ligature of the limb. Homer also tells how wounds sustained in the heat of battle may pass unnoticed till later.

Hippocrates

The 'divine Hippocrates' was born on the island of Cos in 460 BC, the first year of the 80th Olympic Games and died at a great age around 370 BC. He was a contemporary of Socrates and is treated respectfully in the *Dialogues*. He epitomizes the rational as opposed to the mystical and religious in Greek medicine, and may be regarded as in the line of the 'philosophers', i.e. the natural scientists, through Thales, Pythagoras and Alcmaeon; for these fore-runners medicine was just part of their activities and did not become a specialized profession until the advent of Hippocrates himself. Early Greek medicine had not been systematized; anyone was free to practise; there were herbalists and charlatans of all kinds. Only the gynmastic trainer was a respected figure, and one important to medicine, for the wrestlers often dislocated their opponents' shoulder joints and inflicted other injuries, and someone had to be able to deal with them. Before Hippocrates, Democedes of Croton, himself a gymnastic surgeon when a Persian slave, cured King Darius: 'his foot was twisted rather violently, for he got his astragalus dislocated from its joints' – it was reduced by manipulation.

Was Hippocrates a real individual? There seems no doubt about this; there are well known portrait busts and, above all, a very definite personality shines through his writings. These took the form of a Corpus of some sixty books ranging from 430 to 330 BC, evidently the work of more hands than one, obviously the work of a school and not just the man himself, and even of the rival school of Cnidus in Asia Minor. Hippocrates did two things: he ran a busy and competitive private practice and he formulated this practice in a series of monographs and aphorisms dealing with different diseases and

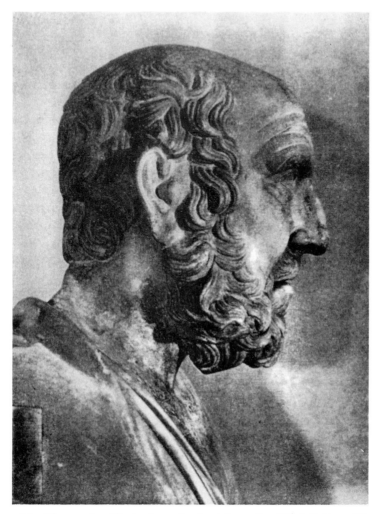

Figure 14 Hippocrates. Illustration of a bust from the Uffizi Gallery, Florence. Reproduced from *A Short History of Medicine* by Singer and Underwood (1962). Published with kind permission from the Clarendon Press

parts of the body that reveal an astute and acutely observant clinician. In doing this, he introduced systematization, developed a proper medical science, and established a proper independence and social standing for the physician. Nor should we forget that he worked for gain; and he never fails to stress the importance of being seen to do the right thing and of not making mistakes likely to incur public obloquy – a hint of the defensive medicine that has arisen in our own times.

He was also very caustic in his comments on incorrect or adventurous methods of treatment, the ignorant use of 'marvellous methods' to impress

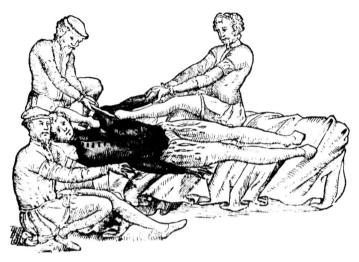

Figure 15   This figure, from the English translation of Paré's works, 1678, shows Hippocratic reduction of a dislocated shoulder with the operator's foot in the axilla and an assistant pulling up the humeral head with a cord and also applying counter pressure with his own heel. Vidus Vidius, *Chirurgia é Graeco in Latinum Conversa,* 1544. Reproduced from Oribasus, *De Machinamentis* (4th C AD)

patients, and this reminds us of another perfectionist in the 19th century in England, Hugh Owen Thomas, who was equally scathing about adventurous methods and also preferred the simplest effective methods. Because Hippocrates knew little anatomy, apart from that of the skeleton and that gained by the priests from sacrifices, he was reluctant to expose himself to criticism through audacity. The later Greeks of Alexandria and Asia Minor did know more and were more audacious.

Greek bandaging was complex and expert and is much stressed by Hippocrates. For fractures, he used an inner and outer layer sandwiching splints and compresses. The inner layers were soaked in 'cerate', which was either white, consisting of wax liquefied in olive oil or oil of roses, or dark, with added pitch, used as a prophylactic in open wounds and to promote suppuration. With resin added as a stiffener, it was used for club-foot.

If Hippocrates ever really existed, and we must assume that he did, and if he ever wrote anything himself, he must have written the volumes of the *Corpus* on *Fractures* and on *Joints* (*De Articulis*); *Fractures* contains a lot about joints and *Joints* much on fractures. Finally, there is an odd little volume, *Mochlicon* (*On Levers*), which is a sort of ragbag of orthopaedic items[26].

De Articulis

As to dislocation of the shoulder, Hippocrates only recognized dislocation into the armpit and had never seen a forward displacement. As Paré put it in 1564, 'Now Hippocrates sayeth that he hath only seen one kind of dislocation of this bone, which is downwards into the armpit'[27]. The signs of a dislocation were that the humeral head was obvious in the axilla, the upper outer arm contour was flattened, the acromion stood out, the elbow was prominent and elevation of the arm was limited. Thin persons with slack ligaments dislocated easily, even voluntarily, and reduction was correspondingly easy; muscular persons dislocated, and were reduced, with difficulty. When reduction was easy, there was no inflammation and the patient could use the arm freely, and might redislocate it if not cautioned by

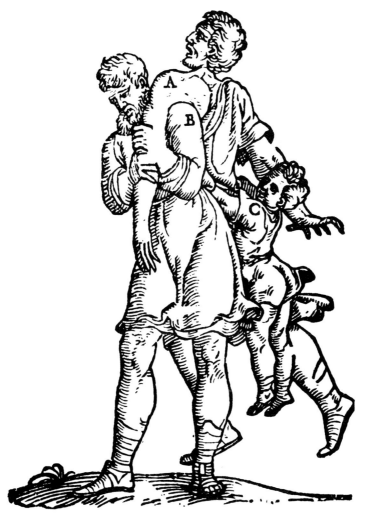

Figure 16 The Hippocratic method of reduction over the operator's shoulder, from the Venice edition of Galen's works, 1625. The addition of the child may not be authentic. (Vidus Vidius)

the physician (this also applied to the knee). Hippocrates says that the knee and shoulder are the joints most likely to dislocate, but the former must have been cases of internal derangement.

There were many methods of reduction, and these have been preserved in a wonderful series of illustrations whose provenance we shall discuss later. Patients with recurrent dislocation could usually reduce it themselves by pushing up with a fist in the armpit and adducting the elbow to the chest-wall; the surgeon could do likewise, thrusting the elbow in with his knee and using his head for counter-pressure at the shoulder-tip. He also describes bringing the forearm behind the back, i.e. into internal rotation, flexing the elbow and pushing in the shoulder from *behind*, which seems rather an account of reducing a posterior displacement.

Another classical method was for the patient to lie supine on the ground, when the surgeon would sit by his side with his foot in the axilla and pull the arm down, an assistant fixing the sound shoulder as counter-traction to prevent the body swinging round. As the tendons at the front and back of the axilla stand out in a conscious patient, and obstruct the heel, an intervening leather ball was inserted to give purchase and held by a strap round the axilla in a north-south line which was steadied by a third person who pressed *his* foot against the top of the shoulder, also as counter-traction. This was the common gymnastic technique.

There was also the shoulder lift, in which a surgeon taller than the patient took him by the hand on the injured side and hoisted him over his back so that the body-weight aided reduction, with the optional extra of a small boy clinging to the victim to add to the pull. Reduction could also be effected by pulling over a pestle or the rung of a ladder, but the most powerful method was with a long piece of wood strapped to the whole arm, its upper padded end forced up between the humeral head and the ribs to act as a lever with the arm over a beam and the patient on tiptoe. The leverage was enormous and effective even for old unreduced cases, 'for what could not correct leverage move?' As well as the ladder rung, there was also the 'Thessalian chair' or the lower half of a double door: one wonders about the radial nerve. What will not be found is any account of a procedure resembling Kocher's method.

Recurrent dislocation was treated with the cautery right down to the front of the joint, avoiding the nerves and artery, then binding the arm to the side for a long time to allow the recess into which dislocation occurred to cicatrize: 'It deserves to be known how a shoulder which is subject to frequent dislocation should be treated. For many persons owing to this accident have been obliged to abandon gymnastic exercises though otherwise well qualified for them; and from the same misfortune have become inept in warlike practices, and thus have perished. The cautery should be applied thus: taking hold with the hands of the skin at the armpit it is to be drawn into the line in which the head of the humerus is dislocated, and then the skin thus drawn aside is to be turned to the opposite side ... the cauteries should be red-hot, that they may pass through as quickly as possible ... throughout the treatment the sores are to be treated so as to avoid any marked extension of the arm ... and when the sores are proceeding to cicatrization, then by

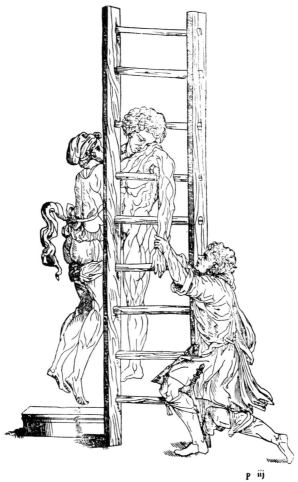

p iij

Figure 17 Reduction over the rung of a ladder, from Vidus Vidius, 1544. Paré pointed out that, if the upper rung were not removed, the patient risked a dislocated neck. (Vidus Vidius)

all means the arm is to be bound to the side night and day, and for a long time even after the ulcers are completely healed: for thus it is more likely that cicatrization will take place, and the wide space into which the humerus used to escape will become contracted.'

It is doubtful whether this procedure was actually carried down to the joint capsule; rather, the contracture of the skin and loose subcutaneous tissue prevented the lateral rotation which leads to recurrent dislocation. (There is no reason to suppose that this was not effective; the writer recalls having to abandon an operation after exposure of the joint because of an anaesthetic complication – the soft tissue scarring led to cure.)

Hippocrates recognized Erb's palsy and described the patients as 'weasel-armed'; he thought it a dislocation, congenital or due to suppuration. He

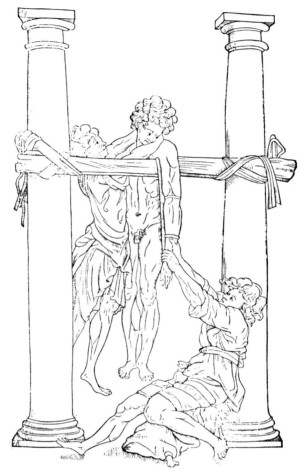

Figure 18   Reduction over a beam with a wooden splint at the inner side of the arm
providing enormous leverage. Hippocrates' favourite method. (Vidus Vidius)

notes that acromioclavicular dislocation, which he calls 'avulsion of the
acromion', is deceptive as the hollow beneath may be mistaken for a shoulder
dislocation and lead to wrong treatment, 'and I know many otherwise
excellent practitioners who have done much damage in attempting to reduce
shoulders of this kind'. The treatment was by compression pads over the
prominence and an upward lift with the arm bandaged to the side. 'No harm
... happens to the shoulder from this injury, but the part will be deformed';
the bone *cannot* be restored to its original position and this remains true for
nonoperative measures today.

Of fractures of the clavicle, transverse lesions were more easily reduced
than oblique and union was rapid 'as with all spongy bones'. Some
practitioners used elaborate arrangements of pressure pads connected to a

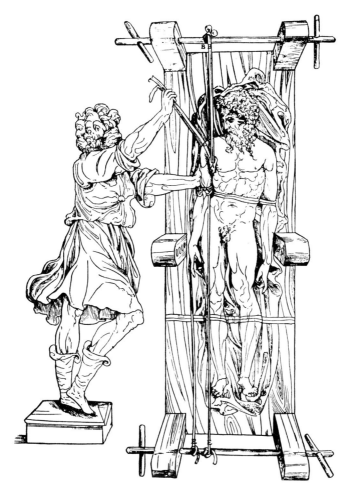

Figure 19   The use of the rack to reduce a shoulder dislocation. (Vidus Vidius)

body-belt or perineal belt, but Hippocrates says that these did not work; bed-rest for 14 days came nearest to full reduction, just as advised in the Edwin Smith papyrus and by Susruta. It was illogical to try to depress the inner fragment; what was needed was to elevate the arm with the outer fragment.

An elbow dislocation, after reduction, was bandaged at a little above the right angle, as the most functional position should ankylosis (presumably myositis ossificans) occur.

The account of wrist dislocation is obscure; we know that this virtually never occurs, whereas Hippocrates describes frequent displacements in four planes. These must have been either fractures of the lower radius or carpal fracture-dislocations.

Reduction of the temporomandibular joint is described. For mandibular fractures, the teeth were fixed with gold wire, bandaging and a leather strap. Much attention is devoted to nasal fractures, probably because the result was such a good or bad advertisement for the surgeon. A depressed fracture could be elevated with a spatula in the nose and held with paste of wheat-flour, stiffened with powdered frankincense or gum. There were also fractures of the cartilages of the ear, presumably from wrestling or boxing.

Spine

When the vertebrae were 'drawn into a hump by diseases', most cases were incurable, especially if the hump were above the attachment of the diaphragm. 'Such persons ... also have, as a rule, hard and unripened tubercles in the lungs, for the origin of the curvature and contraction is in most cases due to such gatherings', a quite extraordinary early appreciation of the relation between pulmonary tuberculosis and Pott's disease. When the hump was below the diaphragm, it was sometimes complicated by lumbar and groin abscesses, persistent and difficult to cure. (One recalls Calot, of Berck-Plage in France, in the 1890s, 'To open an abscess from a tuberculous spine is to open a door through which death always enters[28].')

Lateral curvatures, i.e. scoliosis, had the most satisfactory prognosis. A curved hump-back due to injury was not easy to treat (but these could not really have been traumatic cases, rather adolescent kyphoses) 'attempts at straightening rarely succeed'. Many tried 'succussion' on a ladder, but Hippocrates thought that, though this might sometimes work, it was a matter for charlatans, often done to impress the public, for impressive it certainly was. The patient was bound to the ladder, feet down for high lesions and head down for low ones, and the ladder dropped from a height, steadied by ropes held by assistants. 'Even in the healthy, the spine may become twisted in various fashions: and the spinal cord tolerates such distortions well, for this reason, that the deviation takes place in a curve and not an angle'.

There is a good description of the structure of the spine and its ligaments. He stresses the impossibility of reducing vertebral luxations, for:

(1) If the cord were so injured 'as to produce complete narcosis of many large and important parts', it would be pointless to trouble to adjust the vertebrae, and

(2) One could only do so by cutting the patient open and inserting a hand to exert pressure, 'but one might do this with a corpse but hardly with a living being', a point he returns to from time to time with some regret.

He says that he is writing this because ignorant practitioners deceive themselves, and others, by asserting that they can effect reduction, confusing fractures of spinous and transverse processes with injuries of the bodies and intervertebral joints.

Sharp spinal angulation due to injury could and should be treated, however. The patient was laid prone on the scamnum with windlass traction

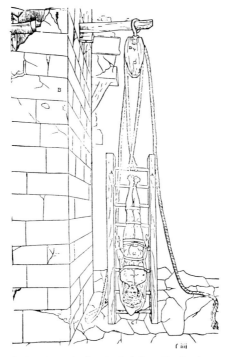

Figure 20 Hippocratic treatment of spinal deformity by 'succussion' on a ladder (Vidus Vidius)

to hips and shoulders, and the operator exerted vigorous manual pressure on the kyphus, very much as Calot[29] did 2500 years later for a tuberculous gibbus (p. 267), or he sat or stood on the hump or walked on a plank across it. Hippocrates had tried having the patient supine and blowing up a bag behind the angulation, but it did not work, 'I relate this on purpose: for those things also give good instruction which after trial show themselves failures, and show why they failed'. As for the method of forcible pressure on the prominence by means of a lever, a board attached to the wall, 'I know of no forcible procedure more applicable or useful.'

He distinguishes between 'inward deviations', causing death or paralysis, and a hump, i.e. a crush fracture, without such complications. It is as if the slighter-appearing injury were the more sinister, which is of course the case in the context of unstable rotary dorsolumbar lesions, which do not have much deformity.

Hip

The hip could be dislocated four ways, 'but far most frequently inward'. This is and remains a mystery. There is no doubt that Hippocrates is talking of

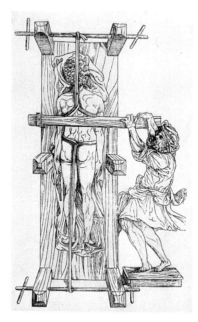

Figure 21   Hippocratic treatment of spinal deformity by traction and leverage on the scamnum. Originally from Oribasius; *De Machinamentis* (Fourth Century AD) reproduced by Vidus Vidius in Paris, 1544

medial displacement, for he describes the lengthened, laterally rotated limb and the hollow in the buttock and the prominence of the femoral head in the groin; and he specifically states that the head lies on the ischiopubic region. He also states that backward dislocation is rare, yet he knew its exact physical signs: shortening, instability, buttock prominence, internal rotation. How can this be? The writer has seen only one obturator dislocation in a lifetime. Were these wrestlers' injuries?* He carefully analyses the gait and the details of crutch support and the changes in the limbs in unreduced dislocation of either kind. And he makes this point, 'All parts of the body which have a function, if used in moderation and exercised in labours to which each is accustomed, thereby become healthy and well-developed: but if unused and left idle, they become liable to disease, defective in growth, and age quickly. This is especially the case with joints and ligaments, if one does not use them.'

---

* We may recall that anterior dislocation may occur in the hip that is hyperextended behind the body during weight-lifting[49]. Also that when Jacob wrestled throughout the night his opponent put out his hip, so that Jacob limped for the rest of his life.

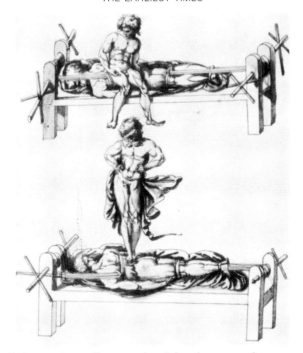

Figure 22 Sitting and standing on the deformity were also recommended by Hippocrates, the patient under traction on the scamnum. (Vidus Vidius)

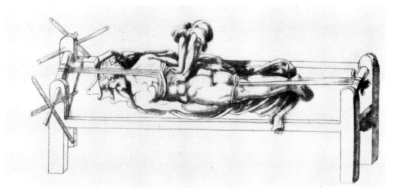

Figure 23 Manual pressure for spinal deformity. (Vidus Vidius)

Club-foot

Congenital club-foot was for the most part curable (we seem to be past the age of exposure of infants with this deformity) if it were not too severe or growth too advanced. After manipulative correction, the foot was dressed with cerate stiffened with resin, pads and bandages, a soleplate of lead or leather applied, and bandaged from within out to maintain correction. The last turn of the bandage was sewn to the outer side of the foot covering and pulled up tight on the outer side of the calf and fixed round the upper calf to act as a valgus retaining strap. 'This then is the treatment, and there is no need for incision, cautery or complicated methods, for such cases yield to treatment more rapidly than one might think. Still, time is required for complete success, *till the part has acquired growth in its proper position.*' (My italics, DLV) When ready for footwear, rather rigid 'mud shoes', used for walking on mud or clay, were supplied, as the feet yielded to these rather than vice versa.

Fractures and dislocations

A compound fracture-dislocation at the ankle or higher with bone protruding through the skin should not be reduced; let someone else do so if he wished, for death ensued in a few days due to tetanus or gangrene. Yet, even if reduction were not attempted, most survived. Treatment was with pitch cerate and wine compresses, but without forcible bandaging or plastering: 'Those thus treated are saved, but if the joint is reduced and keeps its place, they die.' This also applied to compound forearm fractures with protruding bone and to compound injuries at the knee and elbow; proximal injuries were the most dangerous, distal ones less so. Also, the first few days were the most dangerous for reduction; if it were to be done, it should be on either the first or second day or after the tenth; the intervening days, especially the fourth, were dangerous.

Gangrene, death and separation of bone were not necessarily alarming and quite compatible with survival, even if part of the thigh came away. In gangrene following a fracture ('strangulation with lividity'), demarcation and separation were rapid because the bone was already fractured, but in gangrene without fracture, though the soft parts soon died, separation of bone was very slow. In such cases, amputation should be done through a joint at a level of dead tissue to avoid pain and shock. Loss of soft parts meant great delay waiting for the underlying bone to separate; yet these wounds were 'more formidable to look at than to cure, and mild treatment is sufficient, for they determine their own process.' However, there was always the danger of secondary haemorrhage.

The reduction of a dislocated hip was as follows; the patient was suspended by the feet from a beam and the surgeon inserted his forearm between the thighs and between the perineum and the dislocated bone. He then grasped one hand with the other and suspended himself from the patient with the whole of his weight and so levered the head out of the perineum into its socket. This again indicates a medial dislocation. True, the suspension in itself would tend to reduce a posterior dislocation, but Hippocrates' manoeuvre, if it did anything at all, would redisplace it. Yet he did recognize posterolateral dislocation, and that this method could only make it worse, and that abduction and leverage on the buttock were required. Still, 'in some, the thigh is reduced without any apparatus by the aid of slight extension, such as can be managed with the hands and a little jerking: while in many, flexion of the leg at the joint and making a movement of circumduction is found to reduce it'. And this 2000 years before Bigelow![30] Another method of hip reduction was by inserting a bag between the thighs at the perineum and inflating it to push the femoral head outward: but this was not easy. Any dislocated joint was best reduced as soon as possible, 'while the parts are still warm', before swelling set in. Finger joints were reduced by traction and countertraction, or using 'lizards' of plaited palm tissue like Japanese fingerstalls. 'Dislocation' of the knee was easily reduced: it was usually an inward displacement, reduced by flexion, or by a sharp kick, or by squatting over a rolled bandage in the popliteal fossa. Obviously, these were internal derangements or patellar dislocations. A fall from a height on the heel with contusion carried the risk of necrosis and lifelong trouble due to dislocations (of the talus?) with mortification of the heel.

The Hippocratic bench, or *scamnum*, was of the greatest importance in orthopaedic practice for some 2000 years, being modified and reinvented down the centuries. It was 'a quadrangular plank, 6 cubits long and about 2 cubits broad', with a windlass at each end and an adjustable perineal post, or *priapiscos*, for countertraction and outward leverage of the femoral head. There were five or six longitudinal grooves in the lower part of the plank for the placement of wooden levers to exert pressure at either side of the hip, and other modifications were available – props at either side of the perineal post, crossbars, etc. It is all very like the fracture table of the ancient Hindus.

The general management of fractures is marked by considerable ignorance of the anatomy of the skeleton, emphasis on reduction by traction and manual moulding of the parts, bandaging with compression, and – though given a rather secondary place – splintage. Also by a great deal of commonsense and an obviously wide acquaintance with the natural history of skeletal injuries.

Forearm

'In dislocations and fractures, the practitioner should make extension in as straight a line as possible, for this is most conformable with nature; but if it incline at all to either side, this should be towards pronation rather than supination, for then the error is less.'

Hippocrates uses forearm fractures as a model for the management of all fractures: the theorising doctors were the very ones who made mistakes, for the patient spontaneously presented with the arm in the proper position; here he was wrong. Continued traction with the elbow extended was condemned, 'If one bandages it when extended, then the positions of the fleshy parts are altered by bending the elbow'. Further, 'the elbow cannot be kept extended for long since it is unaccustomed to that position, only to that of flexion. And besides, since patients are able to get about after injuries of the arm, they want it flexed at the elbow.' So the joint should be held at a little above the right angle.

A fracture of the radius was easier to treat than one of the ulna (can he really have meant this?) but required stronger traction. Fractures of both bones called for powerful traction and moulding into place with both hands, followed by overlapping bandaging and compresses, the object being uniform compression of the soft parts and pressure over the site of angulation. This principle of soft part support was dear to Hippocrates, dearer almost than splintage, and we shall return to it. 'These are the indices of good treatment and proper bandaging; that is, when the patient is asked if the part is compressed, he says that it is, but only moderately, and that mainly at the fracture site.' Rebandaging was done at three days and again at the seventh day, with increasing pressure as the soft part oedema subsided, and splints were not applied until after the first few days. These were on the dorsal and volar aspects of the limb, and not in the line of the radial and ulnar styloids: if they did have to be applied laterally, they should not extend as far as the bony prominences at the wrist 'for then there is a risk of ulceration and baring of the tendons.'

It was the dressings that were meant to adjust the fracture, and the splints were applied 'to maintain the dressing, and not bound in for the sake of pressure.' A soft broad scarf was added as a sling. Nevertheless, once on, the splints were left in place for 20 days or more. 'It takes about 30 days in all usually for the forearm bones to join, but this is in no way exact since constitutions and ages vary widely.' In any case, 'if splints are used, and it seems that the bones are not accurately adjusted or that something else may be troubling the patient, you should remove the dressing and reapply it at the middle of the interval or a little earlier ... if any of the results are not as laid down, it is certain that there has been some defect or over-zealousness in the surgical management.'

Humerus

The patient sat with the axilla over a suspended rod, with heavy weight-traction on the arm or elbow, so that he was almost suspended on the stool while the surgeon manipulated the fracture. The arm was then bandaged and splints applied at 7–9 days. Union took around 40 days and bandages and splints were readjusted as required during this period. It was important to preserve the natural curvature of the bone. However, 'all bones, when fractured, tend to become deformed during the cure towards that side to which they are naturally curved', so 'if you suspect anything of that kind, you should pass an additional broad bandage round the limb binding it to the chest.'

Tibia and fibula

The account of the anatomy is not quite accurate. 'The leg has two bones, one much more slender at one end than the other, but not so much at the other end. The parts adjacent to the foot are joined together and have a common epiphysis. In the length of the leg they are not united, but the parts near the thighbone are united and have an epiphysis, and that epiphysis has a diaphysis' (this probably refers to the apophysis of the tibial tuberosity).

'Of the two bones, the inner or so-called shin is the more troublesome to treat, needing stronger extension, and if the fragments are not accurately reduced it cannot be hidden, for it is visible and entirely without flesh. When this bone is broken, patients take longer to be able to use the limb, while if the outer bone is fractured ... they can soon stand. For the inner shin-bone carries the greater part of the weight, since the alignment of the femur and the general disposition of that side of the body are as they are.'

Strong extension was required for these fractures, in the natural line of the leg and thigh; but, 'if extension by manpower does not suffice, then call in some of the mechanical aids, whichever may be useful', though 'to resort to machines when not required is rather absurd.' A caution that moderns might bear in mind. After the conventional manual moulding and bandaging, the leg was placed on a smooth soft pillow to avoid distortion. 'As for the hollow splints which are placed under fractured legs, I am uncertain what to advise as to their use, for they do not do as much good as their users suppose.' Splintage could not enforce immobilization of the fracture because of the patient's movements in bed, and it was distressing to have wood under the limb unless padded. 'But it is very useful when changing the bedclothes and getting up to go to stool. It is therefore possible to manage affairs well or awkwardly, with or without the hollow splint; yet the vulgar have more faith in it and the practitioner will be less open to blame if a hollow splint is applied, though it is rather bad practice.' However, splints (presumably lateral) should be applied at the 7th, 9th or 11th day and rebandaging was done as the oedema subsided, with extension repeated on these occasions.

Ankle fractures

'The bones are occasionally dislocated at the foot end, sometimes both bones with the epiphysis, sometimes the epiphysis is displaced and sometimes only one of the bones ... most dislocations are outwards' (i.e. the foot outwards on the leg).

Reduction was by extension, 'Generally, two men suffice, one pulling one way and one the other.' More powerful devices were available; ox-hide thongs round the foot could be attached to a rod inserted into a 'wheel-nave' that was pulled on; or traction could be concentrated by having the upper trunk fixed to a post in the ground with adjustable pegs in the armpits and the arms at the side; or straps from the knee and thigh could be taken to a post above the head; or the patient could be laid on planks and a foot-strap pulled over a fulcrum at the end of the plank; or windlasses could be used at either end of the body. When the traction had done its work, the displacement was reduced by the palms of the operator's hands, 'pressing on the projecting part with one palm and with the other making counterpressure below the ankle on the opposite side', an exact account of the reduction of a Pott's fracture. Bandaging began, and applied most pressure over the projecting part, followed by rest and elevation; there is no mention of splintage.

The foot

'Consists of many small bones ... all of which are completely healed in 20 days, except those that are connected with the leg-bones in a vertical line.' These were larger than the others and, when displaced, healing took longer. Here, we are concerned mainly with the os calcis. 'Those who jump from a height and land heavily on the heel have the bones separated ... swelling develops and severe pain, for this bone is not small, it extends beyond the line of the leg and is connected with important vessels and cords. The back tendon is inserted into this bone ... It is not everyone who can bandage such cases properly ... there is a risk of necrosis of the heelbone; and, if such necrosis arises, the condition may persist throughout the patient's life. Indeed, necrosis from other causes, as when the heel blackens due to lack of care for its position while the patient is confined to bed ... or when there is some other disease requiring prolonged rest on his back – all these necroses are equally chronic and troublesome and often recur anew if not given the most skilful attention.' Recovery might be expected after 60 days with bed-rest and elevation of the foot.

Femur

'It is essential that the extension applied should not be inadequate, whereas any excess can do no harm. Indeed, even if bandaging be done while the bones are held apart by the force of the traction, the dressing would be powerless to keep them apart and they would come together as soon as the assistants relaxed their pull, for the fleshy part, being thick and powerful, will prevail over the bandaging and not be overcome by it.'

Hippocrates was very conscious of the importance of public recognition of successful reduction, or, at any rate, of avoiding obvious evidence of insuccess, 'for the disgrace and harm are great if the outcome is a shortened thigh. It is true that the arm, if shortened, may be concealed and the defect not great, but a shortened leg leaves the patient lame and the sound leg, being longer, exposes the defect; so that, if a patient is going to have unskilful treatment, it would be better for him to have both legs broken rather than one, for then he will at least be level'. (This notion persisted, even to the extent of deliberate fracture of the sound side, in connection with femoral fractures and the treatment of congenital hip dislocation, up to the 19th and 20th centuries (p. 515).)

With bandaging and splintage the fracture was 'firm' in 40 days. The knee was to be held straight, if necessary by a hollow back-splint for the whole limb, and the splints must not be allowed to press on bare skin, tendons or bony prominences. The normal anterior and lateral bowing of the femur should be respected, but not to the point of exaggeration. 'More injury than good results from placing under the thigh a splint which does not pass further down than the ham and has a tendency to produce what of all things must be avoided, namely flexion at the knee.' It had to extend to the ankle.

In all leg fractures, the positioning and support of the foot were important;

if allowed to dangle, there would be convexity at the fracture, if over-supported, concavity. 'All bones unite more slowly if not placed in their natural position and immobilized in the same position, and the callus is weaker.'

Compound fractures

The bones might or might not protrude, splinters might or might not work their way to the surface, various applications (compresses of pitch or wine) could do some good and no great harm. There is a round condemnation of the contemporary equivalent of the windowed plaster, of those who apply bandages to either side 'while leaving a gap at the wound itself and let it be exposed and dress it variously ... This treatment is bad, and those who use it are likely to show the greatest folly in their management of other fractures also. For what matters most is to understand the benefits of proper application of the bandages and of applying the main pressure at the proper place, and the harm of not applying the bandage properly and of applying pressure, not where it ought to be, but at one or other side ... for in a patient so bandaged the swelling is bound to arise in the actual wound, since even if healthy tissue were bandaged on either side and a gap left in the middle, it would be just at this gap that swelling and discoloration would occur. How, then, could a wound fail to be affected in this manner? For it is bound to happen that the wound is discoloured, with everted margins, and has a watery discharge lacking pus and, as for the bones themselves, even those come away that otherwise would not have done so. The wound becomes hot and throbbing, so they finally remove the dressings and treat it thereafter without bandaging. Nevertheless, faced with other similar wounds, they use the same treatment, for they cannot conceive that it is the peripheral bandaging and exposure of the wound that are to blame, but some mishap. However, I should not have written so much about this had I not fully recognized the dangers of this dressing and that many use it, and that it is vitally important to unlearn the habit.'

It is a habit that is still having to be unlearned all over the world, especially in wartime. Not long ago, in an African country ravaged by war, the present writer found wards full of civilians with gunshot fractures of the tibia which did not and could not heal because they were in neatly windowed plasters; healing took place when the plasters were closed and the patients sent home.

Incidentally, the impression gained from 17th and 18th century western European writings that a compound fracture, especially of the tibia, was virtually a sentence of death, or at least of amputation, is not at all the view of Hippocrates. Perhaps the sun and soil of Greece were more propitious for survival, 'If those who contract tetanus do not die within four days, they recover' (*Aphorisms*).

In compound fractures, the fracture itself was to be treated exactly as if there were no external wound, the wound anointed with 'pitch cerate' as a compress and entirely covered and overlapped by a wide pressure bandage, 'for bandages narrower than the wound ligate it like a girdle and should be

avoided.' The dressings were changed on alternate days, the hope being for
suppuration, and splintage was postponed longer than usual. Simple fractures
might become compound, either from piercing from within or undue external
pressure, and such wounds were treated similarly. Blackened muscle or
tendon came away easily with bland applications of 'white cerate' and the
extrusion of bone was heralded by profuse discharge.

Maintenance of length and alignment were essential and to be secured
primarily by bandaging, but 'it is especially convenient to use mechanical
treatment for the leg.' Tying it to the bedpost or other fixed support was
useless or even harmful as movements caused displacement, 'If it were not
so fastened, there would be less displacement, as it would not so much lag
behind the movement of the rest of the body.'

Therefore, and quite remarkably, Hippocrates describes a method based
on exactly the same principle as the external fixator of today, but two
millennia ahead of time. He used tight leather cuffs at the knee and ankle
containing sockets for springy wooden rods that were rather too long and
inserted when bent to apply distraction, three or more pairs of these. 'This
mechanism, if well arranged, will make the extension both correct and even
consistent with the normal alignment, and will cause no pain in the wound

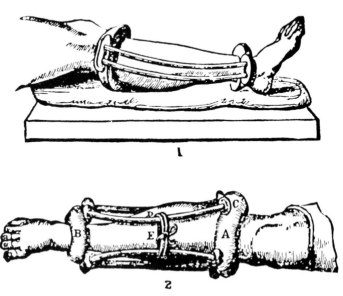

Figure 24   The essential principle of the external fixator for tibial fracture, as applied
by Hippocrates. The wooden splints are under great compression. (Bick, E. M.
[1968]. *Source Book of Orthopaedics*. (New York, Hafner)

since the external pressure, if any, will be diverted partly to the foot and partly to the thigh ... and the wound is both easy to examine and easy to handle.' But, if it be not well arranged, it will harm rather than help, 'for it is shameful and contrary to the art to construct a machine and obtain no mechanical effect.'

The third or fourth days were the very last on which a lesion should be actively interfered with, and all probings as well as anything else that might irritate the wound should be avoided on those days, 'for, in general, it is at the third or fourth day that exacerbations arise in the majority of lesions.' There is here an implicit recognition of the fragility of the lymphatic barriers that were being laid down against the spread of inflammation and infection. But, if bandages were applied at the outset and left relatively undisturbed, then at the seventh day there would be no inflammation and dressings and splints could be safely applied. If the fracture ends projected and could not be reduced by traction, they could be brought into place by an iron lever inserted between the ends; and if it were an overriding oblique fracture that would not engage on the lever, 'cut a step in the bone to form a secure lodgment'; but this must be done on the first and second day and not at 3–5 days, for then disturbance could cause inflammation or 'spasm' (tetanus) with little hope of recovery. Interference was less hazardous after the seventh day.

'As for bones that cannot be reduced ... these will come away, as will those that are completely laid bare ... some separate early while others are exfoliated only after desiccation and corruption.' Bone was eliminated more rapidly where suppuration and the growth of new flesh (granulation tissue) were more rapid, 'since it is the growth of new flesh in the wound that usually elevates the fragments ... the more porous bones coming away more quickly and the solider ones more slowly.' A protruding piece of bone could be resected if necessary, but this was not usually very important as bone entirely deprived of soft parts would inevitably come away entirely. If both bones are broken and heal with overlap, or if a 'circle' of bone (i.e. an annular sequestrum) is extruded, shortening is inevitable.

'Cases where the bone of the thigh or upper arm protrudes rarely recover, for these bones are large and contain much marrow, while the cords, muscles and vessels involved in the injury are many and major ... it also matters greatly whether the bone projects at the inner or outer side of the thigh, for many important blood vessels run along the inner aspect and it is dangerous if some of these are injured.'

Hippocrates says that dislocations of the knee are less severe than those of the elbow, and commoner, easily reduced without much ensuing inflammation; but he must have meant patellar subluxations and meniscus tears. Elbow dislocations were difficult to reduce, especially if left late, with complications due to inflammation and excessive callus; but, from his detailed accounts, some at least of his dislocations seem to have been supracondylar fractures. As a rule, fractures are always less difficult than cases where there are no bones broken but there is extensive contusion of blood vessels and major cords in that region – perhaps the first enunciation of the adage that it is better to break an ankle than to sprain it. Dislocations must be reduced at once because of the rapid onset of inflammation of the tendons and ligaments, which might contract and restrict the natural range of movement for some considerable time. The injured elbow was best treated at a right angle, for 'if ankylosis should eventually develop, an arm ankylosed in the extended position would be better away (i.e. amputated) for it would be a great hindrance and of little use to the patient.' Hippocrates was very reserved about elbow injuries. Indeed, 'sometimes the head of the humerus itself is fractured at the epiphysis, yet this, though it may seem a very serious injury, is much less so than injuries of the elbow joint.' We should add that he does not seem to have used any angled splints; if it was necessary to fix the elbow, it was by overlapping arm and forearm splints.

There was also the practice of inducing venous stasis to promote union in sluggish fractures, by proximal or proximal and distal ligation of the limb, rediscovered at intervals and practised assiduously in modern times by Thomas[31] and Bier[32].

Mochlicon (levers or instruments of reduction) is a book that is a ragbag of orthopaedic oddments, with a reasonably accurate review of the anatomy of the skeleton and a recapitulation of material from *Fractures* and *Joints*.

If bilateral temporomandibular dislocation were not reduced at once, death was usual in ten days. The shoulder was dislocated downwards, 'I have no knowledge of any other direction' and methods of reduction were as has been described. Again, we have the puzzling detailed description of 'wrist dislocations' and the insistence that hip dislocation was nearly always inward, which increases the conviction that this was a wrestling injury. Hippocrates recognized that dislocation of the hip could be due to suppuration, or congenital, noting that bilateral displacement was not very troublesome. 'Those suffer the greatest injury in whom, while still in the womb, this joint has been dislocated ... it sometimes happens that an outward dislocation of both hips is found in one case from birth and in another as the result of disease.'

At the ankle, the leg bones ended in a common epiphysis, at which movement of the foot took place, but this epiphysis is not defined and there is no mention of the talus. When Hippocrates says that the commonest dislocation is of the leg inwards and the foot outwards, he is describing Pott's fracture and, as before, it is advised that compound injuries with protruding bone be best left alone. Suitably treated, they may survive badly maimed and with a thin scar. The only hope of safety for dislocations in general, save those of the fingers, when compound, was not to reduce them; and if reduction were attempted, the risks should be explained to the patient and it was on no account to be tried between the second and tenth days. Otherwise, 'one must bear in mind that reduction means death, the quicker and more certain the larger and higher they are.' In compound dislocation of the foot, spasm (tetanus) and gangrene were to be expected; but amputation at a joint or not too high in a bone could be expected to lead to recovery.

Gangrene was due to (1) constriction in wounds swollen with haemorrhage, (2) compression in fractures, and (3) mortification from bandages, presumably blood-soaked and stiffened. Even when part of the arm or thigh fell off and bones and flesh came away, many survived. Cases with soft tissue loss not immediately affecting the bone looked terrifying, but were not really so dangerous, 'so one should take on these cases.'

Spinal curvatures 'after a fall' (but whose traumatic origin was really spurious) were not easy to correct, especially if above the diaphragm, 'Many patients spit blood and get an abscess.' Hippocrates was frustrated by internal curvatures of the spine, 'not reducible by sneezing, coughing, injection of air or cupping: a mode of restoration is wanting.' As stated, at one or two places he hints that he would dearly like to open the body cavities and reduce them from within. He recognized that fractures with angulation could simulate inward dislocation, but were not so serious and healed rapidly.

As to fractures, 'the most spongy bones consolidate quickest, and vice versa.' Of dislocations, 'the most distal are the most easily put out: and those most easily put out suffer least inflammation, but where there is least heat and no aftertreatment, there is greatest liability to another dislocation ... oft-repeated dislocations are more easily reduced and they are due to the disposition of the bones or ligaments ... or to flatness of the socket.'

Again, we have the extraordinary account of the principle of external fixation for compound fractures of the leg bones with protrusion: the circular thongs at knee and ankle with pockets for the insertion of rods of cornel wood, over-long so that they sprang out and straightened the limb under tension, 'making extension both ways'. If need be, projecting bone could be sawn off later.

The *scamnum* is described in detail by Hippocrates himself, by Rufus (Heliodorus) and by Paul of Aegina, but later restorations are unreliable. The best known are those of Vidus Vidius (1544), with a row of square holes down the middle and a pointed *priapiscos*, and that of Littré (1844) with grooves in the distal half. Littré's seems to correspond more closely to the

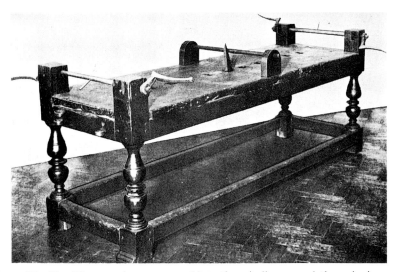

Figure 25   The Hippocratic scamnum. Note the windlasses and the priapiscos. A mediaeval reconstruction

original description.

The influence of Hippocrates, on medicine as a whole and on orthopaedics in particular, never completely died away and is indeed still pervasive. We may not always now take the Hippocratic Oath, but traction and countertraction, the traction table, the method of reducing a shoulder dislocation, are still with us; also, more important than details, the tradition of careful clinical observation and objective assessment of results. His teachings were continued through the Hellenistic Period, preserved through the Dark Ages by the Arabs, and emerged into the daylight of the Renaissance.

AFTER GREECE

As Greek power declined, her academic and practical medical achievements spread in three main directions: to Asia Minor, especially Byzantium; to Alexandria, already the seat of a university and a medical school from 3–200 BC; and to Rome. This may be described, in general terms, as the Hellenistic Period.

With other aspects of Greek culture, Greek medicine was adopted and adapted by the Romans, though Greek physicians practising in Rome were at best colonials and usually also slaves. Sometimes such a surgeon was known as a *vulnerarius* or wound-healer, entirely analogous to the mediaeval German *Wundarzt*. An early Greek arrival was Asclepiades of Bithynia (124–40 BC) and a member of his school became one of the most famous figures at around the beginning of the Christian era, a Roman: Aurelius Cornelius Celsus (25 BC–50 AD). Celsus was not, in fact, a medical specialist, but a layman, an encyclopaedist – a sort of Roman Diderot – whose wide publications included several works on medicine. These contain a description of the four cardinal signs of the inflammatory process, of the treatment of fractures and dislocations and the use of bandages made stiff with starch, and an account of spinal injuries and paraplegia which is accurate enough but no better than is given in the Edwin Smith papyrus. We know that he advised refracture of the soft callus for malunited fractures, and that he used ligatures, for the surgical techniques described include ligature of varicose veins. There was also a bone-drill operated by the recoil of a twisted thong, which was still in use in the Middle Ages. Yet, like so much else, his *De Medicina* or *De Re Medica*, written about 30 AD, was not original but a compilation from Greek sources, was lost in the Dark Ages and was republished in Italy in the 15th century (1478). He resumed the dental wiring of Hippocrates for jaw fractures and advised remedial exercises after fractures had healed.

The medical services of the Roman armies were well organized, but in the hands of very subordinate staff, rather like modern sick-bay attendants; but there were infirmaries, or *valetudinaria*, and these institutions were perpetuated in civil life. Yet Rome itself produced no scientific or theoretic system of medicine, though it did house the great Galen, who contributed so much to medicine as a practical art.

Galen (129–199 AD), of Pergamon, studied in Asia Minor and Alexandria and was therefore greatly influenced by the writings of Hippocrates. As a young man, from AD 158–161, Galen had been a gladiatorial surgeon in the Pergamon arena in Asia Minor, where he must have acquired a mass of useful information; he has been styled 'the father of sports medicine'. He was called to Rome by Marcus Aurelius and wound up with an enormous practice. According to Singer and Underwood[33], his works provided the theoretic basis of medicine for the next 1500 years. He gives a good account of the skeleton as a whole and of individual bones and joints, but is particularly interesting on muscles, not merely in terms of dissection but also in describing their innate tendency to contract, noting that the principle of voluntary movement originated from the brain and travelled through the nerves. He also coined the term 'tonus' as applied to sustained contraction and analysed the reciprocal components of locomotion in *De Motu Musculorum*. He studied bone destruction, sequestration and regeneration in osteomyelitis, which he sometimes treated by resection, and coined, or first used, the terms kyphosis, lordosis and scoliosis for the deformities described by Hippocrates; and he treated scoliosis by traction, local pressure and breathing exercises – the first, it seems to recognize the relation of spinal curvature to respiratory function. In animal experiments he noted the varying effects of section of the cervical cord at successively lower levels. He devised a pressure bandage to control haemorrhage in limbs. He thought that rheumatic diseases were due to discharge of the four humours of the body in unbalanced amounts into the joints (hence gout = *gutta*, a drop).

Galen was an opinionated man, not one to brook contradiction, without a school, followers or disciples. Yet, as has been well said: 'On his death in AD 199 the active prosecution of anatomical and physiological enquiry ceased absolutely. The curtain descends at once ... the Dark Ages have begun[33].'

Gradually, after Celsus and Galen, and catastrophically after its fall in AD 476, Rome declined in the West and the transmission of Greek thought was left to the Eastern Empire in Byzantium, and after that to the Arabs. We must remember that there had long been a flourishing school, or schools, in Greek Asia Minor from at least the time of Hippocrates, and that Alexandria, though its influence, too, dwindled, was later to house Paul of Aegina. By some unlikely chances, valuable teachings and illustrations of orthopaedic treatment reaching back to Hippocrates have been preserved. Apollonius, whose life spanned the birth of Christ, was a teacher in Alexandria who wrote a book on diseases of the joints which is largely a transmission of, and a commentary on, the *De Articulis* of Hippocrates, with figures of the methods of treatment, the oldest illustrated surgical text. This later formed part of a collection of ancient Greek manuscripts made for the Emperor Constantine (913–939) by a Byzantine court physician, one Niketas. Again, Oribasius (325–403) was a native of Pergamon and became personal physician to the Emperor Julian the Apostate (331–363); two of his manuscrips, *De Laqueis* and *De Machinamentis* were also based on tradition. In 1492, Lorenzo de Medici sent an agent to Greece to purchase some of the literary treasures dispersed after the fall of Constantinople 40 years earlier, and on Crete this agent located the works we have described, and others, which were to form the famous collection in the Laurentian Library in Florence.

Here it was mislaid for several decades. Then it was translated into Latin. There was a Florentian surgeon, Guido Guidi or Vidus Vidius (*c.*1500–1569) who went to Paris to serve as a professor at the *Collège de France* from 1542 to 1548 at the request of Francis I, and he took with him a copy of the collection, which he used to produce a magnificent gift edition – the manuscripts in Latin translation plus the illustrations, the famous Manuscript 6866 of the Bibliothèque Nationale, the *Chirurgia, è Graeco in Latinum conversa* of 1544. The illustrations, which still exist and are frequently reproduced (see pp. 22–30), give us what must be a very close approximation to an accurate representation of the treatment of shoulder dislocation and spinal deformities as carried out in Hippocrates' own time.

From these and other sources, we find that the apotheosis of ancient surgery was reached at the end of the first century AD. A great figure, often referred to simply as 'The Surgeon', was Meges of Sidon, who practised in Rome shortly before Celsus and taught Celsus. Two other figures, Archigenes and Leonidas, were amputating very much as we do now. Heliodorus (who lived just before Celsus in the first century AD), used a type of flap amputation and, with his pupil Antyllus, operated for hernia and fistula and resected bone. They divided contracted bands to correct joint flexion and even, it is thought, did sternomastoid tenotomy. Two hundred years later, Oribasius said they had removed the entire humerus and part of the scapula and regarded resection of the mandible as an easy operation, that he could find no better surgeons in his own time; but one must always be cautious about laudatory references to great figures of the past.

One point relevant to orthopaedics may be mentioned here. Bick[34] says that, from the 5th to the 15th centuries, there was a utter lack of any sense of responsibility on the part of society for those who suffered from visible deformities (one supposes the counterpart of the ancient Indian attitude to cripples as evil incarnate). This may have been true for Central and Western Europe; but we are also told that 'a truly satisfactory social welfare system for crippled children and adults did not exist before the era of the Byzantine Empire, when it assumed great importance in accordance with Christian principles ... the Emperor founded a hospital for war invalids, the blind, crippled and handless veterans[35].' We also know that the Christian Church was committed to the care of the sick and the handing down of medical manuscripts; it is unfortunate that disease and deformity were considered to be the punishment for sin. Still, it was the Church Fathers who were the guardians of medical tradition; quite early, there was a line of healing saints, the foremost of whom were Cosmo and Damien, the patron saints of medicine, martyred under Diocletian in AD 303. They it was who miraculously performed the first (and still the only) limb transplant, amputating a gangrenous leg below the knee and replacing it with one removed from a dead patient; as the latter was a negro, the healed man had limbs of two colours. This has been depicted by many artists.

Next in importance after Oribasius was Paul of Aegina, of the 7th century (625–690 AD), who worked for a period in Alexandria. Because this city was

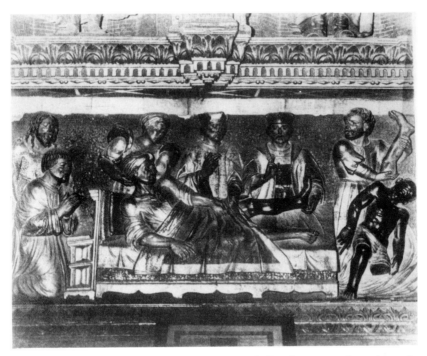

Figure 26 The miracle of Saints Cosmo and Damien: transplantation of a lower limb

caught up in the Moslem invasion which spread over North Africa and the near East at this time, Paul's *Seven Books*, which he acknowledged were mainly due to Hippocrates, became a prime source for the Arab translators as a medical authority valid for centuries. The *Sixth Book* treats fractures and dislocations. Here, he conceives that paraplegia due to spinal fracture may be relieved by removing the compressing bone, and, since he devised scissors for laminectomy, we must assume that he actually carried this out, especially as he says, 'When cutting or sawing the bone, if any vital parts are situated beneath, such as the pleura, spinal cord or the like, we must use the instrument called the meningophylax (literally: membrane-protector) to shield them.' He also wrote on ganglia, but not distinguishing those around the small joints of the limb from sebaceous cysts of the scalp. He treated patellar fractures by cramming the fragments together by bandaging with the knee extended, exactly like Hugh Owen Thomas 1200 years later, and fractures of the clavicle much as Hippocrates had done, advising several weeks' recumbency if necessary. He was not always orthodox, 'When bones heal distorted by callus, no little lameness ensues ... The method of breaking them again is not acceptable as it may be dangerous, but if the callus be newly formed we must have recourse to medicines for dissolving callus, and we may also dispel it by friction with the hand and bending it one way or another. If stony hard, one must separate the union of the bone with chisels.'

For several centuries after Paul, the Arab – better, the Mohammedan – empire and culture extended from Spain along the southern shore of the Mediterranean and into areas of Asia Minor that had once been Greek, and beyond. We have to regard Islamic medicine, not as a natural Arab growth, but as the medicine of later Greek antiquity reformulated in the Arabic language from the 9th century, a Hellenization of the newcomers[36]. The Arab conquest of the Persian Sassanid empire found Greek medical traditions already established there and was followed by the Abbasid Caliphate of 750–

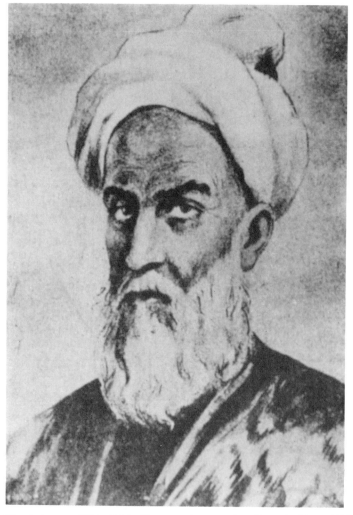

Figure 27 Avicenna (980–1036) (Source: *Avicenna* by Czerminski, published by Wiedza Powszechna, Warsaw, 1953)

1250 AD which laid the foundations of Persian medicine[37,38]. This was the period of the translators, of the great Rhazes (850–932) who first described spina ventosa and the recurrent laryngeal nerve, of Avicenna (Ali ben Sina)[39] (980–1036) with his *Qanum* or Canon of medicine which advises the freshening of ununited fractures, of the Jew Maimonides in Cordova, and of Averroes who influenced Europe via the Moorish occupation of Spain.

The *Medical Aphorisms* of Moses Maimonides, originally published in Arabic in Cordova around 1497[40], are distinctly antagonistic to Galen in many places. Aphorism 10 says that a limb which is anaesthetic will become gangrenous and should be amputated forthwith through healthy tissue next to the demarcation site. (Since Orthodox Jews were forbidden to handle dead tissues, the Talmud advises leaving the limb attached by a shred of tissue so that the patient could wrench it off himself.) Aphorism 12: if the limb were already putrefied or necrotic, the stump should be cauterized. Aphorism 17: nerve punctures were very painful; the wound should be left open and warm water was dangerous. Aphorism 64: 'One should not attempt to reduce any broken bone until four or more days have passed, lest one cause the patient much harm.' This counsel was not unique; and a school of deliberately delayed reduction persisted in the USA even after World War II. Aphorism 68: 'Fractures of the leg require the application of a cast, lest the leg move and the limb crepitate ... one should closely reflect whether the damage that might arise from the cast will be greater than its benefit.' But what type of cast? We are not told.

Some fairly recent writers have been almost ecstatic about medicine in the pre-Muslim and Muslim Persian empire. Elgood[38,41] says even that the Hippocratic system must have derived from Persia, since it emerged full-fledged so rapidly between 700 and 500 BC, and since one book of the *Corpus* is almost identical with a Persian text. He says that Avicenna was one of the greatest men this world has ever seen. The cleavage between physicians and surgeons became complete in the post-Mongol period: the great physicians would not operate except in extreme emergency and would not describe details of operations or bonesetting. 'Since bonesetting is a form of surgery and is a dangerous practice, a skilled Master is necessary to watch and learn from.' Additionally, there was a school of barber-surgeons.

There was also a surgery of punishment. A verse in the Koran says: 'And as for the man who steals and the woman who steals, cut off their hands as a punishment for what they have earned, an exemplary punishment from Allah.' The public executioner did so and applied burning pitch or oil (but then, so did the Elizabethans, p. 479). There was also blinding, burning, castration. Yet, though once common, the Persians lost the art, and by the 18th century considered therapeutic amputation as done by Europeans impossible because of the mortality. Elgood also refers to the beautiful illuminated illustrations in *Le Premier Manuscript Chirurgical Turc*, now in the *Bibliothèque Nationale* in Paris.

However, there was a religious prejudice against animal dissection or experiment, and little surgical enterprise except for Avicenna, in Bokhara, who was vigorous in the treatment of kyphosis, and Albulkasim (Albucasis) in Cordova in the 11th century. The latter's treatise, *Tractatus de Operatione*

(a)

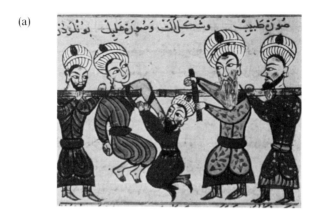

(b)

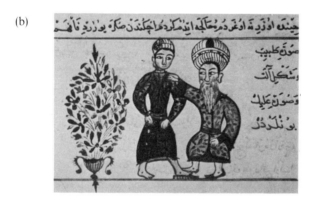

Figure 28 From *Le Premier Manuscrit Turc* of 1465 (Editions Roger Dacosta, Paris) (a) is stated to be a shoulder reduction but appears more like that of an elbow (b). shows reduction of a dislocated toe by standing on the foot

menus seu de Chirugia Albucasis, was for long an authoritative if not very original text, one volume of which dealt with fractures and dislocations. 'Surgical operations are of two kinds: those that benefit the patient and those that usually kill him.'

Albucasis[42] recognized fractures and dislocations from the deformity, protrusion and crepitus and his management was very Hippocratic: first careful bandaging and then splints of halves of cane, palm-branch ribs, fennel stalks, but this was delayed for a few days if there was swelling: also hollow gutter splints. His initial venesection, purging and starvation were not of Greek derivation. His 'plasters' used a variety of elements: fine dust from the flour-mill with egg-white; pulse, gum-mastic, acacia, clay (Armenian bole), myrrh, aloes; wool soaked in oil and vinegar; pulped fig and poppy leaves; or other vegetable mixes. If there were no pain and swelling, the part was left alone for up to 3 weeks, a very general conservatism at this and later periods. He condemns the 'ignorant bonesetters' who refracture for malunion as mistaken and dangerous, 'If it were right, the Ancients would undoubtedly have spoken of it in their books ... but I have not found a trace of it in a single one of them, and the right course is not to use it.' He was wrong; many of them had so practised.

He treated fractures of the clavicle by reduction with pressure, using a ball of wall in the axilla to give leverage to the bandaging when the arm was at the side; but the patient could be treated supine on a bolster. If a movable splinter were felt, 'you must cut down on the splinter and gently remove it, and if it sticks to the bone you must contrive to cut it with one of the chisels ... having first put behind the clavicle the instrument to protect the membrane (meningophylax).' A figure-of-eight bandage with axillary pads was much the same as used today. He also removed rib fragments which might damage the pleura. In neck injuries, if both hands were powerless and insensitive, 'he's doomed'; and if the feet were in similar case after a back injury without control of the sphincters, 'his case is hopeless, so do not concern yourself with his treatment.' We are back to the Edwin Smith papyrus. On hip dislocation he was with Hippocrates: there was medial shift and a longer leg; posterior dislocation was rare, but he also states that the heel is never fractured, something that the Greek did recognize. For toe fractures, he got the patient upright and stood on his feet. He says something that I can find nowhere else, 'When a man's organ is fractured, take a goose's neck and introduce the penis into it, then let it be wrapped and bandaged and left for about three days until it be healed.'

There were the great hospitals of Baghdad, especially the Bimaristan Al-Azudi, founded in 981, with its specialized wards and departments, regularly visited by physicians and specialists in surgery and orthopaedics. The last were rapidly recognized: 'Orthopaedic surgeons had a further examination in the Sixth Book of the Pandect of Paul of Aegina, which Hunain had translated, and were compelled to have a special knowledge of bones.' One Al-Jurgani, born at the mid-11th century and dying at Merv around 1140, wrote a compendium of nine books, the seventh of which has two splendid sections on fractures, dislocations and bonesetting, the details being such as to make it clear that orthopaedics as a discipline and orthopaedists as a class were well-recognized.

Plaster-of-Paris was used at a very early date in the East for the treatment of fractures (see p. 567).

In Europe, so long benighted – and how one agrees with Charles Lamb in thinking of the Dark Ages as literally without sunlight – the period of the Awakening is that of the foundation of the great universities, hospitals and medical faculties in the 10th–12th centuries: the great medical centre of Salerno in the 9th century, Paris, Oxford, Bologna, Montpellier, Padua (both the last two with medical schools), the Faculty of the *Collège de St. Côme* in Paris which was later to be so unwelcoming to Paré when he applied for admission. All these either arose as monastic establishments or were subservient to religion; and, at a later date, medicine in some schools was allied or subject to legal instruction – not always a disadvantage as there is some evidence that medicolegal requirements promoted dissection.

To a great extent this upsurge in intellectual life was stimulated by Latin translations of the Arab translations of the Greeks, including Hippocrates. The Moslems had been a European Empire, by virtue of their occupation of Spain, for hundreds of years; they had extended as far north as Poitiers. The relevance of this process to orthopaedics lies in its attention to dissection though this was initially confined to animals, while human dissection had to await the 13th–14th centuries. Nevertheless, the rebirth of anatomic studies inevitably led to a rebirth of surgery.

Three mediaeval figures of successive apprenticeship are of interest. *Hugo of Lucca* (1160–1237) was educated at Salerno and Bologna. His spiritual (if not actual) son was *Theodoric* (1205–1298), Dominican Bishop of Cervia, who wrote a book on surgery in 1267; and Theodoric's pupil was *Henri de Mondeville* (1260–1320). Their views are so similar that they may be epitomized jointly. The first objective in fracture treatment was true and correct realignment, with restoration of the intervening flesh to its proper state. The second was maintenance by proper binding, using bandages or pads of tow soaked in egg-white, or padded splints made from the staves or branches held together by such bandages, and these staves were also dipped in egg-white and care taken to ensure that their ends did not rub on exposed skin. Splintage was not disturbed for 20–25 days, except for pain, and the part was then rebandaged and resplinted for another 14–20 days. Patients with leg or hip fractures were kept constipated to lessen movement. (Hippocrates and Galen had delayed splintage for 5–6 days.)

In compound fractures, all layers were to be individually apposed: bone to bone, muscle to muscle, skin and flesh; but only the skin and subcutaneous tissue were sutured; the wound was bound up with the fracture and not disturbed for 10 or more days. A divided nerve could be reapposed if the adjacent layers were carefully brought together. A malunited fracture, if the callus were still soft, was to be treated by fomentation, manipulation, refracture and resetting; if the callus were old and hard, it was best to make an open incision and refracture with a chisel, for if manipulation were used the bone might break elsewhere.

The 'knotting' which followed fractures might prevent normal function if near a joint (*myositis ossificans*); when hard, excess callus should be scraped away after incision. Limbs must be kept in the functional position.

Projecting fragments of the clavicle were to be removed, while protecting the important deeper structures with the meningophylax used in head injuries. Crush fractures of the spine with angulation were reduced by manual pressure, or by sitting on the patient, or by the classical method of leverage with a board.

The signs of dislocation were lack of firmness of the joint and an abnormal cavity, or a cavity might appear on one side with a bulge on the other; and reduction was by drawing out the ends of the limb in each direction until the two extremities were opposed at the point of dislocation and the dislocated part turned to the point from which it had emerged, reduction often being indicated by an audible snap; and then it was to be bound up. Dislocations of the elbow were the most troublesome, 'dislocation of the wrist' (i.e. Colles' fracture) easily reduced. Shoulder dislocation was reduced by pressing with hand or foot on a ball of wool in the axilla and then rotating the head of the humerus internally for a moment, 'and when this is done, the humerus falls into its joint', an anticipation of Kocher. Mondeville gives the first description (from personal experience) of an infallible sign of shoulder dislocation: inability to touch the opposite ear with the hand if the elbow is kept to the side. It is unequivocally stated that dislocation of the hip, for the most part, occurs externally, and very seldom internally, which is not the Hippocratic teaching (p. 29) but observational.

Roger of Palermo (active in 1170–1200), a Salerno surgical graduate or *magister*, wrote his *Practica chirurgiae* in 1180, the first surgical text of Western Europe, much of it based on Greek tradition. It deals extensively with fractures of the skull, trephining for depressed fractures, the reduction of dislocations. Roger thought suppuration necessary for proper wound healing, the old concept of 'laudable pus', but the teachers at Bologna later insisted on the possibility and desirability of healing 'by first intention' based on cleanliness, gentleness and avoiding cautery in favour of the scalpel.

So wrote William of Salicet (1210–1280), whose excellent treatise, *Cyrurgia*, of 1275 dealt with anatomy and surgery and contains the first mention (in Europe) of crepitus as a sign of fracture and describes the reduction of cervical dislocation. The practice of nerve suture has been ascribed to William, though it had been suggested by Avicenna two centuries earlier and was performed sporadically by later practitioners, though with the difficulty that nerves were not clearly distinguished from tendons before the time of Vesalius, whose *De humani corporis fabrica* appeared in 1543. But nerves are still sutured to tendons, and not only in the Third World!

Guy de Chauliac (1300–1368), professor at Montpellier and advocate of traction in suspension for femoral fractures, is discussed at p. 221 and his near-contemporary in England, John of Arderne, at p. 63. In his *Chirurgia Magna*, de Chauliac refers to the frequent use in the Middle Ages of narcotic inhalations for operations; and Singer and Underwood, in their *Short History of Medicine*, quote from Middleton's *Women Beware Women* of 1622:

> I'll imitate the pities of all surgeons
> To this lost limb, who, ere they show their art,
> Cast one asleep, then cut the diseased part

Many great hospitals were founded during this period, as developments of the Roman *valetudinaria* or religious-based centres of care. Some survive, in far from their original form, such as the London hospitals of St Bartholomew's (founded in 1123) and St Thomas's (1200).

We have referred to the role of Vidius in the collection and republication of Byzantine texts and illustrations going back to Hippocrates. Not only do these include illustrations made very early in the Christian Era of Hippocratic methods of treatment, but they also illustrate or describe the traction appliances of Oribasius and Niketas, the *glossocomum* of Nymphodorus, the *trispastum* of Apellis, the famous *scamnum* of Hippocrates himself.

Elsewhere, we refer to the acceleration of orthopaedic evolution produced by the invention of gunpowder, marked by the first use of cannon at the Battle Crécy in 1346. As Bick points out: 'As Western Civilization emerged from its "Dark Ages" and attained the glorious culture of the Renaissance, there appeared throughout Europe more broken limbs, more distorted spines, and hence better orthopaedic surgery.' One result was that, for a long time, surgery was generally equated with the treatment of war wounds: in Germany, *Wundartznei* was often carried out by unqualified paramedics, a sort of medical underclass, battlefield hangers-on. The greater part of this seems to have taken place in Central Europe, in short to have been Teutonic.

Thus, Hieronymus Braunschweig (1450–1512) is known for his belief that gunshot wounds were poisoned and needed to be purified by cleansing applications or having silk threads (setons) drawn through them. He was also an early advocate of osteoclasis, for in his *Buch der Chirurgia* or *Buch der Wund-Artzney*, published in Strassburg in 1497, he says that a broken bone crookedly healed must be 'readjusted'. The readjustment consisted of the surgeon's standing on the fracture, positioned between two wooden wedges, after some preliminary softening-up with poultices or ointments. This is, of course, no more than Celsus had advocated nearly 1500 years earlier. His book contains the first detailed account of gunshot wounds in the literature, though he was run very close by John of Arderne in England; but such wounds had been mentioned in a book on military surgery by a Bavarian surgeon, Heinrich von Pfolspeundt, in 1460 and were dealt with in great detail in the 17th century by Matthäus Gottfried Purmann (1648–1721) in 1692, including an account of the removal of a bullet from the brain. Richard Wiseman (1622–1676), Thomas Gale (1507–1587) and William Clowes (1544–1604) were British army or navy surgeons who wrote on the subject. Clowes, a fleet surgeon who was also surgeon to St. Bartholomew's Hospital, wrote at length on gunshot wounds in his *Proved Practise for all Young Chirurgians* of 1588. Alfonso Ferri (1515–1595) is stated by Singer and Underwood to have written the first book dealing exclusively with such wounds, in 1552, his practice being conservative and favouring the removal of clothing and foreign bodies from the depths of the wound.

In 1517, Hans von Gersdorff (1455–1517) wrote his *Feldtbuch der Wund-Artzney*. This advised a gentler than usual treatment of gunshot wounds: the oil was warm and not boiling, the amputation stump was covered with a musculotaneous flap. Gersdorff used screw traction for shoulder dislocations and a combination of metal splints, screws and turnbuckles to stretch out flexion contractures of the joints. These are called 'appliance for the crooked arm' or, significantly, 'armour appliance' (*Harnesch instrumentum*) to straighten the knee: significant because it was precisely the recognition by the armourers that their products were no defence against gunpowder and cannon that led many to the manufacture of surgical appliances.

Thus, in 1592, the *Opera chirurgia* of Hieronymus Fabricius ab Aquapendente (1533–1619), a Paduan anatomist and surgeon and teacher of William Harvey, with an interest in spinal curvature, wry-neck and club-foot, has a famous illustration of the *hoplomochlion*, or surgical cuirass. This is simply a model or compendium of all the possible splints that could be applied to the different parts of the human body for deformities and contractures, in the form of a knight's armour. The 16th century was a time when the armourer's art made every capable locksmith a constructor of surgical

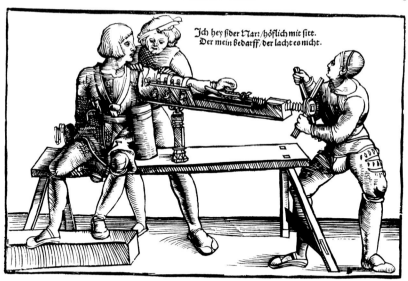

Figure 29   Hans von Gersdorff: *Feldtbuch der Wund-Artzney* (1517). Screw traction for reduction of shoulder dislocation

appliances.

Fabricius' book was translated into German by Johannes Scultetus (1595–1645) as *Wund-Artznei*[43]. Scultetus, like Gersdorff, advocated gradual correction for scoliosis and joint contracture. He also excised the shaft of a long bone for chronic osteomyelitis. His other book, the *Wund-Artzneyisches Zeug-Hauss*[44], rendered into English in 1674 as *The Chyrurgeon's Storehouse*, catalogues contemporary surgical instruments, including many employed for operations on bone, and describes their employment. Scultetus also used correction by screw traction for reduction of the dislocated shoulder. He had been the son of a sea-captain of Ulm, his unlatinized name Schulthess, also to be the name of a very famous Zürich orthopaedist of the late 19th century. He studied in Padua, dissecting there for Adrian Spiegel, during a period (1564–1630) when Padua was resorted to for academic teaching by thousands of students from north-west Europe: Dutch, Swiss, Germans and English. He used the Hippocratic bench and ladder for reduction of fractured arms and legs and shoulder dislocations and for scoliosis, exactly as had Hippocrates.

Lorenz Heister (1683–1758) was professor of medicine and surgery at the Julius University of Helmsted, had a library of 12 000 volumes and 500 instruments, partly silver. His very well illustrated *Chirurgie*, published in Nuremberg in 1719, contains a chapter stating 'Dislocation of the head with the uppermost vertebrae of the neck is very dangerous and often precipitates death, because the spinal cord (which is very fragile here and quite close to the brain), together with the brain and nerves, is severely injured, torn, damaged and crushed. This dislocation readily occurs if one is plunged on the head or neck. If anyone falls violently on the head or neck from a high

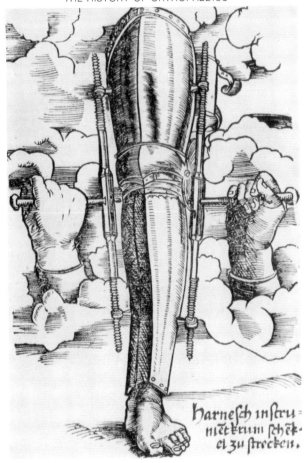

harnefch inftru=
mettrum fchck-
el zu ftrecken.

Figure 30   Hans von Gersdorff: turnbuckle correction of knee flexion contracture

place, ladder, stair or horse, and perishes, he is usually said to have broken
his neck, though normally this is nothing but this dislocation.'

The victim, if living, was to be laid supine on the ground, the surgeon
straddling him with both knees on the patient's shoulders and the head
between his feet. He was to grasp the head with both hands and pull
cautiously but firmly, moving it to and fro and from side to side until there
was a click and the natural shape was resumed or the patient himself said
it was back in place. Or else an assistant could pull down on the shoulders
while the surgeon did the reduction. Heister also did sternomastoid tenotomy
for torticollis, but is most famous for his 'iron cross' for scoliosis (Figure 34).
According to Theodor Billroth[45], Heister, albeit greatly influenced by Sharpe
of London, was the first entirely independent German surgeon, and his
Handbook of 1719 was still in use in Vienna in 1838. It was translated in
Japan in 1822, where for a time it was the basis of teaching.

At about this same time, another Fabricius – Guilhelmus Fabricius

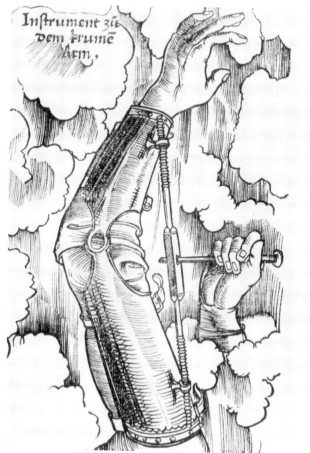

Figure 31   Hans von Gersdorff: turnbuckle correction of elbow flexion contracture

Hildanus (1560–1634), also of Frankfurt – gave the first illustration of a scoliotic spine[46] and describes an operative procedure which seems to have consisted – if it was ever carried out – of dividing the tight soft tissues on the concavity and reefing the structures on the convexity, together with the usual mechanical correction. Hildanus is usually considered as having introduced the practice of amputation through healthy tissue, rather than below the upper level of gangrene as advised by Hippocrates. In 1641 he published a series of case reports which include an account of the first astragalectomy – or the first account of an astragalectomy – for a compound dislocation; the wound healed and the patient walked without a stick. There is also a description of the post-mortem appearances of the spinal cord affected by Pott's disease. His appliances for joint contracture resemble those of Gersdorff 150 years earlier, but his splints for club-foot are a significant advance for they incorporate a turnbuckle for gradual correction[47].

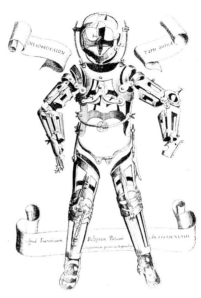

Figure 32   Hieronymus Fabricius ab Aquapendente: the *Opera chirurgica* of 1592.
The *hoplomochlion* or surgical cuirass

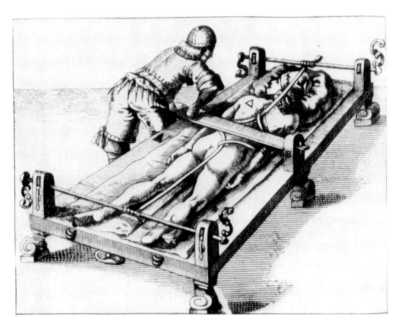

Figure 33   Johannes Scultetus: the *Wund-Artzneyisches Zeug-Hauss* (Frankfort
edition of 1666) 'How to correct and straighten the outwardly deviated spine'

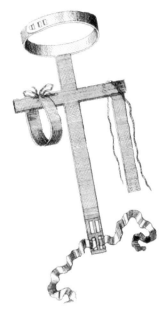

Figure 34 Lorenz Heister: the *Chirurgie*, Nuremberg, 1719. The 'iron cross' for correction of spinal curvature

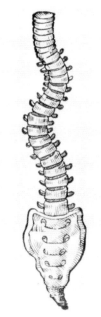

Figure 35 Guilhelmus Fabricius Hildanus: *Wundartzney*, Frankfort, 1652 (posthumous edition). The first depiction of a scoliotic spine

Of Ambroise Paré (1510–1590) we have written at length elsewhere (p. 222) and need only note here that this most famous of 16th century surgeons had been trained as an apprentice barber–surgeon, and that this led to his rejection by the Paris Faculty of Physicians and to his admission by the ancient surgical fraternity of the College of St Côme only when his achievements made it no longer possible to deny him. This was, however, in an era when barbers and surgeons were being formally integrated, in France, England and Ireland, an integration that elevated the barbers but kept the surgeons academically and socially below the level of the university-graduated physicians until the union was dissolved centuries later.

An account of subsequent developments in the 17th and later centuries is given in each of the sections devoted to individual countries.

REFERENCES

1. Moodie, R.L. (1921). Status of our knowledge of Mesozoic pathology. *Bull. Geolog. Soc. Am.*, **32**, 321

2. Moodie, R.L. (1923). *Palaeopathology.* (University of Illinois Press)

3. Petersen, K., Isakson, J.I. and Madesn, J.H. (1972). Preliminary study of palaeopathologies in the Cleveland-Lloyd dinosaur collection. *Utah Acad. Proc.*, **49**, 44

4. Campbell, J.G. (1966). A dinosaur lesion resembling avian osteopetrosis. *J. Roy. Microscopic Soc.*, **35** (Pt. 2), 163

5. Bartels, P. (1907). Tuberkulose (Wirbelkaries) in der jüngeren Steinzeit. *Arch. Anthrop. Braunschweig*, **34 NF6**, 243

6. Hamada, G. and Rida, A. (1972). Orthopaedics and orthopaedic diseases in Ancient and Modern Egypt. *Clin. Orthop.*, **89**, 253

7. Gurlt, E.J. (1898). *Die Geschichte der Chirurgie.* (Berlin)

8. Smith, G.E. and Ruffer, M.A. (1910). In Sudhoff, K. and Sticker, G. *Zur historischen Biologie der Krankheitserreger.* (Giessen)

9. Smith, G.E. and Ruffer, M.A. Pott'sche Krankheit an einer ägyptischen Mumie aus der Zeit der 21 Dynastie. In Sudhoff, K. and Sticker, G. *Zur historichen Biologie der Krankheitserreger.* (Giessen)

10. Smith, G.E. and Jones, F.W. (1910). *Archaeological survey of Nubia: Report 1907–8* Vol. 2. (Cairo)

11. Smith, G.E. and Dawson, W.R. (1924). *Egyptian Mummies.* (London, Allen & Unwin)

12. Smith, G.E. (1912). *The Royal Mummies.* (Cairo)

13. Smith, G.E. and Dawson, W.R. (1924). *Egyptian Mummies.* (London)

14. Hussein, M.K. (1968). Kocher's method is 5000 years old. *J. Bone Jt. Surg.*, **50B**, 669

15. Beasley, W.A. (1982). The origins of orthopaedics. *J. Roy. Soc. Med.* **75**, 648

16. Slomann, H.C. (1927). Contribution à la paléopathologie égyptienne. *Bull. Mém. Soc. Anthropol*, 8, 62

17. Smith, G.E. (1908). The alleged discovery of syphilis in prehistoric Egyptians. *Lancet*, **2**, 521

18. Duraiswami, P.K. and Tuli, S.M. (1971). 5000 years of orthopaedics in India. *Clin. Orthop.*, **75**, 269

19. Le Vay, D. (1956). *The Life of Hugh Owen Thomas*. p. 44 (Edinburgh and London, Livingstone)
20. Morse, W.R. (1934). *Chinese Medicine*. (New York, Clio Medica)
21. Huard, P. and Ming Wong (1968). *Chinese Medicine* (trans. Fielding, B.). (London, World University Library)
22. Wong, K.C. and Lien-Teh, W. (1932). *History of Chinese Medicine*. (Tientsin)
23. Fujikawa, Y. (1934). *Japanese Medicine*, in *Clio Medica* series. (New York, Paul B. Hoeber)
24. Beasley, A.W. (1972). Homer and Orthopaedics. *Clin. Orthop.*, **89**, 10
25. Flaubert, G. *Madame Bovary*
26. The Loeb edition of Hippocrates (1928). (Heinemann, London and Harvard University Press, Cambridge, Mass.)
27. Paré, A. (1678). *The Works of that famous Chirurgeon, Ambrose Parey* (translated Th. Johnson). (London)
28. Calot, J.F. (1909). *L'Orthopédie indispensable aux praticiens*. (Paris, Masson)
29. Calot, J.F. (1897). *Note sur quelques modifications apportées a la technique du redressment des maux de Pott*. (Paris)
30. Bigelow, H.J. (1869). *The mechanism of dislocation and fracture of the hip*. (Philadelphia)
31. Le Vay, D. (1956). *The Life of Hugh Owen Thomas*, p. 88. (Edinburgh & London, Livingstone)
32. Bier, A. (1903). *Hyperämie als Heilmittel*. (Leipzig)
33. Singer, C. and Underwood, E.A. (1962). *A Short History of Medicine*, 2nd edn. (Oxford, Clarendon Press)
34. Bick, E.M. (1968). *A Source Book of Orthopaedics*. (New York, Hafner)
35. Hartofilakidis-Garofalidis, G. and Papathanassiou, B.T. (1972). Orthopaedics in Ancient Greece. *Clin. Orthop.*, **88**, 308
36. Ullmann, M. (1978). *Islamic Medicine*. (Edinburgh University Press)
37. Elgood, C. (1934). *Medicine in Persia*, in Clio Medical Series. (New York)
38. Elgood, C. (1951). *A Medical History of Persia*. (Cambridge University Press)
39. Krueger, H.C. (1963). *Avicenna's Poem on Medicine*. (Springfield, Illinois, Charles C. Thomas)
40. *The Medical Aphorisms of Moses Maimonides, Vol II*. (1971). (New York, Yeshiva University Press)
41. Elgood, C. (1970). *Saffavid Medical Practice*. (London, Luzac)
42. Albucasis: *On Surgery and Instruments* (eds. Spink, M.S. and Lewis, G.L.). (University of California Press, 1973)
43. Fabricius ab Aquapendente, H. (1673). *Wund-Artznei, übersetzt durch Joh. Scultetum*. (Nuremberg)
44. Scultetus, J. (1666). *Wund-Artzneyisches Zeug-Hauss*. (Frankfort)
45. Billroth, T. (1876). *Lerhen und Lernen der Medizinischen Wissenschaften*
46. Fabricius Hildanus, G. (1952). *Wundartzney*. (Frankfort)
47. Fabricius Hildanus, G. (1646). *Opera observationum et curationum Medico-Chirurgicarum quae extant omnia*. (Frankfort)
48. Kerényi, C. (1960). *Archetypal Images of the Physician's Existence*. (London, Thames and Hudson)
49. Smith, E.J. (1934). Traumatic anterior dislocation of the hip. *Proc. Roy. Soc. Med.*, **27**, 579

Section 2

National Histories

CHAPTER 2

National Histories – Great Britain

In the 14th century, **John Arderne** was a surgeon with a special interest in osteomyelitis and, in this disease and infected compound fractures, advised sequestrectomy as Hippocrates had done[1].

One of his contemporaries, **John of Mirfield** (d.1407), a friend of Adam Rous, surgeon to the Black Prince, was a cleric without formal medical education who lived at St Bartholomew's Close in Smithfield, London, and was chaplain to the hospital there. He wrote a *Breviarium Bartholomei* of 1380–95 which, though admittedly an unoriginal collection of medical data, is a valuable mediaeval scholastic work based on Galenism and therefore on Greek, Arab and Salernian sources and which also quotes William of Salicet, Lanfranc and Henri de Mondeville[2].

Lanfranc, in his *Chirurgia Magna* of 1296, had deplored the division in medical practice: 'Good God! Why this abandoning of operations by physicians to lay persons, disdaining surgery ... because they do not know how to operate ... an abuse that has reached such a point that the vulgar begin to think that the same man cannot know medicine and surgery ... I say, however, that no man can be a good physician who has no knowledge of operative surgery.' This sentiment was echoed by de Mondeville in his *Cyrurgie* of 1320, and now by John of Mirfield, 'But today a great distinction is made between surgery and medicine. And this, I believe, stems from arrogance because [the physicians] disdain working with their hands ... because they have learned nothing of the method of operating which is the proper business of all physicians ... and it is believed impossible that one man could learn a mastery of each. But he will not be a good physician who does not know the basic practice of surgery. And on the other hand, a surgeon who does not know medicine ought to be considered worthless.' (*cf.* Wilfred Trotter in the 20th century: a surgeon is a physician who uses his hands.)

On wounds, John stresses the importance of removing 'dirt and decay' from damaged muscles and makes certain points that appear again and again in surgical history: that longitudinal wounds are more benign than transverse (for obvious anatomical reasons); that wounds in the vicinity of the knee and elbow and more dangerous than those more proximal or distal (for the same reasons); that wounds with loss of substance ('concave' or saucerized wounds) should be cleansed and encouraged to fill up from the base by granulation. He agrees with John of Gaddesden (?1280–1361) in his *Rosa anglica medicinae* that very fresh wounds exposing bone should be brought together at once: bone to bone, flesh to flesh, the skin sutured; but for late compound fractures he was at one with Hippocrates in delaying interference (for eight days in winter and five in summer) until the danger of infection was passed, though, unlike the Greek, he advised a windowed bandage for inspection. This delay 'does not please some modern surgeons', who advised immediate closure; but he himself was cautious, sometimes treating a deep wound with a tent – a rolled-up linen scroll, and suturing, but not cauterizing, transverse muscle wounds. it was always wise to dilate a small wound or puncture and use oil of roses and a tent 'to let the humours breake out'. An arrow head stuck fast in the bone should be freed by trephining all round; and if the marrow cavity were opened by a wound so that 'unctuous blood' flowed, this was always an indication of death or the loss of the limb.

'Bone can never be consolidated, if lost, with a true consolidation because its material is the sperm of the parents. But in place of the lost bone there develops a certain reparative material which is called sarcoid callus ... but if the bone is not completely cut through transversely ... try to reduce that portion to where it was with instruments to force it into position. And try to consolidate it with healthy bone by using consolidative powder.'

Wounds were to be sutured layer by layer, recognizing that transverse wounds might sever nerves and produce distal paralysis. 'But if the nerves of feeling or other nerves have been cut transversely, it is not unsuitable that the severed nerves be brought together with sutures. For when Nature has found this bringing together done by the physician, it will be better and more gently reknit the parts of the severed nerve and will preserve the ligaments in more noble fashion.' (The reader must decide whether this means that the nerves themselves should be directly sutured, or only approximated by suture of the adjacent tissues.)

We quote this lay author at some length because he obviously epitomizes the practice of the period.

English surgery of the 16th century was more military than civil: we think of Thomas Gale (1507–87), who wrote a book on gun-shot wounds in 1563, and of William Clowes (1544–1604)[3], for long surgeon to St. Bartholomew's Hospital in London, who served in both the army and the navy, treated femoral fractures with sword scabbards as emergency splints and then by extension with towels, served in the fleet in the year of the Armada, 1588, and wrote in that year *A profitable and necessarie booke of observations for all that are burned with the flame of gunpowder*. At the turn of the century, a Scot, Peter Lowe (1560–1610) produced in 1597 a book entitled: *The Whole Course of Chirurgerie, compiled by Peter Lowe, Scotchman, Arellian, Doctor on the Facultie of Chirurgerie in Paris and Chirurgien ordinarie to the most victorious and christian King of France, whereunto is annexed the Presages of Divine Hippocrates.* In this he writes of the treatment of fractures by traction with cords or cloth, of splints made of 'cards, wood or white iron' (probably tinplate), also of 'splints made hollow, the first which is biggest shall embrace all the under part of the fracture as fundament, the other two shall be put on both sides a little space from one another.' Lowe also founded the Royal Faculty of Physicians and Surgeons of Glasgow in 1599. The 17th century began auspiciously with a Poor Relief Act, the first European legislation to allow for the needs of cripples and make some provision for their care. This century is associated with several names of immediate interest to us: Sydenham, Glisson, Havers, Wiseman.

Richard Wiseman (1622–1676) was the most eminent British surgeon of the period, served with the Royalists in the Civil War (in which he amputated for gun-shot wounds) and took a special interest in skeletal tuberculosis. Thus, in his *Severall Chirurgical Treatises* of 1676, the first volume, on *Tumours*, applies – it seems for the first time – the term *tumor albus* or 'white swelling' to tuberculosis of the knee and other joints. 'These tumours are without alteration of colour in the skin, or pain ... they are most difficult to cure, and not to be opened without mature deliberation.' They were related in some way to scrofula (cutaneous tuberculosis, the 'King's Evil', because it was cured by the royal touch) and they might present as collections of fluid and cause caries of the adjacent bone, due to the 'rotting' effect of 'acid serum' on the bone marrow. He noted a connection with initiating trauma, which caused 'crude tumours' manifested in the skin or glands or within the bones, 'which arising in the body of them make the *spina ventosa*'. True, Hippocrates had related spinal tuberculosis to lung disease but Wiseman's conception was more unifying.

William Croone (1633–1684) gave a series of lectures to the Company of Surgeons of London on the anatomy of muscles and speculated on the nature of contraction[4].

Thomas Sydenham (1624–1689), 'the father of English medicine', was a great clinician with scant training before graduating at Oxford, who studied subsequently at Montpellier. He is worth noting here because of his enormous influence on Hugh Owen Thomas, who, two centuries later, found their views identical. It was not that there was any deliberate modelling, it was a matter of resonance; they echoed each other across the centuries, the one's traits reflected the other's. As Thomas was to become a cardinal figure in orthopaedics in Britain and the world, we must consider what these traits were: an intolerance of authority, an almost paranoid feeling of rejection amounting to arrogance, yet blended with a humble trust in natural process and an emphasis on clinical observation that ignored pathology.

Both looked back to Hippocrates, who taught that Nature was the physician of our diseases. 'Nature,' wrote Sydenham, 'by herself determines diseases and is herself sufficient in all things against them. It is by joining hands with Nature ... that we are enabled to destroy the disease.' Thomas: 'Nature can be subdued only by obeying, that is by knowing, it.' The doctor's task was to supplement, not to supplant, Nature. Both demanded (and expected) invariable success for their methods. Both felt that their writings

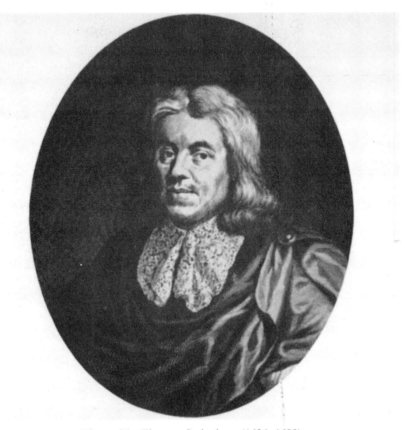

Figure 36   Thomas Sydenham (1624–1689)

were ignored or impugned, their findings considered not new or not true. Both were of exceeding polemic temperament, combative, convinced victims of calumny and ignominy. They lived their lives in permanent opposition.

Sydenham, himself a sufferer, wrote feelingly of the gout in 1683[5], detailing the exquisite torment of the attack, the changes in the urine, the link with renal stone. 'It makes life worse than death and finally brings in death as a relief.' In 1676 he described acute rheumatism and chorea, but did not relate the two, and gave a good general account of the rheumatic disorders. He also described the articular manifestations of scurvy and dysentery[6].

The 17th century was also that of Glisson, a physician we must note because of his concern with rickets and its deformities. **Francis Glisson** (1607–1677) graduated as a Doctor of Medicine at Cambridge in 1634 and was appointed Regius Professor of Physic only two years later, a chair he occupied – often in absentia – until his death 40 years later. He was President of the Royal College of Physicians and a founder-member of the Royal Society. He was a morbid anatomist (Glisson's capsule) and a clinician, but also a physiologist, emphasizing the fundamental irritability of cells and

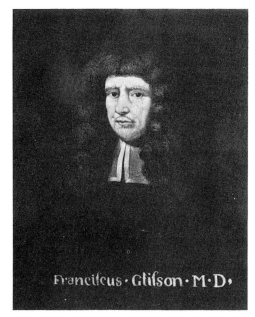

Figure 37   Francis Glisson (1607–1677)

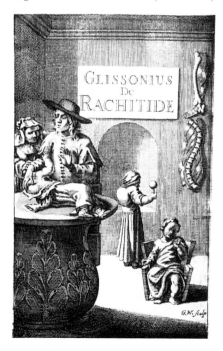

Figure 38   Glisson: title page of *De Rachitide*, from the 1671 Leiden edition (the first Leiden edition was in 1650)

tissues. His great work on rickets: *De Rachitide*, was first published in Latin, at Leiden in 1650; but it was based on discussions with two other Fellows of the College, George Bate and Ahasuerus Regemorter, and the English translation of 1651 bears all three names as *A Treatise of the Rickets. Being a Disease common to Children. Translated into English by Phil. Armin, London 1651.* (It appeared in Latin in London in the same year, as *De rachitide, sive morbo puerili, qui vulgo The Rickets dicitur Tractatus.*)

We shall come to the matter of nomenclature in a moment. Meanwhile, let us note that Glisson accurately described the deformities of the disease, especially of the spine – which he regarded as cardinal – and attributed these to unequal bone-growth due to uneven distribution of nutrients, illustrated by ingenious biomechanical figures showing why this must give rise to curvature. He also described infantile scurvy and achondroplasia (which he thought was foetal rickets).

In Glisson's time, and before and after, few doctors were much interested in spinal curvature, nor were the quacks or charlatans since there was no quick and profitable cure. It was the preserve of the smiths, mechanics and appliance-makers. Thus, we have *The Memoirs of the Verney Family during the Civil War*[7], which tells how Edmund Verney, aged 16 in 1653, was sent to Utrecht to be treated for scoliosis by one Skatt, and had to wear quilted iron corsets day and night. 'Thousands flock to Skatt,' wrote the boy's tutor, 'and young people have been brought to him from further than the utmost parts of Shetland or the Orcades, even from Svedland, Denmark, Holsteyne, etc.' Yet Skatt was not regarded as a proper doctor.

Glisson's management was purely orthopaedic: exercises and massage to counter the weakness, braces and splints for the limbs, and suspension of the spine several times a day by slings pulling on the head, arms and under the armpits. From the Latin: 'By artifice, the body is held suspended by an appliance, hanging by a bandage made in such a manner as to clasp the chest under the armpits, and the head is enveloped by another bandage under the chin, and the two hands caught in a loop, whereby the body is held swinging in the air ... so that with assistance it is impelled not unpleasurably to and fro ... rather than any harm resulting, the children become accustomed to the pleasure of this exercise.' But he provides no illustrations.

THE DERIVATION OF THE NAME 'RICKETS'*

The writer may now exercise his hobby-horse. Let Glisson himself state the problem, bearing in mind his title-page: *De rachitide ... qui vulgo The Rickets dicitur* (popularly known as The Rickets).

'The most receaved and ordinary Name of this Disease is, The Rickets:

---

* This section is largely based, by kind permission, on an address given by the present writer to the Section of Orthopaedics of the Royal Society of Medicine in London in 1975[8].

But who baptiz'd it, and upon what occasion, or for what reason, or whether by chance or advice it was so named, is very uncertain ... But it is an accident well worth our admiration. That this Disease being new, and not long ago nameless, at least not being known by this Name ... yet no man hitherto could be found who knew, or could shew, either the first Author of the Name, or the Patient to whom the appellation of the Disease was first accommodated, or the peculier place where it was done, or the manner how it came to be dispersed among the common people; for the inhabitants having gotten a Name for the Disease, receave it with acquiescence as a thing done with diligence and deliberation, and are not at all further solicitous about the Name, or the Author of the Name.'

Thus Glisson, in 1651 states the essential paradox of the situation. For him and his clinical contemporaries, rickets was an absolutely *new* disease; yet it was one already familiar to the common people of England, and endowed by them with a name whose origin was inexplicable. There is ample evidence of its newness. Glisson again:

'If we examine all the diseases of Infants and Children described either by the Ancients or Modern Writers in their Books of the Diseases of Infants, we shall meet with none with a sufficient exactness doth delineate the condition and Idea of this evil ... He who will accurately contemplate the signs of this affect ... may most easily persuade himself, That this is absolutely a new Disease ...'

Again, Sir Thomas Browne, in 'A Letter to a Friend' of 1657, wrote: 'In the Years of his Childhood he had languished under the Disease of his Country, the Rickets; after which notwithstanding many I have seen become strong and active Men; but whether any have attained unto very great Years, the Disease is scarce so old as to afford good Observation ... but too certain it is, that the Rickets encreaseth among us.'[9]

That the disease was not only new but was becoming commoner was also pointed out by one of the fathers of medical epidemiology, John Graunt, in his *Observations on the Bills of Mortality*, of 1676: '... of the rickets we find no mention among the casualties until the year 1634, and then but of 14 for that whole year. Now the question is, whether that disease did first appear about that time, or whether a disease, which had been long before, did then first receive its name? ... It is also to be observed that the rickets were never more numerous than now, and that they are still increasing!' This refers to the annual Bills for the City of London, where the peak incidence was in 1684, with 576 cases reported, after which the figures slowly subsided to 11 in 1752.

Glisson was not the first to write about the rickets, so-called; but all the other mentions fall within the fifth decade of the 17th century. It was mentioned by a West Country cleric, the Rev. Thomas Fuller, in 1647. The earliest book, that of Daniel Whistler, published in Leiden in 1645, was *De morbe puerili Anglorum quem patrio idiomate indigenae vocant The Rickets*, which makes the essential points: it was a disease of children, it was a disease

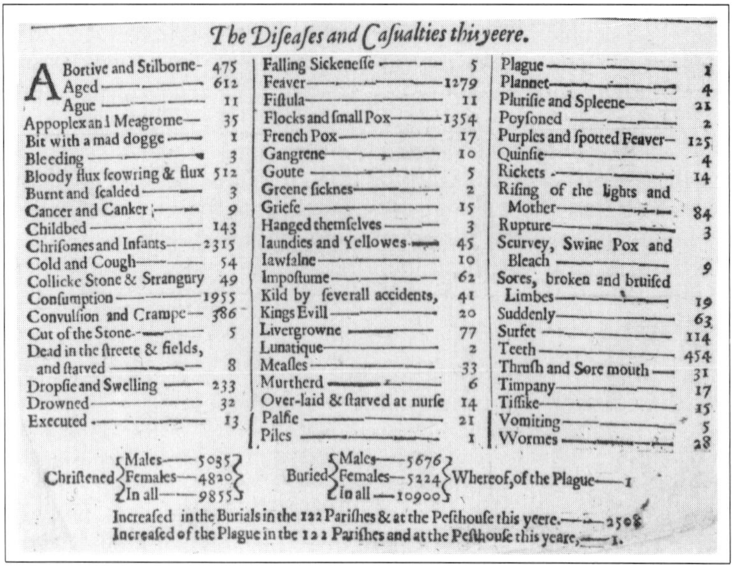

The Diseases and Casualties this yeere.

Abortive and Stilborne— 475	Falling Sickenesse — 5	Plague — 1
Aged — 612	Feaver — 1279	Plannet — 4
Ague — 11	Fistula — 11	Plurisie and Spleene — 21
Appoplex and Meagrome— 35	Flocks and small Pox — 1354	Poysoned — 2
Bit with a mad dogge — 1	French Pox — 17	Purples and spotted Feaver— 125
Bleeding — 3	Gangrene — 10	Quinsie — 4
Bloody flux scowring & flux — 512	Goute — 5	Rickets — 14
Burnt and scalded — 3	Greene sicknes — 2	Rising of the lights and Mother — 84
Cancer and Canker — 9	Griefe — 15	
Childbed — 143	Hanged themselves — 3	Rupture — 3
Chrisomes and Infants — 2315	Iaundies and Yellowes — 45	Scurvey, Swine Pox and Bleach — 9
Cold and Cough — 54	Iawfalne — 10	
Collicke Stone & Strangury 49	Impostume — 62	Sores, broken and bruised Limbes — 19
Consumption — 1955	Kild by severall accidents — 41	
Convulsion and Crampe — 386	Kings Evill — 20	Suddenly — 63
Cut of the Stone — 5	Livergrowne — 77	Surfet — 114
Dead in the streete & fields, and starved — 8	Lunatique — 2	Teeth — 454
	Measles — 33	Thrush and Sore mouth — 31
Dropsie and Swelling — 233	Murtherd — 6	Timpany — 17
Drowned — 32	Over-laid & starved at nurse 14	Tissike — 15
Executed — 13	Palsie — 21	Vomiting — 5
	Piles — 1	Wormes — 28

Christened { Males — 5035 { Females — 4820 { In all — 9855

Buried { Males — 5676 { Females — 5224 { In all — 10900 } Whereof, of the Plague — 1

Increased in the Burials in the 122 Parishes & at the Pesthouse this yeere. — 2508
Increased of the Plague in the 122 Parishes and at the Pesthouse this yeare, — 1.

Figure 39 Part of the Bill of Mortality for the City of London 1634, containing the first known written use of the word 'rickets' in the English language (column 3). Published with the kind permission of the Guildhall Library, London

of English children, and it was popularly known as 'the rickets'. Arnold de Boot in 1649 stated that the common appellations of the disease in England were 'doubling of the joints' and 'the rickets'[10].

How are we to account for this shock of recognition? It is manifestly impossible for a vitamin-deficiency disease not to have coexisted with the race. Evidence in neolithic skeletons shows that it existed in prehistoric times. Sigerist deals with its incidence in Ancient Egypt[11], and Soranus of Ephesus in AD 110 described a deforming disease of Roman children which is probably its first mention. Valentin[12] quotes a little-known epigram of Martial, who died around AD 102:

Cum sunt crura tibi simulent quae corbuae lunae
In rhytis poteras, Phoebe, lavare pedes
(Since, Phoebe, your legs are bent like half-moons,
You might wash your feet in a drinking-horn.)

In the Middle Ages, Coiter refers to 'the luckless children who fall into the unfeeling hands of incompetent and arrogant barbers, butchers and old women, and return with monstrous heads, many hunchbacked, bow-legged, knock-kneed and with limbs strangely contorted.'[13]

In 1582, Hieronymus Reusner published in Basel a *Dissertatio de tabe infantum* on a disease of children familiar in Holland and Switzerland, often called simply The Varus, marked by weakness and deformity of the ribs and legs. So, if it was not new, it must have been newly recognized. There is much evidence that the disease suddenly became prevalent in England during the first twenty years of the 17th century. But it is obscure why this should have been so. If there was an explosion, it seems to have taken place in the south-west of the country, and Glisson was a Dorset man; but why in a part of the country better endowed with sunshine and dairy products than most? When Glisson's book was published in Latin, in London, it was necessary to find a scientific name for the disease, and here he threw a formidable spanner into the etymological works:

> 'Because they which are expert in the Greek and Latin tongues may peradventure expect a name from us, whereof some kind of Reason may be given ... one of us fell upon a Name which was complancenceous to himself, and afterwards pleasing to the rest; now this was Rachitis [in the Greek form in the original], the Spinal Disease ... for the Spine of the Back is the first and principal among the parts affected in this evil ... besides, the Name is familiar and easy, and finally, the English Name *Rickets*, received with so great a consent of the people, doth by this name seem to be executed, yea justified, from Barbarism; for, without any wracking* or convulsion of the Word, the name Rickets may be readily deduced from the Greek word Rachitis.
>
> Objection: You will say, that they which imposed first the English name Rickets, were peradventure altogether unskilful in and ignorant of the Greek tongue, or that they never thought of the Greek word Rachitis, at least understood that the Spine of the Back was the principal among those parts which were first affected in this Disease.'

He then argues backwards with extraordinary casuistry, without the slightest foundation, that 'rachitis' must have been the original name used by the learned, and that:

> '... the common people might by the error of pronunciation somewhat pervert the name so given and express it as to this day they retain it, by the word Rickets. But whether it were so or not, we are not at all solicitous ... suppose, if you please, that we now newly devised the English name of this Disease, and deduce it from the Greek word Rachites, the English word resulting from thence would be the Rachites, and how little is the difference between that and the ordinary word Rickets? ... But we trifle too much in staying so long upon these trifles ... And thus much, if not too much, of the Name.'

So *rachitis* it became, and soon acquired an additional 'h' as *rhachitis*, and was so accepted throughout Europe as a condition, primarily spinal, often known simply as 'the English disease', a rare use of a national eponym for a disorder that was not venereal. The etymologic puzzle as to where the English derived their common expression has never been solved. Valentin mentioned that Trousseau had pointed to an old French word, *riquet*, signifying a hunchback. It was also suggested that French and English terms

---

* A Freudian slip, as we shall see.

might have a common origin in the German *Rücken*, the back or spine.
'Rack' did mean the backbone in Old English and a 'rackbone' is a vertebra.
It has also been suggested that there is no problem at all, that around 1620
a Newbury doctor had acquired a reputation for treating the disease, that
his name was Rickets, and that the disease came to be called by his name.
There is, however, only one source for this belief – John Aubrey, the dilettante
author of *Brief Lives*:

> 'I will whilst tis in my mind insert this Remarque, viz. – about 1620 one
> Ricketts of Newberye, a practitioner in Physick, was excellent at the
> Curing Children with swoln heads and small legges: and the Disease
> being new, and without a name, he being famous for the cure of it, they
> called the Disease the Ricketts: as the Kings Evill from the King's curing
> of it with his touch: and now tis good sport to see how they vex their
> Lexicons and fetch it from the Greek *rachis*, the backbone.'[14]

It is clear that Aubrey had made this up to tease Glisson, for Aubrey was
writing only a few years after Glisson's book had been published, Glisson
was a founder-member of the Royal Society, and Aubrey was elected in 1662.
More important, no trace of a Dr Ricketts exists in any of the Church or
administrative archives of the region relative to the period. If there is
eponymy here, it is eponymy in reverse, the doctor named after the disease.

We could dispose of the doctor altogether if the word could be shown to
have been in use in the written language before the 17th century; unfortunately,
we cannot. The etymology is clear enough, and Glisson himself gives us
unwittingly the clue when he says '... without any *wracking* or convulsion
of the Word, the name Rickets may be readily deduced from the Greek word
Rachitis.' The obvious thing about a sufferer from rickets is that he is *twisted*;
the word *wrong* itself means twisted, and the children on Glisson's title-page
are manifestly wrong. *Rick* as equivalent to a sprain or twist of a limb goes
back a very long way, and is cognate with rack, wrench, wreak and wreck: all
deriving from the old Scandinavian root, *rykk*, meaning tug, twist, pull or jerk.
It does seem that we got the word *rickets* from our Norse and Low German
ancestors, and that the good Doctor never existed, and that the Greek
does not come into it at all. However, we shall never be able to prove it.

Although the 17th century was that of William Harvey, he has no place here
except for a link to a figure who is important to us, that of **Clopton Havers**,
educated at Utrecht at a time when Antoni van Leeuwenhoek (1632–
1723) was active there in tissue microscopy. Leeuwenhoek had sent a
communication to the Royal Society in London in 1674, describing, among
other things, the vascular channels entering the bones and the longitudinal
channels within the bones[15]. Havers also applied microscopy to the structure
of bones and joints, and in 1689–91 gave a series of lectures to the Royal
Society dealing with the fine architecture of bone[16]. These gave the first
good description of the Haversian canals, and of the fibres connecting

periosteum and cortex and the vessels traversing them (though he did not uphold Harvey's theory of the circulation.) The periosteum he saw as a limiting membrane; there is no mention of osteogenesis but, unlike the bone, it was sensitive. He failed to detect the presence of capillaries in his canals, but describes fatty lobules in the yellow marrow, each with its arterial pedicle, expelling 'medullary oil' into the canals, also the metaphyseal vascular plexuses. He noted the mucin-producing cells in the synovial membrane, but was wrong in regarding the fat-pads as mucin-producing glands and was corrected for this by Bichat (p. 259). He did not clearly understand function, but he made a wealth of observations. As Bick says: to the question 'What?' Havers often found the answer, to the question 'Why?' he sometimes failed.

We add that **Sir John Pringle** (1707–1782), a Scot, greatly influenced military hygiene[17], speculated on the role of putrefaction in disease, and gave a paper to the Royal Society in 1750 on *Experiments upon septic and antiseptic substances, with remarks relative to their use in the theory of medicine*, which may have presaged Lister's discoveries. A similar service for naval hygiene was provided by another Scot, James Lind (1716–94), notably in prevention of the scurvy.

Before pursuing the purely medical aspects of orthopaedics, it is useful to refer to Valentin's classification of those classes in England who treated 'disorders of the human frame' over the centuries. He divides these into the bonesetters, the truss-makers (orthopaedic mechanics or appliance-makers) and the doctors.

THE BONESETTERS

Bone-setting goes back for thousands of years, and bonesetters practised long before there was an organized medical profession and in parts of the world where no profession exists. Or they were in rivalry with that profession, or were delegated, half-contemptuously, with the mysteries of their art by the doctors, or have evolved into modern osteopaths or chiropractors. In Europe, the English bonesetter was matched by the French *rhabilleur, rabouteur, bailleul or remetteur*, the German *Knocheneinrenker*, the Spanish *algebrista* or *ensalmador*. Bick equates him with the German *Wundärzt* of the Renaissance, but this is inaccurate for the latter was a surgical practitioner and the bonesetters never cut their patients like the wandering mountebanks. They could not move on, leaving their mistakes behind; they had to stay in place to build a reputation; and their patients came to them, often in the spirit of a religious pilgrimage as a cripple might visit Lourdes. The English bonesetters had a much higher reputation, for they dealt with orthopaedic disorders long before the doctors, as a whole, took any interest. The secrets of their art were unpublished, kept within the family and handed down from father to son (or daughter), and for the same reason that the obstetric forceps were kept a secret within the Chamberlen family in the 17th century: their livelihood was at stake and would have suffered by dissemination[18].

In England, these families included the Huttons, Taylors, Crowthers, Masons, Bennetts and Thomases. The Taylors practised for over 200 years at Witworth, in Lancashire. A Welsh family migrated to America and their descendants practised on Rhode Island until 1917[19]. They also tended to live and work in remote rural areas, rather than in the cities where they would have been directly exposed to medical rivalry and rancour. Yet the archives of St Bartholomew's Hospital in London first mention payments to bonesetters in 1583 and continued to do so until 1628[20], and we know that unqualified men helped with the fracture clinics of the great London teaching hospitals until well on in the 19th century. Until the 18th century, if not later, the bonesetters treated not only fractures, dislocations and sprains but also congenital disorders. The great William Cheselden (1688–1752) (p. 83) related how he learned to treat club-feet from two 'professed bonesetters', Presgrove and Cowper, obviously regarded as legitimate, if unqualified, practitioners. Again, in 1787 a London surgeon, William Jackson, wrote a critique of the use of irons for foot deformities, in which he recommended 'a much more agreeable and effectual mode of treatment' which he had to keep secret since he had learnt it from a bonesetter who made him promise secrecy[21].

To go back, in 1539 one Friar Moulton published in Tudor English a book called *This is the Myrrour or Glasse of Health*, often reprinted, which included a chapter on fracture treatment. In 1654 a medical doctor, R. Turner, wrote *Microcosmos: a description of the Little World*, which had a chapter on 'the manner of reducing and curing dislocated and fractured bones.' Two years later, there appeared *The Compleat Bone-setter, wherein the Method of curing Broken Bones and Strains and Dislocated Joints, together with Ruptures, commonly called Broken Bellyes, is fully demonstrated*. This was alleged to have been written originally by Moulton, but 'revised, Englished and enlarged' by Turner. In fact, it contained little of the original. Turner denied any intention of inducing cobblers to lay aside their lasts 'and straightway turn Doctors', but he did aim to instruct 'those godly Ladies ... who are industrious for the improvement of the talent God has given them in helping their poor sick neighbours.' He also refers to the age-old fracture bandage, soaked in egg-white and oil of roses.

A famous caricature by Hogarth, *The Company of Undertakers*, shows a group of Fellows of the Royal College of Physicians with their gold-headed canes, but among them is a woman holding a bone. This was the famous Sarah Mapp, an Epsom bonesetter and contemporary of John Hunter. The daughter of a bonesetter, she was very much in vogue around 1736 and attended on the Queen. Hostile surgeons tested her by sending her a man with an uninjured bandaged wrist, which she is said to have promptly dislocated, telling him 'to go back to the Fools who sent him and get it set again, or if he would come to her that day month she would do it herself.'

The Thomas dynasty in Wales began with Evan Thomas (d.1814), one of two boys rescued from the sea off Anglesey around 1745, whose innate skill was promoted by a local medico and is referred to on his memorial. His son, Richard (1772–1851) continued the tradition; as with his four brothers, this was a sideline to farming and he did not always exact a fee. Two of Richard's daughters settled in the USA, one in Waukesha, Wisconsin, where she was locally famed as a bonesetter. Richard's eldest son, Evan Thomas II (1804–

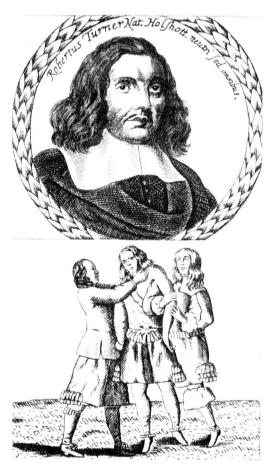

Figure 40   Robert Turner: title page of 'The compleat bone-setter. Written originally by Friar Moulton. Englished and enlarged by Rob. Turner'. 2nd edition. London 1665

1884), the father of Hugh Owen Thomas, adopted bonesetting as a wholetime vocation and moved to Liverpool in 1830 and after a hesitant start established a practice in the docklands. He was a dour, very skilled man.

What happened next in the Thomas family epitomizes the friction between the bonesetters and the doctors in mid-19th century England, and this in turn exacts a look at the emancipation of the surgeons. In 1745, two years later than in France, they finally rid themselves of any link with the barber–surgeons' guild. In Keith's words, 'they seceded from the Mystery and Commonalty of the Barbers and Surgeons of London to become the Commonalty of the Art and Science of Surgeons of London.' Then, the Apothecaries Act of 1815 compelled surgeons – for centuries the lower caste drudges ordered about by the proper doctors – to follow the same course

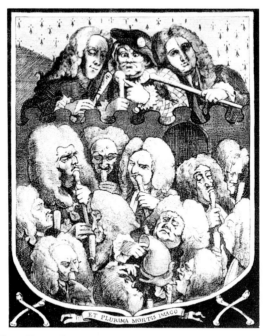

Figure 41   William Hogarth 'The Company of Undertakers' (1736). Mrs Mapp, in
the back row, holds a bone instead of the physician's gold-headed cane

of higher study; and in 1858, when the Medical Register became law, both
surgeons and physicians were forbidden to collaborate with the unqualified.
This embittered both groups: the bonesetters felt looked down on and
ostracized, while the doctors saw men without professional training or status
making a good income by curing patients whom they could not.

This was largely the doctors' own fault. They did not know how and did
not really want to know. So that, in the 1820s, John Shaw (1792–1827) (p. 95)
thought the 'rubbers' and manipulators got better results with scoliosis than
the doctors and admonished his colleagues to concern themselves with the
pathology and treatment of the cases bonesetters cured; this did not happen.
Byron had to submit to painful and inefficient treatment for his congenital
club-foot at the hands of unqualified mechanics, and we shall see that Little
gained nothing from the lay practitioners for his paralytic equinus before he
was operated on by Stromeyer in Hanover in 1836 (p. 499).

In 1867, in an essay on *Cases that bonesetters cure*, and in his *Clinical
Lectures and Essays* of 1875, Sir James Paget (1814–1899) warned his
colleagues that few were likely to practice without a bonesetter for a
rival, that bonesetters sometimes obtained better results by massage and
manipulation than the conventional rest and neglect, and that the doctors
should absorb the good and reject the evil of their methods. 'Without doubt,
their remedy, rough as it is, is often real. Yours may be as real with much

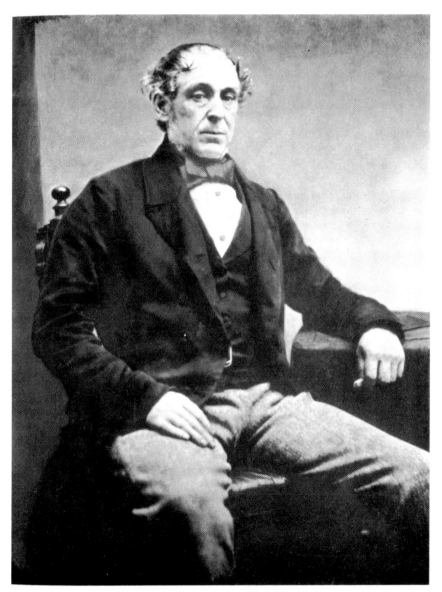

Figure 42   Evan Thomas II (1804–1884)

less violence[22].' *Fas est ab hoste doceri* was his maxim: it is good to learn from the enemy.

However, this was not easy when the bonesetters jealously guarded their secrets and published nothing. Then, in 1865, a London doctor called Peter Hood treated without fee a wellknown bonesetter, Richard Hutton, scion of a northern bonesetting family, who in gratitude taught his methods to Hood's son, Peter Wharton Hood (1833–1916), provided the recently qualified young man revealed nothing in Hutton's lifetime. This was observed. Hutton died in 1871 and that year Hood published *On bonesetting (so-called) and its relation to the treatment of joints crippled by injury, rheumatism, inflammation, etc.* Other revelations followed: *The Bonesetter's Mystery*, by J M Jackson, in Lincolnshire in 1882, Bennett's *The Art of the Bonesetter* (London 1884) and Dacre Fox's *On Bonesetting* of the same year, Fox having been an assistant to a member of the Taylor family for three years.

The essence of these teachings was that every damaged joint, for the bonesetter, was 'put out' and must be 'put in' again by jerky passive manipulation. Thus, an internal derangement of the knee due, as Hey and other doctors later found, to a meniscus tear or jammed loose body, was rectified by sudden flexion, extension and rotation with firm pressure on the tender spot: there was a snap, free painless movement was restored and the bonesetter would assert that the 'displaced bone' was restored to its proper place. This notion was embedded in the popular consciousness. When Hugh Owen Thomas was attempting to reduce an old dislocated hip, 'there was an audible snap as the femur suddenly fractured and the bystanders cried out "It's in its place!" Dr Bruce and I exchanged glances and placed the injured extremity in line with its fellow.' (Since it was a subtrochanteric fracture, the patient was greatly benefited and Thomas subsequently sometimes deliberately fractured the femur to correct fixed flexion–adduction deformity.)

There is an echo of bonesetting doctrine in Thomas's classification of joints in their passage through disease as 'sound' or 'unsound' and of course it has lingered on into osteopathy and chiropractice, where it is unfortunate that the elaboration of 'joint displacement' into a system of pathogenesis involving the spinal nerves has tended to obscure the very real value of manipulation, always best approached from the empiric standpoint, as by Timbrell Fisher[23,24] and the Cyriax clan[25-27]. It is sad that so many orthopaedic surgeons still lack the interest – and, more important, the 'feel' – for manpulative treatment, which can yield such dramatic improvement in low back conditions, for adhesions at the knee (the 'frozen' medial meniscus or coronary ligament strain), the shoulder and ankle. It is obvious that the transmitted notion that manipulation is somehow the preserve of charlatans lingers on.

The growing breach between bonesetters and doctors caused family strains in the former, well reflected in the Thomas family. Evan Thomas II found it politic to give his five sons a medical education, but they were then confronted with an unqualified father resented by their own profession, whose hostility drove him into a series of legal confrontations, sometimes in the coroner's court, from which he always, and irritatingly, emerged triumphant to the plaudits of the public. Worse, Evan exploited his sons to provide medical cover, a situation that was not only embarrassing but actually illegal under the Medical Registration Act and which led to Hugh's rift with his father and entry into independent practice.

This strange and strained relationship lasted until between the two world wars, when a London osteopath like Herbert Barker became famous enough to be knighted and enjoy royal favour while the wretched doctor who anaesthetized for him was struck off the register for 'collaboration'.

THE TRUSS-MAKERS

This generic term refers to a group of unqualified practitioners active in England from about 1750 to 1850, who might equally be labelled surgical or orthopaedic mechanics or appliance-makers. In Europe they were called *bandagistes* or *chirurgiens herniaires*; the latter, like Borella in Italy, might even be proper doctors (*chirurgo-ernista*). Before the advent of tenotomy in 1825, even the most eminent surgeons, like Sir Astley Cooper (1768–1841) left the treatment of club-foot and other deformities to these technicians. So did Paget (1814–1899). Richard William Tamplin (1814–1874), Little's brother-in-law, who founded what was to become the Royal National Orthopaedic Hospital in London, acknowledged in 1846 that 'until recently, deformed patients were left almost entirely in the hands of mechanists.'[28] This is in no way to be deplored. At a time when most doctors were not much interested in deformities, the appliance-makers rendered signal service; they were masters of their craft, superior to their fellows in other countries, intelligent as clinicians and authors. If they were motivated by profit, they were not more so than the doctors.

An early leading figure was **Timothy Sheldrake**, 'truss-maker to the Westminster Hospital and Marylebone Infirmary', established at No. 50 in the Strand, not to be confused with his younger brother, William, who, said Timothy, had bungled the treatment of the schoolboy Byron's club-foot. He patented all his devices, most of which were activated by leaf-springs, a true novelty, as for the correction of knee deformities. Some of his appliances cost as much as £200–300, an enormous sum for those days, though this merely enhanced his reputation. In 1783 he wrote *An essay on the various causes and effects of the distorted spine*, figuring traction from chin and occiput via an overhead rod to a girdle, and in 1791 he produced *Observations on the causes of distortions of the legs of children*. Sheldrake began his career with reverent references to William Hunter, Percival Pott and Astley Cooper; he ended it by abusing the doctors – Chessher and Harrison – and even members of his own family.

The instrument-makers, like the bonesetters, sometimes founded dynasties. Sheldrake's partner was **Henry Bigg** and the tradition was carried on by his son, Henry Bigg (1826–1881) and by his grandson, Henry Robert Heather Bigg (1853–1911), this last prudently following the example of the Thomas family and other paramedicals of the era by securing a medical qualification, that of a Fellow of the Royal College of Surgeons of Edinburgh. Like other mechanics, the Biggs made real contributions to the science of orthopaedics. Henry Heather Bigg wrote: *On artificial limbs* (London 1855); *Mechanical appliances necessary for the treatment of deformities* (London 1858–62); *Orthopraxy: the mechanical treatment of deformities* (1865) and *Curvature of the spine and its mechanical treatment* (1871). For a brief period he treated Garibaldi for a foot deformed after a wound in one of his campaigns. Henry Robert Heather Bigg, like Hugh Owen Thomas, was marked by the

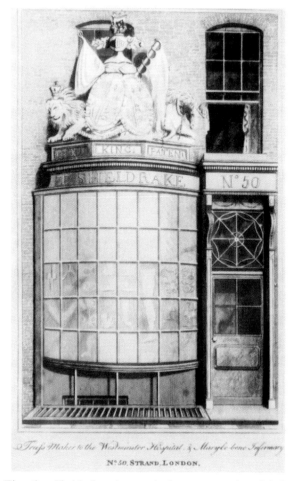

Figure 43   Timothy Sheldrake: A practical essay on the club-foot and other
    Distortions in the Legs and Feet of Children. London 1798. Frontispiece

arrogance – perhaps compensatory, perhaps defensive – that seemed to afflict
the first medically qualified scions of a long line of unqualified practitioners.
He sharply criticized Sayre, when he came from New York for a lecture tour
in London in 1877 – it takes an egotist to know one – but he did write
cogently on spinal disorders: *Orthopragms of the spine* (London 1880); *Spinal
curvature* (1882); *Caries of the spine* (1902); *An essay on the general principles
of the treatment of spinal curvature* (1905). He also wrote *A short manual of
orthopaedics*. The lineage of Sheldrake and the Bigg family extends for well
over a century.

It is worth bearing in mind that the appliance-makers of the 19th century
had a cordial and publicly acknowledged relationship with their medically
qualified colleagues. Chessher had his ideas put into practice by men called

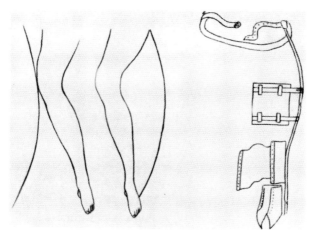

Figure 44   Timothy Sheldrake: the use of springs as splints for correction of lower limb deformities. (Monthly Magazine, London 1797, Vol 4)

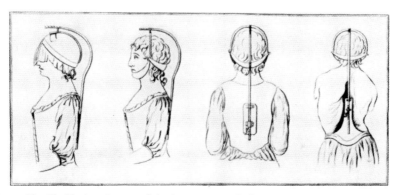

Figure 45   Sheldrake: the use of the jury-mast and sling, mounted on a pelvic girdle, to treat spinal deformity. The left hand appliance is by Levacher, the other figures illustrate Sheldrake's improvement.

Reeves and Felton; Benjamin Bell's leather splints were made by Wilson Gavin; John Shaw names Callam, 'truss-maker in Great Queen Street'; W J Little mentions a Mr D Ferguson, 'surgical instrument-maker of Giltspur Street', employed at St Bartholomew's Hospital. This was at a time when everything was on more of a one-to-one basis; the mass market did not really exist. With the expansion of orthopaedic surgery and of the provision of its benefits at public expense we are in an era where a successful (and patented) new device has become very lucrative and the introduction of new equipment highly competitive. When orthopaedic surgeons and patients are very numerous, the potential gains from manufacture can be enormous; and this may mean that the relations between surgeons and instrument-makers can be tainted by a degree of venality and by premature and perhaps ill-founded claims. Too much takes place behind the scenes. On the other hand, there are those surgeons who patiently elaborate their techniques, even over decades, in a cordial partnership with commercial interests activated by enlightened self-interest.

MEDICAL ORTHOPAEDISTS

In Britain, as elsewhere, orthopaedics was intially the surgery of war, and fostered by war, and the province of general surgeons: only the bonesetters took orthopaedics as their exclusive province. Some early figures of the 18th–19th centuries made notable contributions – Percival Pott, Charles White, Hey, Astley Cooper, Syme, are among the names that come to mind – but they remained general surgeons. Even when it is only their orthopaedic contributions that are remembered, they were not orthopaedists. William John Little may have founded an orthopaedic infirmary in London, but officially he was the senior physician to the London Hospital. However hard one looks, there were only one or two true orthopaedists in the 18th century and no more than a handful even a hundred years later. Even when the operative situation had been transformed by Listerian principles, and even when orthopaedics had emerged as a speciality, it was not practised by specialists. An attempt at specialist organization in the form of the British Orthopaedic Society lasted only from 1894 to 1898 and was not renewed until the foundation of the British Orthopaedic Association in 1918.

It was World War I plus Robert Jones that put orthopaedics squarely on the map and some of the hospitals created for treating the wounded, often staffed by men who had been colleagues of trainees of Jones, remained open for peacetime civilian orthopaedic patients. At the old Hammersmith workhouse in West London, which Robert Jones converted into the Shepherd's Bush Military Hospital, many future leaders worked and trained: Sir Thomas Fairbank, George Perkins, Jenner Verrall, Blundell Bankart, St John Dudley Buxton, Naughton Dunn, RC Elmslie, SAS Malkin and many others.

Still, even by World War II there was nothing approaching universal coverage. Over the larger part of the country there were no services at all and therefore little demand, for in medicine it is supply that creates demand. Consultation with a specialist required a journey to an often remote city. This situation was mitigated by the existence of a few specialized centres, like the Robert Jones and Agnes Hunt Hospital at Oswestry in North Wales and the Wingfield Orthopaedic Hospital at Oxford under GR Girdlestone, the staff of which made regular 'pastoral' visits to the general hospitals in their diocese, admitting the more serious cases to the parent unit. In London itself it was almost always necessary, between the wars, to visit one of the great central teaching hospitals; and even here, one of these, University College Hospital, appointed no designated orthopaedic surgeon until the 1960s. From the consumers' point of view, the orthopaedic map was still largely a blank until this was changed by the introduction of the National Health Service in 1948. This made reasonable allocations of orthopaedists in all areas, men who were mostly young and back from the wars, and now there are very few inhabitants of these islands who cannot depend on seeing a trained specialist within a few hours.

It must not be forgotten that all this has been built on earlier, voluntary, i.e. charitable, exertions. Societies of well-meaning citizens had been formed back in the 19th century for the care of cripples, especially crippled children, and we see, over and over again, in various parts of the country, alliances between energetic, wealthy or aristocratic philanthropists and surgeons with driving energy who were gifted organizers. One thinks of William Morris, the millionaire car manufacturer, and Girdlestone at Oxford, of the Duchess of Portland and Malkin at Nottingham, and many other examples. The groundwork had already been laid before the State placed its hand – too often a dead one – on orthopaedic activities and the flame that flourishes in the famous centres was lit a long time before the politicization of medicine.

The specialized centres usually treated mainly 'cold' orthopaedic cases — congenital deformities, skeletal tuberculosis, tumours – and only sometimes the late results of trauma. The ordinary orthopaedist, practising with the few beds grudgingly allocated him by the general surgeons in a district hospital – a situation that persisted long after World War II in many places – inevitably had to include trauma in his work: the general surgeons were usually glad to hand over the treatment of fractures. Every British hospital after 1948 had a fracture clinic, but there was – and remains – only one institution wholly devoted to injury, the Birmingham Accident Hospital (see p. 145). (It is often argued that it is right and proper to combine orthopaedics and trauma. This is not the opinion of the present writer. The tempo of the two disciplines, the mental attitudes called for in the therapists and their technical and mechanical skills, are entirely different. The one is mechanical, the other is – or should be – biological. It is the fact that both happen to relate to the musculoskeletal system that confuses the issue.)

It must be added that, until a few decades ago, very considerable contributions were still being made by general surgeons: some, like Denis Browne (p. 165) because of their attachment to paediatric hospitals in the French tradition, others – like the charismatic Walter Mercer in Edinburgh – because they could not resist a challenge. While it is never safe to claim priority in surgery, it does seem that Mercer was the first to operate for spondylolisthesis through the abdomen (though mesenteric thrombosis and ileus soon discouraged him.)

Let us now go back and look at **William Cheselden** (1688–1752), surgeon and anatomist[29]. Cheselden was a general surgeon, probably best known for his operation for bladder stone. He was apprenticed at the age of 15 to a London surgeon for seven years and learned his anatomy from William Cowper (1666–1709). He was approved as qualified by the Barber–Surgeons' Company in 1710 and taught the first regular course in anatomy in London. His *Anatomy of the Humane Body* first appeared in 1713 and lasted nearly a century, for the 13th British edition was in 1792 and American editions appeared in 1795 and 1806. He was appointed to St Thomas's Hospital in 1718, but resigned in 1738 to join the Royal Hospital in Chelsea and was largely instrumental in the separate incorporation of the surgeons, as distinct from the barbers, in 1745. His great work was the *Osteographia, or the*

Anatomy of the Bones of 1733, with 56 fine copper plates showing the bones life-size, though a financial failure. Of his work he wrote: 'If I have any reputation in this way, I have earned it dearly, for no one ever endured more anxiety and sickness before an operation, yet from the time I began to operate all uneasiness ceased', a feeling fully shared by any surgeon of sensibility who has ever been unable to sleep the night before a difficult list.

It is a well known story that he was treated in childhood for an elbow fracture by a bonesetter using linen strips soaked in egg-white and flour, and that he later referred his own cases of club-feet to another bonesetter who used sticking-plaster until he recalled his early experience and began to use that method for both fractures and congenital deformities. 'There is no better way than this ... for it preserves the position of the limbs without strict bandage, which is the common cause of mischief in fractures.' Children with club-feet were brought to him from all over the country. Cheselden also seems undoubtedly to have operated for congenital torticollis if we are to judge from an illustration of tenotomy in 1768 and from the remarks of his pupil, Samuel Sharpe (1700–1778), who used a button-ended knife to divide

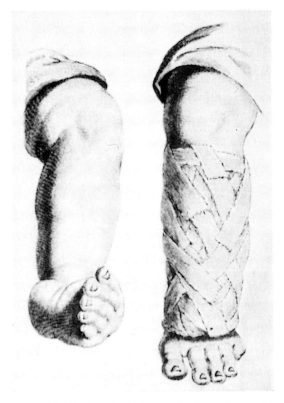

Figure 46   Treatment of club-foot. In: Le Dran *The Operations in Surgery*, translated by Gataker, with remarks by William Cheselden. (4th edn. London 1768, p. 452, Tab. VII)

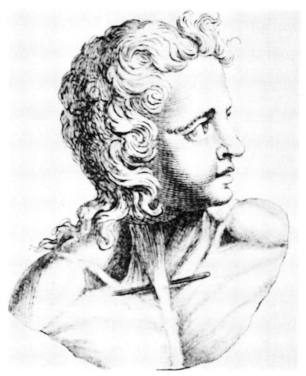

Figure 47   Cheselden: tenotomy for torticollis. In: Le Dran *The Operations in Surgery*. Translated by Gataker, with remarks by William Cheselden. (4th edn. London 1768, p. 454 Tab. X)

the sternomastoid tendon from within outwards. 'After the Incision is made, the wound is to be ... dressed so as to prevent the Extremities of the Muscle from reuniting; to which end they are to be separated from each other as much as possible by the assistance of a supporting Bandage for the Head during the whole time of the Cure, which will generally be about a Month.'[30] Cheselden himself wrote of 'part of a director passed under the tendinous part of the mastoid muscle, which is inserted into the sternum, being as I appreciated, all that is necessary to be cut in the operation of the wry-neck, the thin muscular part of this muscle that is inserted into the clavicle being capable of stretching after the operation. I have formerly divided the muscle near the middle, thinking it would answer better, the whole muscle being divided in that case (but I have altered my opinion)[31].

Cheselden asserted that bones grew by the supply of material into them via the periosteal vessels, thus aligning himself firmly on one side of a controversy about the existence, or not, of osteogenic properties in this membrane that was to last 150 years and was fought as fiercely as the struggle between the Big-endians and the Little-endians. One of his pupils was John Belchier, whose madder experiments on bone growth are discussed elsewhere (p. 260). Another was Samuel Sharpe. A third, greatest of all, was John Hunter.

Samuel Sharpe (1700–1778) was a distinguished London surgeon whose *Treatise on the Operations of Surgery* (London 1769, 9th edition) was dedicated to Cheselden. He was a chauvinist: 'It is true, we have a few Translations from the Writings of Foreigners, but besides that they are unacquainted with these Improvements, their manner of describing an operation is so very minute, and in general so little pleasing, that could nothing new be added or nothing false exploded.' He knew that cut tendons were capable of healing and could be sutured; hitherto, partial division had been treated by complete section and suture, but Sharpe preferred relaxing the damaged tendon by positioning the joint and holding this until healing, which would have been necessary even if suture had been done and is equivalent to the modern treatment (by some) of even complete ruptures of the Achilles tendon. A separated tendon had to be sutured and 'the parts kept steady with Pasteboard and Bandage' for three weeks with small tendons and at least six for the Achilles tendon. 'Cutting the Wry Neck' was done only if the sole contracture were in the *mastoideus* muscle, and not if others were affected, or in longstanding cases where vertebral growth had been compromised. A probe-ended razor was passed under the muscle, which was cut outwards with due care for the vessels, and reunion prevented by cramming the wound with dry lint and bandaging the head. Sharpe preferred not to amputate for 'spreading mortification' as formerly, but to wait until 'the mortification was not only stopped but advanced in its separation', especially for vascular gangrene in the elderly. He amputated immediately, however, for gunshot wounds and compound fractures, closing the vessels by circumferential muscle suture rather than by artery forceps and ligation. He recognized that the guillotine operation could lead to a conical stump and sequestration and attempted to sew up the skin. He wrote that gunshot wounds at the shoulder really required disarticulation, though this was never generally done for fear of haemorrhage; yet he had heard of more than one successful case and seems to have operated himself, starting with ligation of the great vessels. He quotes a traumatic forequarter amputation in a miller hoisted by his own tackle in which there was no bleeding (as one notices so often after avulsion of the fore- or hind-quarter). A century later, the great Billroth stressed how much the development of German surgery had been influenced by Sharpe[32].

We now come to an eminent precursor, almost the only instance of a purely orthopaedic surgeon in the 18th century, 'the English Venel', **Robert Chessher** (1750–1831) of Hinckley in Leicestershire, perhaps the only European figure of that age to specialize in the treatment of deformities from the outset of his career[33,34]. Chessher's father died when the boy was young and his mother married a Hinckley surgeon, a Mr Whalley, who was interested in fractures and sometimes left their treatment to his stepson while still a schoolboy. He came to London at the age of 18 to live as an apprentice with Dr Thomas Denman, a well-known obstetrician. He was also house-surgeon at the Middlesex Hospital and attended John Hunter's lectures. Hunter

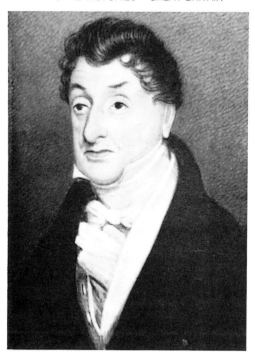

Figure 48 Robert Chessher (1750–1831). From a miniature in the Hinckley Public Library, Leicestershire

introduced him to a stay-maker named Jones, who had invented an appliance for spinal curvature. 'You see, gentleman,' said Hunter, 'that the mechanical contrivance not only takes off the superincumbent weight, but extends the spine in a constant gradual progression, and this continued for a time might by proper deposition of ossific matter into the mollified vertebrae they become firm and compact bones: hence the subject will be made straight and remain in that situation, for there is a disposition always in nature to help herself when oppressed if she is assisted or relieved by art.' But Chessher thought that 'a more surgeon-like method of treating such cases' might be adopted and Denman, told of this, suggested that Chessher take up this subject, prejudicial as it might be to a regular surgical career; and when the lad returned to Hinckley in 1778, he devoted himself after a short period in his late stepfather's practice to the management of spine and limb deformities, and to coal-mining accidents. (We note that, when the Leicester Infirmary was founded in 1771, the prime mover, Dr William Watts, had referred to the 'foul bones and stiff joints' resulting from even the commonest accidents.)

By 1810, there were 200 patients under treatment, mostly children, many boarded out locally in houses built for them, and he had a workshop in his own home for splints and appliances and half a dozen workmen, and made his daily rounds accompanied by his foreman. Treatment was by friction, massage, motion and splintage, also by 'monitoring machines' activated by the patients. A contemporary, Edward Harrison, also concerned with spinal curvature[35], wrote that Chessher's methods 'had gained for him a greater degree of reputation than has attached to any other individual in the same walk of practice. The little town of Hinckley ... was constantly filled with patients attracted to the spot by the character of Mr Chessher ... Persons in the highest ranks of life did not hesitate to commit their children to the professional care of the eminent surgeon.' (They included Henry Edward Fox, the son of Lord and Lady Holland, and that of Canning, the politician).

There were other views: 'I remember Mr. Cheshire (sic), with his irons, trying to make people straight when the Almighty had made them crooked.' 'No, no,' said Mr Toller, 'Cheshire was all right – all fair and above board.' So we read in George Eliot's Middlemarch of 1872.

Like Hugh Owen Thomas, Chessher often reduced or dispensed with his fees when treating needy patients. He operated for compound fractures, and was noted for saving the limb of a young women with a serious open ankle fracture by sawing off the projecting tibia and applying a splint. Perhaps his main technical achievement was the double inclined plane for support and axial traction of the fractured femur and tibia (unless credit is given to Jean-Louis Petit, p. 229), also described and illustrated by Sir Astley Cooper in his Treatise on dislocations and fractures of the joints (London 1824), an appliance also used by Pott. This was angled at the knee, the thigh was held down at the groin by a strap, and the lower (tibial) half of the splint could be pulled distally by a ratchet to exert traction on a tibial or femoral fracture. Chessher used a similar plane like a convex frame for spinal disorders and bought the bodies of hanged men for their skeletons. He died, unmarried, at 79, having declined to return to London and a knighthood, and his institute died with him.

Though a surgeon, Chessher did no tenotomies. However, he invented appliances and gave continuous care to residential patients at the very time that Venel was doing the same in his institute in Switzerland, which is usually – but erroneously – considered the first of its kind in the world. He published nothing. His collar was used to relieve the weight of the head on the spine by the Milwaukee or halo-pelvic principle of traction during ambulation in scoliosis – the 'Hinckley collar' illustrated by the mechanician John Shaw in 1824, some 40 years after its introduction. This had pelvic bearing, but no cap or cuirass or jury-mast; it was applied in suspension and worn for years and lengthened the patient, and must have been effective as it caused pressure sores on the pelvis and jaw; indeed, Shaw thought it might affect the growth of the lower jaw and teeth and damned it with faint praise as conducive to muscle wasting and dependency on the appliance[36].

Thus, Chessher's treatment was essentially ambulant, while others, like Thomas Baynton and David in France, advocated complete bed-rest. Baynton was aware of the association between diseased mesenteric glands and disease of the spine and thought that vertebral softening and deformation were due to lymphatic obstruction. 'Nor could it be expected ... that restoration of bone should be properly performed while the body was erect and in action.' Therefore he designed a narrow crib on castors which confined the patient and allowed him to be easily moved. Baynton also noted that in lateral curvature the vertebrae were not diseased and paraplegia did not occur. Thus the management of Baynton, a Bristol surgeon (1761–1820), as described in *An account of a successful method of treating diseases of the spine* (London 1813), was quite contrary to that of Chessher.

Chessher died in 1831, the year of Stromeyer's first tenotomy. It can hardly have been a coincidence that the first orthopaedic institute in England officially recognized as such was founded in Birmingham, only 40 miles from Hinckley in Chessher's lifetime, in 1817. This was 'The General Institute for the Relief of Persons Labouring under Bodily Deformity', the surgeon a Mr Freer. This remained an outpatient institute until 1862, when it became the Birmingham Orthopaedic Institution, renamed the Royal Orthopaedic and Spinal Hospital in 1925, and later merged with the Birmingham Cripples' Union to become the Royal Birmingham Orthopaedic Hospital.

The **Edward Harrison** mentioned above (1766–1838) is a rather obscure figure who set up an 'Institute for Diseases of the Curvature of the Spine' in Lincolnshire and wrote his *Pathological and Practical Observations on Spinal Diseases in 1827*. The sulcus round the lower chest in rickets is eponymous. He treated spinal deformity by manual pressure on the hump with leg and shoulder counter-traction by assistants, and strapped on pads or plates to maintain correction. 'It was during this operation while the articulations were forcibly separated that I undertook to rectify the vertebrae by driving them again into the column.' He did not accept Pott's concept of primary vertebral erosion in tuberculosis, but thought the disease originated in the ligaments. A remarkable case was that of Sarah Hawkes, with grotesque contractures of the lower limbs. Harrison cured this 14-year-old hysteric with pillows and padding over a year[37].

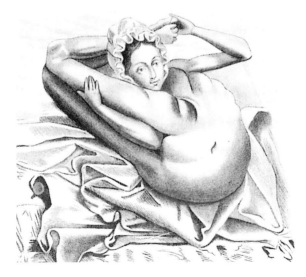

Figure 49   Edward Harrison: the extraordinary case of Sarah Hawkes, cured by a method founded upon simple principles. London 1832

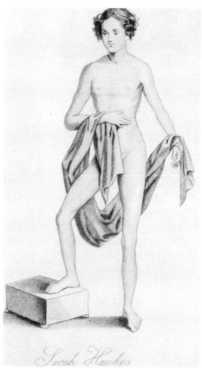

Sarah Hawkes

Figure 50 Edward Harrison: the extraordinary case of Sarah Hawkes; one of extreme deformity, cured by a method founded upon simple principles. London 1832

It is impossible to consider the foundations of bone physiology and pathology, and therefore of modern orthopaedic surgery, without reference to the immortal **John Hunter** (1728–1793). There are few better accounts of the life of this remarkable man than that to be found in *Menders of the Maimed*, by Sir Arthur Keith (London 1919), itself a remarkable book, too little read today, that was based on a series of lectures given by this gifted Scottish anatomist at the Royal College of Surgeons of England during World War I to young surgeons called on to treat and rehabilitate wounds far more serious than experienced before in military history. Keith being a Scot, and connected with the College so closely linked with Hunter and still housing the Hunterian Collection that was to be partially destroyed by bombing in the second world war, inevitably begins with his fellow Scot. We may add that Keith did not didactically lay down methods, only principles for his audience to build on. He did insist on aiding natural mechanisms of repair and not replacing them, 'to supplement but not supplant Nature', as Hugh Owen Thomas had put it in the previous century and Sydenham much earlier. Keith echoed Andry when he said, 'If we had followed Hunter, we should never have made the mistake of supposing that elaborate batteries of gymnastic machines (much in vogue in World War I) could take the place of the thinking brain of the surgeon and the willing response of the disabled soldier.'

This was a reaction to the often very passive treatment of the time, it reechoes Barton's comments in aiming at neoarthrosis of the femur (p. 381) it was consistent with Robert Jones's promotion of active rehabilitation and found its apotheosis in Sir Reginald Watson-Jones's achievements in the rehabilitation of injured airmen in World War II. We cannot begin our discussion of Hunter better than by quoting some remarks that always formed part of his last lecture in his Leicester Square course:

> 'This last part of surgery, namely operations, is a reflection on the healing art. It is a tacit acknowledgement of the insufficiency of surgery. It is like an armed savage who attempts to get by force that which a civilised man would get by stratagem. No surgeon should approach the victim of his operation without a sacred dread and reluctance.'

John Hunter, one of Pott's pupils, the founder of philosophic surgery with a mind much like Leonardo's in his exploration of the possible, has had an enormous influence on our concepts of biologic and pathologic process, particularly as this affects bone. His pupils were many and distinguished. This is not the place to resume his life and work in detail[38]: we shall touch mainly on the orthopaedic implications, the most important of which was his concept of the essentially plastic nature of bone, which, far from being 'stedfast and enduring' as Housman called it, was actually subject to continued remodelling by simultaneous laying down of new bone and reabsorption – all this under the influence of growth, repair, muscle pull, stress and strain. The new bone, he thought, was laid down via the arterioles (his elder brother, William, had described the vascular circle of the metaphysis.) 'A bone, although completely formed, yet is changing its earth and probably every other part ... the new matter that is deposited in an old bone is to make up for the waste that is daily going on in it, but in a very old bone the waste is more than the repair.' Other aspects of Hunter's work on both growth are given in connection with the Lyons school at p. 259.

How did Hunter go about his work? A late developer, who idled on a Lowland farm until he was 20, he then became a pupil and house surgeon at St George's Hospital in London, and until the age of 32 also worked in the dissecting-room of his brother in Covent Garden. He served as a military surgeon from 1761 to 1763 in the Seven Years' War and the expeditions to Belle-Isle and Portugal in 1763–8, and was Surgeon-General to the British Army in the last three years of his life, but these were interludes. He set up his own centre for research and experiment in London's Golden Square and at the age of 40 his professional arrival was marked by appointment as surgeon to St George's and a practice at 42 Jermyn Street, off Piccadilly (William's old house). From 1783 to 1793, the leading British surgeon of his time, he taught and lectured at his rooms in Leicester Square until his death from angina on 16 October 1793.

Hunter's animal experiments were performed at Earl's Court, then a rural area outside the city. He noted that subcutaneous tenotomy led to healing by fibrous tissue. He describes how to assess the 'minimal load' a weak muscle can bear, allowed to perform under favourable and relaxed conditions, as by eliminating gravity (grade 2 of modern times). Anticipating Thomas, he notes that, in joint injury and disease, premature motion before recovery from inflammation promotes contracture and that motion, preferably voluntary, is permissible only later, when the joint is what Thomas would have called 'sound'. Muscles atrophied with joint disease and disuse but could be educated and coaxed, so there was a place for friction, passive motion, heat and cold, and even for the then novel electricity. He recognized, without defining it as such, the mental alienation of the injured patient from his muscles, as from the quadriceps after a displaced patellar fracture. He himself at 39 ruptured an Achilles tendon while dancing and noted the total loss of voluntary action in the calf muscles. He treated such cases by bandaging, a night splint and walking with a raised heel.

He emphasized the important influence of muscular action on skeletal structures, though not to the point of obsession with 'convulsive muscular contraction' as the cause of most deformities that gripped many French surgeons after Andry (p. 233). He saw that rehabilitation was a matter of muscle recuperation, and that the brain was concerned with actions produced by synergist groups, rather than with individual muscles. In general terms, he saw that recovery depended on the innate powers of living tissues: 'The only rational means of treatment are those which are based on the natural recuperative power of the body.' It was the surgeon's task to aid these. Of soldiers with severe gunshot wounds, he remarked that 'their wounds were dressed superficially, and they all got well', rather like Paré's famous: '*Je le pansais, Dieu le guérit.*' Believing, like Lucas-Championnière, that activity favoured repair, he cured nonunion of the femur by making the patient take weight on the limb.

Intensely speculative, all his speculation rested not on ossified systems of thought, but on what he had actually seen and what had happened in his experiments; his ideas on natural process were as plastic as the bones he studied. Bone disease and its treatment did not essentially differ from that of the soft parts, but the bones could not swell and often required mechanical management. He studied everything: loose bodies in joints (which he thought formed from extravasated blood), pseudarthroses (which he treated by removing the eburnated surfaces and rawing the bone-ends so that irritation stimulated bone growth, plus splintage) and the healing of fractures. He traced, before Dupuytren, the histologic sequence in the transformation of the fracture haematoma through fibrocartilaginous callus, the deposition of new bone, trabeculation, reestablishment of the medullary canal and reabsorption of the excess bony tissue. He recognized that ossification in vertebrates is by extension from a bony centre within a cartilaginous model: 'Wherever Nature intended bone, she first made a cartilage of the shape of the intended bone.'

His observations and experiments on the nature and behaviour of the arteries, partly based on his military experience, appeared in *A Treatise on the Blood, Inflammation and Gunshot Wounds* (London 1794). Hunter also made many attempts at tissue grafting, notably by implanting a human tooth into a cock's comb. He found that cock's spurs survived when transplanted to the legs of other cocks, but not to those of hens; but it was too early to see that this was a matter of hormonal control. Basically, his endeavours in grafting were frustrated by sepsis.

Hunter's influence on the profession was immense: both by his direct example of principles and by his inspiration of a brilliant cluster of pupils which included Chessher, Jenner, Abernethy and Philip Syng Physick, 'the father of American surgery'.

Percival Pott (1714–1788) was a Londoner, apprenticed to a surgeon at St Bartholomew's Hospital, received the diploma of the Barber–Surgeons' Company in 1763 and joined the staff of the hospital in 1744. In 1756, he sustained a compound fracture of the tibia when thrown from his horse in what is now the Old Kent Road, and with admirable presence of mind refused to be moved until he had purchased a door to be laid on and had two chairmen nail their poles to it, for the jolting of a coach would have exacerbated the injury. Amputation, then the standard measure for such an injury – at that time a compound fracture was very often a death sentence, and amputation not much better – was rescinded at the last moment (it was evidently an oblique fracture of the lower third, with a spicule which had penetrated the skin at a distance and then retracted.) Before his injury, he had written only *An Account of Tumours which render the Bones soft*[39]; now he had leisure to embark as an author. He wrote on hernia, head injuries, and, in 1796, *Some few general remarks on fractures and dislocations*, in which he introduced, or reintroduced – for Chessher had used it – the double inclined plane for leg fractures.

His most famous work is on the paraplegia of spinal tuberculosis, *Remarks on that kind of palsy of the lower limbs which is frequently found to accompany a curvature of the spine and is supposed to be caused by it* (1779). It was not, he said, a true flaccid palsy but a spasmodic condition, nor was it due to any dislocation or pressure on the cord. The spinal lesion was often associated with 'strumous disorders' in the lungs and a distempered state of some of the abdominal viscera; it was part and parcel of the scrofula, which also caused cervical adenitis, mesenteric obstruction and chronic arthritis. 'Although there can be no true curve without caries, yet there is, and that not unfrequently, caries without curve.' The essential lesion was a caries of the bone which gave rise to deformity and cold abscesses and might end in ankylosis. His treatment included creating a sinus with a seton and keeping it open for months with powdered Spanish fly – which is odd, considering the dire results of secondary infection.

Pott also wrote *Further Remarks on the useless State of the Lower Limbs in consequence of a Curvature of the Spine (London 1782)*. We have noted that his observations were anticipated by Dalechamps in Lyons 200 years earlier (p. 221). Also, in the very same year as Pott, Jean-Pierre David of Rouen described the deformities – though not, it seems, the paraplegia – of spinal tuberculosis, and their treatment by recumbency[40].

In his *Remarks on Fractures and Dislocations*, Pott describes his eponymous ankle fracture, 'which ... gives infinite pain and trouble both to the patient and surgeon, and very frequently ends in the lameness and disappointment of the former and the disgrace and concern of the latter.' The compound Pott's fracture 'not infrequently ends in a fatal gangrene, unless prevented by early amputation', a view considerably ameliorated when Astley Cooper wrote of this condition 30 years later. Pott said of splints that they must be extensive enough to fix the joints above and below the fracture; a splint that did not was 'an absurdity and, what is worse, a mischievous absurdity,' and, as Hippocrates had stressed, it must not compress the fracture, a rooted idea which underlay the 19th century opposition to plaster-of-Paris. Pott was deeply concerned about the functional outcome of fracture treatment. 'Is it not notorious,' he asked, 'that often, very often, broken legs and thighs are left deformed, crooked and shortened?' His successor, a Mr Skey, also spoke of 'the numerous examples of distorted and contracted members, which have cast a reproach on the surgery of Great Britain'[41].

William Hey (1736–1819) was a Leeds surgeon trained at St George's Hospital, much interested in joint disorders, particularly internal derangement of the knee, so named by him[42]. This was a condition that bonesetters could cure by manipulation and Hey studied the pathology of the lesion by dissection, discovering displacements or tears of the menisci, and worked out a method of reduction by gradual extension and sudden complete flexion of the joint. For Hey, the paradox was that the articulation was so stable that true dislocation was a rarity, 'yet this joint is not unfrequently affected with an internal derangement of the component parts, and that sometimes in consequence of trifling accidents. This disease is indeed, now and then, removed as suddenly as it is produced by the natural motions of the joint without surgical assistance ... I am not acquainted with any author who has described either the disease or its remedy[43].' (This is not true, and Hey must have known it was not true, for his own teacher, William Bromfield (1713–1792), a London surgeon, wrote in 1773, 'I have seen a temporary lameness happen from one of the semilunar cartilages within the joint of the knee having slipped out of its situation, the knee immediately becoming swelled and very painful ... while I was examining the joint the cartilage slipped into its place and the patient soon became easy.' Bromfield had also removed loose bodies from the joint[44].)

Hey thought this was due to some change in the condition of the cruciate ligaments altering the relationship between the femoral and tibial condyles, thus approaching the true pathology as nearly as Goldthwait approached that of the invertebral disc in the early 20th century, when he thought in terms of intermittent mechanical shifts in the lumbosacral joint. 'Still,' wrote Hey, 'whatever may be thought of my theory, my practice proved successful, for the patient was immediately able to walk without lameness, and on the third day after reduction she danced at a private ball.'

Sir Astley Cooper (1768–1841)[45] was apprenticed to his uncle, William Cooper, senior surgeon at Guy's Hospital, but was influenced more by Henry Cline at St Thomas's and by John Hunter and soon transferred to Cline. As a young man, he watched Chopart operating in Paris in 1792 during the Revolution. In 1800 he was on the staff of Guy's. Cooper must have been an early skin grafter when, in 1817, for a young man whose thumb he had amputated at the interphalangeal joint, he 'cut off a healthy piece of integument from the amputated part and applied it to the piece of the stump', where he secured it with adhesive slips. It survived. His interest for us lies mainly in the field of vascular surgery and the treatment of compound fractures. In 1817, though perhaps not the first, he ligated the abdominal aorta for iliac aneurysm (the patient died) and also most of the main vessels, thus influencing Valentine Mott, who was a postgraduate visitor from the new United States and a pupil at Guy's for six months in 1807, to pioneer arterial surgery in America. Cooper used catgut long before Lister, though Galen had advised it for vessel ligature (in those who could not afford silk!) in 201 AD. The *Lancet* of 16 January 1824 reported his disarticulation of a hip; it was not the first, or even the first successful case and Cooper took his time (35 minutes, carefully tying the great vessels first). In typical Scottish rivalry, Syme repeated the procedure in Edinburgh in the same year, taking only one minute, but his patient had torrential haemorrhage and eventually died whereas Cooper's patient convalesced happily in Cooper's own country home. In compound fractures, Cooper showed an advance on Sharpe 70 years earlier; he tried to avoid the conventional amputation by applying lint, bandage and a splint and then leaving the limb absolutely undisturbed like Trueta. He ascribed the pathogenesis of nonunion of the neck of the femur to the poor blood-supply via the *ligamentum teres*, the tearing of the *retinacula* and the lack of apposition produced by muscle pull.

The brief-lived **John Shaw** (1792–1827) was a brilliant shooting-star of early British orthopaedics. He was surgeon to the Middlesex Hospital in London and lectured on anatomy at the 'Windmill Street School' behind Piccadilly Circus, built by William Hunter. In 1823 its director was Charles Bell and Shaw was Bell's brother-in-law and junior partner. His main interest lay in spinal deformities[46]. He distinguished between rickety and other curvatures and thought scoliosis was due to muscular weakness. He rejected treatment by prolonged rest or suspension and went in for activity, friction, massage, exercises and elaborate machines, which, as related elsewhere (p. 247), could be employed during such everyday activities as piano-playing or carriage excursions and were an inspiration to Delpech in Montpellier. Shaw was an enthusiastic advocate of Chessher's 'Hinckley collar', which he adapted for his own purposes: 'No single method of treatment is so effectual in counteracting or curing slight distortions of the spine as properly regulated exercises ... the child should be in the open air for at least three hours in the day, and while out be skipping about ... instead of walking sedately.'

Shaw warned that lay therapists practising without medical supervision failed to distinguish between lateral curvatures and caries. A sharp critic of uninformed manipulators, he was one of a series of 19th century surgeons anxious to recover patients from the hands of the bonesetters, and some of his remarks are still applicable to some aspects of modern osteopathy and chiropractice; 'The proposal to cure distortions by replacing vertebrae alleged to be dislocated is founded on so mistaken a notion of the structure and physiology of the spine ... that it scarcely deserves a serious refutation ... Happily, it is scarcely possible to alter the position of a vertebra without a degree of violence that is not likely to be used.' In the context of the crude

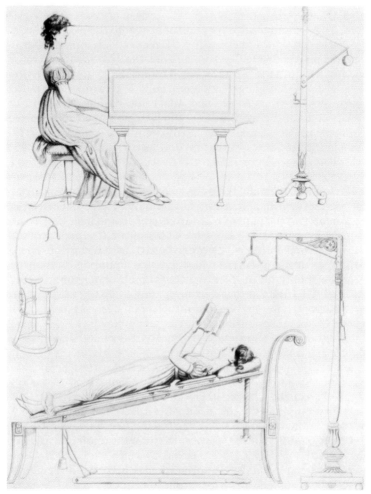

Figure 51   John Shaw: engravings illustrative of a work on the nature and treatment of the distortions to which the spine and the bones of the chest are subject.
London 1824

attempts of charlatans (and, he might have added, some doctors) to correct the kyphosis of Pott's disease by pressure, 'If it were possible to push them in and out, the operation would certainly be fatal to the patient[46].' Bony ankylosis, even in angulation, was the desired outcome. He also, in an almost throwaway remark with an obvious bearing on poliomyelitis, said, 'Certain paralytic affections of the muscles are sometimes so instantaneous that we must consider them as depending on a change which has suddenly taken place in the brain, or spinal marrow, or in the nerves which supply the affected parts.'

True pathological observations on torn menisci began with **John Reid** (1808–1848) in Edinburgh. 'The fibrous tissue connecting the outer margin of the external semilunar cartilage to the edge of the head of the tibia was torn through in its anterior half, and the semilunar cartilage was found thrown inwards and backwards ... the cartilage on the anterior part of the tibia, which had been exposed to the free motion of the condyle of the femur, had become rough.' Reid noted the development of fibrocartilaginous metaplasia at the periphery of the torn meniscus[47].

By 1867, **Bernard Edward Brodhurst** (1822–1900) at St George's Hospital could report on 36 arthrotomies of the knee for loose bodies of meniscal or other origin[48].

In his 1845 *Traité des maladies des articulations*, Amédée Bonnet of Lyons described the ease of experimental production of medial meniscus tears in the cadaver by external rotation of the tibia with the knee flexed, also the possibility of reduction of the displaced fragment by manipulation.

Peltier[49] points out that, in England in the middle half of the 19th century, before Listerism, while operation was largely avoided because of the fear of sepsis, it was difficult to distinguish between internal derangement and tuberculosis or other chronic infections, and this was unfortunate as the treatment of the two conditions was entirely opposite: the unoperated meniscal tears would languish with immobilization while manipulated or operated joint infections would suffer harm, so that doctors and bonesetters probably both created iatrogenic disability. After Lister's innovation, **Thomas Annandale** at the Edinburgh Royal Infirmary began to open knees for mechanical troubles and sutured detached menisci back in place[50]. On 16 November 1883, he operated on a miner with an internal derangement, 'having decided that the case was one of displaced semilunar cartilage and not likely to be cured by ordinary treatment.' Through an incision at the inner side of the joint he found the medial meniscus completely separated from its anterior attachment and sewed it back in place. The patient was back in the pit in two months[51]. In 1884, he operated on three further cases. Margary of Turin, very active in operative orthopaedics in Italy in the late 19th century, was removing menisci by 1882[52], and German surgeons did not lag behind[53,54]. Robert Jones, in 1909, reported no less than 500 operations for knee derangement[55]. Argument whether to remove the whole meniscus or only the displaced part was rife well before the end of World War I.

A group of men concerned with the physiopathology of bone includes Havers (discussed at p. 72), John Belchier (1706–1785) of Guy's Hospital, famous for his observations on the madder staining of growing bone (p. 260), and two Scots – Redfern and Goodsir.

John Goodsir (1814–1867), one of Syme's dressers and curator of the museum at the Royal College of Surgeons in Edinburgh in 1841–44, described the osteogenic activities of certain 'corpuscles' in a soft hyaline membrane within the bone in the *Anatomical and Pathological Observations* published by his brother in London in 1845. (It was not until 1867 that Segenbauer called these osteoblasts.) This important observation of the contribution of cellular function to tissue elaboration was acknowledged by Virchow, who dedicated his epochal *Die Cellularpathologie* of 1858 to Goodsir, calling the uncalcified soft component of bone 'osteoid' and linking this with cartilage, connective tissue and formed bone.

Goodsir's essay, in his *Observations on the Structure and Economy of Bone* is elegant and acute; yet he was an adherent of the school that conceded the periosteum no bone-forming properties. It was because Goodsir could study ossification with the microscope, as Hunter could not, that he discovered ossification to be a *cellular* process in the linings of the Haversian systems, and not just an arteriolar deposition as Hunter had thought. Absorption was also cellular, and not lymphatic. He focussed (in both senses) on the role of the corpuscles and found an analogy with the cellular formation of the spicules of sponge skeletons and their stress-related arrangement. He also noted, in 1842, that in diseased joints the articular cartilage was invaded and destroyed both from the periphery, i.e. by synovial pannus, and subchondrally from the underlying bone[56].

One is repeatedly struck by the work done on bone in Scotland, and by the way it was followed up in successive generations, perhaps because the profession was more closely knit in a smaller community. Thomas Annandale, already mentioned, was an anatomist at Edinburgh under Goodsir, became house surgeon to the Royal Infirmary, and succeeded Lister as Professor of Clinical Surgery in 1877. Goodsir himself had been interested in the screw-home mechanism of extension of the knee described by Meyer of Zürich around 1859, and thought that the menisci helped to produce an exact fit. Another Edinburgh man, W Scott Long, wrote his MD thesis in 1886 on internal derangement of the knee, noting the essential role of rotation in producing tears of the menisci, and which type of rotation tore which meniscus. We have seen that the growth of operation for this condition was exponential. In 1889, at St George's Hospital, HW Allingham collected 19 cases; in 1900, also at St George's, Sir William Bennett reported 53 personal operations; and in 1912 A M Martin of Newcastle reported a series of 509 operations[57].

Peter Redfern (1821–1912) was another student of Goodsir's. He was, first, professor of anatomy and physiology at Aberdeen, and later professor of anatomy at Queen's University, Belfast. He showed in animal experiments that breaches in articular cartilage either remained patent or were excellently healed by fibrous tissue, but were never repaired by the same substance, and that there was little reaction beyond the edges of the injury; also that cartilage cells are very susceptible to pressure and rapidly die. The fibrous healing process was activated by softening of the matrix, release of cell nuclei and fibre formation within the matrix or by elongation of the nuclei. Lost or damaged cartilage was never replaced by the original tissue, only by fibrous tissue: 'Such a process has peculiar interest as occurring in a tissue which has no blood-vessels and in which, therefore, the reparative material is furnished by transformation of its own substance, not by exudation from the blood.'[58]

To complete the catalogue of Scottish achievement – or at least to arrest it at this point – for Lister is still to come, and Macewen was also a pupil of Goodsir's – we must now discuss James Syme.

Syme (1799–1870), Edinburgh born, was professor of surgery in that city from 1833 until his death*, with a brief interlude in 1847 when he occupied

---

* Having paid his elderly predecessor an annuity to resign.

Liston's vacant chair at University College Hospital in London. At the height
of his powers he was probably the leading surgeon in Europe. Hugh Owen
Thomas was one of his students; the future Lord Lister was his assistant
and married his daughter. In 1825 he resected a tuberculous shoulder with
sinuses in a woman of 39, who did well, and seems to have been influenced
in this by the French surgeon, Moreau, who had been advocating excision
in place of amputation towards the end of the 18th century. Syme's *Treatise
on the excision of diseased joints*, published in Edinburgh in 1831, referred
to 14 elbow resections at a time when infective arthritis often occasioned
sacrifice of the limb, and when amputation, 'though a measure very
disagreeable to both patient and surgeon, has been regarded as the only safe
and efficient means for removing diseased joints which did not admit of
recovery.'

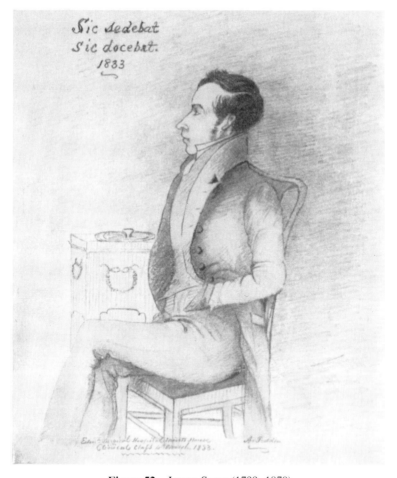

Figure 52   James Syme (1799–1870)

He was, of course, speaking of the *tumor albus* or white swelling, 'the precise seat and nature of which has not yet been satisfactorily ascertained.' While stressing the importance of rest and splintage and supporting the general health, he opened cold abscesses when necessary and noted that 'though the use of the red-hot iron was introduced by myself, I have never been prevented from employing it by prejudice on the part of the patients.' Because the disease was usually secondarily infected and might destroy the patient, amputation was commonly performed, but Syme now proposed the moderate alternative of excision. This was not original. Besides Moreau, it had been performed by **Charles White** of Manchester in 1768 and by **Henry Park** of Liverpool in 1783. White had been a student with Hunter at the Covent Garden school; his patient was a boy of 14 with osteomyelitis of the upper humerus and White's excision of several inches left a very serviceable limb. He reported the case to the Royal Society in 1769. Park gave an account of his 'new method of treating diseases of the joints of the knee and elbow' in a letter to Pott, 'The resource I mean is the *total extirpation of the articulation* ... with the whole, or as much as possible, of the capsular ligament; thereby obtaining a cure by means of Callus or by uniting the femur and tibia when practised on the knee; and the humerus, radius and ulna, when at the elbow, into one bone, without any movable articulation.'

It is clear that Park's operations were carefully designed and contoured to leave a solid fusion, whereas the later excisionists often left a mobile pseudarthrosis: that was certainly the result when Larrey performed excision for fresh gunshot wounds in Napoleon's *Grande Armée*. Park had hesitated because of the risk of injury to the great vessels and of suppuration, doubts as to sound ankylosis and the subsequent usefulness of the limb, and the uncertainty of removing the whole of the carious disease and hence of recurrence. But, after some cadaver trials, he resected a tuberculous knee-joint, not quite ankylosed at right angles, in a Scottish sailor and the joint was straight and solid enough for the patient to return to sea after six months, and to be shipwrecked and eventually drowned in the Mersey. This was exactly 100 years before Eduard Albert (1841–1900), of Vienna, usually considered the father of arthrodesis, did his first operation: 'I have tried the idea of making paralysed legs, especially those incapable of bearing weight due to poliomyelitis, more usable and more independent of appliances by artificial ankylosis.'

To return to Syme: 'I have cut out 14 elbow joints and the operation had been performed three times by other practitioners; of all these 17 cases, only two terminated fatally. The result of 17 amputations in similarly unfavourable constitutions would not be so satisfactory.' This last was an understatement for the period, when the mortality for amputation was at least 50 per cent. Syme's operation left a remarkably useful limb.

In 1842, Syme described the amputation at the ankle that bears his name[59]. His first case was a lass of 16 with a chronic, probably tuberculous, infection of the hindfoot, too extensive for a Chopart's amputation, which he had otherwise found very satisfactory. 'It would have been necessary, in accordance with ordinary practice, to remove the leg below the knee, but as the ankle-joint seemed to be sound, I resolved to perform disarticulation

there.' This was a true disarticulation plus removal of the mall
juxtarticular section of the tibia was introduced later by others; ⸜
original Syme's amputation was not that practised today, though h
that, if the tibiotarsal rather than the subtaloid joint were diseased, 'it would
be easy to remove all of the bone that is essential for recovery by sawing off
a slice from the articulating extremities of the tibia and fibula.' The patient
did well – 'any degree of pressure can be borne by the stump' – and Syme
thought it could replace higher amputations for certain diseases and injuries
of the foot, particularly compound dislocations or caries of the talus. In its
later form, Syme's amputation was frequently performed in the American
Civil War (p. 424) and in the two world wars, especially in the British and
Canadian armies (the Americans were not enthusiastic) to the extent that
the great Canadian orthopaedist, R I Harris, wrote in 1944: 'This is the most
useful of all amputations of the lower extremity because of the perfection of
its weight-bearing properties[60].' Some limb-makers have been prejudiced
against it, however, and this has discouraged some surgeons; and it is not
the easiest operation to do well.

We may just look ahead to Hugh Owen Thomas's reaction to excision. With
typical extremism, he recognized no halfway house between conservatism and
amputation: 'If these cases do well after excision, they would have done well
without it; and, if not, amputation is better. We have resources at our service
which enable safe and simple treatment to gain better results than high
operative skill.' These resources, available to Thomas and not to Syme 30
years earlier, took the form of a precision of early diagnosis, of splintage
applied with a relentless efficiency unknown to preceding generations of
surgeons, and an insistence on a diagnosis of recovery. Thomas (see p. 115)
condemned and abandoned every meddlesome practice of local interference
with the diseased joint.

Robert Liston (1794–1847) was Syme's cousin, trained at the Edinburgh
Royal Infirmary and St Bartholomew's in London. With Syme, he founded
a school of anatomy and surgery which lasted for five years and ended in a
quarrel and separation. A jealous surgical staff denied him appointment to
the Edinburgh Royal Infirmary until 1827. In 1833 he was defeated by Syme
for the Chair of Clinical Surgery, but in the following year gained the chair
at University College Hospital in London, where, in 1846, he did the first
major operation under ether, a thigh amputation, making the famous remark:
'Gentlemen, this Yankee dodge beats mesmerism hollow!' – a reference to
contemporary efforts by Elliotson to introduce hypnosis for surgical procedures at that same hospital. Liston was an impressively tall, handsome
and powerful man. His long lateral splint was the standard treatment for
femoral fractures for nearly a hundred years. It was Liston's premature death
that led Syme to replace him in the London chair, only to return to Edinburgh
after a few months.

Sir Benjamin Brodie (1786–1862) was a student at the Windmill Street
school, surgeon to St George's at 24 (at a later date than Hunter) and a
national figure. He was also a friend of the Thomas family and therefore a
formative influence on Hugh Owen Thomas. His book, *On the diseases of
joints*, was first published in 1819 and editions followed until 1850; it must

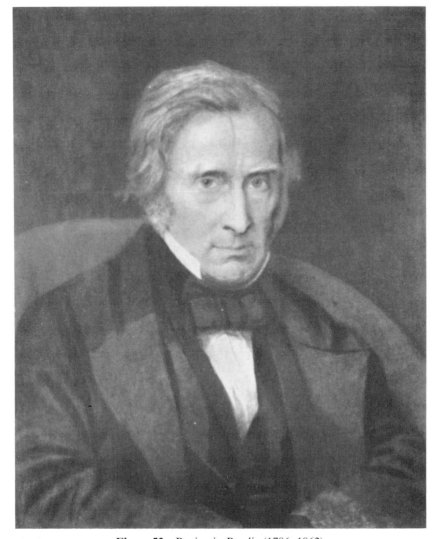

Figure 53   Benjamin Brodie (1786–1862)

have been an important source of reference until well beyond the mid-century and made a valuable contribution in stressing the constitutional aspects of tuberculosis – still referred to as scrofulous – joints. 'The disease is always indicative of defective bodily powers and whatever tends to their further depression is injurious.'

Brodie condemned bleeding, leeching and other interference as mischievous, and valued country or seaside air and a good diet. (The notions which had to be unlearned were such useless and irritating procedures as the production of an issue, or sinus, with caustic; but Brodie still believed it helped a painful tuberculous hip to apply a blister or run a seton through the groin.) What counted was rest. 'Although different diseases of joints may require different modes of treatment, there is one rule equally applicable to all of them: the diseased joint must be kept in a state of absolute and complete repose.' Arthrotomy of a septic joint was ineffective and dangerous. Brodie's splints were not very efficient and he did not specifically describe a diagnosis of recovery, but he realized that most cases could not recover without ankylosis and emphasized the importance of sound fusion, of fusion in good position and of continued protection of the ankylosis. He also made Thomas's own comment: that the prognosis for saving the limb was largely determined by social class, usually possible in the rich, rarely in the poor, for whom amputation might well be done sooner than later to permit earlier return to work. He always bore in mind that the fate of the patient was determined more by the systemic than by the local manifestations of the disease. It is interesting that Brodie nowhere refers to Syme's practice of excision, perhaps an instance of the antipathy between Edinburgh and London.

In 1832, Brodie described the chronic bone abscess known by his name[61]. His first case was a man of 24 who had recurrent symptoms above the ankle and requested amputation, but when Brodie examined the specimen he found a pus-filled cavity: 'It is evident that if the exact nature of the disease had been understood, and the bone had been perforated with a trephine … a cure would probably have been effected without the loss of the limb and with little or no danger to the patient's life' – poignant words since the young man died of haemorrhage and sepsis on the fifth day, whereas Brodie was now able to trephine and cure two other similar cases. He recognised the association of arthritis with gonorrhea; also that some cases of hip disease in children never suppurated and healed with excellent function: these must have been either transient synovitis or Perthes' disease.

John Hilton (1807–1876) was an anatomist and then a surgeon at Guy's Hospital. His famous book, *Rest and Pain*, was based on lectures given at the Royal College of Surgeons in 1862. For him, it was 'Pain the monitor and Rest the cure.' Dissection had shown him that joints were supplied by branches of the nerves to their motor muscles, hence the fixed flexion of diseased joints. Hilton used extensive splintage over extensive periods, up to three years for a tuberculous hip (at a time when three months was the maximum stay the poor were allowed in public hospitals!) He minimized the constitutional aspects and was more aware than Brodie of the local indices of activity: limp, tenderness, warmth and spasm, and felt that the longest immobilization did not tend to ankylosis. 'The surgeon will be compelled to admit that he has no power to repair directly any injury … it is the prerogative of Nature alone to repair … his chief duty consists of ascertaining and removing those impediments which thwart the effort of Nature.'

Sir James Paget (1814–1899), first a surgical apprentice at the East Anglian seaside town of Yarmouth, became surgeon to St Bartholomew's Hospital in London and an outstanding clinician and lecturer. In his *Clinical Lectures and Essays* of 1875 he warned his readers that few were likely to practise without a bonesetter for a rival, and that they should imitate the good and avoid the bad of these practitioners. 'Without doubt, their remedy, rough as

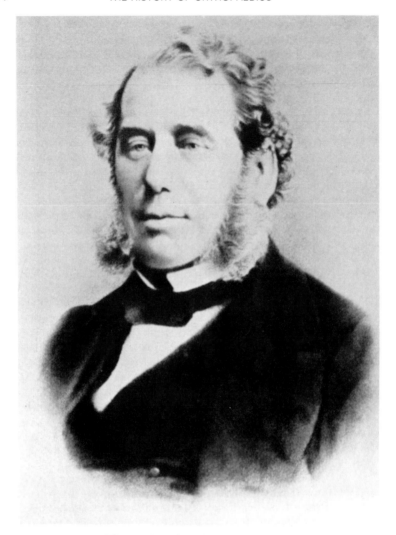

Figure 54   John Hilton (1807–1876)

it is, is often real. Yours may be as real with much less violence.' Like his
predecessors, Paget found it difficult to assess the moment when rest, from
having been beneficial, became injurious, for overlong rest stiffened and
damaged joints. Overcaution risked loss of time, yet rashness risked recurrence; like Hilton and Brodie, he relied mainly on the temperature of the
part. He operated only when essential and personally supervised every detail
of dressing and splintage. In 1877 he gave the first description of what he
thought a rare disease of bone, one he labelled 'osteitis deformans', but which
is usually eponymous[62]. He noted the increasing deformities and head size
and the incidence of sarcoma (and, in a footnote of a few lines, refers to a

similar attitude in 'a rare form of what I suppose to be general chronic rheumatic arthritis of the spine involving its articulations with the ribs, causing stiffness and bending but without deformity of head or limbs, obviously ankylosing spondylitis.)

In his *Lectures on Surgical Pathology* of 1853[63], he quotes a case of Hilton's with compression of the median nerve after a fracture of the lower radius, a severe carpal tunnel syndrome, and in 1891 he described the condition subsequently known as Schlätter's disease of the tibial tuberosity as a 'periostitis' due to strain in young persons given to athletic pursuits, who got well of themselves. Incidentally, Paget had little sympathy with the mollycoddling school: 'So many of the injuries of which I have spoken occur in athletic sports that I may be expected to write urgent protests and even claims for some sort of legislation. I am not disposed to do anything of the kind. The advantages, both moral and muscular, of free and self-managed games in our schools are immeasurably greater than the disadvantages of the occasional damages done in them.'

Paget was fascinated by reparative osteogenesis. In one of his lectures on surgical pathology to the Royal College of Surgeons in London around 1850, he said that no other example of repair presented so many features of interest and referred to 'the abundant illustrations of the general principles of recovery present in every stage of the process, or the perfect evidence of design which it displays – design that seems unlimited ... in the way it is adapted to all the possible diversities of accident.' In 1854, he gave an account of the clinical and pathological features of giant-cell tumour of bone and also described the process of fracture healing in general agreement with Dupuytren (p. 258), distinguishing between the essential or definitive callus between the bone-ends and the circumferential callus which could be and was dispensed with. Paget had also suggested the possibility of primary union of severed nerve trunks after end-to-end apposition with restoration of function in two weeks! Obviously because of ignorance of the distinction between protopathic and epicritic sensation and of nerve overlap; but he also believed in secondary healing, as in tendons, with recovery, if any, in no less than a year.

Paget was also interested in congenital pseudarthrosis of the tibia and describes three cases[64]. One was a 5-month-old girl, whom he splinted, and who had ivory pegs inserted (in Australia) at the age of two. At three-and-a-half there was no union, and when Paget next saw her, at age 30, she had been amputated and preferred to be so. The second case was a baby just walking, after a fall, with nonunion after splintage, excision and wiring, also amputated. The third case was one of congenital bowing, broken by a bonesetter at age three and ununited despite excision and wiring, also amputated. Paget saw that this was not fragilitas ossium because only one bone was involved and the fractures of fragilitas always united, nor did it resemble rickets or syphilis. He wondered whether it was like the 'osteitis deformans' described by Czerny in Vienna in 1873[65], though Paget had coined this term himself in 1877 before seeing Czerny's paper.

Joseph Lister (1827–1912) must be mentioned here because his application, first of antisepsis and then of asepsis, made him the father of safe surgery, and made it possible for orthopaedic surgery to evolve from 'methods of adventure', bound to be ill-fated in many cases, into an enormous expansion of safe elective technique. All this was correlated with the work of Koch and Pasteur on the germ theory of infection.

Lister was not a Scot, though later much associated with Scotland. It must have been important that his father was a distinguished amateur microscopist. He began as a student at University College Hospital in London in 1844 at age 17, had smallpox and a nervous breakdown, attended the first operation under ether by Liston in December 1846, and graduated in 1852. He visited Syme at Edinburgh, was impressed with the surgical facilities there, became Syme's house surgeon in 1853, married his daughter, and was appointed assistant surgeon to the Royal Infirmary in 1854. There, *in loco parentis* to Syme's dressers, he must have been well known to the student Hugh Owen Thomas, who was well acquainted with Listerian antisepsis from its earliest days, casually accepting its central tenet of asepsis as consistent with his own cossetting of natural process while others continued to drench wounds with powerful chemicals. Later, Lister became Regius Professor at Glasgow, and in 1877 returned to London as surgeon and professor at King's College Hospital.

Lister made his first application of carbolic acid to a compound fracture on 12th August 1865: it was in the form of creosote and the patient was a girl of 11 with a fractured tibia. It was not published in the *Lancet* until 16th March 1867: 'On a new method of treating Compound Fracture, Abscess, etc., with observations of the conditions of suppuration[66].' He was able to say: 'Since the antiseptic treatment ... wounds and abscesses no longer poison the atmosphere ... my wards, though in other respects under precisely the same conditions as before, have completely changed their character, so that during the last nine months not a single case of pyaemia, hospital gangrene or erysipelas has occurred in them.'* How did this arrive? It was because Lister came to appreciate the role of bacterial infection in parallel with Pasteur. 'It occurred to me that if, in a compound fracture, before decomposition of the blood set in, a material were applied to the wound which, though it might allow the gases of the air to penetrate, would destroy its living germs, all evil consequences might be averted. For this purpose I selected carbolic acid.' Again, 'The disastrous effects of compound fractures as compared with the freedom from all danger of simple fractures, evidently depends essentially on the fact that in the former the blood effused around the fragments, being in communication with the external air through a wound undergoing decomposition ... produces more or less death of tissue and suppuration ... we know now, thanks to the beautiful researches of Pasteur, that the active agents are not the gaseous elements in the air, but minute living organisms suspended in it.'

When Lister arrived at the Edinburgh Infirmary in 1854 the amputation mortality was 43 per cent; later, that part of the mortality due to infection fell almost to zero. He first introduced his spray in 1871, and abandoned it

---

* This was partly because he resolutely refused to accept the over-crowding of patients.

for asepsis in 1887, even regretting his earlier endeavours. Antisepsis met with an enthusiastic reception in France and Germany, vituperation at home, but that is about par for the course.

Taking only his orthopaedic work, it is relevant that he developed (but did not invent) the sterile absorbable catgut ligature. In 1862 he contributed the chapter on amputations to Holmes's *System of Surgery*, reviewing the subject from Hippocrates to Larrey, including Morel's 'invention' of the tourniquet in 1674 (Paré had used it a century earlier). His original contributions were amputation through the knee and the use of an abdominal tourniquet for disarticulation at the hip (though it seems that Joseph Pancoast in the USA may have done this in 1860). Before Esmarch, he had obtained a bloodless field by elevation of the limb[67], and he was an excisionist in a mild way, reporting excision of the tuberculous wrist[68]. In 1876, Lister witnessed the performance of resection of a tuberculous hip at the International Medical Congress in Philadelphia, saying that this alone would have been sufficient reward for crossing the Atlantic.

His orthopaedic operations were numerous, and regarded by some as adventurous. In 1868 he operated for a recent fracture of the femoral neck, freshening the surfaces (there was haemorrhage, he had to use a carbolic pack, but the result was successful). In the same year he did a meniscectomy. In 1873 he wired a fractured olecranon, and in 1877 a patella, creating a furore by his audacity in converting a closed fracture into an open one, albeit temporarily, though he had been anticipated by Cooper in the USA in 1861[69]. He reported 7 cases of patellar wiring in 1883–4. A leading London surgeon said, of his first case: 'When this poor fellow dies, it is proper that someone should proceed against that man for malpractice.'

Lister was made a baronet in 1883. It is a truism that he made modern operative orthopaedic surgery possible. This does not mean that we may saddle him with responsibility for the excesses that have followed, mitigated as these may be by the discovery of antibiotics. In this latter context, it is fascinating, and little known, that in his later years Lister made a trial of the *Penicillium* mould, applied directly to wounds, in his wards at King's College Hospital.

It is tempting to portray the course of orthopaedics in England during the latter half of the 19th century as a development coincident in time, but not in geography or philosophy, conducted by William John Little (1810–1894) and his disciples at the orthopaedic hospital he founded in London, and by Hugh Owen Thomas, who had no hospital and no disciples, except for Robert Jones in later life, in Liverpool. This portrayal is not entirely justified by fact, for there was much work proceeding elsewhere, but it affords a useful basis for discussion. Little was relatively famous and accepted; he was at the centre of things and in orthopaedics his fame rested initially on operative methods, the introduction of subcutaneous tenotomy into Britain. Thomas was geographically as well as psychologically eccentric, isolated in both senses, never accepted in the profession – though this was largely a self-exclusion – and with a convinced opposition to operative 'methods of adventure', not because he could not operate – he was skilled and enterprising when necessary and introduced the massive transverse exsection of the secondarily infected tuberculous hip that Girdlestone was to develop in the next century as the basis of his pseudarthrosis – but because he would not, preferring to act with and not against Nature.

Hugh Owen Thomas (1834–1891)

'*Nature by herself determines all diseases and is herself efficient against all of them.*' Sydenham
'*Nature can be subdued only by obeying, that is, by knowing it.*' Thomas

If not the father, Thomas is the grandfather of British orthopaedics, counting Robert Jones as the proximate parent. This is fair, since Thomas trained Jones, while Jones made Thomas's principles acceptable to the profession where his combative senior had been unable to do so.

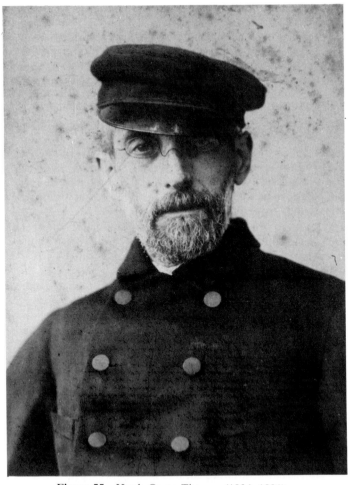

Figure 55   Hugh Owen Thomas (1834–1891)

Thomas must be seen as a giant, one of the immortal triad whose other members are Jean-André Venel and Jacques-Mathieu Delpech. But this is a retrospective appraisal; he was not seen so in his own time; he was hardly seen at all in his own country. Others who were famous in their own time are often now forgotten; Thomas, who was not famous, has become so over the years, as a mountain looms larger in the distance.

Why was this so? Largely, it was because of his peculiar temperament. The fourth generation scion of a line of Welsh bonesetters, the son of an unqualified practitioner who had settled and prospered in Liverpool against the venomous opposition of the doctors, even the possession of a regular medical qualification and an unparalleled orthopaedic experience never abolished the defensiveness which was manifested in bitter attacks on those, however eminent, who denied his certainty that his principles were right. Such a polemic temper could never gain popularity among the suave; if he was excluded, it was a self-exclusion; and yet, in the busy west coast port, he was linked across the Atlantic with like-minded solitaries: Louis Bauer, John Ridlon, Pendleton, Gibney and others, men who came to Britain either specifically to meet Thomas or because Liverpool was conveniently where they disembarked before going on to London. Even patients came from America and returned there. Let Ridlon speak (it is 1887);

'Thomas seemed to me to feel keenly ... that he was ostracised professionally, and this appeared to be true. I visited Macewen in Glasgow, William Adams in London – the most well-known orthopaedic surgeon of his time – Chance of the City Orthopaedic Hospital, Noble Smith, successor to Chance, Howard Marsh, Muirhead Little and many others, and not one of them had a kind word to say of Thomas. But I was able to compare their work with his. One could gain more useful knowledge following Thomas round for an hour than anyone else in Great Britain for months. ... He insisted on right principles, not on this or that mechanical appliance, and the soundness of his teaching is substantiated by the verdict of experience and time[70].'

Thomas was an apostle of rest in the management of joint disease, at that time largely tuberculous. In his copy of Hilton's *Rest and Pain* he had underlined this passage;

'It will be well if the surgeon can fix his memory ... the physiological truth that Nature has a constant tendency to repair the injuries to which her structures have been subjected, and that the reparative power becomes more conspicuous when the disturbing cause has been removed.'

Hence his insistence on rest – 'enforced, uninterrupted and prolonged.' Hence his dismay at the frequent performance of amputation and excision, his abhorrence of methods of adventure whose main indication was impatience. Here he was totally identified with Sydenham in insisting on the importance of unhindered natural process.

Thomas separated violently from his father's practice in 1859, soon after the Medical Registration Act imperilled collaboration with an unqualified man, and removed to 11, Nelson Street, retaining a house in Hardy Street for eight patients which was the sum of his hospital practice for his entire life. He had his workshops and examination rooms in his own home and

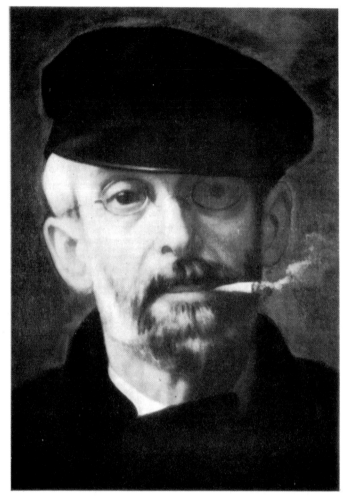

Figure 56   Fleury's portrait of Hugh Owen Thomas. Reproduced with permission
from the Curator of the National Portrait Gallery

began his rounds at five or six in the morning, driving a phaeton of his own
construction, a sailor's cap always pulled down over a damaged eye, a
cigarette constantly in his mouth. Then he had a hurried breakfast at eight,
consulted till two, visited again, operated at Hardy Street (which might
include a mastectomy, oöphorectomy or lithotomy), did an evening surgery,
and often spent half the night working on his splints or writing his books.
He never left home for other than professional purposes and never took a
holiday. An average week included some 20 major fractures, several compound, several cases of intestinal obstruction (managed conservatively with
morphia) and many cases of joint disease and deformity, all in addition to

an enormous general medical and surgical practice; perhaps 80 outpatients daily and as many home visits, all treated by Thomas himself and supervised in every detail. Sunday was the 'free day', when hundreds of patients from the country around besieged Nelson Street.*

Thomas was often thought – and is still sometimes thought – to have been an unqualified bonesetter like his father, because he was isolated, was never on the staff of a hospital and never used his degrees. He had been apprenticed to a general practitioner uncle in Wales, a friend of Brodie's, and was then a medical student at Edinburgh with his brothers, a dresser to Syme when Lister was his house surgeon, but influenced mainly by Hughes Bennett, professor of medicine, an outspoken man, sharp in diagnosis, intolerant of meddling. He then spent a year at University College Hospital in London, attended Hilton's lectures, and spent a short time in Paris studying operations for bladder stone which he always liked to perform. He attended only three or four medical meetings in his life, and the British Medical Association, meeting in Liverpool in 1883, had to visit his house, where, in 30 children with hip disease, 'the limb had been brought down straight and the children looked well and happy, though some had been in as bad a condition as could well have been conceived', and in whom, though scarred with the sinuses of tuberculosis, there was an astonishing freedom of movement when Thomas removed the splints after years of fixation. He was not interested in the pathology of the conditions he treated and openly expressed his indifference to differential diagnosis, concerned only with symptoms and signs and their response to rest.

A feature of his practice consisted of sailors returning from the ends of the earth with old ununited or malunited fractures or unreduced shoulder or elbow dislocations, the shoulder reductions performed by traction through a padded ring fixed to a chair without anaesthesia, the forces of up to ten men brought in from the street, timed at three minutes for a month-old displacement with a minute added for every subsequent month. He had an amiable habit of succeeding where his colleagues had failed, and telling them so.

Thomas wrote freely and uninhibitedly, dogmatic and damning as required, but his books were published locally and largely unread. In 1867 he published a method of wiring the mandible allowing daily tightening to preserve coaptation. Although not the first of his *Contributions to Medicine and Surgery*, his volume on *Intestinal Disease and Obstruction* in 1883 clearly establishes his orthopaedic principles. Diagnosis is unimportant, because

---

* It may be difficult for present-day orthopaedic surgeons in the west to envisage such conditions. Yet they still exist in the Third World; and only 40 years ago, in a London suburb where no orthopaedist had practised before, the present writer many times struggled singlehanded with clinics of 150 or more patients – and twice as many after retirement to Africa. Thomas's secret lay in economy of effort, immediate accurate diagnosis and the essential precise minimum of treatment. The present writer sometimes found it useful to remove the patient's chair; later, he removed his own chair.

symptoms and treatment are always much the same. The irritated or obstructed or paralysed bowel must not be coerced with purges or enemas, but rested by starvation and opium in a long-drawn-out battle which might last for weeks. Robert Jones: 'As a boy of 17 or 18 I used to go to different quarters of the town armed with a hypodermic syringe ... some who recovered were so bad that no surgeon of today would do more than rapidly make an artificial anus as last resort ... we should despair of their recovery, yet a large proportion of such cases lived. By following them we became conversant with the natural resolution of obstruction, before Thomas probably never seen.' And Thomas, 'In the treatment of this case 45 grains of morphia were consumed and treatment extended over 32 days. *Altogether 100 visits were made* (my italics, author). Most of the morning and evening visits were made by my nephew, Mr R Jones, who very efficiently assisted me.'

In one case he trocared the bowel 40 times, as often as five times a day. Thomas was aware that many of these patients were suffering from appendicitis (typhlitis then) and his treatment was a remarkable anticipation of the expectant regime laid down by Ochsner in 1913 for late cases. 'Diseased localities cannot respond to the physiological stimulus of remedies.' We may think that we can do better than this now, but Thomas agreed with Horace that Nature will return even though we expel her with a pitchfork. It was not that he could not or did not perform laparotomy or operate on the bowel; he could and did, but his natural and family bias and the conservatism adopted in his overwhelmingly orthopaedic practice inclined him to abstention. 'It is better to do nothing if we are in ignorance, either of what we do, or of the train of consequences that follows what we elect to do. To enable us to judge of the value of any innovation in treatment it is essential to see, first, what course the disease would run if not interfered with and, second, the success attendant upon previous methods of treatment.' We need to know the natural history of untreated disease, and this knowledge is largely denied us today.

In a pendant to this book, *The Collegian of 1666 and the Collegians of 1865, or What is Recognised Treatment?* (where the collegian of 1666 was Sydenham) Thomas indignantly refuted the claim of Treves of the London Hospital and others that his method was already standard. He conceded that an operation, 'wanted or not', at least put an end to noxious medication; and 'Nature always operates late', i.e. a spontaneous faecal fistula was always possible. One feels that he knew he was wrong in opposing urgent surgery for strangulation; but he also knew that many patients died because the surgeon did not know how to deal with the postoperative ileus and flogged the bowel to collapse. When he admits that 'we have not yet come to a remedy for every disease', this may be taken as a hint that modern specific therapy has supplanted Thomas's principles. It has not; and when it fails, patient and surgeon are flung back into the primitive conditions that govern disease and injury.

In *The Principles of Treatment of Diseased Joints*, Thomas laid down the foundations of orthopaedic practice, defining for the first time the terms 'sound' and 'unsound', soundness being the ability to move the joint freely without exciting the last reflex muscle spasm. He defined true and false ankylosis and the position of function should ankylosis develop, and practical *avoidable* defect or deformity. He laid down as a test of recovery that the joint could deviate increasingly from the position of fixation after release from the splintage of the acute phase, without return of spasm.

Complementary to this, sound fixed deformities were to be rendered unsound and kept so until correction was obtained; most deformities could be corrected without recourse to tenotomy. (The present writer recalls being shown by the late E P Brockman many years ago how almost any deformity of the wrist can be corrected by serial plasters.) 'Eccentric forms that cannot be altered in the dead body without rupture of fracture can, during life, be altered by mechanical influences as time and physiological action commode the part to the direction of the employed force', an independent anticipation of Wolff's Law on the relation between form and function.

To diagnose early cases of hip disease, he devised his famous test to reveal concealed flexion by first eliminating lumbar lordosis: the earliest diagnostic sign, a quantitative as well as qualitative index, applicable to bilateral disease, negative in hysteria and Charcot's arthropathy, valuable as a test of recovery. If joint disease ended in ankylosis, this was never due to immobilization, however protracted, but to destruction of joint components by the inflammation; then it was unavoidable, even desirable. 'Other surgeons made the mistake of supposing the muscles able but obstinate, whereas their actual condition was that they were unwilling, being cognisant of the disease in the joint and of the damage that might accrue if they relaxed their intelligent control. No matter what the cause of primary disease in a joint … rest cannot be dispensed with … arrest of motion is the one thing needful, in man's evolution it was the only chance of recovering from joint inflammation.' Thomas was a Darwinian. Of course, he never spoke of tuberculous arthritis as such, any more than Hilton; the bacillus was not discovered by Koch until 1882, X-rays not until 1895. Joint disease was a largely undivided entity marked by irritation, spasm, effusion and deformity; sometimes trauma featured, sometimes the condition was quiet and abscesses formed; there was no clear differentiation within the gamut of the arthropathies. Thomas did see that there were favourable cases with a history of injury and little diathesis and unfavourable ones with severe constitutional malaise, but rest was the treatment for all and the origin of the disease a pointless speculation. The typical problem of the tuberculous hip is shown in Figure 58. Thomas vehemently denounced the 'North American tractionists' and the 'American system' of combining traction with movement, also their fears that rest caused ankylosis. There was a great variety of contemporary solutions (Figure 59). Thomas's ambulatory hip splint with a patten on the sound side – still sometimes used for Perthes' disease – is shown in Figure 60. It also fixed the spine and knee; it was modelled on the sound side and the diseased hip was gradually brought down from flexion in a few sessions of remodelling. Rushton Parker, a leading Liverpool surgeon, was so impressed by seeing a lad so splinted in the street that he persuaded Thomas to write *Diseases of the Hip, Knee and Ankle Joints*. These patients were not admitted to hospital, they remained active and at home, the splints were *cheap* and

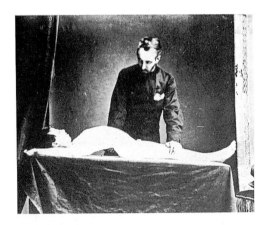

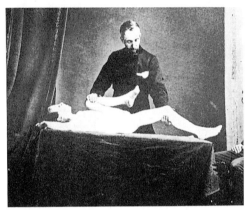

Figure 57   Thomas demonstrating concealed flexion of the left hip joint. (Le Vay, D. [1956]. *The Life of Hugh Owen Thomas*. [Edinburgh and London, Livingstone])

therefore more available than grander appliances and – most important – they satisfied the principle of rest. Bick says it was ischial bearing, but this is not borne out by the illustration. The better-known Thomas splint for femoral fractures, which revolutionized the transport and treatment of these fractures in World War I, was a modification of this splint. Thomas offered it to the French in the Franco–Prussian War in 1870 but it was declined. It has been much modified, given a half-ring or a knee flexion piece, combined with plaster of Paris as the Tobruk splint for transportation of the wounded in the British desert campaigns of World War II, altogether dispensed with by some, like George Perkins and the Chinese.

When the hip splint was removed, the flexion test confirmed or disproved recovery. The principle of splintage was not new; what was new was uninterrupted splintage in the optimum functional position, no matter how stormy the passage; any accompanying stiffness or wasting was almost welcome as an aid to recovery. Thomas never hesitated to aspirate or lay

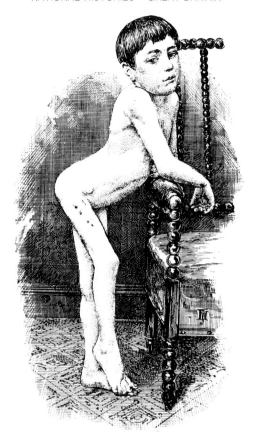

Figure 58 The problem. (Le Vay, D. [1956]. *The Life of Hugh Owen Thomas.*
[Edinburgh and London, Livingstone])

open an abscess, and in very severely secondarily infected cases he reflected
the great trochanter and radically excised the femoral head and neck. In
general he had nothing but contempt for excision and amputation. His
experience in Syme's wards and again in Liverpool, where Park had pioneered
excision in the previous century, was reinforced when excised patients came
to him from the city hospitals still uncured. 'Early in my practice I began to
deviate from the ordinary paths of treatment which induced surgeons to
perform amputation or excision ... but as I dwell in a large town endowed
with several large hospitals in charge of enterprising surgeons who, inspired
by the spirit of the times, prefer to cut mechanically what can be unloosed
physiologically, my observations have been ample and confirmatory of my
opinion.'

Oddly, for one so concerned with function, he left rehabilitation to
take its own course after removal of splintage, advised no exercises or
manipulations. Like Brodie, he noted that 'many cases (of hip disease) have
a strong tendency to recover. These are the cases that sometimes recover

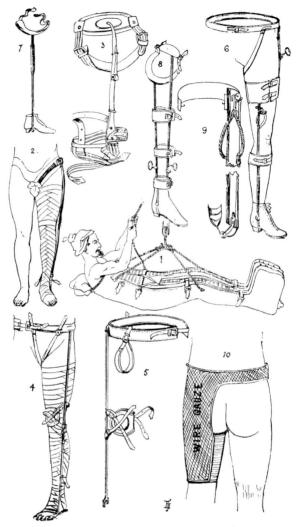

Figure 59   Some contemporary solutions in 1875, most of them condemned more
or less scathingly by Thomas. (Le Vay, D. [1956]. *The Life of Hugh Owen Thomas.*
[Edinburgh and London, Livingstone])

spontaneously (an extremely rare occurrence), never reaching the destructive
stage though neglected,' i.e. cases of transient synovitis or Perthes' disease
or slipped epiphysis.

In his *Principles of Treatment of Fractures and Dislocations*, the stated
aims are restoration of length and symmetry, using absolute rest obtained
by splintage taking its purchase on the healthy parts and not compressing
the circulation at the fracture site. Hence his denunciation of plaster-of-Paris,

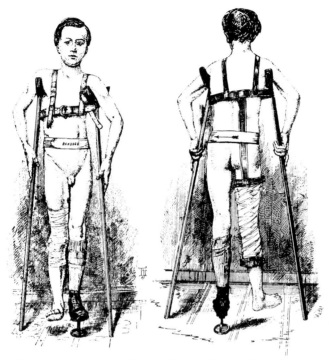

Figure 60 Thomas's solution to the problem of Figure 58 – the ambulatory hip splint with a patten on the sound side. (Le Vay, D. [1956]. *The Life of Hugh Owen Thomas.* [Edinburgh and London, Livingstone])

especially, it seems, in the hands of Sayre in New York. 'It is my belief that hitherto a too mechanical view of treatment has prevailed. Since the discovery of antisepsis ... even recent fractures are at once drilled or pegged in the surgery of fractured bones. If we are thoughtful of the fact that it is living matter we have to influence, interference will seldom be required. Such operations are sometimes a hindrance, rather than an aid, to repair.'

If we wish to know what Thomas would have thought of the AO system, he has already said it: 'Most practitioners are too prone to look upon bones as mere machines, like watches, possessed of no automatic repairing quality.' It is not the present writer's duty to do more than hint at the possible iatrogenic disasters inherent in modern fracture management, and to contrast these with Thomas's conservatism. But no-one can fully appreciate this who is unfamiliar with conservative methods and who, perhaps afraid of litigation, tends to operate on the X-rays. The brilliant results of operative treatment should not conceal that many occupants of orthopaedic wards are being treated for the failure of previous treatment. Thomas exactly echoes Hunter's polemic against operations: 'Any knowledge which enables us to dispense with them is welcome ... true antisepsis is the conservatism which obviates the need for operation. We can introduce a little more physiology with gain.'

The Treatment of Fractures, Dislocations, Diseases and Deformities of the

Bone of the Trunk and Upper Extremities is largely concerned with dislocation of the shoulder and elbow, blending arrogance towards authority with humility towards natural process. The diagnosis of recovery is as important a that of defect. Treatment is often brusque, even cruel: Thomas whips out the wrench he has modified from an engineer's monkey wrench and refractures a malunited Colles fracture in his rooms before the woman knows what is happening. He percusses ununited fractures with a hammer and also treats them by 'damming' – local venous stasis induced by ligature. The elbow is managed in the famous 'gauge halter' or collar-and-cuff sling, sealed with wax to prevent interference, and it is the elbow which must not be coerced by manipulation or operation and in which the test for recovered soundness most readily applies. For a dislocation unreduced after three months, a 'sham reduction' with attention to rest and recovery is better than anatomical reduction strenuously secured (old unreduced elbow dislocations are common in the Third World and, in the present writer's experience, open reduction always fails to restore function).

The final volume of the *Contributions* is *Fractures, Dislocations, Deformities*

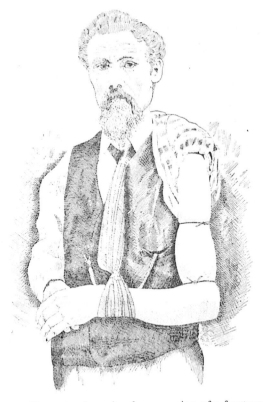

Figure 61　Thomas: illustrates damming for nonunion of a fractured humerus, also the collar and cuff or 'gauge halter' sling. (Le Vay, D. [1956]. *The Life of Hugh Owen Thomas*. [Edinburgh and London, Livingstone])

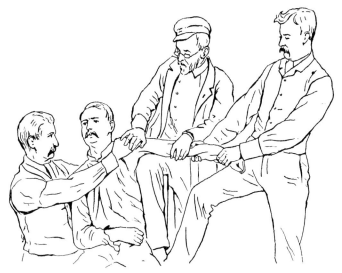

Figure 62 'We put on the collar and back extension movement'. The burly figure on Thomas's left is that of Robert Jones. (Le Vay, D. [1956]. *The Life of Hugh Owen Thomas*. [Edinburgh and London, Livingstone])

and Diseases of the Lower Extremities (1890). Here, 'Mr R Jones' is frequently mentioned: Thomas had adopted his wife's nephew into his practice;* and it emerges that surgeons from all over the world – but not from Britain – are now visiting the little clinic in Nelson Street.

Thomas applied splints from his stock, converted bed-splints into calipers, all very rapidly. 'This day I left home to visit Dr Symons of Ormskirk, who had fractured a patella the previous day. On arrival at his home at 3.15 pm my various appliances were unpacked, heel-plates screwed, boot tied, bed-splint converted into caliper, then placed in position, and the patient got out of bed and walked in his room 15 minutes after my arrival. I was able to leave by the 3.55 train.'

Thomas was obsessed with the importance of the blood-supply to a fracture and used percussion or flagellation to induce hyperaemia. He was willing to inflict a few days' pain and strain to bring a diseased joint into correct position rather than waste weeks on traction. He introduced the metatarsal bar for forefoot disorders and the crooked elongated heel for flat-foot to support the ligaments that he thought more important than the muscles: 'A few pennyworths of leather on the sole of a boot will do more than any expensive appliance to make a bad foot behave like an excellent one.' Rigid flat-foot was treated by tenotomy of the peronei and extensors. Talipes was treated by repeated manipulation, yielding 'better correction

---

* It is a common error to suppose that Robert Jones was Thomas's flesh and blood nephew.

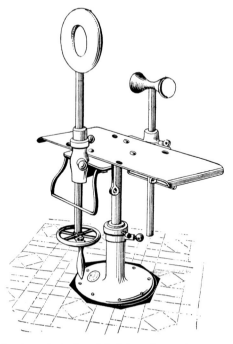

Figure 63   The reduction chair for old dislocations of the shoulder. (Le Vay, D. [1956]. *The Life of Hugh Owen Thomas.* [Edinburgh and London, Livingstone])

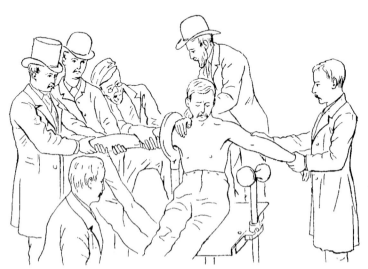

Figure 64   A reduction in progress. (Le Vay, D. [1956]. *The Life of Hugh Owen Thomas.* [Edinburgh and London, Livingstone])

than by knife or saw', but always begun with an Achilles tenotomy, then using his wrench but with intermittent bandaging in an iron shoe and stress on overcorrection while the lengthened muscles shortened.

He was against trying to correct the curvature of Pott's disease: 'Keep the patient in the shape you find him and be willing to sacrifice some symmetry to the curtailment of the period of recovery' – the main-stem of the treatment of spinal tuberculosis in Britain and one observed in the next century by Girdlestone at Oxford, only adding the development of secondary curves close to the kyphosis. Thomas vindictively opposed the plaster jacket for this or for scoliosis.

He recognized the hazards of the dislocated talus and removed it if necessary and stressed the aftertreatment of Pott's fracture. Patellar fractures well illustrate his principles. By the 1880s, wholesale operation by wiring had followed Listerism, especially in America, where Cooper's operation of 1861 antedated Lister's of 1877. Thomas crammed the fragments together in a knee splint and in half an hour the patient walked off to his usual occupation. Visiting a patient in Wales who had been bedridden for three weeks, 'we fixed the fracture by the indirect method and at the end of the operation the surgeon, patient and myself went downstairs and enjoyed dinner. From that moment he resumed his duties of commander of a steamship and recovery was perfect.' What did it matter whether it was a bony or a firm fibrous union? Can we say more of present-day treatment? Many of his patients returned to work on the day of their injury. His compound fractures of the tibia were rarely admitted: the wound was trimmed, an antiseptic pad and a caliper applied, and the patient went home. His hip fractures – and he was able to categorize them – were all treated in the same way in his hip splint and his nonunions seem to have been rare.

On traumatic dislocation of the hip he paid generous tribute to Bigelow (p. 388). On hip disease in general, he inveighed against a gamut of surgical sectaries pulling on a femur 'which is providentially hooked into the acetabulum to resist them.' He did not splint young children unless his test showed increasing flexion, thus avoiding the overtreatment of transient synovitis. He discussed every detail of treatment with the parents, who were allotted due responsibility, and stressed that such discussion was a valuable exercise for the clinician. Thomas asserted, a century ago, that 'every case of hip disease can be cured without leaving a fraction of deformity of flexion, and with no shortening except that arising from arrest of growth where the epiphysis has been affected, or from erosion, and no matter whether the case goes on to suppuration or not, or is even presented for treatment in advanced suppuration.' Antibiotics apart, this was a routine achievement of which a modern orthopaedic surgeon might be proud, and which he obtained by unremitting attention to detail, with the briefest exposure to devitalizing hospital life, without the shortening of years in plaster, without immobilizing the whole patient, and without radical and hazardous surgical intervention.

An Argument with the Censor of St Luke's Hospital, New York was first published in 1876 as a review of hip disease, but given its aggressive title in 1889 as a counterblast to Shaffer's treatment of his friend Ridlon (p. 402), and reissued as *A Review of Orthopaedics* in 1890 just before his death. It apotheosizes his feelings about American orthopaedic surgeons, whom he vilified, either for disregarding his methods in favour of traction with motion, or for pirating his views. A few, like Bauer, he respected. Shaffer was repeatedly attacked, his results mercilessly dissected and rejected. Sayre and Taylor also suffer. However, the management of chronic hip disease in the third quarter of the century was as chaotic as Thomas alleged, and he thought it his duty to castigate the 'extensionists, posterior fixationists, anticoncussionists, distractionists, plaster of Parisists, profrictionists and do-nothingists'. He introduced order into this chaos to such a degree that any unannounced visiting surgeon could be sure of an overwhelming demonstration of the truth of his views, seeing cases of serious disease treated as outpatients which, in his rivals' hands, came too often after long hospitalization to amputation, excision, even death.

In 1891, after visiting a country patient in the depths of winter, Thomas caught pneumonia and was dead in a few days. His funeral was marked by an unparalleled display of spontaneous homage from the population of a great city.

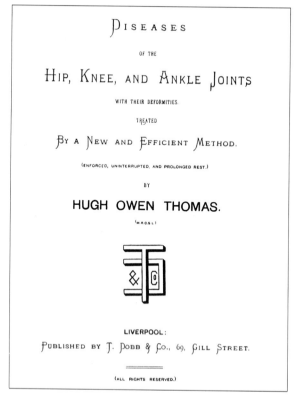

Figure 65 Title page of *Diseases of the Hip, Knee and Ankle Joints*. (Le Vay, D. [1956]. *The Life of Hugh Owen Thomas*. [Edinburgh and London, Livingstone])

Thomas's appliances were widely adopted in his lifetime, but his theories found only limited acceptance. Other schools arose, including the 'movement treatment' of fractures associated with Lucas-Championnière (p. 269), in direct opposition to the principles of rest. Bick points out that the two are not as antithetic as may appear. Championnière had X-ray controls, Thomas did not; fixation is essential as long as it is indicated, mobilization as soon as it is safe.

Looking at fracture treatment in historical perspective, and if one has to choose between those, like Thomas, who rely on biological process, and the 'meccano men' – not that the two are necessarily incompatible, since everything is finally settled by the osteoblasts – the choice must lie with the former. Principle is more important than detail. The present writer is not ashamed of his devotion to Thomas. 'He is the Hero we must all follow.'

To return to London, and to Little, Rocyn Jones has rightly emphasized that it was here that orthopaedics began to exist as a speciality in England, since Thomas founded no hospital or institute and his principles were made widely known only after his death in 1891 through the gentler influence of Robert Jones, whereas Little, at Stromeyer's instigation, had founded the 'Infirmary for the Cure of Club Foot and other Contractures' in Bloomsbury Square in London in 1838.

William John Little (1810–1894) was educated partly at the Jesuit seminary at St Omer. His personal saga, the story of his own paralytic club-foot and his successful search for a cure by tenotomy in Germany at the hands of Stromeyer in Hanover because nothing but amputation was available at home, his foundation of what was to become the Royal National Orthopaedic Hospital in London, are related elsewhere (pp. 499–501). We must always remember that Little saw himself, and was seen, as the senior physician to the London Hospital, with a neurological bent, and an attending physician at obstetric hospitals and at the Asylum for Idiots at Earlswood (which led to his account of the eponymous congenital spastic palsy), and must have regarded orthopaedics as only a part, and probably a minor part, of his work.

His famous paper: 'On the influence of abnormal parturition, difficult labour, premature birth and asphyxia neonatorum on the mental and physical condition of the child, especially in relation to deformities' was in fact founded on these extra-orthopaedic activities, so that the first definitive account of Little's disease was published in an obstetric journal and based on 63 case reports[71]. The pathology of the foetus *in utero* was already established. Now Little turned to the pathology of birth, 'which does occasionally imprint upon the nervous and muscular systems of the nascent infantile organism very serious and peculiar evils.' He had previously pointed out in his *Treatise on Deformities* of 1853 and elsewhere that 'in premature birth, difficult labours, mechanical injuries during parturition to head and neck, *where life had been saved*, convulsions following the act of birth were apt to be succeeded by a determinate affection of the limbs of the child which I designated spastic rigidity ... from asphyxia neonatorum ...' The italics are mine because until then obstetricians and others had concerned themselves with the life or death of these children and had not reported the fate of the survivors. Little,

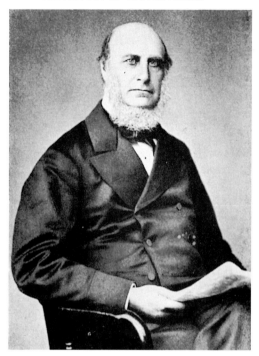

Figure 66　William John Little (1810–1894)

however, had seen 200 cases in 20 years of orthopaedic practice and wanted
to report these to his obstetric colleagues. Whatever the actual circumstances
of the labour, the primal and proximate cause was interruption of the
placental relation of mother to foetus, unsubstituted by pulmonary respir-
ation. Autopsies had shown 'capillary apoplexies' in the central nervous
system[72,73] and Little attributed spasticity to these, and hence to neonatal
asphyxia, rather than to mechanical injury (there may be a presage here of
the vogue for 'hyperphlebaemia' as a universal pathology of the newborn in
some quarters in the 1930s). He then describes classical diplegia and its
variants, the typical speech and gait, absence of sensory deficit, the choreiform
(athetotic) type, the convulsions and retardation. It may not be appreciated
that Little ascribed this spasticity to lesions of the cord, rather than the
brain, and never thought or spoke of it as cerebral palsy; and he also thought
that not more than one in twenty cases of spastic contracture in young
children were of obstetric origin, and was in this mistaken. His outlook was
far from pessimistic: '... treatment based upon physiology and rational
therapeutics effects an amelioration surprising to those who have not watched
such cases. Many of the most helpless have been restored to considerable
activity and enjoyment of life. Even cases which exhibit impaired intellect
may be benefited in mind and body to an unexpected extent', a sympathetic
and constructive approach echoed and developed by Winthrop Phelps in
the USA in the next century.

As Little's work on club-foot is dealt with elsewhere, we need only state that he was apprenticed to a local apothecary, a Mr James Sequeira, while graduating at the London Hospital. He taught comparative anatomy there but was passed over for a place on the staff at that time. He decided to devote himself to medicine; membership of the Royal College of Physicians required two years at a university and, partly because of this and partly because he was unable to find anyone willing or able to treat his club-foot in England (where it was considered outside the legitimate scope of surgery) and had been refused tenotomy by Delpech for fear of sepsis, went to Berlin in 1834 (the year of Hugh Owen Thomas's birth). There, as Keith says, 'he stepped into the centre of the most productive and progressive medical movement then in Europe', led by Müller, Schwann and Henle.

Little's personal operation by Stromeyer (who had been trained partly in Britain) is described elsewhere. Stromeyer suggested that he found a hospital in England to perform this treatment in the poor, and Little returned to London to practise in Finsbury Square in 1837 and did his first tenotomy on 20 February of that year – the first, as he thought, to do so in Britain, though he later discovered that a Mr. Whipple of Plymouth had done so in two cases the year before. Whipple reported these to the Royal Medical and Chirurgical Society on 28 March 1837, on which occasion Little described his own experience as patient and surgeon and generously acknowledged Whipple's priority. At the meeting at his house in 1839 to set up the new Infirmary, it was stated that 'this committee, duly appreciating original Genius, desires to record the fact that J W Whipple of Plymouth performed the successful operation on the Tendon Achillis for the cure of Club Foot in this country before any other practitioner.'

Little wrote, in 1853: 'The principal reasons assigned ... for establishing an additional eleemosynary institution in London were the dispensation of that relief to poor persons afflicted with deformities which they were unable to obtain in the existing hospitals, the formation of a school for studying deformities, and instruction in the art of remedying them[74].' We have noted elsewhere that John Ball Brown, who did the first subcutaneous tenotomy for club-foot in America in 1839, founded the first orthopaedic hospital in the USA at almost exactly the same time, and for the same reasons: that 'deformities of the human frame cannot be conveniently and judiciously treated, except in a hospital or institution expressly devoted to this object[75].'

Little's Infirmary opened its doors on 1 July 1840, and soon changed its name to that of Orthopaedic Institution. Little was elected physician and R W Tamplin, his brother-in-law as surgeon (they had married each other's sisters). Little resigned only four years later, in 1844, because of incompatibilities with lay governors and administrators. An early committee member had been a Mr Quarles Harris, a city merchant, who later declared himself to have been the founder and Little of no consequence. Little wrote much of orthopaedic interest: *A Treatise on the nature of Club-Foot* (London 1839); *On Ankylosis or Stiff Joints* (London 1843); *On the Nature and Treatment of the Deformities of the Human Frame* (London 1853); *Medical and Surgical Aspects of In-Knee (genu valgum)* (London 1882); his famous paper on congenital spastic palsy in the *Transactions of the Obstetric Society of London*

in 1862; a contribution to Holmes's *System of Surgery* in 1870. We note that
he recanted somewhat in later life, for he wrote on *Unnecessary orthopaedic
operations* in the Lancet of 1857[76], admitting that he had operated too freely
in his earlier years, and pleading for the nonoperative treatment of club-foot.
He had, for instance, persuaded Solly, in 1857, to remove the cuboid for a
late deformity and the operation failed[77]; it sounds like midlife depression.

The Orthopaedic Institution became the Royal Orthopaedic Hospital in
1845 and moved to Hanover Square in 1855.

William Adams (1810–1900) was Little's major colleague at the hospital
and his successor and became the most eminent London orthopaedic surgeon
of the mid-Victorian epoch. A St Thomas's graduate, apprenticed to his
father, a City surgeon, he failed to gain appointment at St Thomas's and
joined the staff of the new hospital. He studied the healing of divided tendons
in animals and also in those dying for various reasons at varying periods
after subcutaneous tenotomy at the Royal Orthopaedic Hospital, concluding
that the tendon sheath played a decisive role as matrix and guide for bridging
tissue[78]. He also wrote, in 1857, an excellent book, *The Principles and
Practice of Subcutaneous Surgery*, an interest now extended from tendons to
bones, and at a time, before the advent of Listerian antisepsis, when entry
of outside air into the wound was thought noxious. He therefore devised a
special keyhole or 'pistol-shaped' saw to divide the femoral neck in vicious
ankylosis of the hip[79], and gave a Smithsonian Lecture on this theme in
1877[80]. This was to correct flexion–adduction deformity and not, like Barton
(p. 381), with the deliberate intent of creating a pseudarthrosis. His book,

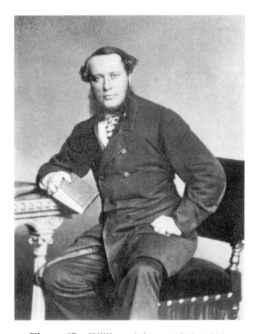

Figure 67   William Adams (1810–1900)

Club-Foot: its Causes, Pathology and Treatment, of 1866, received the Jacksonian Prize of the Royal College of Surgeons. Like Pravaz (p. 248), he claimed to have succeeded in reducing congenital dislocation of the hip by traction and he treated hip disease by combining traction with motion – the 'American method', though he did not designate it as such[81]. Like Little, he retired prematurely because of friction, and died, either a bachelor aged 90 or a married man aged 80 with three children, depending on the authority consulted.

In 1845, William Lawrence of St Bartholomew's Hospital, became consultant surgeon, with Richard William Tamplin (1814–1874) as surgeon and Edward Francis Lonsdale and Edward John Chance as assistant surgeons. By 1849, the hospital had 36 beds, mothers were admitted with their young children and there was occupational therapy. But all was not sweetness and light. Tamplin was very authoritarian and allowed his two assistants little or no independence. Chance was forced to resign in 1851 (though appointed to the City Orthopaedic Hospital founded in that year), and Bernard Edward Brodhurst and William Adams elected. Tamplin, an unfriendly aggressive individual, remained in dictatorial charge, with an effective veto on new procedures and on the simultaneous attendance of his staff at other hospitals. There was so much ill feeling that, in 1872, both Tamplin and Adams were constrained to resign. Tamplin died two years later, and Adams joined the staff of the new National Orthopaedic Hospital (where Little was consultant physician) in 1873.

We leave this institution for the moment to turn to the City Orthopaedic Hospital, founded in 1851, largely because of the long waiting-list at the Royal, and with Chance as surgeon. A year later there were 799 patients on the books, mostly with club-feet and rickety deformities. In 1893, Chance, now 86, was still surgeon-in-charge; Noble Smith was elected and Chance died two years later. In 1897 the medical staff consisted of Smith and John Poland as surgeons, Chisholm William and Jackson Clarke as assistant surgeons, plus some ancillaries.

The National Orthopaedic Hospital was a third institution, and there is often confusion as to its origins. A 'Society for the Treatment, at their own homes, of Poor Persons afflicted with Diseases and Distortions of the Spine, Chest, Hip, etc.' had been founded in 1836, based on the use of a special couch invented by a Charles Verral, surgeon at Seaford in Sussex. Chance had worked with Verral for a time from 1839. In 1850, the Society moved to 84 Norton Street (later Bolsover Street), adjacent to Great Portland Street, near London's Regent's Park, and in 1856 became the Spinal Hospital for the Cure of Deformities with 12 beds, staffed by Verral and Thomas Carr Jackson as surgeons and William Brinton as physician, and renamed in 1865 the National Orthopaedic Hospital. Other staff were added, including Little's son, Louis Stromeyer Little, Henry Dick, who excised the cuboid for club-foot, William Adams in 1873, and Little *père* himself, as consulting physician, in 1874. In 1865, the younger Little performed the first osteotomy for knock-knee in Britain (Mayer had done this in Würzburg in 1853), a wedge excision of the tibia and fibula on both sides at an interval of six weeks, with a good result. He left for China in 1875 and returned 30 years later to serve on the committee of what was now the Royal National Orthopaedic Hospital.

By 1881, the staff of the National included W J Roeckel and Little's youngest son, Ernest Muirhead Little. Roeckel went to Australia to practise in Melbourne around 1890, but is not mentioned in Barry's *Orthopaedics in Australia* (p. 341). He was succeeded by A H Tubby, who became very famous indeed (p. 149).

Ernest Muirhead Little (1854–1935) was not only an orthopaedic surgeon in his own right, on the staffs of both the National Orthopaedic Hospital and the Royal National Orthopaedic Hospital, but a formidable medical historian. He was one of the founders of the British Orthopaedic Association and its first president. He wrote on the history of spinal curvature and its treatment, on Glisson, on pre-Stromeyerian orthopaedics, and on the dawn of recognition of skeletal tuberculosis. He was a colleague of Robert Jones in World War I, surgeon to the Royal National from 1888 to 1919, in charge of the amputation centre at Queen Mary's Hospital in Roehampton in the first world war, and subsequent adviser to the Ministry of Pensions on artificial limbs.

The National Orthopaedic Hospital expanded considerably into Great Portland Street in the 1890s to a total of 62 beds, and really provided the basic physical structure for the amalgamations of 1903 and 1907, after T H Openshaw had joined the staff in 1894.

The 'amalgamations' involved much jockeying for position, as these procedures usually do. Everyone was sensitive of his dignity. The transient

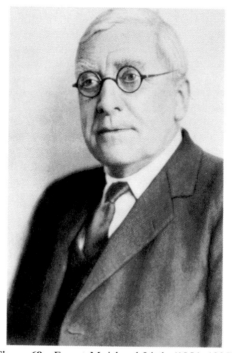

Figure 68   Ernest Muirhead Little (1854–1935)

British Orthopaedic Society of 1898–1901 had had its first meetings at the Royal, the new discipline was on the upgrade, position was paramount. In 1903 a preliminary meeting agreed on the desirability of uniting all three hospitals – the Royal, the National and the City Orthopaedic Hospitals – at the Great Portland Street site of the National. The first two did fuse, in 1905, but the City hung back until 1907 when financial difficulties forced its hand. The Royal seems never to have had an X-ray department of its own, the films being made by contractors.

The newly united institution was now known as the Royal National Orthopaedic Hospital, with its base in Great Portland Street and a rural outpost at Stanmore, to the north of London. In 1913, it provided facilities for the International Medical Congress in London in August, which marked the first recognition by that body of orthopaedic surgery as an independent subject. There was a dinner; operations were demonstrated by Bankart (A S Blundell Bankart had been appointed registrar to the National in 1911 and rapidly rose to full surgeon), Openshaw, Tubby, Laming Evans (house surgeon to the Royal in 1898 and surgeon to the Royal National until 1936), and Jackson Clarke. Fred Albee read a paper on 'Original uses of the Bone Graft as a treatment for the Ununited Fracture, Certain Deformities and Pott's Disease', and actually used his electrically powered twin-bladed saw on a boy of three with spinal tuberculosis, assisted by Rocyn Jones. Other visitors included Murphy from Chicago, Lovett from Boston, Rollier from France.

In 1904, R C Elmslie was appointed house surgeon to the Royal, and in 1919, when he became the first orthopaedic surgeon at St Bartholomew's Hospital, he was made full surgeon at the Royal National with Sir Robert Jones and H O Trethowan. (All these individuals are discussed at greater length later.) In 1921, Openshaw retired and H A T Fairbank declined an invitation to replace him.

Before we go further with the story of the Royal National Orthopaedic Hospital, we must complete our account of Victorian figures. **Richard Barwell** (1826–1916) wrote *On the Cure of Club-Foot without Cutting Tendons* (2nd edn. London 1865), opposing the use of tenotomy and favouring his own employment of rubber springs to substitute for the weakened muscles, though he seems to have plagiarized this from the famous orthopaedic mechanic, Henry Heather Bigg, who protested vigorously[82]. Barwell's conservatism also showed in his *Treatise on Diseases of the Joints* (Philadelphia and London 1861), in which he stressed the function of the epiphyseal plates and the risks of retardation of growth from knee-joint resection in youth: 'It is evidently of extreme importance to preserve the epiphyseal junction in all patients below 18 years of age.' Nevertheless, he osteotomized the femur as well as the leg bones for severe knock-knee[83] and he also divided the muscles attached to the great trochanter in attempting to reduce congenital dislocation of the hip.

The other members of this Victorian London group deserving mention are Lonsdale and Brodhurst. **Edward Francis Lonsdale** made a valuable statistical evaluation in 1855 of 3000 cases of various deformities from the Royal Orthopaedic Hospital, giving a good overview of the types of disorders treated at such a hospital in the mid-19th century[84]. **Edward Bernard Brodhurst** (1822–1900) is known for his work on congenital dislocation of the hip[85] and claimed to obtain manipulative reposition of unilateral cases as a routine in children under two years of age, though whether the improvement was really due to reduction is impossible to say in the absence of X-rays. We recall that he had also removed a medial meniscus in 1866.

Let us now complete the story of the Royal National Orthopaedic Hospital before turning to a detailed study of some famous figures. The country branch, which housed a residential school for physically handicapped children, was based on the rebuilding of a Shaftesbury Society convalescent home at Stanmore, in Middlesex, and was opened in 1922. Robert Jones retired in 1924, at age 65, to become an honorary consultant, a sort of emeritus status, but had to resign even from this in 1927 because of an unfortunate clash of interests involving double loyalties to Stanmore and to the Chailey orthopaedic hospital for children in Sussex, founded in 1903. Both hospitals had peripheral clinics and poaching was suspected, and indeed inevitable, as those of the RNOH covered a large part of south-east England. In 1928, Sir Thomas Horder (later Lord Horder) became honorary physician. H J Seddon (p. 154) became registrar, visited Michigan for a year in 1931, and returned to Stanmore as resident surgeon in 1931 but was not allowed private practice.

In 1929, E P Brockman became assistant surgeon, George Perkins, who had been on the staff, resigned and was replaced by R Y Paton, and V H Ellis of St Mary's Hospital was made consultant. In 1931, various registrar appointments were made, including A T Fripp and H Jackson Burrows, both eventually to become surgeons. In 1936, Karl Nissen joined the junior surgical staff. J A Cholmeley became assistant resident surgeon in 1937 and did an enormous amount to run the hospital smoothly, as well as much later writing the superb history of the institution from which most of the present material is drawn[153]. Seddon left in 1940 to become Nuffield Professor of Orthopaedic Surgery and Director of the Wingfield–Morris Orthopaedic Hospital at Oxford. Before this, in 1933, he had used the clinical material at Stanmore for a distinguished essay on Pott's paraplegia, written with Weeden Butler of Cambridge, which gained the Robert Jones Gold Medal of the British Orthopaedic Association.

In 1941, Bankart, of the Middlesex Hospital, had become senior surgeon. The patients were evacuated to Scotland at the flying bomb stage of World War II in 1944. In 1945–6, a Postgraduate Institute of Orthopaedics, based on the hospital, was founded as part of the University of London to retain a degree of independence before the implementation of the National Health Service in 1948, as it was well-known that the authorities were inimical to specialized hospitals. In 1946, the war over, a number of surgeons were appointed: Jackson Burrows, David Trevor, Karl Nissen, Philip Newman, J I P James. In 1947, J T Scales joined the permanent staff at Stanmore and became the first British professor of biomedical engineering. In 1948, Cholmeley became a part-time surgeon and E J Nangle, a junior colleague of Seddon's at Oxford, became resident surgeon before emigrating to Rhodesia.

We should add that Rocyn Jones (see p. 157), who had been on the junior staff for many years but had had trouble with his higher examinations, became a full surgeon in 1924. In the same year a Mr R Watson-Jones was appointed house surgeon at Great Portland Street.

The late 1940s and early 1950s saw the establishment of special clinics: for scoliosis (James, then Charles Manning in 1958), leg equalization (Nissen), poliomyelitis (Donal Brooks), vascular surgery (Seddon and Bonney). In 1949 Hubert Sissons from the Antipodes, arrived to build up what was to become one of the leading departments of bone pathology in the world, while from 1956 to 1977 R O Murray achieved a comparable development in the radiology department. Seddon returned from Oxford in 1948 to direct the new Postgraduate Institute and became Professor in 1965, was knighted in 1964 and retired in 1967. He was succeeded in the Chair by R G Burwell, who resigned in 1972.

But the administrators eventually caught up! The Great Portland Street hospital was closed in 1983 and its urban clinical activities amalgamated with those of other London hospitals such as the Middlesex. The library and other departments of record moved to Bolsover Street. The Middlesex Hospital itself amalgamated with University College Hospital.

The present writer has given this account of the Royal National Orthopaedic Hospital at what may seem inordinate length. The formal reason is the outstanding position of this institution in the history of orthopaedics in Britain. The private reason is that, for a season, he was a very small part of it.

Now let us turn to the opposite pole, to Scotland. **Sir William Macewen** (1848–1924)[86,87] was a student at Glasgow under Syme and Lister and became surgeon to the Glasgow Royal Infirmary at 28. The new antiseptic surgery enabled him to develop as routine procedures that would previously have been unjustifiable risks. In 1875 he did a wedge osteotomy for a knee ankylosed at right angles, in 1877 subcutaneous femoral osteotomy for genu valgum, in the same year an open wedge osteotomy for bilateral knock-knee which suppurated somewhat but ended well, and seven years later reported 1800 cases of osteotomy (mainly for rickets) without serious infection. For these he devised a one-piece osteotome, i.e. without a separate wooden or bone handle which might absorb corruptible material, sharpened on both sides unlike a chisel, and is usually credited with this innovation though Heine, of Würzburg, had introduced his *osteotom* (admittedly constructed on quite different principles) in 1830. Macewen acknowledged that the stimulus to his first operation came from a report of two similar cases by Volkmann, of Halle[88]. Macewen did much research into bone growth in animals and did his famous pioneering bone-grafting in 1879, on a four-year-old boy who had had the whole shaft of the right humerus removed the previous year for osteomyelitis. Fifteen months later, Macewen inserted small fragments from two bone wedges removed from a case of tibial correction; further grafts were inserted three and eight months later, and 16 months after the first procedure the bone was consolidated from end to end and only half-an-inch shorter than the left. When Macewen saw the patient again 30 years later, in 1909[89], he had worked all that period as a carpenter;

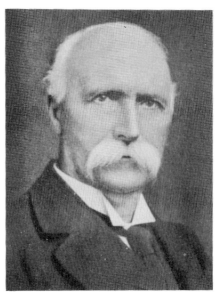

Figure 69   William Macewen (1848–1926)

and he subsequently served in World War I. This Macewen took as absolute proof that osteogenesis was not a function of the periosteum, but may have erred in this if he had really been working within an intact periosteal sleeve. And where the excisionists often left a flail limb, albeit with a useful hand, Macewen had taken the logical next step in filling and consolidating the gap.

However, in *The Growth of Bone: Observations on Osteogenesis* (Glasgow 1912) he reported experiments in which he stripped the shafts of the long bones of dogs and filled the gaps with chips devoid of periosteum; the shafts regrew. This seemed to show conclusively that the periosteum was not osteogenic and that, when it appeared to be so, it was because it was a limiting membrane investing bone arising more deeply, the same view as Goodsir's 79 years before. Osteogenesis was the function of the osteoblasts alone; when a shaft regrew, it was from the growth-plates. Here we are involved in almost theological arguments over dogma; as Keith says, both the periosteal and the shaft schools were right. Macewen had succeeded with his humeral graft in 1889 because he was operating in the same institute where Lister had introduced antisepsis in 1866, because of his preconception of bone as a survivable graft, and because he placed his grafts where they were subject to muscle stresses. Sepsis had ruined Hunter's attempts at grafting, and Ollier's periosteal grafts (p. 261) often failed because of sepsis and because they were placed in the soft tissues and not subject to stress. The literature on artificially induced ectopic bone is too enormous to review here.

Macewen was truly a general surgeon interested in orthopaedics, and is more properly regarded as the founder of neurosurgery in Britain through his work on cerebral tumours and abscesses. He was the leading European surgeon of his time and was offered the Chair of Surgery at Johns Hopkins in 1889 (it was only his refusal that led to the appointment of Halsted). He did the first pneumonectomy. In 1911, Fred Albee acknowledged Macewen's role as a precursor to his own work on massive bone-grafting[90]. Overall, Macewen has to be seen as a pioneer in thoracic surgery and neurosurgery.

Also in Scotland, **Alexander Ogston** of Aberdeen (1844–1929), almost an exact contemporary of Macewen, had the idea, or adopted it from Annandale, in 1876, of doing an oblique osteotomy of the medial femoral condyle in knock-knee and allowing it to shift upwards to produce correction. This he did on a bilateral case under the carbolic spray, with success[91]. Ogston was also interested in physiopathology, believing that the synovial fluid was formed by the attrition of articular cartilage and of little primary importance[92]. He was also something of a pioneer in the operative treatment of flat-foot, for in 1884 he performed a talo-navicular arthrodesis and inserted ivory pegs in subsequent cases to maintain apposition[93]. He also, in 1881, published a case of suture of the ulnar nerve[94].

Another Scot, **Sir William Arbuthnot Lane** (1856–1938), from Inverness, trained at Guy's Hospital in London, whose staff he later joined, and spent his early years trying to relate skeletal form and function. He noted how fracture malunion impaired joint function if there was malalignment, and how this and shortening caused depreciation of the patient's 'relative financial value as a machine, both before and after the accident.' This led him to try internal fixation of fractures, starting with silver wire, which had been used intermittently for at least a century before, but he found it unsuitable for firm coaptation. He moved on to fixing oblique fractures of the lower tibia with ordinary (oxidizable) steel screws, doing his first case on 8th January 1894 and two similar cases a week later, and employing an elaborate 'no

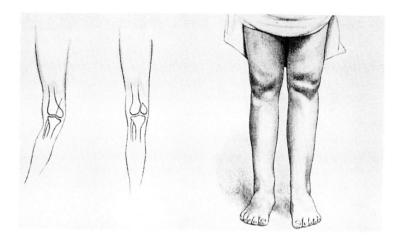

Figure 70   Alexander Ogston: The operative treatment of genu valgum. (Edinburgh Med. J. [1877] **22**, 782)

touch' technique, at much the same time as Albin Lambotte in Belgium and a little later than Gluck and Hansman in Germany. (In fact, Lambotte had operated on these fractures in 1888, 1889 and 1890, calling his procedure 'osteosynthesis'.) Lane then moved on to plates and screws for transverse fractures, always with the earliest active and passive mobilization. In 1910, he visited the USA and encouraged American surgeons to use his methods, not that they needed much encouragement. It is not widely known that, in 1892, following Hadra's wiring for cervical displacements (p. 589), Lane used silk sutures for spinal stabilization[95]. He also tried animal grafts, including the substitution of a sheep's joint for an artificial elbow. Partly because of Lane's work and that of his followers, in 1912 a commission of the British Medical Association reported on a two-year study of fracture treatment, concluding that young patients were best served by simple reduction and splintage, with operation reserved for adults; the worst results were with massage and mobilization, but this may have been cross-Channel chauvinism[96]. Lane, we note, regarded his patients as machines, and so must be held responsible to some extent for the later spread of this attitude. He was of course an eccentric, and the last part of his career was spent as an enthusiast for total colectomy as a cure for 'auto-intoxication'. He resigned from the Medical Register to further health propaganda[97].

Lane's summing up of his work in his 1905 *Operative Treatment of Fractures* is excellently produced and illustrated with X-rays of his results and has a description of his principles and instruments. But David Lloyd Griffiths says: 'In many ways it is a sad book; if its principles had been appreciated and followed, and indeed if the pages had even been read carefully, the disasters that followed its publication might not have happened. Lane made everything look so easy that his methods were thrown into undeserved disrepute when bad plating produced bad results.' That the bad results of surgery are the results of bad surgery may not be entirely true, but is a good working axiom. And, of course, his methods encountered enormous initial opposition. The then President of the Royal College of Surgeons said that anyone who converted a simple into a compound fracture was guilty of malpractice and should be arraigned before the General Medical Council, and any student who expressed even cautious approval of Lane's methods at an examination was failed and cautioned to avoid such criminal procedure! Lane is often regarded as the model for Cutler Walpole in Shaw's *The Doctor's Dilemma*, but this is not so; GBS had written the play before ever meeting Lane, of whose ideas he heartily approved.

Ernest William Hey Groves (1872–1944) was a somewhat larger than life figure of England's west country, a Bristolian[98]. He qualified at St Bartholomew's in 1895, was first a village general practitioner, then moved to Bristol, where he operated, first in his own home and then in a nursing-home, without any surgical training. He became general surgeon to the Bristol Infirmary in 1903 and a Fellow of the Royal College of Surgeons in 1905. He travelled twice a week to University College Hospital in London to research on fracture union in animals, devising external fixators, bone-pins and clamps and plates and screws[99]. In 1916 he won the Jacksonian Prize of the College for an essay on *Methods and results of transplantation*

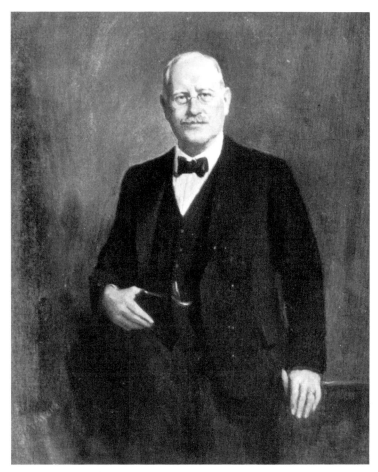

Figure 71   E W Hey Groves (1872–1944). (Reproduced with permission from the British Journal of Surgery)

of bone in repair of defects caused by injury or disease, and his book *On Modern Methods of Treating Fractures*, published in Bristol in the same year, refers back to Ollier, Axhausen and Macewen. In this, he relates the use of accurately fitted full-thickness bone-grafts and of intramedullary bone pegs for subtrochanteric fractures and of medullary metal nails for femoral shaft fractures, inserted retrograde at the fracture site and hammered back into the lower fragment, this a quarter of a century before Küntscher. He anticipated the now accepted finding that really rigid fixation could actually delay union.

He founded the *British Journal of Surgery* in 1913 and was its editor for 27 years. In World War I he worked at the military orthopaedic centre in Bristol in collaboration with Robert Jones and wrote a book on *Gunshot Injuries to Bones*.

Hey Groves was an immensely energetic and inventive surgeon. He devised a revolving spinal bed before Stryker produced his frame, and was repairing cruciate ligaments as early as 1917[100,101]. He constructed substitutes for the anterior cruciate from the iliotibial band, and for the posterior cruciate from the semitendinosus, retaining the upper attachment in each case and passing the graft through drill-holes in the femur and tibia. He even created an artificial ligamentum teres by passing a ligament through the acetabulum and attaching it to the joint capsule.

When the British Orthopaedic Association was founded in 1917, Groves was not invited to join as he was regarded as a general surgeon, but this was soon remedied and he served as President in 1928, having been Professor of Surgery at Bristol from 1922. His paper on *Some contributions to the reconstructive surgery of the hip* of 1927[102] includes references to the internal fixation of hip fractures under X-ray screening, capsular arthroplasty for hip ankylosis (at about the same time as Willis Campbell in Tennessee) and ivory femoral head replacement arthroplasty. His paper in the *Robert Jones Birthday Volume* of 1928 (p. 655) precisely anticipates the Colonna capsular arthroplasty for congenital dislocation of the hip. He made the work of Böhler and Lorenz on fracture treatment available to English-speaking surgeons by translating their *Modern Methods of Treating Fractures*. When Smith–Petersen did an open reduction of a femoral neck fracture and fixed it with a flanged nail in 1925, he was repeating Hey Groves' technique of nailing under direct vision. Groves, like Thomas, stressed that 'the more the importance of principle and the relative subordinate character of detail are recognised, the better will be the results of fracture treatment[103].' In 1933 he described approaching the hip from behind and removing the lower acetabular rim to correct the disproportion in osteoarthritis[104]. Hey Groves' life exemplifies the thesis that it is possible to have the right ideas at the wrong time, that is, too early, in this case before suitable metals and other materials were available.

The state of orthopaedics in Britain at the turn of the century, around 1900, is set out in detail elsewhere (p. 623). We have noted that the infant British Orthopaedic Society of 1894 lasted only a few years, and that its major items of interest were the operative treatment of club-foot and congenital dislocation of the hip, together with the new, or newish, tendon transplantation.

The subsequent half-century, 1900–1950, has been well reviewed by the late **Sir Henry Osmond-Clarke** (1905–1986)[105]. He was born in Fermanagh in Northern Ireland, studied anatomy at Trinity College, Dublin, and trained in orthopaedic surgery at Manchester under Harry Platt. In World War II, with Watson-Jones, he was orthopaedic consultant to the Royal Air Force as an Air Commodore and later joined the staff of the London Hospital, where he served for 25 years, though still continuing to visit Oswestry. His legend and work are still bright enough not to need recapitulating here. We need only stress his contributions to fracture services development and postgraduate orthopaedic education.

Osmond-Clarke says that this period was marked as much by the development of orthopaedics as a social service as by advances in technique, though the two are of course complementary, and also by inevitable specialization within the speciality in fields such as hand and disc surgery.

As we have said earlier, the temptation to juxtapose, or oppose, the Liverpool school of Hugh Owen Thomas and the London school of W J Little must be resisted, for Little was born 25 years before Thomas (though they died in the same year of 1891) and founded an orthopaedic hospital in London in 1838, whereas Thomas founded no hospital at all and the Liverpool school did not really get going until Robert Jones was at the Southern Hospital there at the end of the 19th century, after which it is linked with his name, and those of McMurray, Norman Roberts, Diggle and, eminently, Watson-Jones. We may note, in passing, that Thomas told Ridlon that, fond as he was of Robert Jones, he considered him far less able than the American to carry on the teachings for which Thomas had been contending. Winnett Orr, of Nebraska, recorded that 'Sir Robert was never so consistent or emphatic as he might have been in his enunciation ... of the functional principles which dominated the life and practice of Hugh Owen Thomas ... He relaxed considerably the technical details of Thomas's regime and even the apparatus essential to the kind of rest Thomas demanded for the correct treatment of bone and joint disease. But the very dogmatism which prejudiced Thomas's contemporaries against him adds to the value of his writings.' These fears proved quite unfounded. As Ridlon was to remark much later, the greatest service Robert Jones did was to render Hugh Owen Thomas's principles acceptable to the profession, a much easier task after the departure of their craggy originator.

Robert Jones (1857–1933) was not only a great man, quite possibly the greatest orthopaedic surgeon the world has ever seen, and a splendid operator – the clock seemed to stand still while he was working – he was also a good man and a kind man and a great organizer, as shown in World War I. He helped usher in the characteristic 20th century cooperation between orthopaedic surgery, charitable care and governmental action for crippled children and then adults. It should, however, never be forgotten that this cooperation flourished long before the foundation of the British National Health Service in 1948 and still underpins it. In 1900, for instance, private philanthropy made it possible for Robert Jones to help found the Royal Liverpool Country Hospital for Children at Heswall. A few months later a nursing sister with vision, Agnes Hunt, herself crippled, opened the Baschurch Home, enrolled Robert Jones in 1904, and in 1921 it was moved to Gobowen as the Shropshire Orthopaedic Hospital at Oswestry, renamed the Robert Jones and Agnes Hunt Orthopaedic Hospital after Jones's death in 1933. What was to be the usual British pattern now developed, one of peripheral clinics visited from the centre by orthopaedic surgeons, nurses and physiotherapists, with admission of patients to the central institute and the addition of educational and vocational training facilities; and this pioneer work led to the formation of a national Central Council for the Care of Cripples, to the Invalid Children's Aid Association and similar bodies – nongovernmental organizations with access to and influence on the ministries of health and education.

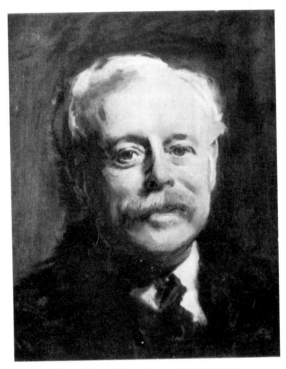

Figure 72   Robert Jones (1857–1933)

The aims of centres like Oswestry have never been more clearly set out than by G R Girdlestone when he was visiting South Africa in 1937 to plan orthopaedic services there for the Nuffield Fund. The essentials were early detection, efficient treatment and proper aftercare. It was easier for the surgeon to go to the patients rather than the reverse, so there should be a central orthopaedic hospital with peripheral clinics in general hospitals, visited by the specialists from the centre with their aftercare and plaster sisters. He wanted 'a living organization which aims at preventing crippling, a well-knit central organization with decentralized clinics that runs like a machine. The vast majority of patients need never come into hospital but are cured as outpatients ... Easy cure by early treatment is a salvation to these children and an actual economy to the state[106].'

It is difficult for us to appreciate now that, at the start of World War I, Robert Jones, like Hugh Owen Thomas, was better known to his friends in the USA than in Britain, where he was sometimes sneered at as a mere bonesetter[107]. Even when his outstanding work in the war earned the following eulogy from Sir William Osler, we can still detect a faintly patronising echo of the attitude of physicians to surgeons which is as old as medical history:

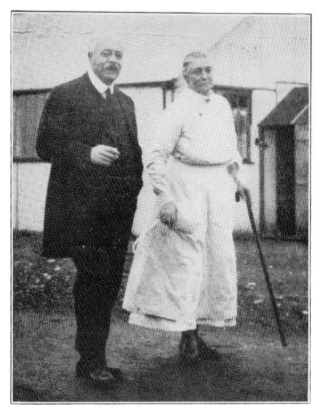

Figure 73   An early photograph of Robert Jones and Agnes Hunt

'There has grown up a department of surgery, the branch known as orthopaedics … now widely applied to the relief of deformities and disabilities of all kinds. The orthopaedic surgeon is a teacher, a personal teacher and in two directions, of the patient's mind quite as much as of his muscles and joints. It is not simply a surgical matter, but an individual human problem requiring prolonged attention and study in each case. The new specialists in this branch are as much superior to the half-educated osteopaths and bone-setters as are our ophthalmic surgeons to the old vendors of eye-salves.'

To sketch Robert Jones's life very briefly, family poverty sent him as an apprentice to Thomas, whose wife was his aunt, and he qualified in 1878 and worked with Thomas until the latter's death. He became general surgeon to the Royal Southern Hospital in Liverpool in 1899 and confined himself to orthopaedics from 1905. In the last decade of the century, from 1887 to 1894, he organized the casualty service for the building of the Manchester Ship Canal between the two cities, obtaining the sort of experience in traumatology that Imhotep had acquired during the building of the Pyramids. The work at Oswestry came to serve a large area in Wales and midland

England. Initially, his surgical technique was still much influenced by his pupillage with Thomas, relying heavily on reduction under general anaesthesia, traction, alignment and immobilization, in splints rather than plaster. He did then begin to operate on difficult tibial fractures, initially a simple open reduction rather than plating or screwing, and he also operated for fractures of the olecranon, patella and radial neck. Though he observed Thomas's admonition to leave healing to Nature, he thought it wise to give her the best conditions to work in. Even so, at the end of World War I the Liverpool school still thought that manipulation and splintage was best for most fractures. Robert Jones saw at once the importance of Roentgen's discovery in December 1895 and immediately sent to Würzburg (in May 1896) and obtained a machine. With Thurston Holland, he took probably the first X-ray in Britain, of a bullet in a boy's wrist, but thought it initially no more than an adjunct: 'It has done little if anything to perfect or even alter our treatment of fractures[107].' Early in the century, Robert Jones introduced the immediate reduction of fractures.

Of his organizing abilities we have already had evidence. He opened the first British hospital for the long-term treatment of crippled children in 1899, the West Kirkby Convalescent Home; later he was connected with the Royal Liverpool Country Hospital for Children at Heswall. He was 57 at the outbreak of the First World War, with an established international reputation. The enormous number of casualties in 1914 led the army medical services to ask for help. He joined the Royal Army Medical Corps as a major, toured the military hospitals, and sent a blistering report on their shortcomings to the War Office.

The problem was that there were still very few trained orthopaedic surgeons in Britain. From the start he resisted the idea that soldiers unlikely to become fit to fight again should just be discharged into civilian life: 'It would involve the discharge of half our wounded in the most critical stages of disease, many of them to die, and most of them destined to deformity and functional disability ... no soldier should be discharged until everything is done to make him a healthy and efficient citizen.' Early in 1915, Alder Hey Hospital in Liverpool was opened with Jones in charge of the surgical side. One of his aides was a Captain T P McMurray. The hospital was soon entirely reserved for orthopaedic cases. Jones preached the urgency of specialist care, patient segregation (even by type of fracture), rehabilitation, surgical training. He showed at the front how the immediate use of Thomas's bed knee splint for femoral fractures could reduce mortality from 80 per cent to 20 per cent. In 1916, the Hammersmith Workhouse at Shepherd's Bush in West London (later to become part of the British Postgraduate Medical School) became the South-East Military Orthopaedic Hospital with 800 beds; and similar institutes arose throughout the country, with, as Jones insisted, workshops for active rehabilitation rather than the passive motion machines favoured by the French and Italians. By the end of the war there were nine military hospitals with 30 000 beds, with continuity of treatment by the same surgeons throughout. After the war, with the help of Girdlestone, 26 centres continued in existence as civilian orthopaedic hospitals.

Jones emerges as a man of immense stature, inevitably Inspector of

Military Orthopaedics and an eventual Major-General, a man of great vision, energy and tact, always tact. The great general surgeons of the time, like Berkeley Moynihan, had the sense to acknowledge that this was an orthopaedic war and to give him their support. The younger men who worked with Jones at Shepherd's Bush and elsewhere were a band of brothers; as with the pupils of John Hunter, that work was a forcing-house for talent which came to dominate British orthopaedics for the next generation and after. We repeat some of the names given at several places elsewhere because they are so important: Blundell Bankart, Sidney Higgs, H A T Fairbank, St John Dudley Buxton, Naughton Dunn, McCrae Aitken, Harry Platt and others, many others – Americans, Canadians, Australians, New Zealanders, Egyptians.

Because there were not enough British orthopaedists, Jones turned to his American friends for help in 1917. There, Joel Goldthwait had already been quietly organizing for the inevitable for a year or two and had a list of young men, and sailed off with twenty of these to arrive in Liverpool on 28th May 1917. He returned in October with 42 more and 12 trained nurses. These men were initially assigned to Jones for work and training and then passed on to the American Expeditionary Force in France as needed, there to train the general surgeons actually treating the wounded for there were too few orthopaedists to do much of the work themselves. The pattern developed and some 400 US surgeons trained and worked under Jones. It was a very tangible manifestation of the 'special relationship' which was revived in World War II, which persists somewhat improbably and despite Europeanization even today, and which is perpetuated by the interchange of young orthopaedic surgeons as visiting Fellows between the USA, Canada and Great Britain. The American contingent of the first war was sometimes referred to as the 'Goldthwait unit', or the Division of Orthopaedic Surgery of the American Expeditionary Force.

We may add here, though it is not strictly pertinent, that the American base hospitals in France, where the policy was for immediate repatriation wherever possible, were enormous, up to 35 000 beds in some cases. Peltier tells us, for instance, that Winnett Orr was called up from a small orthopaedic practice in Nebraska, worked for a time at the military hospital in Cardiff and ended up in charge of 18 000 patients at Savenay in France.

In 1918, Robert Jones instigated the foundation of the British Orthopaedic Association, which proved as permanent as the earlier British Orthopaedic Society had been impermanent. He moved to London (an occupational hazard for famous Liverpudlians) to St Thomas's Hospital and died, full of years and honours, in 1933. He touched nothing that he did not adorn.

The Oswestry pattern spread over the country. There arose, for instance, the Chailey Heritage in Sussex in 1903, the Lord Mayor Treloar's Cripples' Hospital in Alton, Hampshire in 1908, a famous open-air institution directed by Sir Henry Gauvain, and many others. The partnership between philanthropic aristocrats and orthopaedic surgeons is exemplified by the joint work of Dame Georgina Buller and Norman Capener at Exeter, by the Duchess of Portland and S A S Malkin at Harlow Wood, Nottingham. Orthopaedic hospitals arose at Plymouth, Wrightington, Black Notley,

Birmingham, Bath. One of our very few women orthopaedic surgeons*, Maud Forrester-Brown (1885–1970) came to run an enormous service in the west of England for children with neglected tuberculosis, poliomyelitis, rickets and cerebral palsy, based on the Bath and Wessex Orthopaedic Hospital, founded in 1924.

All these developments took place at a time when orthopaedic specialists and nurses were very thin on the ground, and when tuberculosis, poliomyelitis and rickets were widespread. Often it meant starting from scratch and training ancillary staff at all levels. Later, after the mid-century, these diseases disappeared and the centres were able to turn to other fields, particularly chronic arthritis. Thus the Wrightington Hospital, originally a tuberculosis sanatorium, became Charnley's hip surgery centre.

Some of the benefactions were enormous. At Oxford, the Wingfield Hospital had been a hutted first war establishment and was used for orthopaedics afterwards by Girdlestone, Professor of Orthopaedic Surgery at Oxford. He was treating the then Sir William Morris, the car manufacturer millionaire, for backache and one day his patient asked him casually how much it would cost to rebuild the hospital. Girdlestone had the plans and costs ready later that day and the new building became the Wingfield-Morris Orthopaedic Hospital, later the Nuffield Orthopaedic Centre when Morris became a peer. Nuffield also gave very large sums to aid academic and clinical orthopaedics throughout the British Commonwealth.

In some areas, the orthopaedic services had an occupational basis, like those organized for miners in Nottinghamshire (associated later with E A Nicoll) and in Wales. Inevitably, a division tended to arise between the long-stay country hospitals, purely orthopaedic and dominated by skeletal tuberculosis (and, often, by their autocratic surgeon–superintendents) which sometimes, as in the case of the Royal National and others, came to acquire independent postgraduate academic status, and the urban orthopaedic centres, originally based on the teaching hospitals, to which specialist orthopaedic surgeons began to be appointed before and after World War I, and in which there were often ferocious running battles for beds and services with the general surgeons. Later still, after World War II, the National Health Service brought an orthopaedic department to every major district hospital. There is no doubt that, for a considerable time, the staffs of the sanatoria felt themselves the poor relations of their city colleagues with their private practices, but the former had some advantages. With time on their hands and an X-ray machine, they could make new observations, as Calvé had at Berck-Plage, while the teaching hospital stars remained ignorant of large areas of their speciality. But, inevitably, the two became intermingled.

Now we have to make some detailed references to Robert Jones's methods

---

* Another was Erna Henrietta Jebens (1900–64), an ambulance driver in World War I who was one of the first women to graduate at St. Mary's Hospital in London after the war. She taught anatomy at the Royal Free Hospital for 30 years and became orthopaedic surgeon to Battersea Hospital in the 1930s, the only woman, to my knowledge, then practising orthopaedics in London.

and publications. At an early stage he shared Thomas's aversion to plaster-of-Paris as 'barbarous', but this had to be recanted when it came to the postoperative fixation of corrected feet. He was also very conservative around the turn of the century: 'Never do an arthrodesis in a child under the age of ten, or a tendon transplant under four.' He preferred manual correction for talipes equinovarus to bone operations which left the foot painful, otherwise using a Thomas's wrench plus an Achilles tenotomy, with an occasional internal rotation osteoclasis of the tibia. However, he did operate when necessary and was doing astragalectomy and wedge tarsectomy even in 1900[108]. Club-foot was not cured until and unless the child could voluntarily assume overcorrection in valgus[109]. In 1908 he was doing fusion for paralytic calcaneo-cavus[110]. He made full use of general anaesthesia and the new X-rays for fracture reduction. Like Thomas, he was strenuously opposed to forcing stiff joints by passive motion[111].

He was an early and keen exponent of knee meniscectomy, done through small anteromedial or anterolateral incisions, and reported 100 cases in 1906[112,113]. However, his treatment of recurrent dislocation of the patella by coronal splitting of the lateral femoral condyle and forward wedging of the anterior portion was less successful[114]. Hip ankylosis in vicious position was treated, if unilateral, by a transtrochanteric abduction osteotomy; but in bilateral cases he tended to excisional pseudarthrosis or sheathing the femoral head in foil or film, and one case of bony ankylosis treated by interposition of gold foil in 1902 had good function 21 years later[115].

Jones was an early enthusiast for tendon transplantation and reported 253 cases at a meeting in France in 1908[116]. He did this to reinforce or replace weak or useless groups, to alter a line of pull, or to supplement a fusion. Maximum preoperative correction was essential, and the tendon was routed in a straight line and sutured to bone or periosteum. He often completed

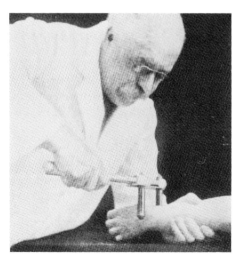

Figure 74 Robert Jones using Thomas's wrench to correct a malunited Colles fracture (*Orthopaedic Surgery of Injuries*, Oxford Medical Publications, 1921)

the operation by excision of an oval of skin on the dorsum of the foot on the weak side, and it is fascinating to see this very procedure illustrated in a Japanese text of 1837 in connection with the treatment of club-foot. The foot was held overcorrected in plaster. For paralytic calcaneus he moved the peronei to the Achilles tendon, and in congenital equinovarus the tibialis anterior was transferred laterally; in spastics the hamstrings were taken to the patella. It is interesting that, at this period, and untypically for him, he thought exercises and reeducation quite valueless for spasticity and employed tenotomy from the start, even in the mildest cases[117].

Another oddity is that he visited Calot at Berck in France and was impressed by the forcible correction of Pott's kyphosis under general anaesthesia and used the method for a time. Also in 1901, he described a case of 'multiple enchondromata' which is clearly one of congenital myositis ossificans; indeed, he thought it much like a myositis – it is a very early report[118].

In 1903, with A H Tubby, he wrote *Modern Methods in the Surgery of Paralysis* (Macmillan, London) and, during World War I, several instructional manuals. One of these was *Injuries of Joints*, reissued in 1922, one of the Oxford War Primer series for young army surgeons. In this book he stressed avoidance of passive movements in physiotherapy, but manipulated under anaesthesia, noting the importance of rotation at the knee. He had abandoned operation for Volkmann's contracture in favour of progressive stretching. All elbow fractures (except of the olecranon) were treated in full flexion to limit the space for callus or myositis at the front of the joint, and his test of recovery was Thomas's test, i.e. the ability to hold the joint in progressively increasing extension while retaining the power of full active flexion. He gives a good early description of myositis ossificans after elbow dislocation and excised displaced fractures of the head of the radius. He gives what is possibly the first account of the sabre-cut incision through the acromioclavicular joint and acromion for repair of supraspinatus rupture and/or exploration of the subdeltoid bursa, long before Codman made it popular later in the century. He disposes of the myth of the sprained wrist and fixed the responsible scaphoid fractures in dorsiflexion, removing any blocking fragment. In reducing Colles fractures he stressed the importance of pronation and used two tin gutter splints applied spirally to maintain this position.

He stressed the dangers of moving patients with neck fractures and reduced atlantoaxial displacements under general anaesthesia. He says, strangely, that 'fractures of the bodies of the dorsal vertebrae are practically unknown'; this was, of course, before the age of universal motoring. He gives a clear clinical account of slipped upper femoral epiphysis, which he attributed to injury, or a succession of injuries, and treated by reduction under anaesthesia and a hip spica plaster. Hip fractures were all treated in abduction frames, with no mention of operation. There should, he said, be no hesitation in operating for torn medial menisci if they imperilled the patient's livelihood, but 'the surgeon who operates upon a healthy knee-joint should be clean beyond reproach. He should have an antiseptic conscience. His finger should never enter the wound, however scrubbed or thickly gloved, as an infection would prove a tragedy.' He did not much favour operating on the cruciate ligaments, and operated for patellar fractures only in young adults, otherwise using a Thomas splint with the fragments crowded together as the inventor of that splint had taught him.

In 1917 there came *Notes on Military Orthopaedics* (London, Cassell) and in 1921 he edited *The Orthopaedic Surgery of Injuries* (London, Henry Frowde and Hodder and Stoughton), a two-volume work much of which he wrote himself, and which contains his famous preface stating that orthopaedic surgery is based on principles of treatment, whether operative or other, leading to restoration of function. In 1923 there appeared the *Orthopaedic Surgery* by Jones and R W Lovett, of Boston, which was really a continuation of the original wholly American text by Bradford and Lovett, the 1890 *Treatise of Orthopaedic Surgery* (New York, William Wood). This remained a standard text for English-speakers for many years and was valuable to the present writer in the 1940s. It was revised with Harry Platt's help. Lovett died while visiting Jones's home in Liverpool in connection with this work in 1924. The important and influential *Robert Jones Birthday Volume* of 1928, with its markedly European orientation, is reviewed at length elsewhere (p. 655).

Perhaps the longest lasting 'orphan' of orthopaedics was traumatology. Only a few general surgeons had been really interested in the treatment of fractures and other injuries; it had been regarded as a troublesome chore, often delegated to juniors, without much attention to function or rehabilitation. There were exceptions, like Harold Stiles at Edinburgh, who took a real interest. With the advent of the National Health Service, most gratefully abandoned this work to their new orthopaedic colleagues. The idea of segregated fracture clinics was originally seen as unnecessary and unwelcome, despite Robert Jones's experience with the Ship Canal, despite the first organized clinic of Harry Platt at Ancoats Hospital, Manchester, in 1913–14, even despite the experience of segregated treatment in World War I, whose lessons tended to be forgotten.

In the 1930s, however, stimulated by a British Medical Association investigation which reported in 1935, and based on the success of Platt's clinic and that of Watson-Jones at the Liverpool Royal Infirmary, government accepted that organized casualty services were required, and although this was overtaken by the war, the very experiences of that war reinforced the recommendation. In 1943, The Fracture and Accident Services Committee of the British Orthopaedic Association set out the case in detail. The effect has not been quite what might have been expected, nor what the originators had in mind. The regional orthopaedic centres do not deal with trauma, or only with some of its late results. The departments of the district urban hospitals deal with both elective orthopaedics and trauma, regarded as axiomatically desirable by some (but not by the present writer); and there are effectively only two specialized trauma centres, the Birmingham Accident Hospital and the Stoke Mandeville Centre for Spinal Injuries. After World War I, Robert Jones had urged the development of an accident centre in every major city, but this did not happen. The Birmingham centre is linked with William Gissane (1898–1981), an Australian, influenced by Böhler, who founded and directed it from 1841, always emphasizing prevention. He transformed a hundred year old hospital into a world-famous institution for injuries and burns, stimulated the requisite training and pathological and bacteriological services, and became Professor of Accident Surgery. His work related to occupational and environmental conditions, including road traffic, and stressed rehabilitation. Like Robert Jones, Gissane wanted to segregate trauma from orthopaedics as such, but this has not happened. Some have got very near, like L W Plewes with his accident service at the Luton and Dunstable Hospital, fed from an adjacent motorway and a local car factory. The Stoke Mandeville Hospital pioneered the modern treatment of spine and cord injuries during World War II and after, under the initial guidance of Sir Ludwig Guttmann; this work is described at p. 671.

Rehabilitation had been given immense impetus by Robert Jones in World War I. Later, it gained industrial connotations: with H E Moore at the Railway Rehabilitation Hospital at Crewe, with Sir Hugh Griffiths for dock workers in Greenwich in 1938, for miners in the hands of Miller in Glasgow and Nicoll in Mansfield, Nottinghamshire, and this spread to other industries and vocations. The outstanding work of Watson-Jones as orthopaedic adviser to the Royal Air Force in World War II included rehabilitation services that started in the ambulance and saw the patients back to their original duties wherever possible.

Government legislation from the beginning of the century has aided orthopaedics, whether by regulating working conditions and safety or through the National Insurance Act of 1911 which provided medical treatment for wage-earners. The school medical services checked children for orthopaedic disorders and other measures catered for skeletal tuberculosis, from inspection of milk to the provision of treatment facilities. Various workmen's compensation acts were not always as beneficial as planned, sometimes encouraging compensation neuroses; and, of course, litigation after injury or alleged orthopaedic negligence has grown enormously in recent years and has tended to create 'defensive' treatment, which is not in the best interests of the patient.

Academically, orthopaedic surgery became a recognized subject for under-graduate teaching early in the century, but not until 1937 did G R Girdlestone become the first occupant of a Chair, established at Oxford with the aid of Lord Nuffield, to be succeeded by Sir Herbert Seddon and then by Joseph Trueta. Such chairs are now widespread. Postgraduate training – the most important stage in an orthopaedic career – was originally, and still is to a great extent, by apprenticeship in an orthopaedic department, but there are a number of specialized postgraduate training centres, notably in Liverpool and London.

In Liverpool, T P McMurray, who continued to practise at 11 Nelson Street, home of Hugh Owen Thomas, after the departure of Robert Jones, established the diploma of MCh Orth (Master of Orthopaedic Surgery) in conjunction with Liverpool University, a first-class if still somewhat conserva-tive course which has left its mark in the North of England and on numerous trainees from overseas. Such is English clannishness, however, that it still attracts few from south of the Wash and is not often encountered in the affluent south-east. There is, in fact, more interchange, both orthopaedic and general, between Scotland and London than between the north and south of England.

If we may, at this stage, refer to some peculiarly British achievements that have advanced orthopaedic surgery, there is, of course, Listerian antisepsis and asepsis. Asepsis was rigorously applied by Arbuthnot Lane (p. 133) in his pioneering internal fixation of fractures, recognizing that ordinary standards of surgical cleanliness were quite inadequate when metal foreign bodies were implanted. Lane used a strict no-touch technique, with gloves and carefully sterilized instruments, all resterilized by boiling after each manoeuvre of an operation. Antiseptics were eschewed in favour of care to exclude infection; today the availability of antibiotics tends to reverse this.

Fleming's 'discovery' of penicillin (in quotes because of Lister's work on the penicillum mould at King's College Hospital before 1900), its application by Trueta and Agerholm to osteomyelitis at Oxford in 1946 after its victories in World War II, have transformed many fields of orthopaedic surgery, especially since the search for other antibiotics has been so successful, notably in combating skeletal tuberculosis.

The massive local resection of bone tumours and other lesions and their replacement by endoprostheses was initiated by Seddon, Jackson Burrows and Scales at the Royal National Orthopaedic Hospital (p. 605) before workers in other countries. The first knee replacement in England was devised and performed by Shiers in 1953, using an uncemented stainless steel hinge[119], while in 1954 Burrows and Scales used a hinged replacement for malignant disease and an essentially similar prosthesis is still in use at Stanmore 34 years later[120]. There is no need to rehearse the multiplicity of designs since, nor is there any need to stress the enormous contributions of Sir John Charnley to total hip replacement, partly because they are so well-known, partly because they are reviewed elsewhere. To take just one special field, osteotomy for osteoarthritis of the knee was pioneered in England, before anywhere else, by William Waugh, now Emeritus Professor of Orthopaedic Surgery at Nottingham University. Waugh points out[121] that debridement of the Magnuson type or occasional denervation were the only surgical measures for this condition until the late 1950s. Then Kenneth Pridie, of Bristol, began drilling the eburnated bone and showed that this was followed by fibrocartilaginous repair[122]. Though this work was interrupted by his premature death, Pridie had recognized the importance of malalignment and did a tibial osteotomy in three of his six cases. The only other operation of any use before 1950, before the arrival of osteotomy or joint replacement, was arthrodesis, preferably with compression as popularized by Charnley[123], which in its turn was based on Key's work in the USA in the 1930s[124]. (The present writer was taught by Paul Jenner Verrall at the Royal Free Hospital in London in 1938 to transfix the bone ends and jam them together on a Thomas splint, a method he had used during World War I.)

Supracondylar femoral or upper tibial osteotomy for angulation was far from new; but its first deliberate use for arthrosis was by Jackson and Waugh at Harlow Wood Hospital at Nottingham in 1961[125,126]. Initially, this was just below the tuberosity: Wardle in Liverpool had divided the tibia at a much lower level for some time[127]. The original aim was simply to correct obvious malalignment; but it was then realized that the bone section itself seemed to relieve pain and stimulate cartilage repair, possibly by changes in the intraosseous circulation, that it was best done for unicameral disease, preferably medial, and above the tuberosity. The operation has been well developed by Mark Coventry at the Mayo Clinic; it is an excellent procedure, notably because it does not prejudice subsequent replacement operations.

Writing in 1950, Osmond-Clarke[128] stressed the conservatism of the old British tradition, now so much less marked that the proper application of a Thomas splint or Robert Jones bandage is unknown to many. Manipulation, too, is now much less used than formerly, and not at all by some surgeons, and this is sad because, for the right indications, it is invaluable. Osmond-Clarke called idiopathic scoliosis 'a challenging mystery', it still is. In the early part of the century, McCrae Aitken did valuable work of a nonoperative nature for spinal curvatures. If we have got rid of tuberculosis and poliomyelitis, it is not through the effort of orthopaedic surgeons; they are still there in the Third World, but in Britain the once frequent tendon transplants are now done only for nerve injuries and spasticity.

John Charnley's *The Closed Treatment of Common Fractures* of 1950 shows what can be done with simple measures, scrupulously observed, yet there is an ever-accelerating trend to operation, especially since the arrival of AO osteosynthesis. Medullary nailing, as we have seen, was used by Hey Groves in 1916, and then lapsed until B H Burns and R H Young of St George's Hospital popularized Küntscher nailing after World War II. The publication of Watson-Jones's *Fractures and Joint Injuries* in 1940 ended the prewar dependence on the works of Böhler and Lorenz and give a bible to English-speakers (and many others) round the world. It had its faults; it was possibly over-dogmatic; but it settled for nothing but the best and showed exactly how to achieve this. Anyone who had the good fortune to attend Watson-Jones's wartime lecture course on fractures at Hammersmith left totally enthused. He introduced clarity and certainty, and this is essential to surgeons in training, at least until they discover that clarity is not enough and that certainty does not exist.

Just as European countries remained in the dark ages as far as orthopaedics was concerned during the second war and borrowed avidly from Britain after 1945, so the British, though luckier, found themselves adopting American techniques in the postwar years, particularly in the context of disc surgery, limb equalization and the use of the newer metals and prostheses.

We can note only briefly some of the accomplishments of the first half of the century: Elmslie's work on the skeletal dystrophies, Watson-Jones's procedure for persistent ankle instability, the Bankart operation for recurrent dislocation of the shoulder, among others. H A Brittain, of Norwich, developed the architectural principles of arthrodesis by methods of extra-articular fusion, which were later outmoded by the disappearance of the disease which had called them into being. When spinal tuberculosis with paraplegia was common, Norman Capener of Exeter developed anterolateral decompression of the cord, or lateral rachotomy, though this cannot be said to have been altogether original. The Keller operation for hallux valgus described in New York in 1904[129] had, in fact, been anticipated by Davies-Colley (for hallux flexus) in 1887[130].

In Oxford, at the Wingfield-Morris Orthopaedic Hospital, Girdlestone exquisitely laid down the principles of the treatment of bone and joint tuberculosis before, during and after World War II, and of other fields besides; to work with him was a privilege and an inspiration. Hand surgery required some American stimulation and is referred to in connection with Guy Pulvertaft (p. 163). Elmslie and Platt did valuable work on bone tumours, as did Sir Stanford Cade at the Westminster Hospital in London. It is not commonly recognized that Philip Wiles (see p. 599) was doing all-metal total hip replacement at the Middlesex Hospital in the 1930s, or that Lambrinudi of Guy's Hospital was using intramedullary fixation of forearm fractures in 1940–41. The hindquarter amputation was developed, or at least popularized, by Sir Gordon Gordon-Taylor, also at the Middlesex Hospital, before the war.

The prenatal diagnosis of neural tube defects was made possible by D J H Brock and colleagues at Edinburgh by their testing for alphafetoprotein in the amniotic fluid and maternal blood, so that early antenatal screening could permit termination. The enzyme phosphatase was discovered by Robinson and Kay and work on vitamins by Mellanby and others led to the virtual disappearance of deficiency diseases (though rickets and pregnancy osteomalacia have re-emerged in dark-skinned immigrants in recent years). There are also the immense contributions of nonmedical scientists, notably computerized tomography by G N Houndsfield and of magnetic resonance imaging by J Mullard and G N Holland independently.

SOME PERSONALITIES

We have already discussed **W J Little** at length, and it only remains to add that, in his 1855 Lectures on the *Deformities of the Human Frame*, he described two brothers with pseudohypertrophic muscular dystrophy but did not name it (Duchenne did so 13 years later), and that in 1878 he visited Canada and the United States, where he met Detmold, Stromeyer's pupil, in New York, who introduced subcutaneous tenotomy into the USA. Little did three things: he introduced subcutaneous tenotomy into England; he wrote the first major English book on orthopaedic surgery; and he established the first English orthopaedic hospital.

His sons, **Louis Stromeyer Little** and **Ernest Muirhead Little**, are discussed on pp. 127–8. **A H Tubby** (1863–1930) was on the staff of the National Orthopaedic and the Westminster Hospitals and, next to Robert Jones, was the outstanding genius of his day in British orthopaedics. We have mentioned his literary collaboration with Robert Jones, but the standard British work of the early century was Tubby's *Deformities: a Treatise on Orthopaedic Surgery* of 1896. The first edition did not deal with skeletal tuberculosis (because this was the province of the general surgeon), but the second edition of 1912 did, and was rewritten and retitled as *Deformities, including Diseases of the Bones and Joints, a Textbook of Orthopaedic Surgery* in two volumes, with the still novel 'Roentgen-ray illustrations'. Tubby was a cultured man with a busy practice and took little interest in orthopaedic politics.

T H ('Tommy') Openshaw (1856–1929) was the first surgeon in charge of an orthopaedic department at the London Hospital and also served the Royal National, a great character but uninterested in administration. **E Laming Evans** (1871–1945) was for many years on the staff of the Royal National – a tall, gentlemanly, irascible figure, interested mainly in congenital dislocation of the hip and astragalectomy (see p. 503).

R C Elmslie (1878–1940) was a student and then surgeon to St Bartholomew's Hospital, interrupted in World War I when he was in charge of the Military Orthopaedic Hospital at Shepherd's Bush. He was a founder member of the British Orthopaedic Association and its president in 1930. He had to struggle to get his department at St Bartholomew's properly staffed and bedded, and even in 1928, 16 years after his appointment, he still had only five male and five female beds. Elmslie was of scholarly bent, a good operator and committee-man (not a usual combination), devoted to the organization of cripple care. His classical work was on fibrocystic disease of bone[131], but his total of publications exceeds 200.

W H Trethowan (1882–1934) was the first orthopaedic surgeon at Guy's Hospital in 1912, one of Robert Jones' team at Shepherd's Bush in World War I, then at the Royal National and Queen Mary's Hospital for Children at Carshalton. He was an inspiring teacher who wrote little, concentrated on function and operated like an angel, never ligating a vessel, and was an expert bone-grafter.

Constantine Lambrinudi (1890–1943) was Trethowan's junior at Guy's and died tragically early, but not before producing lasting procedures: interphalangeal fusion for clawed toes and pes cavus, the famous drop-foot operation[132], and the intramedullary fixation of forearm fractures with Kirschner wires.

Naughton Dunn (1884–1939) was Robert Jones' house surgeon at Liverpool and his private assistant until Jones steered him into a post at the Birmingham Cripples' Union, later the Royal Orthopaedic Hospital in 1913. He worked with Jones again in the first world war and at Oswestry afterwards. His main contribution consisted of his fusion operations for paralytic deformities of the feet.

Walter Rowley Bristow (1883–1947), a graduate of St Thomas's Hospital in London in 1907, took up orthopaedics after appointment to Shepherd's Bush under Robert Jones on being invalided from Gallipoli. After the first world war, St Thomas's acquired an orthopaedic department with Robert Jones as its head and Bristow as his assistant, but Jones' position was rather nominal and Bristow was the director in practice, aided by George Perkins. Bristow was particularly interested in peripheral nerve injuries[133] and was to revive this interest as a member of the Medical Research Council Committee in this field when he became brigadier and consultant to the British Army in World War II, as Jones had been in the earlier war. St Thomas's acquired a longstay country branch at Pyrford in Surrey, now known as the Rowley Bristow Orthopaedic Hospital. Bristow attracted many later famous pupils: E P Brockman, George Perkins, R J Furlong. He used to say: 'We treat patients not diseases.'

Thomas Porter McMurray (1888–1949) was an Ulsterman, a 1910 graduate at Queens University, Belfast, who became Robert Jones' house surgeon and private assistant at 11 Nelson Street and worked there with him until Jones left for London. In the first war he worked at the Alder Hey military hospital near Liverpool, a disciple and advocate of Hugh Owen Thomas and Jones, training English, Canadian and American surgeons. After Jones's death in 1933, McMurray was largely responsible for the establishment of orthopaedic surgery as an academic discipline in Liverpool, became professor of orthopaedics in 1938, the second in Britain after Girdlestone at Oxford, and started the MCh Orth diploma course, which influenced orthopaedic surgery throughout the Commonwealth. He remains best known for his displacement osteotomy for ununited fractures of the femoral neck and arthrosis of the hip, and for his famous sign of a torn knee meniscus[134]. His operative dexterity was legendary; he could disarticulate a hip in ten minutes. He also wrote a textbook, not now sufficiently read, which contains the essence of the Liverpool school of thought in orthopaedic surgery.

Sir Harry Platt (1886–1986), a great father-figure in British orthopaedics, a centenarian, one of Robert Jones' last pupils, who received some postgraduate orthopaedic training at the Massachusetts General Hospital before World War I, greatly contributed to raising orthopaedic surgery in Britain from a small and struggling speciality to a level where every general hospital now has its own orthopaedic surgeon, an orthopaedic department and a fracture clinic. Like quite a few orthopaedists, he was himself handicapped, by an ankylosed knee due to childhood osteomyelitis treated by Robert Jones. His year in Boston, at the instigation of Robert Jones and the invitation of Brackett, then chief of orthopaedic surgery, exposed him to the influence of Lovett, Bradford and Goldthwait. He started the first fracture clinic in Britain at Ancoats Hospital, Manchester, in 1913–14, and served as surgeon-in-charge of a Manchester military orthopaedic hospital in World War I, where he was assigned some American surgeons, notably Osgood. It was really the combination of Robert Jones, Platt and Osgood that led to the foundation of the British Orthopaedic Association. Although an orthopaedic surgeon in Manchester and Oswestry, he had no department at the Manchester Royal Infirmary until 1932, to which he moved with Osmond-Clarke as his junior in 1934 to set up an orthopaedic division and, in 1939, to occupy the first Chair in Orthopaedic Surgery in the country after Girdlestone's endowed Chair at Oxford.

Platt was a great traveller and orthopaedic internationalist, a founder-member and sometime president of both the British Orthopaedic Association and of SICOT, first chairman of the editorial board of the British Volume of the *Journal of Bone and Joint Surgery*. He was a great planner of services and encouraged his pupil, John Charnley, in his work on hip replacement, Many of his other trainees achieved eminence – David Lloyd-Griffiths, Roland Barnes and others.

In World War II he was adviser to government on orthopaedic services and collaborated with Philip Wilson of New York to send over young American orthopaedists to staff the American Hospital in Britain. He was

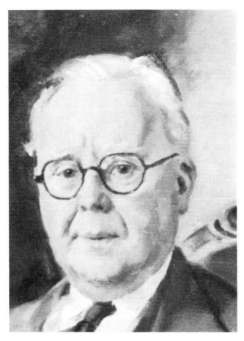

Figure 75   Fourth President of SICOT (1951–1954), Sir Harry Platt

knighted in 1948 and President of the Royal College of Surgeons of England in 1954–7, the first orthopaedic surgeon to be so. He helped found the International Federation of Surgical Colleges and was its first president.

Platt created the first fracture clinic in Britain, possibly in Europe, at a time when orthopaedics was being taught, if at all, by general surgeons resisting this upstart speciality. As David Lloyd Griffiths says[135], its present independence in the UK is owed to him as much as anyone. His help in planning fostered the enormous expansion of services in the National Health

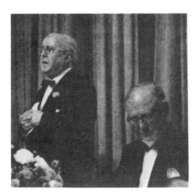

Figure 76   Sir Harry Platt (standing) and Sir Henry Osmond-Clarke (1966)

Service after its inception in 1948, and he nurtured the academic as well as the practical side. He always insisted on the importance of follow-up and hated to discharge a patient. A competent if not a brilliant operator, he was irritable in the theatre, where he literally used to kick the bucket until his nurse filled it with plaster!

Sir Walter ('Watty') Mercer (1890–1971), of Edinburgh, was a charismatic figure, a most remarkable general surgeon and an equally remarkable orthopaedic surgeon, in this way resembling his fellows at Edinburgh, Harold Stiles and John Fraser. He was a surgeon in the British Army in both world wars, and his famous textbook of orthopaedics of 1952 is still going strong under the editorship of Duthie at Oxford. He became Regius Professor of Surgery at the Edinburgh Royal Infirmary and took over all orthopaedic and fracture work after World War I, but retained his wider interests and introduced cardiac surgery in 1946. All his early orthopaedic work was done in the general wards. Thus he pioneered anterior fusion for spondylolisthesis 20 years ahead of others (but gave it up because of mesenteric thrombosis and ileus), did hip arthroplasties and Smith–Petersen pinning, all at the same time that he was developing pulmonary and gastro-oesophageal surgery. In 1948 he was offered a special chair in orthopaedic surgery to establish and direct orthopaedic training and practice in south-east Scotland, and though this meant a great step down in power and prestige he accepted the challenge and produced brilliant young men like Ian Lawson Dick and Ewen Jack. His speed and dexterity as an operator were formidable. He was chairman of the editorial board of the British Volume of the *Journal of Bone and Joint Surgery* for seven years.

Gathorne Robert Girdlestone (1881–1950) went from Oxford to graduate at St Thomas's and, after first going to Shropshire as a general practitioner surgeon, worked at Oswestry under Robert Jones. This shaped his career and gave him the mission of going out from the centre to find those needing treatment, to arrest or prevent crippling disease. He became the apostle of the regional practice of orthopaedic surgery, with a central hospital and peripheral clinics. In World War I he was placed in charge of an Oxford military hospital with 400 beds, which had attached the Wingfield Convalescent Home in the then village of Headington nearby. Robert Jones arranged for Girdlestone to use some army huts in its grounds, and in 1919 this became the Wingfield Hospital under the Ministry of Pensions, with one ward for crippled children. In 1922 the hospital was transferred to a local Wingfield Committee. When Jones and Girdlestone launched the Central Council for the Care of Cripples after that war, Girdlestone was its honorary secretary. He ran his region – Oxfordshire, Berkshire, Buckinghamshire – by being appointed to most of the general hospitals in the region and establishing satellite clinics run by permanent integrated Wingfield staff, as at Oswestry. Here he was well assisted by W B Foley and J C Scott (q.v.)

Girdlestone was a marvellous operating surgeon, despite the loss of an index finger infected from a patient, and devised procedures for Pott's paraplegia, hallux valgus, arthrosis of the hip (the famous pseudarthrosis salvage procedure by excision of the femoral head and neck, still a by no means negligible last resort for many problems), flexor/extensor tendon transfer for clawed toes. In 1930 Sir William Morris, later Lord Nuffield, rebuilt the hospital and in 1937 endowed a Chair in Orthopaedic Surgery at Oxford, the first such in Britain, for Girdlestone. Girdlestone visited South Africa and elsewhere to plan orthopaedic services which Nuffield financed. In 1939 he resigned his chair to devote himself to war work as governmental adviser, planned orthopaedic services in the new National Health Service after the war, and in 1949 integrated the work in the Oxford region in the Nuffield Orthopaedic Centre, the totally refurbished Wingfield-Morris Hospital, the crown of his career.

Girdlestone was worshipped in his hospital and established an esprit de corps which is still very evident. He was a devout Christian and managed to combine humility with an intense belief in his mission that was sometimes alienating. Many contributions, to organizations and individuals, came from his own pocket. He was largely responsible for creation of the American-staffed orthopaedic Churchill Hospital at Oxford in World War II.

Walter Barham Foley (1889–1979) was a 1912 St Thomas's graduate who worked under Bristow after service in World War I and then, in 1927, moved to Oxford as assistant to Girdlestone and was also appointed at the Radcliffe Infirmary and at hospitals at Aylesbury and Windsor. He was in total contrast to Girdlestone – quiet, unassuming, almost dry as dust – yet they had 25 years of harmonious collaboration. He fostered the peripheral clinics and did the bulk of his work there. He pioneered cervical osteotomy for slipped femoral epiphysis and perfected ischiofemoral fusion.

James Christopher Scott (1908–1978), a Canadian and Toronto graduate of 1932, influenced by W E Gallie and R I Harris, went to Oxford in 1934 to work under Girdlestone and Foley and served in the Royal Air Force in World War II. He initiated the accident service at the Radcliffe Infirmary and in 1948 succeeded Girdlestone as director of the Nuffield Orthopaedic Centre and fulfilled academic duties in the University. An excellent committee man and organizer, he was also one of the earliest users of penicillin and introduced the excision of slough and primary suture for hand infections under penicillin cover.

Sir Herbert Seddon (1903–1977) had an immense influence on orthopaedic surgery in Britain and the world. A St Bartholomew's graduate of 1928, he spent some time in 1930 as surgical instructor at Ann Arbor, Michigan, and was appointed Resident Surgeon at the new Stanmore country branch of the Royal National Orthopaedic Hospital near London at a time when poliomyelitis and skeletal tuberculosis were the main longstay problems. He did fundamental work on Pott's paraplegia, distinguishing the early and late varieties and showing that it was not due to the mechanical effects of the kyphosis. Apart from his prize essay with Weeden Butler on the subject before the second war, in 1956 he collaborated in a book, *Pott's Paraplegia*, with Robert Roaf and David Lloyd-Griffiths. In 1940, at the age of 37, he succeeded Girdlestone as Nuffield Professor of Orthopaedic Surgery at Oxford. There, during the war, he developed the peripheral nerve injury unit which has contributed more to this field than any department before or since, developing methods of classification, muscle charting and operative technique which gave clarity to a confusing picture. The work is summed

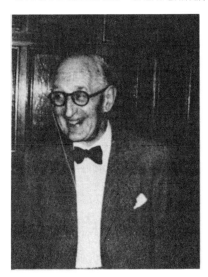

Figure 77 Sir Herbert Seddon (1903–1972)

up in his *Surgical Disorders of the Peripheral Nerves* of 1971.

In 1948 he returned to the Royal National in London as director of its new Institute of Orthopaedics, of which he was the main architect, and made it a great centre for visitors and trainees from all over the world. He became professor there in 1965 and retired in 1967. An academic, scientific surgeon, he gave valuable service to the Medical Research Council, planned the care of poliomyelitis epidemics in Malta, Mauritius and Africa, and (with others) organized a world trial to compare surgery with drug therapy for spinal tuberculosis. He was a man of great moral courage and intellectual honesty, even if, like Gladstone, when found to have an ace up his sleeve, he gave the impression that God had put it there.

A S Blundell Bankart (1879–1951), a Guy's Hospital graduate of 1906, was influenced there by Arbuthnot Lane, and in 1909 became the first registrar at the Royal National Orthopaedic Hospital soon after its formation by amalgamation of the three separate institutions discussed at p. 129. There he operated at a furious rate, especially in the summer holidays when his chiefs were away, and to the end of his career enjoyed an eight-hour session. In 1911 he became assistant surgeon and was also appointed to the Maida Vale Hospital for Nervous Diseases and to various children's hospitals, combining paediatric, orthopaedic and neurosurgery. Like so many others, he was at Shepherd's Bush in the first war under Jones. Even after his appointment in 1920 as the first ever orthopaedic surgeon at the Middlesex Hospital, he continued with neurosurgery at Maida Vale until World War II, in the spinal rather than the cranial field, and was one of the first to perform lateral cordotomy for pain. At the Middlesex he had an uphill struggle against the general surgeons (how often one has to write that phrase, how much the present writer himself so suffered!) and for long had only one weekly outpatient clinic and three male and three female beds and a few children's beds. He had no orthopaedic wards until 1935 and no real fracture service until after the second world war. In 1923 he described the Bankart lesion in recurrent dislocation of the shoulder and his operation for it. There were no bounds to his intrepidity: he sometimes excised the whole of a tuberculous hip, femoral head, acetabulum, capsule and all; he transplanted the upper fibular shaft and epiphysis to replace the femoral head and neck lost in infantile suppurative arthritis, and it survived and grew and adapted itself to the acetabulum[136]. He was the first secretary of the new orthopaedic section of the Royal Society of Medicine in the 1930s, a founder-member of SICOT and the British Orthopaedic Association. Always open to new ideas, he studied the work of the osteopaths and put manipulation on the map in his *Manipulative Surgery* of 1932. He was an intensely shy man, often misinterpreted as arrogant, intolerant of fools.

His successor at the Middlesex, **Philip Wiles** (1899–1967) made the transition from business to medicine and wrote a famous textbook which ran to four editions between 1949 and 1965. Wiles was an audacious surgeon and excised congenital hemivertebrae for congenital scoliosis and, well before World War II, devised an all-metal total hip replacement which had considerable success. His business acumen as treasurer was vital in the infant fortunes of the British Volume of the *Journal of Bone and Joint Surgery*.

Sydney Limbrey Higgs (1892–1977), a St Bartholomew's graduate of 1917, saw naval service in World War I. He became assistant to Elmslie at his parent hospital in 1930 and succeeded him as director of orthopaedics in 1937. He was also on the staffs of the Royal National and Queen Mary's Hospital for amputees at Roehampton, and carried forward the Robert Jones/Elmslie project of converting the Chailey Heritage home for crippled children in Sussex into an active hospital. He shouldered heavy civilian responsibilities in World War II, wrote little, devised a useful peg-and-socket operation for hammer-toe and early recognized the value of the cancellous bone-graft.

George Perkins (1892–1979) was a striking figure. A St Thomas's man, one of the Shepherd's Bush group under Robert Jones, he became assistant to Bristow in the new orthopaedic department at Thomas's after World War I, succeeded Bristow as chief in 1946 and was made professor (of general surgery) in 1948. Perkins *thought* about fracture treatment. He had little or no use for plaster or other immobilization and managed his femoral fractures by traction only without even a Thomas splint; if internal fixation was to be used, it had to be so efficient that no other immobilization was tolerated. He wrote a very short but absolutely masterly textbook of fracture treatment with more commonsense to the line than anyone else has ever achieved. One of the good things about Perkins is that he trained **Alan Graham Apley**, a well known figure and teacher at Pyrford to the present day and author of a textbook far more widely known than that of Perkins.

St John Dudley Buxton (1891–1981), another Shepherd's Bush acolyte, became a consultant at King's College Hospital, London in 1922 (as a general surgeon) and succeeded Fairbank (q.v.) as head of orthopaedics in 1936. He was also at Roehampton and Chailey and was consultant to the Army in France and the Middle East in World War II.

Sir Harold Arthur Thomas Fairbank (1876–1961), a Charing Cross Hospital graduate and civil surgeon in the Boer War, shared with Robert Jones the pioneering work of establishing orthopaedic surgery in the 1920s. He became consultant to King's College Hospital, where he built the first London fracture clinic, and also joined the Great Ormond Street Hospital for Sick Children and the Treloar Hospital in Hampshire. A modest, sincere, courteous man, he acquired the greatest second opinion practice ever known. At Great Ormond Street he worked on congenital dislocation of the hip, and he also produced his epochal *Atlas of General Affections of the Skeleton.* In World War II he was director of orthopaedics for the civilian Emergency Medical Service. He was a founder member of the British Orthopaedic Association and of SICOT, and the first external examiner for the MCh Orth (in which he examined the young Reginald Watson-Jones as one of the first three candidates).

Sir Reginald Watson-Jones (1902–1972), a world-famous figure, was a Liverpool graduate of 1924 and appointed by Robert Jones as assistant surgeon in charge of the new orthopaedic and fracture department at the Liverpool Royal Infirmary in 1926, the year he gained his MCh Orth diploma. In 1928 he was appointed to the Country Orthopaedic Hospital at Gobowen, later known as the Robert Jones and Agnes Hunt Orthopaedic Hospital, and pioneered the peripheral clinics. In 1936 he began an instructional course on fractures at the Infirmary. His *Fractures and Joint Injuries* of 1940 has already been referred to and was published and translated the world over. His position in World War II as civilian consultant to the Royal Air Force was equivalent to that of Robert Jones with the Army in the first war, inspiring and training young surgeons and always stressing rehabilitation. He had ten orthopaedic units of 100–150 beds each, with teams of surgeons, ancillary staff and rehabilitation orderlies, and 77 per cent of injured air-crew resumed full duties.

After the war he became director of the orthopaedic and accident department at the London Hospital with the aid of Osmond-Clarke. His close link with the Americans led him to be the driving force in establishing the British Volume of the *Journal of Bone and Joint Surgery*, which he edited until his death. He was knighted in 1945 and was Sir Arthur Sims Commonwealth Travelling Professor in 1950. Watson-Jones is too tremendous a figure, and still too close to us, to be properly appraised in the historical context. In the treatment of fractures – orthopaedics was less his forte – he was driven by the pursuit of an ideal to which he sacrificed everything, even – but not for long and not for anything but the best of motives – the truth. He had exactly the right personality to do what needed to be done in Britain at war. It is doubtful whether anyone else could have succeeded as he did. He was the right man in the right place.

The name of Jones crops up frequently in this history. **Arthur Rocyn Jones** (1883–1972), who originated from a family of Welsh bonesetters, became the grand old man of British orthopaedics and its best historian. A graduate of University College, London, he was the resident at Cardiff to Sir John Lynn-Thomas (1861–1939), a pioneer in bone surgery. He was attached to the Royal National Orthopaedic Hospital from its earliest days as a house-

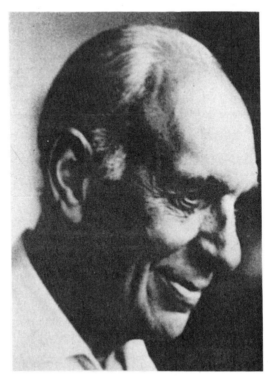

Figure 78 Sir Reginald Watson-Jones (1902–1972) who, among many other accomplishments, was the founder and editor of the British volume of the *Journal of Bone and Joint Surgery*

surgeon in 1913 to end as a consultant and a founder member of the British Orthopaedic Association in 1918. He was much loved, by no means a universal feature of orthopaedic surgeons. He was on the staffs of numerous hospitals in London, East Anglia and South Wales.

Norman Leslie Capener (1898–1975) was initially an anatomist and then chief assistant to the surgical professorial unit at St Bartholomew's from 1924. From 1926 to 1931 he was assistant professor of surgery at Ann Arbor, Michigan, and then settled in as orthopaedic surgeon at Exeter in Devon, where the Devon Association for Cripples' Aid had been founded in 1925 under the influence of Dame Georgina Butler and Robert Jones. The Princess Elizabeth Orthopaedic Hospital was opened in Exeter in 1927 and in 1931 Capener was appointed orthopaedic surgeon, the first such in Devon, where he then created a comprehensive service with peripheral clinics and aftercare services for the whole county, with workshops and a training college, the Oswestry and Oxford pattern all over again. He was president of the British Orthopaedic Association in 1958–9 and did much committee work, such as chairing the British Standards Committee on Surgical Implants from 1956 to 1970. He was a man of parts, a polymath, a great trainer of juniors, the

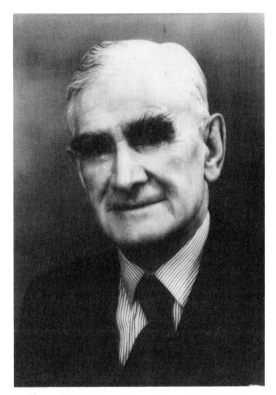

Figure 79 Arthur Rocyn Jones (1883–1972)

developer of anterolateral decompression for Pott's paraplegia and of 'lively' splints for the wrist and hand. It was Capener who initiated the organization of orthopaedic services in Northern Ireland in the 1940s and stimulated the building of the Withers Orthopaedic Centre at Musgrave Park in Belfast.

Harold Jackson Burrows (1902–1981) was assistant to Elmslie and Elmslie's successor, Higgs, at St Bartholomew's Hospital and took over from Higgs in 1952. He was also on the staff of the Royal National from 1946, becoming Dean of the new Institute of Orthopaedics there for 21 years, and he also attended the National Hospital for Nervous Diseases. In 1948 he began a period of many years on the editorial board of the British Volume of the *Journal of Bone and Joint Surgery*. Burrows was a kind and gentle man. He was adviser to the Ministry of Health on artificial limbs, and is well-known for his work with Scales and Seddon at the Royal National on bioengineering and the massive prosthetic replacement of large bone defects (see p. 604). He was a naval orthopaedic surgeon in World War II and had interests in Australia and New Zealand.

Joseph Trueta (1897–1977). If we treat of this man here, it is not to detract from his position as a Spaniard – or, as he would have insisted, a Catalan – but because fate ensured that much of his career evolved in England. He was born in Barcelona, and in 1935, aged 38, became chief surgeon and professor of surgery at the largest Catalan teaching hospital, that of the *Santa Crus i Sant Pau*. He was at once involved in the treatment of casualties of the Civil War, including the first air-raid victims of modern times, and in these circumstances evolved the closed plaster treatment (see p. 661). He escaped to England in 1939, was invited to Oxford by Girdlestone, succeeded Seddon as professor of orthopaedic surgery there in 1949, and remained in the Chair for twenty years.

He reorganized the Nuffield Orthopaedic Centre as one of excellence and of world research in many fields other than those of strict orthopaedics. Thus, he worked with Barnes on the crush syndrome and its relation to renal cortical ischaemia. Always, like Hunter, he stressed the essential role of the circulation in bone disease, and showed that the femoral head was hypervascular rather than hypovascular in osteoarthritis of the hip. He showed that long bone growth was stimulated by occlusion of the medullary and/or metaphyseal vessels (see also Le Vay 1967[137]). He was one of the very first to treat osteomyelitis with penicillin, yet recognized that surgical decompression remained essential if response was inadequate. He established a service for the orthopaedic manifestations of haemophilia, still flourishing under Professor Duthie. He also laid the basis for an orthopaedic service in the Sudan. In his work on war wounds he emphasized drainage, excision of muscle rather than skin, and immobilization in an unwindowed skin-tight plaster cast. This was far from original, but that is not the point: he made it standard practice in the British Army and saved countless lives. He was

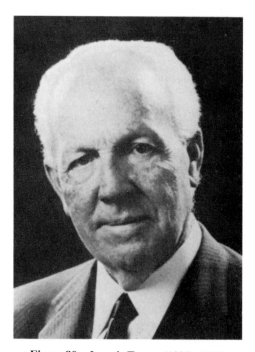

Figure 80   Joseph Trueta (1897–1977)

awarded many national and international honours and retired to Catalonia in 1966.

Trueta was a figure of a type familiar in European surgery but not on the British scene – that of the Great Man – but without the arrogance sometimes seen in France, Italy or Germany. He earns the present writer's respect, not only from personal acquaintance, but because of his respect for natural process, as when he wrote of 'the changing attitude ... from a carpentry approach to orthopaedics to a growing interest in the study and reactions of the living tissues which constitute the skeleton.'

The story of **Sidney Alan Stormer Malkin** (1899–1964) and the orthopaedic service at Nottingham is worth telling in some detail – and has been excellently told by William Waugh, Emeritus Professor at Nottingham University – because it so well illustrates how such services developed in England[138].

It was not that there had been no orthopaedic work in Nottingham earlier, but this had been done at the General Hospital founded in 1781, a Middlemarch type of institution, as part of the work of the general surgeons. The 1868 report refers to numerous amputations, the reduction of dislocated hips and an 'excision of the os calcis'. There were also very many industrial

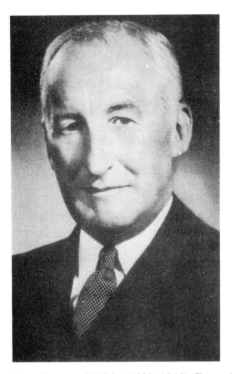

Figure 81   Sidney Alan Stormer Malkin (1899–1964). From *The Development of Orthopaedics in the Nottingham Area*, by Professor W Waugh, published with kind permission from the author

accidents. The Nottingham Cripples' Guild had been formed in 1907 on a private philanthropic basis and was presided over by the Duchess of Portland till 1954. After the first war, Robert Jones with Girdlestone set up a national scheme for crippled children, the Duchess asked his advice, and his recommendations for open-air country hospitals, hospital schools and aftercare clinics were essentially the same as those set out by Girdlestone. 'Whoever be the surgeon appointed, he should be given a free hand to develop his speciality and should have the full responsibility of directing the aftercare treatment. Unless the surgeon appointed to the Cripples' Guild has access to hospital beds, the scheme as outlined cannot be worked.'

This last proviso was – and sometimes still is – important, because it has been notoriously difficult in Britain for orthopaedic surgeons to obtain an adequate bed quota until quite recent years. And yet, Robert Jones was reluctant to abandon the link with the general surgeons that had proved useful during the War – with Moynihan in Leeds, Stiles in Edinburgh, Mayo Robson in Reading; it was as if a growing child were uneasy about letting go of the parental hand.

Malkin, a University College Hospital graduate and one of the wartime Shepherd's Bush coterie, was appointed in 1923 and rapidly ran into the usual difficulties because 'the proper facilities were lacking.' Here again, a driving woman proved invaluable, in this case the formidable nurse–physiotherapist Margaret Wright, whom Malkin very prudently incorporated by marriage. A clinic was built and, in 1929, Harlow Wood Hospital, mainly by private subscription, and Malkin was responsible for fund-raising and administration as well as the actual treatment. The first annual report says: 'The entire voluntary services that have been rendered to the scheme by Mr Malkin... have been invaluable, and indeed may be said to have made the Hospital possible.' Robert Jones helped by acting as visiting consultant. Patients were mainly longstay cases of skeletal tuberculosis and poliomyelitis; but it is worth noting that Malkin was doing osteotomy for osteoarthritis of the hip at least a year before McMurray published his work. Most patients were managed on frames, rather than plaster. Harlow Wood became the centre of a group of peripheral clinics serving the whole of Nottinghamshire and beyond, as far as Chesterfield in Derbyshire. Nottingham is a mining area, and this had repercussions on the work (see below).

All that had been built up by private effort seemed under threat when the National Health Service was established in 1948. Indeed, administrators had an antipathy to special hospitals of any kind and only the strongest of the orthopaedic hospitals managed to avoid closure. Furthermore, official policy veered in quite different directions from year to year (and still does). Harlow Wood has so far managed to survive. After Malkin's retirement in 1957, the work was carried on by Waugh, who gained a university chair, James Campbell and Peter Jackson, Waugh and Jackson developing osteotomy for arthrosis of the knee as described at p. 147, and there was an association with Pulvertaft at Derby and Nicoll at Mansfield (q.v.). It need hardly be said that education, vocational training, rehabilitation, workshops and appliance-making, together with medical postgraduate training, all formed part of the picture.

At the nearby mining town of Mansfield, **E A Nicoll**, who had been a local general practitioner, and was influenced by visits from the great general surgeon Grey-Turner, from Newcastle, possibly also by Sir Arthur Keith, who had also been a general practitioner there at an earlier period, took up general surgery with a special interest in trauma and opened a fracture clinic for miners in the 1930s funded by the mine-owners. After 1948, he became an orthopaedist *pur sang* and became famous for his work with mining injuries, particularly spinal fractures, and their rehabilitation. Berry Hill Hall, opened in 1939, was the first civilian rehabilitation centre in Britain, indeed the first in the world, an example to other parts of the country and other countries. Nicoll showed that stable spinal compression fractures needed no treatment other than exercises, a revolutionary idea at the time and one opposed by Watson-Jones and Böhler. It was Nicoll who was the driving force behind the establishment of the Sheffield Spinal Injuries Unit for paraplegia in the 1950s, a unit built up by Frank Holdsworth and Alan Hardy in international status.

Robert Guy Pulvertaft (1907–1986) was based at Derby but did most of his elective work at Harlow Wood. He was the greatest single influence on hand surgery in Britain, equivalent to Sterling Bunnell in the USA; indeed, Bunnell once said that Pulvertaft got better results than he did himself. Born in Cork, he was an assistant to Platt and Osmond-Clarke at Oswestry and Watson-Jones in Liverpool. He became an orthopaedic surgeon in Grimsby, an east coast port where he repaired the flexor tendons of the women fish-gutters and replaced amputation by tendon grafting. After serving as a consultant in the Royal Air Force in World War II, he joined the Derby and Harlow Wood hospitals and the last nine years of his career were devoted solely to hand surgery. Derby became the Mecca for hand surgeons (and patients!). In 1952 he founded the Hand Club in association with the plastic surgeons, and this amalgamated later with the Second Hand Club to become the British Society for Surgery of the Hand. His fame was international, and after retirement he worked as an adviser on the hand problems of leprosy in Africa and the Middle East.

Ernest Phillimore Brockman (1894–1977) was a St Thomas's graduate and resident, chief assistant to Bristow, and appointed in 1929 as the first orthopaedic surgeon at London's Westminster Hospital, later to the Royal National, St Vincent's Orthopaedic Hospital and others. Brockman was a *sensible* orthopaedic surgeon, stable and old-fashioned in the best and most useful sense of the word. He wrote a small book on club-foot, based on a prize essay for the British Orthopaedic Association (p. 491), which makes fascinating reading though its premise, that there is a primary aplasia of the talonavicular joint, is probably incorrect. He devised an ingenious method of arthrodesing the wrist by converting the lower radius into a wedge plunged into the split carpus, and used peroneus brevis tenodesis for ankle instability. The present writer had the good fortune to work as his junior at the Royal National for two years and learned more from him than from anyone else.

Bryan Leslie McFarland (1900–1963) succeeded McMurray in 1948 as director of orthopaedic studies, later professor, at Liverpool. He was a Liverpool graduate of 1922, one of the first four holders of the MCh Orth diploma, more than anything a children's orthopaedist. He was on the staff of many of the large Liverpool hospitals, a kind simple man, sometime president of the British Orthopaedic Association and of SICOT, a founder-member of the editorial board of the British Volume of the *Journal of Bone and Joint Surgery*, totally frank and democratic in his dealings with juniors.

Kenneth Hampden Pridie (1906–1963) was a Bristolian, at 28 assistant fracture surgeon to the Bristol Royal Infirmary, the first in Bristol wholly devoted to orthopaedic surgery*, who worked closely in his early days with Hey Groves after the latter's retirement. He was lecturer to the University and senior orthopaedic surgeon to the Royal Infirmary and Winford Orthopaedic Hospital, expanding the latter and setting up peripheral clinics. He applied engineering and carpentry to orthopaedics, developing such instruments as a ball-cutter for the acetabulum. He was an innovator, not hesitating to excise the entire os calcis; his articular cartilage drilling at the knee for arthrosis is discussed elsewhere.

Sir John Charnley (1911–1982), the Manchester pupil of Sir Harry Platt, developed the low-friction hip arthroplasty which ranks him with the great benefactors of mankind (and which makes one wonder why it is that surgeons do not receive the Nobel Prize). Before World War II he held junior posts at the Manchester Royal Infirmary and Salford Royal Hospital; and then, as an army orthopaedist in the Middle East, fostered an engineering bent to

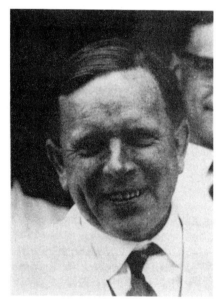

Figure 82   Sir John Charnley (1911–1982)

---

*However, we must allow for **Hubert Chitty** (1882–1966), a general surgeon with orthopaedic interests at the Royal Infirmary and a founder of the rural Winford Orthopaedic Hospital.

produce the adjustable Thomas splint. Later, under Platt, he became university lecturer in orthopaedics and in 1947 consultant at the Royal Infirmary. He early book on *The Closed Treatment of Common Fractures* (Edinburgh and London, Livingstone 1950) showed what could be done by applying simple principles. He became professor of orthopaedic surgery at Manchester in 1972. His work on total hip replacement is discussed in detail elsewhere (p. 601), but we may just say here that he was fascinated by the problem of joint lubrication, moved from teflon to high-density polyethylene (answering an enquiry from the present writer by saying: 'Don't do it just yet – I haven't got it right!') and turned the old Wrightington Hospital into an internationally renowned hip centre to which surgeons had to go to be shown how to do the operation, using the clean air enclosure and body exhaust system.

Hubert Lyon-Campbell Wood (1903–1982) was associated with King's College Hospital in London, where he graduated in 1926, becoming assistant surgeon at 29 and remaining on the staff until 1968. In 1952 he succeeded Dudley Buxton as senior orthopaedic surgeon, though until 1939 he had been half a general surgeon. He was a great civilian organizer in the second war and a great technician. On retirement, he became professor of clinical orthopaedics at the Ahmadu Bello University in Nigeria.

Denis John Wolko Browne (1892–1967), a second generation Australian in England, had an unparalleled influence on British paediatric surgery and was the virtual father of this discipline in the English-speaking world. His work necessarily included the orthopaedic aspects of his field by virtue of his post at the Hospital for Sick Children in Great Ormond Street in London, in this resembling the classical French tradition. He made notable contributions to the treatment of club-foot with his simple and efficient splint, still favoured by many, and to the management of congenital dislocation of the hip, often reducing this in the prone position.

We deal elsewhere with the British Orthopaedic Society and its brief life from 1894 to 1898. We have its *Transactions*, but these give no hint as to why it foundered, but we may judge that it was for the same reasons that made orthopaedic surgeons hesitate to organize as a speciality in Germany and other European countries at the turn of the century. Purely orthopaedic surgeons were very few; most of those practising orthopaedics were also general surgeons and feared to be separated from or ostracized by their surgical colleagues and to risk losing the rewards of surgical practice. They also feared that they would be regarded as no more than 'strap and buckle' mechanicians; and they even hesitated to attempt to take over the care of fractures, possibly because of the fear that this might prove *all* the work allotted to them.

World War I inevitably changed this situation entirely. Orthopaedics was now recognized, even if unwillingly, grudgingly or patronisingly. Many men had spent the war years doing nothing else. However, there had been a forward step between 1900 and 1918 with the creation of a subsection of orthopaedic surgery as part of the section of surgery of the Royal Society of Medicine in London in 1913, with Muirhead Little as president and Bankart and Rock Carling as secretaries. Robert Jones, Tubby, Jackson Clarke and

Openshaw were on the council. By a lucky chance, the International Congress of Medicine met in London in the same year, and the new section was host to famous orthopaedic surgeons from Europe and America discussing their work: Whitman, Lovett, Schanz, Lucas-Championnière, Vulpius, Ridlon, Putti and, inevitably, Fred Albee on bone-grafting. The subsection acquired full sectional status in 1922.

The British Orthopaedic Association, its time now obviously come, was founded in 1917 at the suggestion of Robert Jones, Muirhead Little and Openshaw, with the American Osgood shoving from behind. Little was president, Platt secretary. It has grown enormously since, unhindered – rather accelerated – by World War II. The original members were D McCrae Aitken, T R W Armour, A S B Bankart, W R Bristow, Jackson Clarke, Fairbank, Naughton Dunn, Elmslie, Robert Jones, Laming-Evans, W S Haughton, McMurray and Tubby, plus the officers mentioned. 'Major R B Osgood, of Boston, USA, who had helped very considerably in the preliminary steps which led to the formation of the Association, was present as a specially invited guest.'

The Association not only became larger, it inevitably also became political. It held combined meetings with the Americans and Canadians and the

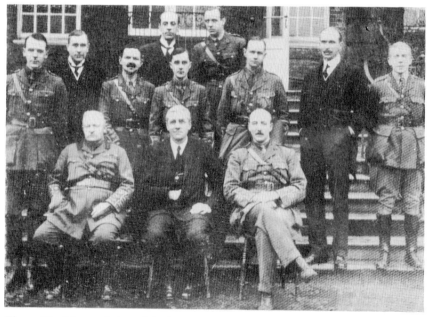

Figure 83   Many of the original members of the British Orthopaedic Association photographed in 1918 outside Queen Mary's Auxiliary Convalescent Hospital, Roehampton, London. *Sitting (left to right)* Openshaw, Muirhead Little (President), Bennett. *First row* McMurray, Blundell Bankart, McCrae Aitken, Harry Platt, Elmslie, Laming Evans, Naughton Dunn. *Back row* Trethowan, Rowley Bristow. Published with the kind permission of the Editor, *Journal of Bone and Joint Surgery,* British Volume

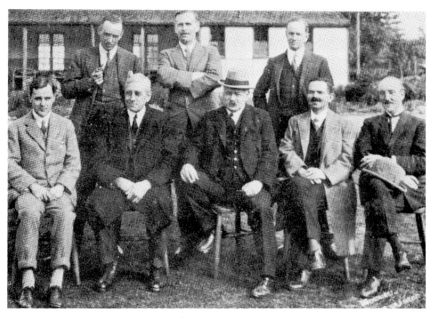

Figure 84 Office bearers of the British Orthopaedic Association in 1921. *Sitting* (*left to right*) Harry Platt (Secretary), Muirhead Little (President), Robert Jones (Vice President) McCrae Aitken, W E Bennett (Treasurer). *Standing* Rowley Bristow, Girdlestone, Elmslie. Published with the kind permission of the Editor, *Journal of Bone and Joint Surgery*. British Volume

resulting exchange system of young travelling Fellows was an outstanding and enduring success. The success of the BOA was a factor in the foundation of SICOT (p. 475). The linkage of the Association with the *Journal of Bone and Joint Surgery* was of great historical importance. The *Journal* in its original form could not provide an adequate medium for the publication of British developments, and a meeting in 1947 between the American Academy of Orthopaedic Surgeons (the AOA) and the BOA agreed that there should be a British Volume as well as the original American one. The new volume first appeared early in 1948 and has been an outstanding success under the inspiration and management of Philip Wiles, Watson-Jones, Jackson Burrows, Alan Apley and many others.

Although it is customary to speak in terms of successive generations of orthopaedic surgeons, this is as fallible as for any other groups of individuals: there are really no clear-cut temporal divisions, everything overlaps. However, there was an approach to one in Britain after the establishment of the National Health Service in 1948 because this created a large number of new orthopaedic posts across the board, in many cases for the first time, and these were filled by young or youngish men, many back from the war, of much the same age and with 25–30 years of specialist service ahead of them. In that sense, there has been a postwar generation of orthopaedic surgeons, and with it a generation gap, in the sense that most of the surgeons we have so far mentioned may fairly be spoken of as the 'Old Guard'.

A useful review of the British orthopaedic scene as it was in the early 1970s has been given by **Arthur Eyre-Brook**, head of the department at the Bristol Royal Infirmary for many years[139]; and, as many of those he mentions are happily still with us, we need not resort to the obituary form.

At that time, **Ian Smillie** was professor at St Andrew's University and an international authority on disorders of the knee[140] and on osteochondritis dissecans[141]. In Edinburgh, the professor was **J I P James** (now retired) formerly at the Royal National in London and specializing in scoliosis and hand surgery. In Edinburgh he developed an integrated clinical and training centre based on the Edinburgh Royal Infirmary and the Princess Margaret Rose Orthopaedic Hospital. One of his associates was **Ruth Wynne-Davies,** known for her work on the genetics of orthopaedic disorders. Her *Heritable Disorders in Orthopaedic Practice* (Oxford: Blackwell 1973) is a mine of information. In Glasgow, the first chair was occupied by **Roland Barnes,** known for his work on bone tumours, fractures of the femoral neck, bioengineering and bone pathology in general. Barnes was succeeded in 1973 by **David Hamblen.** Another leading Glasgow figure was **James Patrick**.

In Newcastle, the university department was long run by **J K Stanger,** and a chair was created in 1972 for **Jack Stevens**, previously Professor of Orthopaedic Surgery at Chicago. The chair at Liverpool was held in 1972 by **Robert Roaf** (now retired), well-known for his work on scoliosis[142] and skeletal tuberculosis[143]. Watson-Jones had left Liverpool for London after World War II, and the then current teachers for the MCh Orth included **Norman Roberts** and **Goronwy Thomas. Robert Garden**, of nearby Preston, greatly contributed to the management of transcervical hip fractures, as by his two-screw fixation. Other Liverpudlians included **F Dwyer** (osteotomy of the os calcis for foot deformities), **Geoffrey Osborne** (hip surgery), **Eric Wardle** (osteotomy of the hip and knee for arthrosis), **Austin O'Malley** (psoas section for hip arthrosis, now outmoded by hip replacement and yet often a simple useful procecure). Another teacher at Liverpool was **Denys Wainwright**, who developed the orthopaedic service at Stoke-on-Trent and is wellknown for his work on internal fixation for hip fractures and arthrosis after osteotomy.

At Oxford, thanks to the generosity of Lord Nuffield, the Nuffield Orthopaedic Centre had been developed by Girdlestone, Herbert Seddon, J C Scott and Joseph Trueta. The Chair was (and is) held by **Robert Duthie**, who arrived there via Edinburgh and the Chair at the University of Rochester. The Centre includes a service for the management of the orthopaedic complications of the coagulopathies, and is linked with an accident service at the Radcliffe Infirmary (now the John Radcliffe Hospital) in Oxford City itself, originally built up by Scott. **Edgar Somerville** was then known for his work on congenital dislocation of the hip, in which he favoured early and rapid management by excision of the limbus followed by rotation osteotomy.

A notable figure in Wales was **Dillwyn Evans** (1910–1974), who joined his old teacher, A O Parker at Cardiff and stayed there. He was known mainly for his work on club-foot, where he stressed the reciprocal differences in length of the medial and lateral columns in equinovarus and calcaneovalgus.

This led to his shortening of the outer column for equinovarus by excision and stapling of the calcaneo-cuboid joint to secure and maintain correction of the varus element. He also formed a personal connexion between British and Brazilian orthopaedic surgeons and organized a training programme for young Brazilians in Britain. In the early 1970s, **Brian McKibbin** was translated from Sheffield to become the first professor of traumatic and orthopaedic surgery in Cardiff, with the typical pattern of an academic department at the city's Royal Infirmary and an orthopaedic hospital outside the city.

In London, although every teaching hospital (and even University College Hospital from the 1960s) had its own department, the centre of excellence was the then still-extant Institute of Orthopaedics in Great Portland Street, with its adjacent town hospital and the main clinical centre at Stanmore in the country. As we have noted, Sir Herbert Seddon became Director and then Professor soon after World War II, the Dean for many years was Jackson Burrows, while the consultant staff included leading figures like P H Newman of the Middlesex Hospital, Charles Manning of St Bartholomew's and Donal Brooks of University College Hospital.

Charles William Stewart French Manning (1918–1982), Dublin born, was always linked with Bart's and became consultant orthopaedic surgeon in 1963. At the Royal National he established a scoliosis clinic and leg equalization clinic and, in effect, took over all the scoliosis cases for many miles around. An obsessive overworker, burdened also with administration, he died too early.

The outcome was that the Institute became a powerful postgraduate training centre which influenced standards and staffing throughout the country. Seddon's best-known work, of course, had been on peripheral nerves and the management of their injuries. The first holder of the Chair had been **Geoffrey Burwell,** but his commitment to research led him to transfer to Nottingham, where he eventually became Professor of Human Morphology and Experimental Orthopaedics. Burwell's contributions to the biological aspects of bone-grafting have been outstanding; references can be made to only a few of his many studies[144-148].

The outstanding research facilities at Stanmore included a bioengineering laboratory, headed for many years by **John Scales**, whose prosthetic replacements for massive skeletal resections were clinically managed by Jackson Burrows. The pathology department of the Royal National was long directed by **Hubert Sissons,** now in the USA, a world authority on bone histology, particularly of tumours. **David Trevor**, recently deceased, had an enormous experience with congenital dislocation of the hip. Other staff members included **Karl Nissen**, from New Zealand, an exponent of osteotomy for hip arthrosis and operation for plantar digital neuroma; **Philip Newman** on the surgery of the lumbar spine and the slipped femoral epiphysis; Charles Manning on scoliosis and Donal Brooks on hand and peripheral nerve injuries.

We have seen how Watson-Jones and Osmond-Clarke made their way from the provinces to the teaching staff of the London Hospital. Other members there were **Alexander Law,** for many years an exponent of the

Smith-Petersen cup arthroplasty of the hip; **Oliver Vaughan-Jackson**; and, more recently, **Michael Freeman,** known for his seminal work on knee prostheses. After the departure of Philip Wiles, the Middlesex Hospital department was led by Philip Newman and **Rodney Sweetnam**, the latter producing the later editions of Wiles's textbook and also writing on bone sarcoma. At Charing Cross, the department was initially directed by David Trevor, and then by **Anthony Catterall**. Westminster Hospital became a national centre for the management of bone sarcoma in the days before chemotherapy, where **Sir Stanford Cade** propounded the virtues of radiotherapy as primary treatment. At St Mary's Hospital, **George Bonney**'s interests were in the neurosurgical (and medicolegal) aspects of orthopaedics, while **John Crawford Adams** was known for his textbooks on fractures, orthopaedics and orthopaedic operations, as well as for his editorial duties with the *Journal.* At the Royal Free Hospital, formerly reserved for women students, the orthopaedic surgeon before World War II was **Paul Jenner Verrall**, an old first war colleague of Robert Jones, to whom the present writer was house surgeon in 1938; after the second war the department was run by **Charles Gray** singlehanded for many years.

At Guy's Hospital, earlier led by Trethowan and Lambrinudi, the orthopaedic department came under **W Crabb** and **Adrian Henry** after a period of direction by **John Batchelor**, whose best contribution is probably the addition of an abduction osteotomy to Girdlestone's hip excision. At King's College Hospital, associated with Lister in the late 19th century, and later with the late Sir Thomas Fairbank and St John Dudley Buxton, direction was for many years in the hands of **Hubert L-C Wood** (see above) and then under **Christopher Catterall,** with **Robert Crellin** and **Christopher Holden**. At St Thomas's after the departure of Rowley Bristow and George Perkins, the department was managed by **Ronald Furlong** for many years, the country branch at Pyrford as the Rowley Bristow Hospital under **Graham Apley**. At the Hospital for Sick Children in Great Ormond Street, the orthopaedic field had been stimulated for many years by the activities of **Sir Denis Browne**, a general surgeon who straddled both fields; under the later direction of **George Lloyd-Roberts** (1918–1986) (also of St George's) the orthopaedic work with children became entirely specialized.

In the provinces, at Sheffield, the late **Sir Frank Holdsworth** was originally a general-cum-orthopaedic surgeon who built up the Spinal Injuries Centre under the stimulus of E A Nicoll and did so much for the operative management of paraplegia. He also created a splendid fracture service in a heavily industrialized area and served on the Royal College of Surgeons training committee, ending with a well-deserved knighthood and a personal chair. His successor, **John Sharrard**, also later professor, is known for his work in paediatric orthopaedics, including leg-lengthening in achondroplastics – a field few venture in – and an interest in the electrical stimulation of osteogenesis; also for his work with the paediatric surgeon, **R B Zachary**, on the prevention and treatment of orthopaedic disability in myelomeningocoele. Another personal chair was that in Leeds, awarded to **Pascoe Clarke**, deviser of a valuable transfer of the pectoralis major to replace the paralysed elbow flexors and editor of successive volumes of *Modern Trends in Orthopaedic Surgery*[149].

Nottingham we have already dealt with at length. At Manchester, the fief of Harry Platt for many years, the orthopaedic department was subsequently managed by **David Lloyd-Griffiths**, who was heavily involved over a long period in international trials which established the value of chemotherapy as the sole treatment for spinal tuberculosis in Third World countries in children as ambulant patients. Manchester really includes the nearby Hip Centre at Wrightington created by John Charnley. The problems and successes of hip replacement are discussed elsewhere. It should be added that, at much the same time that Charnley was developing his programme, **Kenneth McKee** and **Watson-Farrar** in Norwich were obtaining excellent results with a metal-to-metal vitallium prosthesis, also cemented, while **Peter Ring**, of Redhill Hospital near London, was using a metal-to-metal prosthesis, the acetabular component of which had a stem threaded into the ilium towards the sacroiliac joint (lately replaced by a plastic acetabulum, also with a threaded stem and cementless).

The Robert Jones and Agnes Hunt Orthopaedic Hospital at Oswestry, near Shrewsbury, the first real orthopaedic centre in Britain, retained a major place in treatment and training because of its history and traditions deriving from Robert Jones, its enormous fund of clinical material, and its notable weekly teaching and operating sessions conducted by the famous: Harry Platt, T P McMurray, Reginald Watson-Jones, Henry Osmond-Clarke, Bryan McFarland, Naughton Dunn, Robert Roaf, David Lloyd-Griffiths and others. For a time the director of research was **N W Nisbet** of New Zealand. The hospital has always had very strong Antipodean connections (see under *Australia*) and the current director of clinical studies is an Australian, **Brian O'Connor**. Oswestry used to cover a very wide area of Wales and central England; though this has contracted as local facilities have improved everywhere, there is still room for centres of excellence in the special problems of orthopaedics such as scoliosis, spina bifida and many others. And it is in just this context, as Eyre-Brook points out (and as the present writer argues) that insulation from preoccupation with trauma is a positive advantage.

We have mentioned the Birmingham Accident Hospital in connection with Henry Gissane, an experiment not repeated elsewhere, despite the many contributions of Gissane, Peter London[150] and others. Valuable contributions to the pathology and bacteriology of wounds and burns made by Colebrook and others originated from this institution. Elsewhere in Birmingham, at the Woodlands Orthopaedic Hospital, the senior surgeon for many years was **Francis Allan**, who did pioneering work in leg lengthening and internal fixation for scoliosis (long before Harrington). The Lord Mayor Treloar Hospital at Alton in Hampshire, the Bath and Wessex Orthopaedic Hospital at Bath, the Princess Elizabeth Orthopaedic Hospital at Exeter, have all been mentioned elsewhere in connexion with the names of Henry Gauvain, Maud Forrester-Brown and Norman Capener respectively. Because Bath is a spa and attracts patients with chronic arthritis, it houses the National Hospital for Rheumatic Diseases (unless the administrators have managed to abolish it by the time this book is published). There has been much work on chronic arthritis there, recently associated with the names of

Hedley Hall and **Philip Yeoman**, just as there has been at Aix-les-Bains in France.

Bristol we have mentioned as linked with Hey Groves and Kenneth Pridie. The senior orthopaedic surgeon at the Royal Infirmary and the peripheral Winford Orthopaedic Hospital for many years was **Arthur Eyre-Brook**, who pursued a notable commitment in Third World orthopaedics after 'retirement'. At Exeter, besides Norman Capener, the staff included **F Durbin** and **Geoffrey Blundell-Jones**.

At Cambridge, the early days of orthopaedics benefited from the quiet activities of **Richard Weeden Butler** (1901–1982), an unassuming general surgeon who received orthopaedic training under Bristow and Perkins and at the Royal National under Trethowan. With Seddon, in 1933, he won the Robert James Gold Medal of the BOA for a famous essay on Pott's paraplegia. Appointed to Addenbrooke's Hospital in 1932, with only a part initial application to orthopaedics, he then became one of only three purely orthopaedic surgeons in the whole of East Anglia, where there are now about forty. And he always retained his anatomical interests, which is important if the future of academic anatomy lies in its clinical applications as many now maintain. He was succeeded by **John Fairbank**, son of Sir H A T Fairbank.

At Windsor and Heatherwood Hospital, Ascot, **George Arden**, developed the orthopaedic surgery of children crippled by Still's disease, including the use of total hip replacement at a very early age. (It is thought-provoking that Arden, like Blundell-Jones, J I P James, the present writer and many others were graduates of University College Hospital in London where there was no orthopaedic department whatever in their time as students!)

In this rushed journey through modern British orthopaedics, we can do no more than mention the names of **H A Brittain** in Norwich (p. 148), **Denis Dunn** in Colchester, and **St Clair Strange** of Canterbury and the Royal Sea-bathing Hospital at Margate in Kent. Many names have perforce been omitted. Many of those mentioned have left the scene for one reason or another. To come closer to the present time than the early 1970s would deprive us of historical perspective; perhaps we have come too far already. We need only repeat that the birth of the British volume of the *Journal of Bone and Joint Surgery* in 1948 proved an immense benefit to the orthopaedic community in Britain and the Commonwealth and has also provided a platform for workers in other countries. Its very high standards were fostered in the early years by the general editorship of Watson-Jones, the deputy editorship of John Crawford Adams, the chairmanship of Jackson Burrows and the financial acumen of Philip Wiles. No medical journal in the world has better standards of production and editing.

Two final names occur before we leave Britain. **Leon Gillis** (1908–1967) was closely associated with the modern developments in amputations and artificial limbs at Roehampton's Queen Mary's Hospital, London, for many years from 1943, later administered by the Ministry of Pensions as the equivalent of the Veterans' Administration in the USA. Johannesburg born, he wrote *Amputations* in 1945 and *Artificial Limbs* in 1947.

V H Ellis (1901–1953), of St Mary's Hospital, London, had a link with Fleming at the same hospital that gave him early access to penicillin. This he used during World War II at the Park Prewett base hospital for the war injured which treated nearly 16 000 men, 1500 of whom received penicillin. Penicillin permitted earlier repair of tendons and nerves with less risk of sepsis, and allowed delayed primary suture of gunshot wounds. Cancellous grafting and skin flaps were also protected by its local and general use. In the early postwar years he showed, as also did Trueta, that penicillin alone, or in combination with early decompressive surgery, now offered something quite new in orthopaedics – a permanent cure of acute osteomyelitis with preservation of the normal bony architecture[151,152].

REFERENCES

1. Brown, A. (1928). John Arderne. *Ann. Med. Hist.*, **10**, 402
2. John of Mirfield: *Breviarium Bartholomei* (trans. Colton, JB) (1969). (New York, Hafner)
3. Major, R.H. (1932). William Clowes. *Ann. Med. Hist.*, **4**, 1
4. Croone, W. (1667). *De ratione motus musculorum.* (London)
5. Sydenham, T. (1683). *Tractatus de podagra et hydrops.* (London)
6. Sydenham, T. (1749). *Collected Works* (ed. John Swan). (London)
7. Verney, F.P. (1894). *The Memoirs of the Verney Family during the Civil War.* (London)
8. Le Vay, D. (1975). On the derivation of the name 'Rickets'. *Proc. Roy. Soc. Med.*, **68**, 46
9. *Selected Writings of Sir Thomas Browne* (ed. Keynes, G.L.). (1968) (London, Faber)
10. de Boot, A. (1649). *Observationes medicae de affectibus omissia.* (London)
11. Sigerist, H.E. (1951). *A History of Medicine.* (New York)
12. Valentin, B. (1961). *Die Geschichte der Orthopädie.* (Stuttgart, Thieme)
13. Coiter, V. (1572). *Externarum et internarum principalium humani corporis partium tabulae.* (Nuremberg)
14. Aubrey, J. (1656). *Naturall History of Wiltshire.*
15. van Leeuwenhoek, A. (1674). *Phil. Trans.*, **9**, 121
16. Havers, C. (1691). *Osteologia nova.* (London)
17. Pringle, J. (1752). *Observations on the Diseases of the Army.* (London)
18. Fox, R.D. (1882). On bone-setting (so-called). *Lancet*, **ii**, 843
19. Joy, R.J.F. (1954). The natural bone-setters, with special reference to the Sweet family of Rhode Island. *Bull. Hist. Med.*, **28**, 416
20. Thornton, J.L. (1955). Orthopaedic surgeons at St Bartholomew's Hospital, London. *St Bartholomew's Hosp. J.*, **59**, 195
21. Jackson, W. (1787). *Observations on the inefficacious use of irons in cases of luxations and distortions of the ancle joint, and children born with deformed and crooked feet.* (London)
22. Paget, J. (1867). Cases that bonesetters cure. *Brit. Med. J.*, **1**, 1
23. Fisher, A.G.T. (1924). *Internal derangements of the knee joint.* (London, Lewis)
24. Fisher, A.G.T. (1948). *Treatment by Manipulation.* (London, Lewis)
25. Cyriax, E.F. (1909). *Bibliographia gymnastica medica*, Wörishofen 1909; Minor displacement of the vertebrae and ilia. *Practitioner*, **Nov.**
26. Cyriax, R.J. (1914). A short history of mechanotherapeutics in Europe until the time of Ling. *Janus*, **19**, 178
27. Cyriax, J. (1949). *Osteopathy and manipulation.* (London)

28. Tamplin, R.W. (1846). *Lectures on the nature and treatment of deformities.* (London)
29. Cope, Z. (1953). *William Cheselden.* (Edinburgh and London, Livingstone)
30. Sharpe, S. (1739). *A Treatise on the Operations of Surgery.* (London)
31. Le Dran (1749). *The Operations in Surgery, transcribed by Mr Gataker, with Remarks by William Cheselden* (4th edn). (London)
32. Billroth, T. (1876). *Lehren und Lernen der Medizinischen Wissenschaften*
33. Valentin, B. (1958). Robert Chessher, an English pioneer in orthopaedics. *Med. Hist.,* **2**, 3–8
34. Austin, R.T. (1981). *Robert Chessher of Hinckley, first English Orthopaedist.* (Leicestershire County Council Libraries and Information Service)
35. Harrison, E. (1827). *Pathological and practical observations on spinal diseases.* (London)
36. Shaw, J. (1824). *Engravings illustrative of a work on the nature and treatment of the distortions to which the spine and the bones of the chest are subject.* (London)
37. Harrison, E. (1832). *The extraordinary case of Sarah Hawkes: one of extreme deformity, cured by a method founded upon simple principles.* (London)
38. Hunter, J. (1737). *Collected Works* (ed. Palmer). (London); *Medical Observations and Enquiries.* London 1753
39. Pott, P. (1744). *Phil. Trans.,* **41**, 616
40. David, J-P. (1779). *Dissertation sur les effets du mouvement et de repos dans les maladies chirurgicales.* (Paris)
41. Earle, J. (1808). *Life of Pott,* in *Chirurgical Works of Pott.* (London)
42. Pearson, J. (1822). *The Life of William Hey.* (London)
43. Hey, W. (1803). *Practical Observations in Surgery.* (London)
44. Bromfield, W. (1773). *Chirurgical observations and cases.* (London)
45. Brock, R.C. (1952). *The Life and Work of Astley Cooper.* (Edinburgh and London, Livingstone)
46. Shaw, J. (1825). *Further observations on the lateral or serpentine curvature of the spine and on the treatment of contracted limbs.* (London)
47. Reid, J. (1834). Displacement of one of the smaller cartilages of the knee joint. *Edinburgh Med. Surg. J.,* **42**, 377
48. Brodhurst, B.E. (1867). On loose cartilages in the knee-joint. *St George's Hosp. Rep.,* **2**, 141
49. Peltier, L.F. (1987). The lineage of sports medicine. *Clin. Orthop.,* **216**, 4
50. Annandale, T. (1897). Cases of loose cartilages removed from the knee-joint by direct incision with antiseptic precautions. *Lancet,* **ii**, 162
51. Annandale, T. (1885). An operation for displaced semilunar cartilage. *Brit. Med. J.,* **1**, 779
52. Margary, F. (1882). Estirpazione della fibro-cartilagineo semilunare interna del ginocchio sinistro. *Giornale della R. Accademia di Med. di Torino,* **30**, 361
53. Lauenstein, C. (1890). Zur Frage des Derangement interne des Kniegelenks. *Dtsch. Med. Wschr.,* **169**
54. Bruns, P. (1892). Die Luxation der Semilunarknorpel des Kniegelenks. *Brun's Beiträge zur klinischen Chir.,* **9**, 435
55. Jones, R. (1909). Notes on derangement of the knee based upon a personal experience of over 500 operations. *Ann. Surg.,* **50**, 969
56. *The Anatomical Memoirs of John Goodsir* (1868). (ed. Turner, W.)
57. Martin, A.M. (1912). *Brit. Med. J.,* **2**, 1070
58. Redfern, P. (1851). Normal nutrition in human articular cartilage. *Monthly J. Med. Sci.,* **13**, 201
59. Syme, J. (1842). Amputation at the ankle joint. *Edinburgh Med. Surg. J.*
60. Harris, R.I. (1944). Amputations. *J. Bone Jt. Surg.,* **26**, 626

61. Brodie, B.C. (1832). An account of some cases of chronic abscesses of the tibia. *Med. Chir. Trans.*, **17**, 239
62. Paget, J. (1877). On a form of chronic inflammation of bone (osteitis deformans). *Med. Chir. Trans.*, **60**, 37
63. Paget, J. (1854). *Collected Lectures on Surgical Pathology*. (London) (3rd edn, Wm. Turner, London 1870)
64. Paget, J. (1891). *Studies of old case-books*. (London)
65. Czerny (1873). *Wiener Med. Ztschr.*, **Sept.**, 27
66. Lister, J. (1867). On a new method of treating compound fractures, abscess, etc., with observations on the conditions of suppuration. *Lancet*, **i**, 326, 357, 387, 507; **ii**, 95
67. Lister, J. (1879). An address on the influence of position upon local circulation. *Brit. Med. J.*, **1**, 923
68. Lister, J. (1865). On excision of the wrist for caries. *Lancet*, **1**, 308
69. Cooper, E.S. (1861). Fracture of the patella. *San Francisco Med. Press*, **2**, 14
70. Le Vay, D. (1956). *The Life of Hugh Owen Thomas.*, p. 54. (Edinburgh and London, Livingstone)
71. Little, W.J. (1862). *Trans. Obstet. Soc. London*, **3**, 283
72. Hecker, C. (1853). *Verh. der Ges. v. Geburtsk.* (Berlin)
73. Weber, F. (1851). *Beitr. z. Path. Anatomie der Neugeboren.* (Kiel)
74. Little, W.J. (1853). *On the nature and treatment of the deformities of the human frame.* (London)
75. Brown, J.B. (1845). *Reports of cases in the Boston Orthopaedic Institution or Hospital for cure of deformities of the human frame.* (Boston)
76. Little, W.J. (1857). On unnecessary orthopaedic operations. *Lancet*, **ii**, 28, 133, 161, 539
77. Solly, S. (1857). *Med. Chir. Trans.*, **40**, 119
78. Adams, W. (1860). *On the reparative process of human tendons after the subcutaneous division for cure of deformities.* (London)
79. Adams, W. (1871). *A new operation for bony anchylosis of the hip-joint.* (London)
80. Smithsonian Miscellaneous Collections, Washington 1878, Vol. 15, Lecture VI
81. Adams, W. (1885). On the treatment of hip-joint disease by extension with motion. *Brit. Med. J.*, **2**, 859
82. Bigg, H.H. (1869). *Orthopraxy: the mechanical treatment of deformities, debilities and deficiencies of the human frame* (2nd edn.). (London)
83. Barwell, R. (1879). Osteotomy of both thighs and legs for genu valgum. *Brit. Med. J.*, **2**
84. Lonsdale, E. F. (1855). An analysis of 3000 cases of various kinds of deformities admitted at the Royal Orthopaedic Hospital, Bloomsbury Square. *Lancet*, **ii**, 188, 218
85. Brodhurst, B.E. (1866). On congenital dislocation of the femur. *St George's Hosp. Rep.*, **1**, 217
86. Bowman, A.K. (1842). *Sir William Macewen.* (London)
87. Jones, A.R. (1952). *J. Bone Jt. Surg.*, **34B**, 123
88. Macewen, W. (1878). *Lancet*, **i**, 449
89. Macewen, W. (1909). *Ann. Surg.*, **1**, 959
90. Albee, F. (1911). Transplantation of a portion of tibia into the spine for Pott's disease. *J. Amer. Med. Assoc.*, August
91. Ogston, A. (1877). The operative treatment of genu valgum. *Edinburgh Med. J.*, **22**, 782
92. Ogston, A. (1875). *J. Anat. Physiol.*, **10**, 49
93. Ogston, A. (1884). *Lancet*, **i**, 152
94. Ogston, A. (1881). Suture of the ulnar nerve. *Br. Med.J.*, **1**, 391

95. Lane, W.A. (1892). Fracture dislocation of the spine. *Lancet*, **ii**, 661
96. Jones, R. (1912). *Brit. Med. J.*, **2**, 1589
97. Layton, T.B. (1956). *Sir William Arbuthnot Lane*. (Edinburgh and London, Livingstone)
98. Ratliff, A.H.C. (1983). Ernest William Hey Groves and his contributions to orthopaedic surgery. *Ann. Roy. Coll. Surg. Eng.*, **65**, 203
99. Hey Groves, E.W. (1913). An experimental study of the operative treatment of fractures. *Brit. J. Surg.*, **1**, 438
100. Hey Groves, E.W. (1917). Operations for the repair of the crucial ligaments. *Lancet*, **ii**, 674
101. Hey Groves, E.W. (1919). The crucial ligaments of the knee joint, their function, rupture and the operative treatment of the same. *Brit. J. Surg.*, **7**, 505
102. Hey Groves, E.W. (1926). Some contributions to the reconstructive surgery of the hip. *Brit. J. Surg.*, **14**, 486
103. Hey Groves, E.W. (1922). *Modern methods of treating fractures*. (Bristol, Wood)
104. Hey Groves, E.W. (1933). Treatment of osteoarthritis of the hip. *Brit. Med. J.*, **1**, 3
105. Osmond-Clarke, H. (1950). *J. Bone Jt. Surg.*, **32B**, 620
106. Girdlestone, G.R. Unpublished memorandum for Trustees of Nuffield Fund relating to draft outline of a complete orthopaedic scheme, 1938. In Dommisse, G.F. (1982). *To Benefit the Maimed*. South African Orthopaedic Association and National Council for the Care of Cripples in South Africa. (Johannesburg)
107. Watson, F. (1934). *The Life of Sir Robert Jones*. (London, Hodder and Stoughton)
108. Jones, R. (1901). *Trans. Brit. Orth. Soc.*, **4**
109. Jones, R. (1896). *Trans. Brit. Orth. Soc.*, **1**, 20
110. Jones, R. (1908). *Amer. J. Orth. Surg.*, 1908
111. Jones, R. (1910). Fractures in the neighbourhood of joints. *Proc. Roy. Soc. Med.*, **4**, 1
112. Jones, R. (1906). *Clin. J.*, May 9
113. Jones, R. (1909). Notes on derangements of the knee. *Ann. Surg.*, **50**, 969
114. Jones, R. (1916). Disabilities of the knee joint. *Brit. Med. J.*, 696
115. Jones, R. (1901). *Trans. Brit. Orth. Soc.*, **4**, 56
116. Jones, R. (1908). *Rev. d'Orthop.*, 2nd series, **9**
117. Jones, R. (1901). *Trans. Brit. Orth. Soc.*, **4**, 38
118. Jones, R. (1901). *Trans. Brit. Orth. Soc.*, **4**, 25
119. Shiers, G.P. (1954). Arthroplasty of the knee – a preliminary report on a new method. *J. Bone Jt. Surg.*, **36B**, 553
120. Burrows, H.J. (1968). Major prosthetic replacement of knees, lessons learned in 17 years. *J. Bone Jt. Surg.*, **50B**, 225
121. Waugh, W. (1986). *Clin. Orthop.*, **210**, 55
122. Insall, J.V. (1967). Intra-articular surgery for degenerative arthritis of the knee. *J. Bone Jt. Surg.*, **49B**, 211
123. Charnley, J. (1958). Positive pressure in arthrodesis of the knee. *J. Bone Jt. Surg.*, **40B**, 633
124. Key, J.A. (1932). Positive pressure in arthrodesis of the tuberculous knee joint. *South. Med. J.*, **25**, 902
125. Jackson, J.P. (1958). Osteotomy for osteoarthritis of the knee. *J. Bone Jt. Surg.*, **40B**, 826
126. Jackson, J.P. and Waugh, W. (1961). Tibial osteotomy for osteoarthritis of the knee. *J. Bone Jt. Surg.*, **43B**, 746
127. Wardle, E.N. (1962). Osteotomy of the tibia and fibula. *Surg. Gyn. Obst.*, **115**, 61
128. Osmond-Clarke, H. (1950). *J. Bone Jt. Surg.*, **32B**, 620

129. Keller, W. (1904). *New York Med. J.*, **80**, 741
130. Davies-Colley, N. (1887). *Trans. Clin. Soc. London*, **20**, 165
131. Elmslie, R.C. (1935). Fibrosis of bone: generalised osteitis fibrosa cystica not due to hyperparathyroidism. *St Bartholomew's Hosp. Rep.*, **68**, 147
132. Lambrinudi, C. (1927). A new operation for drop-foot. *Brit. J. Surg.*, **15**, 193
133. Bristow, R. (1947). Injuries of peripheral nerves in two World Wars. *Brit. J. Surg.*, **34**, 334
134. McMurray, T.P. (1928). The diagnosis of internal derangement of the knee. In: *Robert Jones Birthday Volume*, p. 305. (London, Oxford University Press)
135. Griffiths, D.Ll (1986). *Clin. Orthop.*, **210**, 3
136. Bankart, A.S.B. (1944). A case of pathological dislocation of the hip, and what happened to an epiphyseal transplant. *Proc. Roy. Soc. Med.*, **38**, 618
137. Le Vay, D. (1967). Stimulation of epiphysial growth in short legs. *Proc. Roy. Soc. Med.*, **60**, 1080
138. Waugh, W. (1988). *The development of orthopaedics in the Nottingham area.* (Published privately)
139. Eyre-Brook, A.L. (1972). *Clin. Orthop.*, **88**, 283
140. Smillie, I. (1970). *Injuries of the knee joint* (4th edn). (Edinburgh, Livingstone)
141. Smillie, I. (1966). *Osteochondritis dissecans. Loose bodies in joints: aetiology, pathology and treatment.* (Edinburgh, Livingstone)
142. Roaf, R. (1966). *Scoliosis.* (Edinburgh, Livingstone)
143. Roaf, R., Kirkaldy-Willis, W.H. and Cathro, A.J.M. (1959). *Surgical Treatment of Bone and Joint Tuberculosis.* (Edinburgh, Livingstone)
144. Burwell, R.G. (1964). Studies in the transplantation of bone. *J. Bone Jt. Surg.*, **46B**, 110
145. Burwell, R.G. (1966). Studies in the transplantation of bone. *J. Bone Jt. Surg.*, **48B**, 532
146. Burwell, R.G., Gowland, G. and Dexter, F. (1963). Studies in the transplantation of bone. *J. Bone Jt. Surg.*, **45B**, 597
147. Burwell, R.G. (1969). The fate of bone grafts. In Apley, A.G. (ed.) *Recent Advances in Orthopaedics.* (London, Churchill)
148. Burwell, R.G., Friedlander, G.E. and Mankin, H.J. (1985). Current perspectives and future directions. Presented at the *1983 Invitational Conference on Osteochondral Allografts.*
149. Clarke, J.M.P. (ed.) (1962). *Modern Trends in Orthopaedics* 3 and 4. (London, Butterworth)
150. London, P.S. (1967). *A practical guide to the care of the injured.* (Edinburgh, Livingstone)
151. Ellis, V.H. (1946). Orthopaedic surgery and fractures. In Fleming, A. (ed.) *Penicillin: its practical application.* (London, Butterworth)
152. Jones, G.B. (1945). The local use of penicillin in war wounds of the knee joint, in *Penicillin therapy and control of 21 Army Group*
153. Cholmeley, J.A. (1985). *History of the Royal National Orthopaedic Hospital.* (London, Chapman and Hall)

CHAPTER 3

National Histories – Germany*

INTRODUCTION

The history of orthopaedics in Germany over the last two centuries is based on two factors. On the one hand, there was the flourishing development, mainly in the first half of the 19th century, of private establishments which were often more finishing schools for girls of families of means than true medical centres, which did not provide for the poor, and which rarely survived their founders, who were often laymen. These institutions, which reflected the increasing *embourgeoisement* of Europe after the defeat of Napoleon and aimed to satisfy the aspirations of the rising middle-class, were commoner in Central Europe than anywhere else, even than in France. In England they hardly existed at all; there may have been schools of deportment, but not informed with the same degree of quasi-medical enthusiasm.

Nevertheless, in a period when few doctors were interested in deformities and a separate discipline of orthopaedics did not exist, these institutes did mark a halfway house to the formal hospital and academic orthopaedic department of the end of the century. We must also remember that, at least till recently, orthopaedic surgery in Germany remained 'pure orthopaedics', uncontaminated by fracture management. Indeed, in 1931 the professors of general surgery issued a statement defining the limits of orthopaedic teaching and practice in the faculties; and one outcome of this was that, at the Bologna meeting of the *Société Internationale de Chirurgie Orthopédique* in 1936, all the German members voted as a minority against the addition of the words '*et de Traumatologie*' to the title of the Society.

The second factor was the growing sense in the latter half of the century of a social responsibility for cripples, of the need for concentrated long-term

---

* For mediaeval German contributions, see p. 52.

179

care, educational and vocational training, and of the need for an academic basis for orthopaedic training. Bismarck may have been responsible for the unification of Germany under Prussian domination and the military consequences thereof; but he was also the architect of modern social insurance.

It must be admitted that initially, at the end of the 18th century and even much later, the segregation of the handicapped was sought almost as if they were lepers: because of the old superstitition that pregnant women catching sight of the deformed might produce similarly afflicted children, because public begging and the exploitation of deformed children – perhaps deliberately deformed – were a nuisance.

> 'Sympathy for cripples and persons suffering from disgusting afflictions has to be limited to arranging for their appropriate sojourn in infirmaries with gardens which, however, *they must not quit* (my italics). The repugnant sight of such infortunates must continue to be excluded from public intercourse, for the impression on the susceptible, or even the pregnant, is extremely serious[1].'
> And this in 1876!

Yet early on, in 1838, Stromeyer saw the essential problem quite clearly:

> 'It would be very sensible for special institutes for the gratuitous treatment of poor children with club-feet to be founded in the larger cities ... the admission of such individuals into general hospitals is inadvisable because the assistant doctors in these places change too frequently, and yet it is on these that the care of such patients especially devolves[2].'

Segregation, for the good of the patients, not that of the public, and continuity of supervision: these were the keys to advance. And in 1841, Dieffenbach had made similarly cogent remarks:

> 'Is it not to be desired that the state should build institutes for the care of club-feet and other curable contractures in large cities in which the children of poor parents could be treated, and to which could be sent those from the country and smaller towns without a doctor conversant with the treatment of the same?'

Here is the prime doctrine of the centralized institute with its peripheral catchment area as put into practice by Robert Jones at Oswestry in Britain 60 years later, and reproduced so often elsewhere. Dieffenbach was draconian about treatment being compulsory: refusal should disqualify for financial aid, education and appliances; the disabled should be forbidden to beg. Some argued that special institutions were unnecessary as general hospitals were freely available. 'But the fact is that in surgical hospitals there are so many other things to do that the necessary attention cannot be devoted to the treatment (of club-feet); for this must be wholly undivided and yet it has to be taken into account that the assistants in such hospitals are always changing and the treatment of difficult cases passes from one hand to another. Yet the treatment requires special measures, great practice and experience, which the rest of surgery does not yet afford[3].'

The details of this picture may have changed. Much more can now be done in the short term in general hospitals, particularly for injuries, but its essence remains. Indeed, the importance of segregation now operates *within* orthopaedics and not just vis-à-vis general surgery, for the management of scoliosis, hand surgery and many other special fields is not now within the competence of the modern 'general' orthopaedic surgeon in a district hospital.

There was also the fact that, in some ways, institutional management was *better* than private treatment, not just because it was available to the poor but because it allowed constant medical observation, day and night[4]. By the end of the 19th century, orthopaedic clinics were attached to the major homes for cripples and these clinics were usually staffed by members of the local faculty. True, the separation of orthopaedics from general surgery at this time caused many pangs and much heart-searching, but this was not at all a peculiarly German problem, it was reproduced the world over.

WÜRZBURG

Germany is a large country and made enormous contributions to orthopaedic science and practice. It is best to follow Valentin's example[5] and consider the different *Länder* separately, and we shall start with Würzburg: because of the very strong orthopaedic tradition there from early days, because Virchow was professor of morbid anatomy there, because so much else originated there, including the discovery of X-rays, and because it has long had an excellent regional orthopaedic hospital which houses one of the finest – if not the finest – libraries of the history of orthopaedics in the world.

Würzburg saw the founding of the first orthopaedic institute in Germany in 1816, by an orthopaedic mechanic, a former cutler's apprentice, **Johann Georg Heine** (1770–1838). He arrived in the city in 1798 and was appointed instrument-maker to the university and the Julius Hospital in 1802. He manufactured instruments and appliances, including instruments to remove bone fragments produced by drilling and a bone-saw; his appliances often operated by spring traction; he discussed the problems of gait and invented a new artificial foot[6]. His institute in the former Stephans-Kloster became famous and with royal approval it was renamed the *Carolinen Institut* in 1822. In 1824 the university appointed him demonstrator of instruction in orthopaedic appliances and assessor (teaching assistant) in the Medical Faculty. His relations with the surgeons of the Julius Hospital were excellent, partly because, as a leading light admitted, surgery was then unavailable against most deformities, Heine had a right to try, and even to be successful[7].

It is clear that the surgeons did not, on the whole, regard Heine as an intruder, for this was a field in which they were not greatly interested and were largely incompetent, but as a valued collaborator. Heine himself does not seem to have been arrogant. In a report on his institute in 1821 he notes that it is the first and so far the only one of its kind, that it admits persons of every class and that it is based on combining the skill of the instrument-maker with the surgeon's science[8]. In 1823, Goethe secured him an honorary

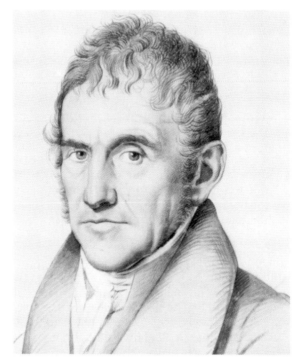

Figure 85   Johann Georg Heine (1770–1838)

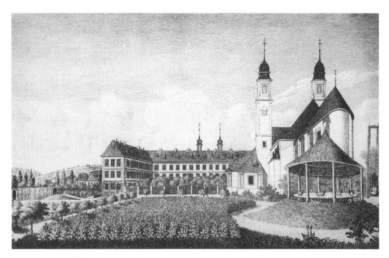

Figure 86   The *Carolinen Institut* at Würzburg

doctorate, though not apparently in medicine, at Jena University. In April 1826 the inpatients included 39 with scoliosis or kyphosis, four with club-feet and one with lower limb curvature.

However, his assertion that his unit was the first of its kind cannot stand: he enthusiastically adopted and adapted the extension bed that Venel was using for spinal curvature at his institute at Orbe, in Switzerland (p. 295), which *was* the first in the world (though we must take Chessher in England into account, p. 86), and the fact that he pointedly makes no reference anywhere in his writings to Venel's world-famous centre may be sufficient evidence of the truth of the situation. Heine created a famous orthopaedic 'model cabinet' which survived until World War II. He took his nephew and son-in-law, Bernhard into apprenticeship and then, in 1828, at the age of 58, in what seems to have been a life crisis, handed over the institute to Bernhard Heine and moved to Scheveningen in Holland, where he established an 'orthopaedic sea-bathing institute'. In fact, he seems to have entered into a confused paranoid state, writing petitions and philosophical ramblings and essays on the treatment of cholera. One is reminded of the last years of W J Little's rural seclusion and his preoccupation with earth closets (p. 501–2).

Bernhard Heine (1800–1846) became famous for his invention of the osteotome and his studies on bone regeneration. Macewen (p. 131) is more generally credited with the osteotome, and it is true that Heine's instrument was far more elaborate and complex. It did not have a single blade but was really a sort of saw constructed to provide an endless segmented cutting band, quite unlike Macewen's double-bevelled chisel. Yet both were designed for the same purpose, and osteotomy was used frequently in the 19th century long before Macewen. Heine certainly foresaw the possibilities of bone surgery and his instrument, produced in 1830–1, made him famous almost overnight, gained him the Montyon Prize of the Paris *Académie des Sciences* in 1834 and earned him a professorship in experimental physiology in Würzburg in 1833. In 1837 he was invited by Tsar Nicholas I to Petersburg to demonstrate his invention, and in 1836 the Würzburg University conferred the degree of Doctor of Medicine, *honoris causa*. In 1838 he became 'Honorary Professor in Orthopaedics and Operative Instruction with the Osteotome devised by him', and in the same year he gained a second Montyon Prize in Paris for a report on bone regeneration. Yet, despite these successes, Bernhard Heine wound up the Carolineum in 1838 to devote himself to scientific studies. He died, of phthisis, in Switzerland in 1846.

Perhaps Heine simply gave up, like his uncle. Perhaps he was dismayed by the activities of a competitor, **Joseph Anton Mayer** (1798–1860), a proper doctor who had trained at Würzburg and served as assistant to von Textor at the Julius Hospital and set up in practice in 1825, when he established a not very impressive orthopaedic institute. Immediately Heine died, Mayer petitioned the King of Bavaria for the succession of the Carolinen Institut but seems not to have been successful and his own institute perished with him.

Würzburg had had a Philosophico-Medical Society from 1827 and in 1844 Mayer reported to it on tenotomy for club-foot[9]. (This body merged with the Physico-Medical Society in 1851 and it was here that Röntgen showed

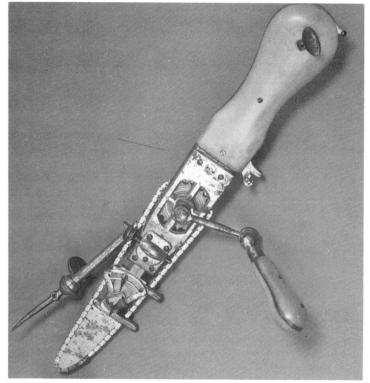

Figure 87   Bernard Heine's osteotome, 1830

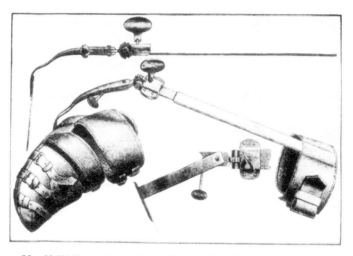

Figure 88   H W Berend: traction splint for club-foot after tenotomy, 1840

his first hand-print at the end of 1895.) He also found other news to communicate to the merged society. Mayer had occasion to treat a patient with a fractured femur who had previously had a fracture of the opposite femur which had shortened the limb, and he deliberately allowed the new fracture to heal with shortening and thus obtained equality of leg-length (Rizzoli in Bologna had acted similarly at almost the same time). He went on to apply this to the shortening of congenital dislocation of the hip, removing an appropriate segment of the healthy femur with the new osteotome[10-12], something that Hippocrates had hinted he would like to do! This quite original procedure, in a nine-year-old girl, was represented as 'the simplest, shortest, safest and most permanent remedial technique'; but other surgeons shrank from operating on a healthy leg. Rizzoli, too, incurred contumely, for he invented a *macchinetta ossifraga*, or osteoclast, for deliberate fracture of the sound femur.

Mayer was enthusiastic about osteotomy[13] and applied it to genu valgum and varum, previously regarded as incurable, removing bony wedges from the upper tibia under chloroform and carefully closing the skin incision to make the procedure effectively subcutaneous. In 1848 he resected a bony fragment in a case of fracture of the 7th dorsal vertebra with cord compression: the patient died[14]. In 1856 he reviewed his osteotomies and resections[15], always insisting on having coined the word 'osteotomy' though he was working in the very city where Bernhard Heine had invented the osteotome in 1830.

After Mayer's death there seems to have been no orthopaedic institute in Würzburg until **Albert Hoffa** (1859–1907), assistant at the university surgical clinic at the Julius Hospital, founded a private remedial unit in 1886. (Hoffa had been born in South Africa, and had persuaded Dr Ernst Simon to emigrate to Cape Town as that country's first orthopaedic surgeon.) Hoffa moved to Berlin in 1902 as successor to Julius Wolff, but died soon after.

Jacob Riedinger (1861–1917) became professor of orthopaedics in Würzburg in 1913. He founded the Lower Francony Society for the Care of Cripples in 1910, and this established a 50-bed institution for the treatment and training of crippled youths. This was the forerunner of the new König Ludwig Haus of 1916, which is now a large modern regional orthopaedic centre, linked with the university and the famous library.

STUTTGART

Johann George Heine in Würzburg had been and remained essentially an instrument and appliance-maker, nominally subordinate to the doctors he was careful to respect. His nephew, Bernhard, received a medical doctorate by virtue of his studies and innovations, but does not seem to have had an orthodox training. However, the other members of the family and their descendants, like the younger members of the Thomas family in England, themselves the descendants of unqualified bonesetters, took care to acquire a regular degree.

Jacob Heine (1800–1879) was a nephew of Johann Georg, a cousin of

Bernhard; his uncle persuaded him to abandon theology for medicine and he graduated at Tübingen in 1829. (The other graduates were Johann Georg's own son, Joseph (1803–1877) and Jacob's son, Karl Wilhelm von Heine (1836–1878) – the prefix of nobility was conferred on Jacob by the King of Württemberg – who was professor of surgery at Innsbruck and Prague.)

Jacob opened an institute at Cannstatt, near Stuttgart, in 1829, and soon had to buy a larger new house, with a garden and a lake for aquatherapy and mud-baths, and with every possible attention from teachers, governesses, clergymen, musicians, drawing and dancing instructors. It was still the era of the orthopaedic institute as finishing school for adolescent girls; but in this case it was much more than that. Perhaps Jacob Heine's greatest achievement was to clarify the condition later to be known as anterior poliomyelitis. Before him, the paralysis had been classified as a group of diseases affecting parts of the body. Heine saw these as manifestations of one and the same pathological process and reported his observations briefly in 1838[16], and more fully in 1840 in a monograph: *Observations on paralytic states of the lower limbs and their treatment*[17]. He was optimistic and reported recoveries with baths and splints, and 20 years later, in 1860, published a revised and enlarged edition using for the first time the title of *Spinale Kinderlähmung* or 'spinal infantile paralysis' as he assumed the site of the disease to be in the spinal cord[18]. His clinical observations were acute, for he not only distinguished the disease from spastic paralysis but noted its epidemic nature, its acute and later phases, the coolness of paralysed limbs, the contractures and deformities and the growth-lag of paralysed extremities. He was a courageous and persistent therapist, using every appliance – and tenotomies if need be – to enable patients to walk, even if they could previously only crawl. Hence it was that the condition was long known in the latter half of the century as Heine-Medin disease (for the Swede, Medin, see p. 332). He also studied congenital dislocation of the hip and devised a reduction apparatus and reported 11 cases, without going so far as to claim evident success[19–21].

The foundation of his institute in 1829 was soon followed by that of another, the *Paulinen-Institut*, two of whose medical staff broke away to set up a rival *Paulinenhilfe* which was to become the oldest continuously functioning orthopaedic institute in Germany[22].

MUNICH

Munich had various institutes from 1833. We mention one to illustrate the *nuances* of the relations between orthopaedic craftsmen and proper doctors. This was founded in 1858 by one Krieger, an unqualified bandagist, with the medical supervision in the hands of the university professor of surgery, Johann Nepomuk Nussbaum (1829–1890). One gets the impression that here, as elsewhere, the building, equipment, appliances and running costs were provided by the lay founder and that the doctor was retained on some financial basis to provide status and medical cover and responsibility. Indeed a Berlin institute of this period was specifically described as being 'under the protection of Herr Dr Dieffenbach'. This must have been irksome at times. At any rate, Nussbaum was driven to remark – but only at the safe interval of a quarter of a century – that orthopaedics, even in 1882, still had an undesirable component of untrained practitioners. 'We still find mechanics and other craftsmen who feel a talent for serving the sick and graduate from craftsmen to bandagists and orthopaedists. It is greatly to be desired that orthopaedics also should soon follow the path traced by those we respect, and that generally trained doctors should devote the whole of their time and powers to it[23].'

While this was true enough, and what actually happened, it was nevertheless the very fear that specialization in orthopaedics might lead them to be grouped with the bandagists and splint-makers by the profession in general, and by general surgeons in particular, not to mention the paying patients, that made many reluctant to take this step at the turn of the century. This fear was correspondingly less marked in countries like the USA where there was no longstanding independent craft of appliance-maker; there the rift that had to be bridged was between the older orthopaedic surgeons who were essentially 'strap and buckle' men and the newer operatively-minded generation.

BAMBERG

To be fair, some of the craftsmen assessed the situation objectively. In Bamberg, in 1863, one **Johannes Wildberger** wrote, 'The possession or manufacture of orthopaedic appliances does not mean more than that one is a possessor or manufacturer of orthopaedic appliances, and does not automatically entitle one to be the director of an institute and, as a quack orthopaedist, to conduct unplanned, often unscientific, and imprudent experiments with the health and lives of the afflicted[24].'

Wildberger had founded his institute in 1849, in a former Benedictine monastery (the 20th century was not the only one to turn churches into health centres). Like J G Heine, he was originally a cutler and instrument-maker and had worked with Heine in Würzburg. And here we see what it was that redeems this class from the charge of being exploiting upstarts. For he became interested in chronic 'spontaneous' (i.e. congenital) dislocation of the hip, devised his own apparatus for reduction by traction and reported his results in publications embellished with photographs at a time when such illustrations were very rare[25,26]. And he was doing this, and developing orthopaedic insights, at a time when few of the doctors were doing so. Indeed, the transition from orthopaedic mechanic to medical status was still possible in the old Germanic states if royal favour was earned; and Wildberger was made a privy councillor by the Duke of Coburg and a medical doctor, *honoris causa*, by Jena University. As long as the doctors did not know or care how to treat deformities, those who did could always count on recognition, and Wildberger attracted a number of medical acolytes. Later in the century, when the doctors were better organized and subject to state requirements, their attitude to the successful mechanic or bonesetter often changed to envious resentment, as was the case in England with Hugh Owen Thomas's father (p. 78).

(p. 78)

BERLIN

An early institute, founded in 1823, was that of a medical doctor, J G Blömer, a capable man who corrected scoliosis with bolster pressure, did tenotomies for squint and had an excellent workshop.

A leading early figure is that of **Heimann Wolff Berend** (1809–1873), a Berlin graduate and Dieffenbach's assistant from 1837 to 1840; this is how he came to know Little when he returned to Berlin after having been operated by Stromeyer in Hanover, and why his name appears as one of the 'opponents' on the title-page of Little's Berlin doctoral thesis of 1837. Berend founded an institute in 1840 which came to have 120 beds and directed it for 31 years; his series of annual reports is a valuable guide to orthopaedic progress over this period[27]. We see the change from mechanical correction to osteotomy and other operative measures under general anaesthesia – he was the first, in 1847, in Berlin to operate under ether and convinced Dieffenbach to do so – and he adopted antisepsis, 'a surgery which encounters the severest obstacles in the large general hospitals', but only as part of a programme that included appliances and exercises (12th report, 1865).

His treatment of club-foot was by tenotomy followed by an ingenious traction splint[28]. He travelled, especially to France, where he was sufficiently

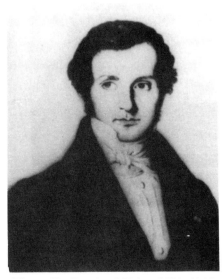

Figure 89   Bernhard Heine (1800–1846)

impressed by Guérin's myotomies for scoliosis to do the same when he returned home[29]. He also endeavoured to incorporate what was good in Ling's Swedish gymnastics in the treatment of scoliosis, having visited Stockholm in the 1850s when the Royal Central Gymnastic Institute was under the direction of Branting, who stressed the value of resisted exercises, the equivalent of modern weight-training. Berend regarded scoliosis as a primarily muscular disorder, the changes in the bones and ligaments being secondary, and its treatment as the most difficult part of orthopaedics. He was keenly interested in congenital dislocation of the hip and not over-sanguine about treatment. He noted, when visiting Duval's institute in Paris in 1842, that the 'reduction' effected by forcible traction was often a transposition of the femoral head into the obturator foramen or sciatic notch, though, as this lengthened and stabilized the limb, it was far from valueless. But he saw the matter as in process of evolution; summarizing 74 cases: 'I have demonstrated from extensive case-series that, even if reduction is not completely achieved, orthopaedics remains effective enough not to abandon this objective.'

We ought to look back at **Johann Friedrich Dieffenbach** (1792–1847), a generous and enthusiastic, if sometimes sardonic, spirit. He wrote eloquently and ironically. Much of this irony was excited by his visits to France and is quoted elsewhere in this book: his account of Guérin's exposure of Hossard's faked cures of scoliosis (p. 536) and his comments on the kangaroo-like progression of the girls on crutches in Bouvier's institute in 1838 (p. 252)[30].

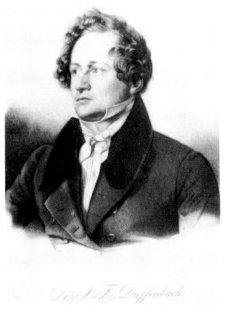

Figure 90   Johann Friedrich Dieffenbach (1792–1847)

He could not restrain himself when Pirogoff advised the injection of blood into the puncture wound of subcutaneous tenotomy to encourage reunion:

'There is nothing so preposterous in conception in science that someone or other will not actually put it into practice. You will find this generally confirmed in the whole history of surgery and medicine. I need only recall, for instance, how this one has tried to restore a sluggish fracture by inserting one galvanic plate in the mouth and the opposite plate in the anus, or how another has aimed at the same by inunction with some kind of narcotic ointment*.'

A theme that could be developed, but not at this place. Dieffenbach did much to further the practice of orthopaedics. He compiled a list of all the varieties of extension beds and chairs in 1829; it ran to 70 pages! He used plaster-of-Paris after the manipulative correction of club-foot. He sent Little to Stromeyer to have his tenotomy, was amazed by the improvement and became an enthusiast, reporting 140 personal cases in a monograph in 1841. He operated for torticollis and was the first to suggest subcutaneous drilling and the insertion of ivory pegs for pseudarthrosis. He wrote, in 1847, a plea for general anaesthesia: *Der Äther gegen den Schmerz* (Ether against pain). In addition, he saw, very clearly, as we have noted, that the care of cripples should be properly and centrally organized.

When Berend visited Stockholm, he was accompanied by **Moritz Michael Eulenburg** (1811–1877). The two wrote a companion to medical studies in 1833[31], and later Eulenburg became an enthusiastic advocate of gymnastic methods for scoliosis, though cooler in later years[32]. He shared the view of Berend and of the French that the basic cause was a disequilibrium of the spinal musculature, and that treatment must therefore be by exercise and galvanism. In 1863 he described congenital elevation of the scapula before Sprengel's account of 1891 gained the latter the eponym (though Eulenburg thought it a dislocation and failed to spot its congenital nature)[33].

In 1890, Berlin saw the opening of a university clinic for orthopaedic surgery. Its first director was **Julius Wolff** (1836–1902), a pupil of Langenbeck, who suggested that Wolff's doctoral thesis should be on the experimental production of bone in animals. He became absorbed in the work of Belchier, Hunter, Duhamel and Flourens on osteogenesis (p. 260). This was interrupted by service in the Franco-Prussian War and by his founding of a private hospital afterwards; but this was incorporated by the university in 1890, which led to his becoming a professor at the age of 54, and in 1892 he produced his famous book, *Das Gesetz der Transformation der Knochen* (The Law of Bone Transformation), which relates form to function.

---

*As given by Meier, in an edition of Dieffenbach's lecture course at the Charité Hospital in Berlin, 1840. The writer was rash enough to employ this quotation in a sceptical manner in a letter to Dr Bassett, of New York, who has so courageously and convincingly championed the electrotherapy of fractures, and was promptly rapped over the knuckles; *of course*, electrodes in the mouth and anus would affect every part of the body, just as the electrocardiogram can be recorded from any part.

There were no X-rays then (there would be three years later) and Wolff developed a technique of thin bone section to study the trabecular structure. Bone deformation, he found, led to changes in internal structure and secondary adaptive changes. The use of normal bone in a new way leads to adaptive changes in form and pattern; if a deformed bone is corrected and its function normalized, the normal shape and form are resumed. The Law formally states: 'Every change in the form and function of a bone, or of function alone, is followed by specific definite changes in its internal architecture and equally definite secondary changes in its external configuration, in accordance with mathematical laws.' Elsewhere: 'Structure is nothing else than the physical expression of function ... under pathologic conditions the structure and form of the parts change according to the abnormal conditions of force transmission[34–36].'

In his *Menders of the Maimed*[37], partly perhaps because it was written during the first world war, Sir Arthur Keith damns this book with faint praise. Admittedly, there were excellent plates illustrating the marvellous remodelling of the internal structure of deformed bones, 'but nowhere does he mention the cunning engineers. His monograph ... is a stage set out with all the necessary fittings for a play, but the actors are never called on to appear ... when we speak of Wolff's Law, we really mean the law of osteoblasts.' It was the osteoblasts, said Keith, which responded to mechanical stress and hormones and biochemical changes and inflammation and alterations in blood-supply. Sir Charles Bell, in *Illustrations of Paley's Natural Theology* (1834) had said: 'The inert and mechanical provision of the bone always bears relation to the living muscular power of the limb'. The flux and remodelling of bone tissue had been observed long before by Hunter: 'The part that seems already formed is not so in reality, for it is forming every day by having new matter thrown into it, till the whole substance is complete; even then it is constantly changing its mattter'. And Flourens: 'If ... new molecules are continuously laid down ... old molecules are as continually absorbed; thus there is a continuous transformation of substance[38].'

In 1838, in his *Human Osteology*, F O Ward, a London anatomist, compared the architecture of the femoral neck with that of a street-lamp in a triangular wall-bracket, the horizontal trabeculae responding to stress and the oblique ones to pressure. (Over a century later, H A Brittain of Norwich, England, used this same analogy in his *Architectural Principles in Arthrodesis* to justify his extra-articular fusions of the hip and shoulder.)

In 1867, von Meyer, a Zürich anatomist, wrote of *The Architecture of the Spongiosa*, and Culmann, an engineer, showed that the structure of the femoral neck was the mathematical solution to the stress of body-weight, as in a crane. In 1883, Hugh Owen Thomas said: 'Eccentric forms, that cannot be altered in the dead body without rupture or fracture can, during life, be altered by mechanical influence, as time and physiological action will commode the part to the direction of the employed force[39].' Most succinct of all, J B Murphy of Chicago: 'The amount of growth in a bone depends on the need for it.'

This long digression, unfair to Wolff, is justified by its illustration of the continuity of orthopaedic thought. The book is worth rereading. Wolff was an enterprising surgeon; he essayed the transplantation of allogenic bone[40], he tried to restore motion to ankylosed joints by simple arthrolysis with a chisel and passive motion[41,42] and he was one of the first to follow Albert in arthrodesing the paralysed shoulder[43]. It may seem now that he was stating the obvious; but that is a recurrent and necessary duty.

In 1902, Wolff was succeeded in his chair by **Albert Hoffa** (1859–1907), born at the Cape in South Africa and educated in Germany, where he established a private orthopaedic clinic in Würzburg in 1886, having been an assistant surgeon at the Julius Hospital, now the university clinic.

Hoffa was the leading orthopaedist of the Berlin school at the turn of the century, but his survival there was pitifully short. He was a thoughtful and forward-looking surgeon, seeing scoliosis as the main problem of the future (p. 529)[44]. Although an enthusiast for the manipulative reduction of congenital dislocation of the hip (which he and Lorenz seem to have appropriated from Paci – see p. 430 – and over which he and Lorenz contested in feats of exhibitionism in Europe and America), he was ready to operate for cases where manipulation had failed or was too late to be safe, and was one of the very first to do so. We should note that German authors, up to and beyond 1900, advocated excision of the femoral head as a routine for the treatment of nonsuppurative hip disease, as Hoffa states in his *Handbook Die praktische Chirurgie* of 1902: so much so that Noble Smith, in London in 1889, urged that, because not every case of hip disease was tuberculous (and this was prescient, since some were to become known as Perthes' disease), excision should *not* be a routine.

Hoffa described chronic inflammatory hypertrophy of the infrapatellar fat-pad, a once dubious lesion that has gained in popularity since arthroscopy[45]. He wrote an excellent textbook of orthopaedic surgery that was reissued posthumously up to 1924[46]. He resected the prominent ribs in scoliosis[47], and suggested reefing of the medial parapatellar tissues for recurrent dislocation of the patella[48]. He performed Achilles tenotomy for severe flat-foot[49], abandoning this on realizing that the contracture was secondary, not primary. He devised machines for derotation and correction of scoliosis. One of his main achievements was the training of Konrad Biesalski. His death at the age of 48 was a tragedy[50].

Roughly contemporary in Berlin with Hoffa, **Friedrich Trendelenburg** (1844–1924) held the chair there in general surgery, in passage between chairs at Rostock and Leipzig. His lifelong interest in orthopaedic disorders may possibly have been related to a period of study in Glasgow before graduating in Berlin in 1866. In 1878, he repeated Langenbeck's attempt to nail a fracture of the neck of the femur[51]. In 1889 he advocated supramalleolar fracture of the tibia and fibula, allowing them to unite in varus, to correct severe flat-foot[52]. In 1900 he anticipated Robert Jones and Albee in treating recurrent dislocation of the patella by splitting the lateral femoral condyle in the coronal plane and wedging the anterior portion forward with an ivory peg, not a very effective measure[53].

He is best known for his famous sign of coxo-femoral incompetence, described in 1895[54]. We need not go into this in detail here, merely note

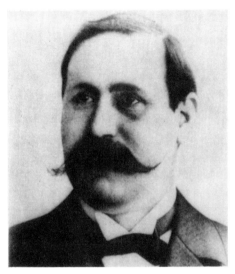

Figure 91   Albert Hoffa (1859–1907)

that the characteristic dip away from the standing side was formerly attributed to sliding of the femoral head on the ilium until Trendelenberg showed by photographic analysis (with the aid of his assistant, Perthes) that the real cause was that the hip abductors were inadequate or their fulcrum unstable. We should also remember that he thought the 'gliding' occurred at the lumbosacral joint.

It may be interesting to note that when, around 1900, Hoffa listed the most important European orthopaedic centres of the earlier 19th century, this was his list: Heine (Würzburg 1812), the most notable; Leithof (Lübeck 1818); Humbert (Bar-le-Duc 1821); Blömer and Hammers (Berlin 1823); Pravaz and Guérin (Paris 1825); Werner (Königsberg 1826); Delpech (Montpellier 1828); Jacob Heine (Canstatt 1829); Langaard (Copenhagen 1834); Hirsch (Prague 1845); Roon (Petersburg 1850).

Konrad Biesalski (1868–1930) greatly developed what had been Hoffa's institute and was very active in organizing aid for crippled children, for he viewed orthopaedics as being sociological as much as surgical. When Leo Mayer came from New York in 1912 to study tendon transplantation with Fritz Lange at München, they found the problem of adhesions troublesome, and it was solved only by fundamental research with Biesalski in Berlin into the nutrition of tendons. This recognized the use of the recipient tendon-sheath and the gentle handling of the transferred tendon with its paratenon, leading to a joint monograph in 1916 from which much of the success in tendon transplantation derives. During 1903–9, Biesalski compiled a famous census of crippled children in Germany: there were 100 000 and only 3000 available beds. He promoted their treatment and education and founded the Oscar-Helene Heim outside Berlin in 1913, where he worked for the rest of his life. He was editor of the *Zeitschrift für orthopädische Chirurgie*, founded in Stuttgart in 1892, until his death; and one of his ambitions was for a history of orthopaedics, which he urged at the 16th Congress of the German Orthopaedic Association in 1921 as the foundation for further advance.

LEIPZIG

The first medical orthopaedist in Germany, **Johann Christian Gottfried Jörg** (1779–1856) worked here, and in 1810 – 18 years before the publication of Delpech's *De l'Orthomorphie* – wrote what is regarded as the first scientific textbook of orthopaedics in the world: *Über die Verkrümmungen des menschlichen Körpers und eine rationelle und sichere Heilarzt derselben* (On the distortions of the human body and a rational and certain method of curing the same). And yet Jörg, like Deventer in Holland (p. 307), was an obstetrician,

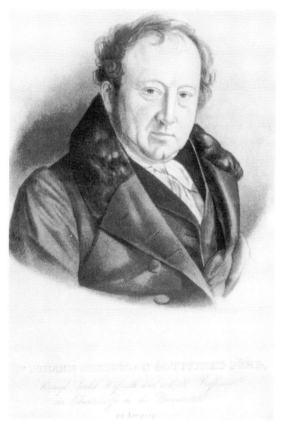

Figure 92   Johann Christian Gottfried Jörg (1779–1856)

a professor of obstetrics, and to some extent a paediatrician. He wrote an excellent account of the morbid anatomy and treatment of club-foot, incriminating the tibial muscles, especially the posterior, as the cause of inveterate adduction[55]. He advocated the mechanical management of deformities with appliances and corsets. He says nothing of the operative treatment of torticollis, except that it might have been suitable for a cruder age, but that every case could be cured by his own ingenious device in which a head-band was connected to a breastplate by a ratchet.

Jörg succeeded in distinguishing between the curvatures of scoliosis and spinal tuberculosis, but was uncertain about the cause of the gibbus in the latter: the proximate cause lay mostly in the bones, less often in the muscles, and rickets, foul air and malnutrition played a part. He laboured to get victims of infantile paralysis on their feet again. He encouraged the chiropodists. He seems to have had an intuition about the cause of rickets, preferring to admit patients to his own home for supervision, so that it virtually became an orthopaedic clinic, since, left to their parents, 'their diet is seldom adhered to as is necessary if rickets is to be avoided thereby.' He made a poignant appeal which indicates how critical for the advance of orthopaedics was a change in medical attitudes at the start of the 19th century:

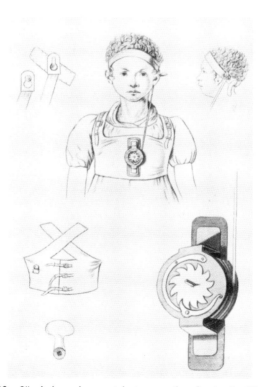

Figure 93   Jörg's ingenious ratchet correction for torticollis, 1810

'I must risk an entreaty, which is that in future the better heads among the doctors should not let themselves be so intimidated by the diseases discussed here ... and rescue these afflictions from the executioners, pastors and the like: for, sad to say ... not only the common man but often also the educated turn to these people because they were occasionally lucky here and there, *and because the patients with these disorders were often rejected outright by the better doctors*' (my italics).

This was why the surgeons in Würzburg were so tolerant of Heine and why lay therapists were so successful in practice, if not in results, until far into the century. Orthopaedics was not a field in which a doctor could count on being seen to be successful or show a rapid benefit, rather the reverse; better leave it to the bandagist, splint-maker, masseur, even the charlatan. Yet there came a point when the financial rewards of the latter excited medical hostility.

An institute opened in Leipzig in 1829 and was later managed by two doctors associated with remedial exercises: **Daniel Gottlieb Moritz Schreber** (1808–1861) and **Karl Hermann Schildbach** (1824–1888). They were influenced by the Swedish gymnastic school and helped create a wave of enthusiasm for the method. The 'Schreber gardens' were private or home gymnasia and his book on medical gymnastics went into 30 editions. Schildbach's reports on the institute show it to have been one where the orthopaedics of the spine were carefully and scientifically developed; he was appointed a university lecturer in orthopaedics in 1875 and opened the first state university orthopaedic polyclinic in 1876.

George Clemens Perthes was professor of surgery in Leipzig from 1903 to 1910, before moving to Tübingen. Perthes' disease is discussed at p. 199 but we should add that he pioneered the use of radiotherapy for malignant tumours, operated for habitual dislocation of the patella and described the Bankart lesion at the shoulder in 1906, 12 years before Bankart.

HANOVER

George Friedrich Louis Stromeyer (1804–1876) was the son of a surgeon and spent a year in London after qualifying. His introduction of tenotomy for club-foot and his operating on Little, referred by Dieffenbach, are discussed elsewhere (p. 499). In fact, his association with Hanover was not a long one; he founded an orthopaedic institute there in 1829 and transferred this to his own home in 1834 – the prospectus emphasizes that one floor was reserved for extension beds and that there was a gymnastic session twice daily in the open air – but he was appointed professor of surgery at Erlangen in 1838. In 1854 he moved to Kiel, where he was succeeded by his son-in-law, Esmarch in 1857. (Stromeyer's first paper on Achilles tenotomy appeared in 1833[56], and his expanded book on operative orthopaedics in 1839[57]. In the preface he says that he intends to use operative measures to speed up the slower treatment of the 'mechanical orthopaedists' and to challenge comparison with general surgery: 'Progress would be made if both methods

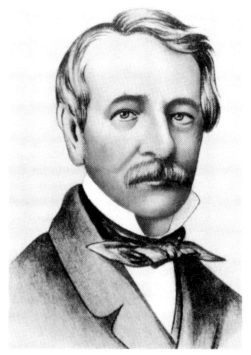

Figure 94 Georg Friedich Louis Stromeyer (1804–1876)

could be followed and perfected by the same artist.')

A very famous hospital, the *Annastift*, was founded in Hanover in 1897 and had an excellent orthopaedic department. From 1924 to 1936 the senior surgeon, until his expulsion by the Nazis, was Bruno Valentin, to whose inspiration this book and orthopaedic history in general owes so much. Under his direction the Institute doubled in size to 400 beds.

DARMSTADT

Darmstadt is linked with the Krauss family. **Gustav Friedrich Mathäus Krauss** (1813–1887) graduated at Bonn in 1834 and was inspired to take up orthopaedics by a chance visit to Heine's clinic at Scheveningen. He was also impressed by Bouvier and Guérin in Paris. In 1837 he began practice in England but friction with Little led to his return to Germany in 1843, where he developed tarsal resection for club-foot[58]. His son, Gustav junior (1846–1910), of little account otherwise, left a fortune to build an institute for the correction of deformities; this was the 'Kraussianum' built during the first world war in München for the free treatment of crippled children and the promotion of research.

MÜNSTER

In Münster, another famous clinic, the *Hüfferstiftung*, was founded in 1889 by Christoph Temmink and funded by Wilhelm Hüffer. Temmink left after three years but the institute came to play an important part in German orthopaedics, showing exactly how these private German institutes provided a stepping-stone to a more rational orgnization, for Temmink wrote, in 1888:

> 'Your task, first and foremost, is to divert orthopaedics into a public hospital whose chief aim is the treatment of the poor. Nowhere ... does the duty to provide help appear so important as here, where the last element of possible self-help has disappeared; and, of any category of persons, the poor cripples have a right to work ... as useful members of the social order. The public orthopaedic hospital is a challenge to humanity ... it should be a school for the training of therapeutic personnel, while simultaneously providing the conditions for the thriving development of orthopaedic science and skill[59].'

So much for the role of the institutes in German orthopaedics. Let us now consider some individuals.

Richard von Volkmann (1830–1889) lived in Halle, Saxony, where his father was professor of anatomy, and became professor of surgery and one of the first in Germany to introduce Listerian antiseptics. His famous paper on ischaemic muscle paralyses and contractures appeared in 1881[60]. This ascribed the cause, not, as had been assumed, to nerve compression but to direct changes in the muscles produced by arterial occlusion, and emphasizes the preliminary weakness, an often overlooked early warning; he noticed its occurrence in the lower limb as well as in the forearm. 'Half a day or less is enough to reduce the fingers to permanent and pitiful deformity.' It is relevant that this paper appeared eight years after Esmarch had popularized his bandage, though Esmarch had certainly recognized its dangers. Volkmann was gloomy about treatment of the contracture; if forcible correction were attempted, 'one would more readily break the bones and rupture the tendons before the muscles would yield.'

Like others, he thought club-foot due to intrauterine pressure[61]. He wrote the section on locomotor disorders in a famous surgical textbook of 1882[62], in which he noted that the improvement after forcible 'reduction' of congenital dislocation of the hip was not necessarily due to actual reposition of the femoral head. He described *caries sicca*, a slow dry tuberculous destruction of bone without caseation[63], he also seems to have described acute transient synovitis of the hip in children, and Key credited him with first distinguishing the joint affections of haemophilia from rheumatism[64].

In 1874 he performed subcutaneous osteotomy for vicious ankylosis of the knee[65]; he resected the first metatarsophalangeal joint for hallux valgus[66] and the rib-hump in scoliosis[67]. He promoted and improved methods of traction in fracture treatment. His thinking about the operative management of joint tuberculosis is interesting. At one time he had been a resectionist. Then, around 1870, he questioned whether this was adequate: the mortality was high and he felt that systemic disturbance and fever after resection were indications for amputation, but did not maintain this position for long. He distinguished the mainly synovial form as more suitable for resection than the type with bone destruction and even came to suggest that, in the former group, removal of soft tissues might suffice, thus heralding the procedure to be labelled synovectomy by Mignon[68] in France, eventually to gain such popularity as it ever achieved mainly in nontuberculous conditions.

Johann Friedrich August von Esmarch (1825–1908) is best known as a military surgeon interested in blood-loss and first-aid. Born in Schleswig-Holstein, he was active in the war against Denmark and in 1857 became professor of surgery at Kiel after Stromeyer, whose daughter he married. In 1866 and 1871 he was engaged in the wars against Austria and France and in 1871 became Surgeon-General to the Prussian Army and wrote a *Manual of Military Surgical Technique*, a copy of which was sent to Bigelow in Boston by the German Empress in return for some service. He was a first-aid enthusiast. His collected works appeared in 1873 and include the famous 1873 paper, *On the Artificial Emptying of Blood-Vessels in Operations*, which was actually an address to students in the operating-room. The limb was exsanguinated with the well known rubber bandage and haemostasis maintained with rubber tubing round the upper part of the limb in place of the older tourniquet which relied on pressure directly over the artery. 'If we now compare the operation of today with that of yesterday, it will at once be evident to you how great are the advantages of this mode of proceeding, both for the patient and for the operator.' Ill-effects were possible rather than probable, but it was important not to use the bandage on infected limbs for fear of proximal dispersion of the infection and to rely on elevation alone.

Another military surgeon, **Georg Axhausen** (1877–1960) became interested in the process of 'aseptic' or avascular necrosis of bone, as distinct from the necrosis so often seen in infections, and this led to pioneer work on bone grafts and to the concept of what Phemister came to call 'creeping substitution'. In an article in 1910[69] he thought that necrosis occurred at the bone-ends in every fracture, and stimulated and was replaced by periosteal proliferation; and he also thought that focal necrosis of subchondral bone caused changes in the overlying articular cartilage which led to 'arthritis deformans'. This was a direct step towards the modern concept of the aetiology of Perthes' disease in children and primary necrosis of the femoral head in adults. The necrosis and sequestration of osteomyelitis he ascribed to septic infarction of the intraosseous vessels[70]. In 1928 he further developed the idea that 'primary epiphyseal necroses' were due to multiple minute epiphyseal or metaphyseal infarcts due to thrombosis or embolism, giving rise to characteristic histologic and radiographic appearances[71]. This was the proximate source of a flood of reports on clinical varieties of 'ostochondritis' in every part of the body, often ill-founded.

Restricting ourselves to German authors, the advent of the X-rays occurred at just the right time in this context. The first pictures of Perthes' disease were made in 1898, but not published by Perthes' assistant, Schwarz, until 1914, in Tübingen. Schwarz, who was killed in the first world war, thought this a vascular disorder caused by loosening of the epiphyseal plate as distinct from the frank detachment of a slipped epiphysis, a fundamental distinction at that time. Köhler, the world's first professor of radiology, in Wiesbaden in 1905, noted a case of flattening and fragmentation of the femoral head which he considered to be not tuberculous, but *infarktähnlich* (infarct-like)[72], and similar observations were made by Preiser in 1907[73] and by Oberst in 1908[74].

In the context of bone-grafting, Macewen's famous success of 1879 stimulated much research, mainly experimental, and in 1908 Axhausen published an exhaustive monograph[75] in which he straddled the conflicting theories by asserting that that part of a free autogenous graft in direct contact with host tissue remained alive while its deeper parts died and served as a scaffolding for invasion by new bony tissue. He also investigated the fate of transplanted epiphyses, but the results were not encouraging[76].

All this is cognate with the fundamental work of **Erich Lexer** (1867–1937) on the transplantation and viability of tissues, including bone-ends and whole joints. Lexer was a Würzburg graduate of 1890 who then studied in Berlin, became professor of surgery at Königsberg in 1905, and occupied chairs at Jena and Freiburg until he succeeded Sauerbruch in 1928. While still in Würzburg he made some classic studies on experimental osteomyelitis by giving staphylococci intravenously after traumatizing a bone, showing that suppuration occurred at the site of injury, i.e. the disease was haematogenous and appeared at sites of least resistance[77]. This research led him to insist on the importance of early drainage. He became interested in the changes in bone circulation in relation to fractures, osteomyelitis and avascular necrosis, and his dye studies showed the formation of new vessels at fracture sites[78].

Like Axhausen, Lexer worked on the fate of bone grafts and epiphyseal transplants, including the transplantation of joints, in whole or part[79]. It must be recalled that attempts at interposition arthroplasty dated back at least to Carnochan in New York in 1840 (wood interposition at the temporomandibular joint), Péan in 1894[80] (metal plates), Chlumsky in Germany in 1896[81] (various metals, rubber, celluloid), Foedre, also in Germany in 1896[82] (pig's bladder, very popular), Robert Jones in Liverpool in 1902[83] (gold foil), J B Murphy in Chicago in 1905[84,85] (fat and fascia) and others. Lexer first used fascia lata with some fat attached, easy to obtain as an autogenous graft, tough and non-irritative. Later, around 1908, he transplanted the articular ends from other individuals and even entire joints, usually after amputations, sometimes from cadavers, but the results were not brilliant. His work was extended to free tendon transplantation after World War I[86].

The entire subject of free autogenous transplants is reviewed in his 1919 book, which led to the work of Gallie and Le Mesurier in Canada, especially on the use of fascial strips to extend transplanted muscles. His arthroplasties were marked by a distaste for inorganic foreign material and he sometimes used cartilage discs cut from the back of the patella to form new joint surfaces. His joint transplants were of three kinds: half-joints; both bone-ends with their articular cartilage; and whole joints with their capsules. These he used after local resection of tumours involving a joint surface and also – rather than osteotomy – to replace joints ankylosed in poor position. These operations never became popular in the West, partly because the results were uncertain, more so because of the availability of resistant metals and plastics just before and after World War II. They did attract attention in Russia, where cadavers were more available than expensive inorganic prostheses and where refrigerated joints or parts of joints were popular in the 1960s and 70s. However, there has been a recent revival of interest in these massive allografts in the USA, in great part due to Professor Mankin at the Massachusetts General Hospital[87]. Such transplants may be intercalary or osteoarticular and can be combined with chemotherapy and banked freeze-dried or frozen or in antibiotic solutions, or a combination of these (see also at p. 552).

Hans von Baeyer (1875–1941) succeeded Riedinger in Würzburg but left to become professor of orthopaedics at Heidelberg until 1933. He investigated muscle action and he devised the bifurcation osteotomy for unreduced congenital dislocation of the hip in 1918. This accepted the displacement and compensated for the instability by a subtrochanteric osteotomy in which the upper end of the shaft was placed in the acetabulum and the small upper fragment allowed to abut against the main shaft, providing two points of support. This was popularized by Lorenz. Von Baeyer also performed rerouting of tendons, e.g. of the flexor pollicis longus for thenar palsy, and a most ingenious translocation of the peroneus longus tendon to replace the tibialis posterior, as well as an operation for recurrent shoulder dislocation similar to the Nicola procedure[88].

Otto Madelung (1846–1926) was a general surgeon with minor orthopaedic interests who became assistant professor of surgery in Bonn in 1881, then at Rostock and finally at Strassburg (then German) in 1894. In 1878 he described his eponymous wrist deformity (it had previously been described by Dupuytren), which he thought was due to a disturbance of growth of the anterior part of the radial epiphysis causing forward angulation[89].

Adolf Stöffel (1880–1937), of Mannheim, later of Heidelberg, introduced partial peripheral neurectomy for spastic paralysis. This was an approach on the efferent side, as distinct from procedures by sensory ramisection or ganglionectomy. In his original technique he sought to identify fibre groups within main peripheral trunks by electrical stimulation and sectioning the appropriate bundles[90], but this proved unsatisfactory and was replaced by division of the actual muscle branches, such as those to the gastrocnemii or the obturator nerve. Selig in 1914 performed obturator section within the pelvis, but extraperitoneally[91].

Themistocles Gluck (1853–1942) is an interesting character because he was so innovative as to be ahead of his time (and of the available materials). He studied in Leipzig, and then in Berlin as Bernhard von Langenbeck's last pupil at the University Clinic, and was appointed professor of surgery at Bucharest in 1883 (he was Rumanian born). In 1890 he returned to Berlin as senior surgeon to the new Kaiser- und Kaiserin-Kinderkrankenhaus. He worked on nerve suture, including the use of synthetic interposition structures as guidelines, and employed synthetic replacements for tendons and other tissues. Here, he may have anticipated Nicoladoni and Lange; the latter certainly acknowledged his precedence. In 1885 he demonstrated fracture fixation with a nickel-coated steel plate and screws, and used this for

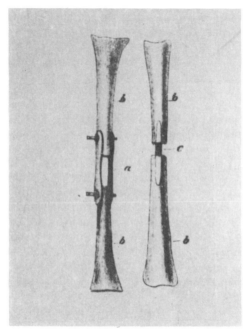

Figure 95　Themistocles Gluck (1853–1942); *left*, fracture fixation with nickel-coated steel plate and screws, 1885; *right*, intramedullary fixation with ivory rod, 1890. (Zippel, J. and Meyer-Ralfs, M. [1975]. *Ztschr. f. Orthop.*, **113**, 134)

compound fractures in the Balkan Wars. In 1890, he used an ivory intramedullary peg and also intramedullary nails.

After animal experiments with inserts of aluminium, wood, glass, celluloid and steel, he began a series of total joint replacements for tuberculosis or tumours, after excision, in the knee, shoulder, elbow, wrist and hip. Some of this is treated at a later page (p. 588). On 9 June 1890, in a 19-year-old patient with severe caries of the wrist, he used an ivory prosthesis with intramedullary fixation in the radius and ulna and 5th metacarpal; and in the same year he inserted a hinged ivory knee-joint. There is, however, no evidence that he used the method electively for arthrosis: only for chronic tuberculosis, after tumour excision and for neglected juxtarticular fractures with poor function. His ankle prostheses were anchored by metal prongs in the shafts of the metacarpals. All his joint replacements eventually suppurated or developed tuberculous sinuses, and he admitted as much as early as 1891. His work was severely criticized by his former teacher, E von Bergmann, as 'a discredit to German science', to be combated by every means. Gluck was simply thinking ahead; if he had had modern plastic cement instead of his primitive mix of plaster, pumice and resin, matters might have taken a different turn. There are still those, naturally in the East, who consider ivory an ideal prosthetic material[164–166].

Fritz Lange (1866–1952) of Munich was an enterprising and innovative surgeon. Platt says that he was probably the first, in 1910, to wire the

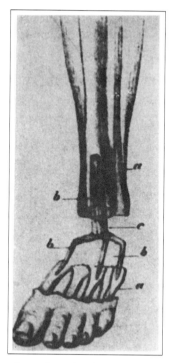

Figure 96   Gluck: ivory and metal total replacement of ankle and tarsal joints, 1890

vertebral spinous processes together, but this is not correct; Hadra had done this in Texas in 1891. Lange also tried inserting steel bars or celluloid plates over the laminae and wiring them to the processes[93]. Hadra's case had been for fracture of the cervical spine; he thought that the method might be useful for tuberculosis and it was for this that Lange, apparently independently, applied it.

Lange performed a biceps transplant into a paralysed quadriceps in 1898 but obtained better results by attaching it directly to the patella and came to insist on the importance of direct subperiosteal attachment of transplanted tendons[94]. In his work on tendon transplanation he became an enthusiast for the use of silk strands to extend short motors, as when the erector spinae was used to replace the glutei, also as a focus for the formation of firm fibrous bands, and reported 200 cases of its use in tendon transplantation in Joachimsthal's *Handbuch der Orthopädischen Chirurgie* in 1905. He also used silk for tenodesis and as a check ligament until this was replaced by fascial strips in the hands of Codivilla and Payr, though this too was eventually discarded. He wrote a book on the orthopaedic management of poliomyelitis in 1930[95] and, in collaboration with others, in 1913, what was to be the standard German text on orthopaedics for many years[96].

Erwin Payr (1871–1946) was a pupil of Nicoladoni and maintained an

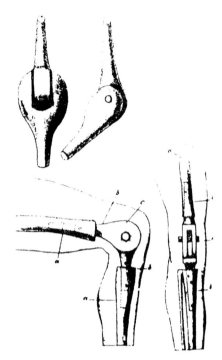

Figure 97   Gluck: hinged ivory knee replacement, 1890

interest in the mobilization of ankylosed joints from an early paper on operative treatment in 1910[97] to an authoritative manual in 1934[98]. His use of fascia late to prolong the insertions of transplanted tendons stimulated all Gallie's work in this field in Canada. Editorially, with Kuttner, he founded the *Ergebnisse der Chirurgie und Orthopädie* in Berlin in 1910. It is odd that Willis Campbell, as an apostle of fascial interposition arthroplasty, has nothing to say of Payr's work in any field in his *Operative Orthopaedics* of 1939.

Alfred Schanz (1870–1932), of Dresden, wrote an orthopaedic text in 1905[99]. He is best known for his low abduction osteotomy of the femur at the level of the ischial tuberosity for ununited fracture of the neck of the femur; also for old irreducible congenital dislocation of the hip, which stabilized both fragments against the side of the pelvis. This is described in his *Praktische Orthopädie* of 1928 and in earlier papers[100], and was based on the recognition that in the bifurcation osteotomy of von Baeyer and Lorenz the shaft rarely remained within the acetabulum; the operation found great favour with Gaensslen in America[101]. Schanz also favoured transplantation of the sartorius to the rectus femoris tendon for quadriceps paralysis, a popular procedure at one time in Germany though patently never as satisfactory as a biceps transplant to the patella. He also attempted derotation procedures in scoliosis.

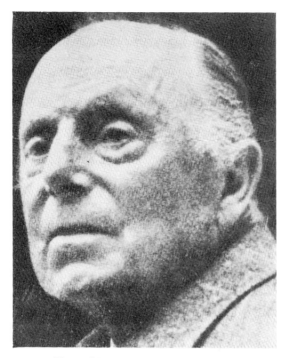

Figure 98   Fritz Lange (1866–1952)

Schanz had a famous pupil, **Friedrich Pauwels** (1885–1980) whose life and work were centred on Aachen. After studying orthopaedics under Lorenz in Vienna and Schanz in Dresden he founded an orthopaedic institute and workshop in Aachen in 1913 and rapidly developed a lifelong interest in biomechanical influences on the growth and behaviour of bone and cartilage, pursuing (and correcting) the earlier work of Julius Wolff. This led to his famous classification of fracture angles at the hip into Pauwels types I, II and III and to the treatment of ununited hip fractures by simple realignment procedures, which, when extended to hip arthrosis, were shown to result in restoration of radiologic joint-space and disappearance of cavities and sclerosis. In 1935 he published *Der Schenkelhalsbruch – ein mechanisches Problem* and summed up his life's work in 1973 in his *Atlas der Biomechanik der gesunden und kranken Hüfte*, translated in 1976 as *Biomechanics of the Normal and Diseased Hip*. In 1934 he became director of the new orthopaedic department at the Aachen city hospital and continued to his retirement in 1960 at age 75, having been made professor in 1942. His work is obviously complementary to that of McMurray in Liverpool and exemplifies a biologic approach to hip disorders which has temporarily been overshadowed by joint replacement procedures but is likely to regain favour.

Georg Hohmann succeeded Lange in the Munich chair and is known for his interest in foot problems[102,103] and for devising the standard operation for tennis elbow in 1933[104].

The name of Langenbeck is confusing, because there were three. The most famous was the Berlin surgeon, **Bernhard Rudolf Conrad Langenbeck** (1810–1887), successor to Dieffenbach, inventor of the famous knee-joint retractor for his medial parapatellar approach[105], and teacher of **Theodor Billroth** (1829–1894). Both engaged in tenotomy for club-foot and used plaster postoperatively, though with some apprehension about gangrene. Langenbeck also corrected rickety deformities by subcutaneous osteotomy, first drilling the bone and then dividing it with a keyhole saw and snapping it through, first in 1852 for ankylosis of the hip and later for ankylosis of the knee, a useful popularization of Barton's technique (p. 381) in the pre-Listerian era[106]. In 1850 he essayed fixation of a fractured neck of femur by driving a nail through the trochanter. He advocated excision of the whole bone in some cases of osteomyelitis. Bernhard's cousin was **Maximilian Adolf Langenbeck** (1818–1877), of Göttingen, who devised a sort of vertical rack for scoliotics in which the victim was fastened upright to a post, with head traction, and pressure applied to the convexity by a board thrust forward by a screw. A Langenbeck of a previous generation, perhaps father of one of the cousins, was **Conrad Johann Martin Langenbeck** (1776–1851), also of Göttingen, who devised an extension bed for scoliotics with lateral traction bands. He worked for a time at the Julius Hospital in Würzburg, where he commented on the excellent services of Johann Georg Heine as instrument-maker.

Franz König (1832–1910), also of Göttingen, is known for his forcible correction of club-foot over a wooden wedge and for developing, in 1891, the construction of an osteoperiosteal shelf for congenital dislocation of the hip (though this had been suggested and practised long before by Guérin)[107]. He was one of the first to definitively establish the relationship between haemophilia and haemophilic arthropathy, previously considered as 'rheumatic' or gouty, though we have noted that Volkmann gave this some attention. And König stressed that misdiagnosis could have fatal results. He noted the three stages of the disease: the acute haemarthrosis, the secondary pan-arthritis, and the late contracture or ankylosis and the resemblance of this last to tuberculosis (two of three patients operated on this supposition bled to death). 'The question what to do for bleeders' joints is completely secondary to the question what *not* to do[108].' In 1875 he repeated Langenbeck's hip nailing[109].

We allude at various pages to the work of **Oscar Vulpius**, of Heidelberg, on tendon transplantation, though he favoured suture to the stub of the replaced tendon instead of subperiosteal attachment like Lange[110]. He wrote many papers on the technique and indications between 1897 and World War I and a monograph on its application to poliomyelitis in 1910[111]. He repeated Albert's arthrodesis of the shoulder in 1888[112], had a fancy for celluloid in splintage[113], and founded the *Zentralblatt für chirurgische und mechanische Chirurgie* in Berlin in 1907.

Extremely important contributions to the radiological study of the normal and diseased spine were made by **Schmorl** in Dresden. He found that Paget's disease was present in three per cent of autopsy specimens[114] and is famous for his description of the cartilage nodes due to disc herniation into the vertebral bodies[115]. In 1932, with Junghanns, he produced a splendid Atlas of the spine in health and disease[116].

We can do no more than briefly mention **Strümpell**'s work on ankylosing spondylitis[117] and that of the neurologist, **Erb**, on his eponymous birth palsy of the brachial plexus[118].

We must not overlook the essential contributions of the pathologists and the radiologists.

Rudolf Virchow (1821–1902), one of the many great men who adorned Würzburg (for a time before his appointment as Professor in Berlin and first director of the Institute of Pathology built for him there by the state) is famous for ushering in the era of cellular pathology, as distinct from morbid anatomy, and for teaching that disease was not so much an invasion of the body by something extrinsic but the total reaction of cells and tissues to an outside influence, to be echoed much later by Hans Selye in his theory of stress disorders. He described and named osteoid tissue, as seen in rickets, as uncalcified bone in one phase of osteogenesis[119] and surmised the fundamental morphogenic identity of bone, cartilage and connective tissue[120]. This illuminated the processes involved in bone healing and bone tumours. He described spina bifida occulta in 1875 and myositis ossificans progressiva in 1894, but it was unfortunate that he used the term 'arthritis deformans' for both rheumatoid and osteoarthritis[121]. Nor did he, at least at first, regard bone sarcoma as a specific form of tumour, merely as a type of metastatic carcinoma[122]. It is interesting that, long before Middleton and Teacher in Glasgow and Goldthwait in Boston reported on intervertebral disc prolapse, both in 1911, Virchow in 1857 refers to disc extrusion due to injury, even though this was an autopsy rather than a clinical finding.

Wilhelm Conrad Röntgen (1845–1923) was professor of physics at Würzburg (and at other times at Strassburg and Munich) and at around Christmas of 1895 reported to the Physico-Medical Society there on a new kind of ray: *Über eine neue Art von Strahlen*. This arose from an accidental observation that a discharge from an induction coil passed through a Crookes vacuum tube surrounded by black cardboard caused fluorescence on paper coated with barium platinocyanide outside the black screen. The agent was shown to penetrate books, wood, glass and thin layers of metal, but not lead sheet 1.5 mm thick, and it exposed photographic films and plates. The skeleton of the hand was cast on a fluorescent screen. These rays were produced by impingement of cathode rays on the glass wall of the tube. Röntgen thought they were due to 'longitudinal waves in the ether' and called them X-rays, but the Society insisted on 'Röntgen rays'. The observation was not quite original, as Lenard and also Hertz had shown similar effects with cathode rays, using an aluminium window in the tube, but Röntgen showed that this was unnecessary as the photoactive rays easily traversed the glass of the tube-wall.

The first observation was on 8th November 1895 and the first radiograph was of Röntgen's wife's hand on 22nd December, a truly original Christmas present. A translation of the paper appeared in *Nature* a month later[123] but its contents had been leaked to the world press only a few days after his address. One effect was that Robert Jones sent immediately to Würzburg and brought back an apparatus; this was installed at 11, Nelson Street, Liverpool and the first X-ray photogaph for clinical purposes there was made by Alan Archibald Campbell Swinton (1863–1930), a London electrical engineer, on 7 January 1896[124].

Röntgen received the Nobel Prize in 1901. There is no need to discuss the importance of this discovery to orthopaedics. But it may be worth noting that this, the most important advance in diagnosis, arose in a laboratory devoted to 'pure' research, in a purely physical study of very limited nature, and that the discovery was made by one man and at very little cost.

Gerhard Küntscher* (1900–1972) was appointed lecturer in surgery at Kiel University in 1938 and extraordinary professor in 1942. He served in the German army from 1941 to 1945, in 1943–4 in Finnish Lappland. After the war he was head of surgery at the Schleswig-Holstein municipal hospital during 1946–1957 (where the present writer studied his methods in 1948) and then at the Hamburg Hafen Krankenhaus until 1965.

He invented his famous nail in the 1930s in conjunction with an instrument-maker, Ernst Pohl, and first described it to the Kiel Medical Society in December of 1939, and soon after at the 64th annual meeting of the German Surgical Society, where, to use his own words, it created 'apprehension, consternation and resentment[125].' With Richard Maatz, he had his *Technik der Marknagelung* ready for publication in 1942 but it was destroyed in air-raids and did not appear until 1945. The great Lorenz Böhler in Vienna was initially enthusiastic[126], but very soon confessed his inability to use the technique presented by Küntscher: 'The risks with marrow nailing are much greater than predicted. We therefore use it as a rule only in femoral fractures … marrow nailing of other long bones … is shown by long-term follow-up to be more deleterious than profitable.' Although Böhler always remained enthusiastic about its use for femoral and certain other fractures, and even wrote a book about it after the war[127], this left Küntscher prejudiced academically for decades and he was never offered a chair. Nor was it warmly received by most of the German military consultants, though the field surgeons liked it: 'The functional results are uniformly good. The social advantage of the method is conspicuously revealed by the saving in time and money from the shortened stay in hospital, easy convalescence and aftertreatment … the physical condition of the patient is better from the beginning[128].'

In 1943 he was posted to Finland, outside the control of the Army medical services, because of the animosity of the profession, but this proved an advantage as his patients remained under his care. Because Germans and Finns were fighting together against Russia, the method came to be used in civilian practice in Helsinki as early as 1944, Swedish articles appeared in the same year[129], the Swedes were using Küntscher nails before the war's end at the Serafimer Hospital in Stockholm, and Küntscher's first article in English appeared in a Finnish journal in 1948[130]. Perhaps not unexpectedly, the method also appeared in the French literature in 1944[131].

---

* Küntscher, not Küntschner; Bankart, not Bankhart.

The first experience of British and American surgeons with this technique was when they encountered prisoners of war so operated in the liberation of Europe; it was rapidly and enthusiastically adopted in the West. But was Küntscher's technique truly original? No more than any orthopaedic technique can be truly original. Gluck had used it in 1890 (p. 202). A Frenchman, P L Chigot, published a paper in 1946 referring to earlier experiences in 1937[132]. Writing in 1950[133], Watson-Jones refers to the work by Hey Groves, in Bristol, England, in 1916, on the massive intramedullary nailing of gunshot fractures of the femoral shaft, by both the retrograde and the direct method: 'It occurred to me therefore to use a long internal peg or strut such as would render unnecessary any further fixation' and then Groves gives a detailed account of the retrograde method of fixation exactly as it is used today[134]. However, the metals he used were not inert and his method had no followers. Even before then, from time to time, an ingenious surgeon like Lambotte or Haglund, faced with a different femoral fracture, would seek to stabilize it with an intramedullary metal or rubber peg – it was an obvious last resort. And at the end of the 1930s, Rush in America was using longitudinal pin fixation for ulnar and femoral fractures[135] and Lambrinudi, in London, was using intramedullary Kirschner wires for fractures of both forearm bones[136]. How far is one to go back? According to Juan Farill[137], ununited fractures were treated by the Aztecs by scraping the wound and insertion of a stick of wood into the medullary canal to set the bone firmly! There is no end to such attributions. The important thing is to be the right man at the right time, which means to have the right materials as well as the right idea, and the opportunity to use it. Küntscher, not particularly likeable, was that man.

AUSTRIA

Valentin tells us that, around 1800, there lived in Vienna one **Sigmund Wolffsohn** (b.1767), 'a physician and orthopaedist, proprietor of the only existing factory for surgical appliances, including artificial limbs.' His catalogue of 1796 gives a list of the 'latest and most useful trusses, surgical machines and bandages[138]'. He was also, of course, a 'hernia doctor', and his workshop was in 'the royally and imperially approved surgical and bandage factory, at the Bauernmarkt, near Petersplatz, No 629, at the Silver Horse, on the first floor.'

To pillage Valentin further, the need to link orthopaedic institutes with remedial exercises and educational training was stressed at the Vienna Congress of German Scientists and Physicians in 1832. If one believes that the travelling showman–surgeon is essentially a 20th century figure, this will soon be dispelled by reading the 19th century literature. In the present context, Dieffenbach visited Vienna for six weeks in 1840 and demonstrated a number of operations: 14 tenotomies for torticollis, 14 for club-foot or equinus, 6 for knee contracture, an unbelievable 158 for strabismus and many others[139].

The first residential institute in Vienna opened in 1838, but lasted only four years. Another was founded in 1850 by **Friedrich Wilhelm Lorinser** (1817–1895) elsewhere and moved to the capital in 1866. As we have often noted with other institutes, this one was of genuine scientific value: Lorinser wrote several useful monographs on such subjects as *The Treatment and Cure of Contractures of the Knee and Hip Joints by a New Method* (continuous traction) in 1848, and on diseases of the spine in 1870[140].

Eduard Albert (1841–1900), 'the father of arthrodesis' (a title more deserved by Park in England), gave much attention to the study of scoliosis[141]. He was born in Bohemia, qualified in Vienna, became professor of surgery at Innsbruck in 1873 and then moved to the capital. He was something of an orthopaedic polymath. As a sequel to his stabilization of the paralytic foot by tarsal arthrodesis in 1878, his 1881 paper dealt with 'artificially produced ankyloses in paralysed limbs'. This related to four cases of poliomyelitis leaving legs unable to bear weight which he wanted to render more useful and independent of appliances. In his first case he did a transpatellar excision of the knee, suturing the bones together with silver wire, and obtained sound fusion despite some infection[142]. (Park's almost exactly similar operation, for tuberculosis, had been in 1781.)

Albert studied the structure of the synovial membrane[143] and was interested in autogenous bone-grafting, with uncertain results, even including transplantation of the entire fibula for congenital absence of the tibia[144]. His main claim to fame originated in 1881, when he performed the first successful arthrodesis of the shoulder and coined the term 'arthrodesis', applying the method to recurrent dislocation as well as paralysis[145].

Albert was the teacher of **Adolf Lorenz** (1854–1946), a name to conjure with in European orthopaedics by the end of the 19th century and one indissolubly linked with the manipulative or 'bloodless' reduction of congenital dislocation of the hip. Lorenz wrote a book on scoliosis in 1884[146], attributing it to a primary weakness of the ligamentous apparatus, and devised his own appliance for osteoclasis and broke club-feet over a padded wedge. His main study was on congenital hip dislocation, on which he wrote three treatises in 1895, 1905 and 1920[147–149], the first of these based on 100 operatively treated cases and the last entitled *The So-called Congenital Dislocation of the Hip*, this because he postulated a 'dysarthrosis iliofemoralis congenita', an arrested development in which the femoral head had never been in its socket so that 'dislocation' was an inapplicable term. His main contribution was the 'bloodless reduction', which now sounds oddly on the student's ear and which gained universal renown when it was first described in 1895[150]. The reduction was rather forceful at times and must often have caused late damage to the epiphysis, especially as Lorenz's upper age limit was higher than elsewhere. It consisted of the following stages: forced extension, flexion, forced abduction to a right angle, external rotation and gradual extension of the limb, followed by immobilization in a frog hip spica plaster in 90° abduction, 90° flexion and 90° external rotation for many months. There was an interesting rivalry and dispute over priority in this field between Lorenz in Vienna, Hoffa in Berlin and Paci in Pisa and occasional revolutionary changes in doctrine. Paci was and remained an advocate of manipulative reduction. Until 1894, Lorenz had held the view

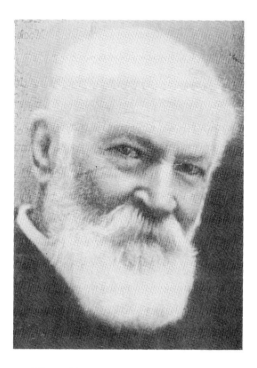

Figure 99   Adolf Lorenz (1854–1946)

that this was impossible; then he suddenly changed tack for a manipulation very much like Paci's and stuck to this, though he did a subcutaneous adductor tenotomy when necessary and, with the new century, began to demonstrate his technique in America and other countries. Thus there was a parting here from Hoffa, who continued to operate for late cases. Lorenz developed von Baeyer's bifurcation osteotomy for late irreducible dislocations. It is not often recognized that Lorenz performed obturator neurectomy for spastic paraplegia in 1891, well before Stöffel in 1911[151].

Carl Nicoladoni (1847–1902), professor of surgery at Innsbruck, is associated with the development of tendon transplantation. This consisted of the report of a single case in which the peronei were transferred to the Achilles tendon of a boy with a paralysed calf and is fully discussed elsewhere (p. 575)[152,153]. The important point is that tendon operations were not new, but that Nicoladoni was the first to apply their transfer for paralytic conditions[154]. He also treated paralytic equinus in 1882 by fusion of the ankle, excising the joint surfaces and wiring the bone ends together, very much as Albert had done a little earlier.

Konrad Büdinger (1867–1944) was Billroth's assistant in Vienna and became professor of surgery. He was interested in injuries and diseases of the knee, describing chondromalacia of the patella and the removal of loose bodies. A 1906[155] paper dealt with fissuring and degeneration of the articular cartilage of spontaneous origin, and a second paper in 1908[156] with traumatic cartilage tears.

Hans Spitzy (1872–1956) held the chair of paediatric surgery with orthopaedics in the French style in Graz, but moved to Vienna in World War I to direct a large military hospital which ultimately became a civilian orthopaedic centre. Spitzy had elaborated König's early hip-shelf operation into a true acetabuloplasty, and was interested in motor nerve anastomosis for paralysis of the arm. He also attempted the treatment of recurrent dislocation of the shoulder by suspending the humerus from the acromion by silk threads, adapting Lange's technique. Also, in 1912, he treated deltoid paralysis by transplanting both the trapezius and the pectoralis major[157].

Lorenz Böhler (1885–1973) made a worldwide impact on fracture treatment between the two world wars, comparable to that of Watson-Jones after the second war. His great textbook, which went into many editions, laid down authoritative and unvarying principles and procedures in utmost detail and, in the present author's recollection, was the young intern's bible before 1939. His life exhibited a remarkable change from that of a country doctor to the

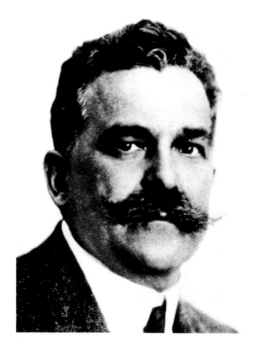

Figure 100   Hans Spitzy (1872–1956)

charge of a military hospital in the first world war; and then, in 1925, he was invited to Vienna to take charge of an accident hospital founded and funded by the Austrian social insurance authorities. His methods included the use of skin-tight plasters and early weight-bearing for leg fractures, together with energetic rehabilitation by unaided active exercises. His attitude to medullary nailing is discussed earlier.

He popularized the Böhler-Braun frame (the lineal descendant of Chessher's inclined plane) combined with routine Steinmann pin or Kirschner wire skeletal traction for femoral fractures. It is not often realized now that before this development skeletal traction was regarded as dangerously risking sepsis, whereas Böhler used the method freely, even in the outpatient department. He also advocated reduction of fractures after injection of novocaine directly into the haematoma. He also established that nonunion and pseudarthrosis of the shafts of long bones were commoner in healthy young men and treated these by drilling the sclerosed bone ends. Not that this was original: Dieffenbach, in 1846[158], had proposed such drilling of the cartilaginous surfaces of a pseudarthrosis and the insertion of ivory pegs, and Detmold, a German-American, had repeated this in 1851[159], but without the use of pegs. Daniel Brainard (1812–1866), professor of anatomy and surgery at Rush Medical College in Chicago, published a book in English and French simultaneously in 1854[160] on percutaneous drilling with a 'perforator' through a single incision and adapted this to the correction of deformities.

Böhler devoted some special attention to the anatomic reduction of fractures of the os calcis by pin traction and countertraction[161], though some, like Bankart in London, thought that the results were bad irrespective of the accuracy of reduction, and that the best primary treatment of a severe fracture was triple arthrodesis[162].

It is not often recalled that **Sigmund Freud** (1856–1939) was initially a neurologist and wrote a book on cerebral palsy before the end of the century in which he contrasted the great clinical interest of the condition with the dispiriting results of treatment[163].

REFERENCES

1. Marx, K.F.H. (1876). *Aussprüche eines Heilkundigen über Vergangenes, Gegenwärtiges und Künftiges.* (Göttingen)
2. Stromeyer, L. (1838). *Beiträge zur operativen Orthopädik.* (Hanover).
3. Dieffenbach, J.F. (1841). *Über die Durchschneidung der Sehnen und Muskeln.* (Berlin).
4. Knolz, J.J. (1840). *Darstellung der Humanitäts- und Heilanstalten in Erbherzogtum Österreich under der Enns.* (Vienna)
5. Valentin, B. (1961). *Die Geschichte der Orthopädie.* (Stuttgart, Georg. Thiene)
6. Heine, J.G. (1811). *Beschreibung eines neuen künstlichen Fusses für den Ober- und Unterschenkel; nebst einer mathematisch-physiologischen Abhandlung über des Gehen and Stehen.* (Würzburg)
7. von Textor, K. (1861) (obituary). *Arch. klin. Chir.,* **1**, 492
8. Heine, J.G. (1821). *Nachricht von gegenwärtigen Stande des orthopädischen Instituts in Würzburg.* (Würzburg)
9. Mayer, J.A. (1844). Einige Wörter über subkutane Operationen überhaupt und

über die unterhäutige Entzweischneidung der beiden Afterpförtner insbesondere. 17. *Stiftungsfeier der philosophisch-medizinisch Gesellschaft Würzburg*

10. Mayer, J.A. (1852). Die Osteotomie, ein neuer Beitrag zur operativen Orthopädik. *Illustr. med. Ztg.*, **2**, 1 and 65

11. Mayer, J.A. (1854). Einige Wörte über die von mir beobachteten Fötalluxationen. *Verh. phys.-med. Ges. Würzb.*, **5**, 246

12. Mayer, J.A. (1855). *Das neue Heilverfahren der Fötalluxation durch Osteotomie.* (Würzburg)

13. Mayer, J.A. (1851). Die Osteotomie als neues orthopädisches Operationsverfahren. *Verh. phys.-med. Ges. Würzburg*, **2**, 224

14. Mayer, J.A. (1848). Die Resektion der Wirbelknochen bei Knochenbrüchen der Wirbelsäule. *J.Chir. u. Augenheilk.*, **38**, **NF8**, 178

15. Mayer, J.A. (1856). Historische und statistische Notizen über die von Dr. A.M. in Würzburg verrichteten Osteotomien. *Dtsch. Klinik.*, **8**, 119

16. Heine, J. (1838). In *Bericht über die Versammlung deutscher Naturforscher und Ärzte.* (Freiburg)

17. Heine, J. (1840). *Beobachtungen über Lähmungszustande der untern Extremitäten und deren Behandlung.* (Stuttgart)

18. Heine, J. (1860). *Spinale Kinderlähmung.* (Stuttgart)

19. Heine, J. (1877). Beiträge zur Kenntnis der angeborenen Luxation des Oberschenkels. *Med. Korresp. bl. Württembg ärztl. Verein*, **7**, 510

20. Heine, J. (1882). Beiträge zur Kenntnis der angeborenen Luxation des Oberschenkels. *Med. Korresp. bl. Württemberg artzl. Verein*, **12**, 132

21. Heine, J. (1842). Über spontane und congenitale Luxation sowie einen neuen Schenkelhalsbruch-Apparat. (Stuttgart)

22. Marquardt, W. (1960). Die Geschichte der orthopädischen Heilanstalt Paulinenhilfe in Stuttgart. *Jb. Fürsorge Körperbehinderte.*, 178

23. von Nussbaum, J.N. (1882). Festrede zu Philipp Franz v. Walther's 100jährigen Geburtstage. (Munich)

24. Wildburger, J. (1863). *Praktische Erfahrungen auf dem Gebiet der Orthopädie.* (Leipzig)

25. Wildberger, J. (1855). *Neue orthopädische Behandlungsweise veralteter spontaner Luxationen im Hüftgelenk.* (Würzburg)

26. Wildberger, J. (1867). *Zehn photographische Abbildungen zum Nachweis der günstigen Heilresultate meiner Behandlung veralteter spontaner Luxationen im Hüftgelenke, mit einer historischen Einleitung über die Fortschritte der Orthopädie.* (Leipzig)

27. The *Berichte über das gymnastisch-orthopädische Institut zu Berlin* extend from 1842 to 1870

28. Berend, H.W. (1840). Beiträge zur Behandlung der Contracturen mittels Sehnen- und Muskeldurchschneidung. *Wchschr. Ges. Heilk.*, p. 54

29. Berend, H.W. (1842). Die orthopädischen Institute zu Paris. *Mag. Ges. Heilk.*, **59**, 496

30. Dieffenbach, J.F. (1838). Einige Bemerkungen über die Orthopädie in Frankreich. *Z. ges. Med.*, **8**, 57

31. Eulenburg, M. and Berend, H.W. (1833). *Situs sämtlicher Eingeweide der Schädel-, Brust- und Bauchhöhle.* (Berlin)

32. Eulenburg, M. (1876). *Die seitliche Rückgratsverkrümmungen.* (Berlin)

33. Eulenburg, M. (1863). Hochgradige Dislocation des Scapula. *Arch. klin. Chir.*, **4**, 304

34. Wolff, J. (1868). Über Knochenwachstum. *Berl. klin. Wchschr.*, **5**, 62, 76, 110

35. Wolff, J. (1870). Über die innere Architektur der Knochen und ihre Bedeutung für die Frage von Knochenwachstum. *Virchow's Arch. f. Path. Anat.*, **50**, 309

36. Wolff, J. (1910). *Über die Wechselbeziehungen der Form und der Funktion der einzelnen Gebilde des Organismus.* (Leipzig)
37. Keith, A. (1919). *Menders of the Maimed.* (London)
38. Flourens, M.J.P. (1842). *Recherches sur le développement des os et des dents.* (Paris)
39. Thomas, H.O. (1883). *Contributions to medicine and surgery, Part II, The Principles of Treatment of Diseased Joints.*
40. Wolff, J. (1863). *Arch. f. klin. Chir.,* **4**, 183
41. Wolff, J. (1893). Über die Operation der Ellenbogengelenks-ankylose. *Berl. klin. Wechschr.,* **43–44**
42. Wolff, J. (1897). Zur Arthrolysis cubitis. *Berl. klin. Wechschr.,* **46**
43. Wolff, J. (1886). Über einem Fall von Schultergelenksarthrodese wegen eine durch traumatische Myopathie entstandenen Schlottergelenks. *Berl. klin. Wchschr.,* **52**
44. Hoffa, A. (1897). Das Problem der Skoliosenbehandlung. *Berl. klin. Wchschr.,* **4**
45. Hoffa, A. (1904). The influence of the adipose tissue with regard to the pathology of the knee joint. *J. Am. Med. Assn.,* **43**, 795
46. Hoffa, A. (1924). *Lehrbuch der Orthopädische Chirurgie.* 6th edn., (Stuttgart, Enke)
47. Hoffa, A. (1896). Operative Behandlung einer schweren Skoliose. *Ztschr. f. orth. Chir.,* **4**
48. Hoffa, A. (1899). Zur Behandlung der habitueller Patellarluxation. *Arch. f. klin. Chir.,* **59**, 543
49. Hoffa, A. (1882). Beiträge zur Lehre und Behandlung des Plattfusses. *Verh. d. dtsch. Ges. f. Chir.*
50. Sperling, O.K. (1960). Die Geschichte der Orthopädie an der Medizinischen Fakultät zu Berlin. *Z. ärztl. Fortbild.,* **54**, 496
51. Trendelenburg, F. (1878). *Verh. d. dtsch. Ges. f. Chir.,* **1**, 89
52. Trendelenburg, F. (1889). Über die operative Behandlung des Plattfüsses. *Verh. d. dtsch. Ges. f. Chir.*
53. Trendelenburg, F. (1900). *Zbl. f. Chir.,* **27**, 1027
54. Trendelenburg, F. (1895). *Dtsch. med. Wchschr.,* **21**, 21
55. Jörg, J.C.G. *Über Klumpfüsse und eine leichte und Zweckmässige Heilart derselben.* (Leipzig and Marburg)
56. Stromeyer, G.F.L. (1833). Die Durchschneidung des Achillessehne als Heilmethode des Klumpfusses. *Mag. ges. Heilk.,* **39**, 195
57. Stromeyer, G.F.L. (1839). *Beiträge zur operativen Orthopädik.* (Hanover)
58. Krauss, G. (1886). Über den Werth der Resektionen der Fusswurzel zur Heilung des Klumpfusses. *Verh. dtsch. Ges. Chir.,* **1**, 114 and 121
59. Temmink, C. (1888). *Aus meiner orthopädischer Praxis.* (Münster)
60. von Volkmann, R. (1881). Die ischaemischen Muskellähmungen und Kontrakturen. *Zbl. Chir.,* **51**, 801
61. von Volkmann, R. (1863). Zur Ätiologie der Klumpfüsse. *Dtsch. klin. Bd.,* **15**, No. 34, 329
62. von Volkmann, R. (1882). Die Krankheiten der Bewegungsorgane; in: *Handbuch der allgemeine und spezielle Chirurgie* (Pitta-Billroth). (Stuttgart)
63. von Volkmann, R. (1879). *Über den Charakter und die Bedeutung der fungosen Gelenkentzüundungen.* p. 168
64. Key, J.A. (1932). Hemophilic arthritis. *Ann. Surg.,* **90**, 198
65. von Volkmann, R. (1874). Zwei Fälle von Diaphysenosteotomien wegen Knieankylosen. *Berl. klin. Wchschr.,* 629
66. von Volkmann, R. (1856). Über die sogenannten Exostosen der grossen Zehe. *Virchow's Arch.,* 297

67. von Volkmann, R. (1889). Resektion von Rippenstücken bei Skoliose. *Berl. klin. Wchschr.*, 50
68. Mignon, M.A. (1900). Synovectomie du genou. *Bull. et Mém. Soc. Chir. Paris*, **26**, 1113
69. Axhausen, G. (1910–11). Kritisches und Experimentelles Bemerkungen zur Genese der Arthritis deformans, insbesondere über die Bedeutung der aseptischen Knochen- und Knorpelnekrose. *Arch. f. klin. Chir.*, **94**, 331
70. Axhausen, G. (1914). Knochennekrose und Sequesterbildung. *Dtsch. med. Wchschr.*, **40:1**, 111
71. Axhausen, G. (1928). Über anämische Infarkte am Knochensystem und ihre Bedeutung für die Lehre von den primären Epiphyseonekrosen. *Arch. f. klin. Chir.*, **151**, 72
72. Köhler, A. (1905). *Atlas der Anatomie und Pathologie des Hüftgelenkes.* (Hamburg)
73. Preiser, G. (1907). Ein Fall von sogenannten idiopathischen juveniler osteoarthritis deformans Coxae. *Dtsch. Z. Chir.*, **89**, 613
74. Oberst, K. (1908). Die Diagnose der Hüftgelenkerkrankungen. *Z. Ärztl. Fort.*, **5**, 513
75. Axhausen, G. (1908). *Die pathologischen-anatomischen Grundlagen der freien Knochen Transplantation.*
76. Axhausen, G. (1912). Über den histologischen Vorgang bei der Transplantation von Gelenkenden, in besondere über die Transplantation von Gelenkknörpel und Epiphysienknörpel. *Arch. klin. Chir.*, **99**, 1
77. Lexer, E. (1894). Zur experimentellen Erzeugung osteomyelitische Herde. *Arch. klin. Chir.*, **48**, 181
78. Lexer, E. (1934). Über den seitlichen Ablauf der Heilvorgänge am Knochenbruch. *Bruns. Beitr. z. klin. Chir.*, **159**, 372
79. Lexer, E. (1908). Über Gelenktransplantation. *Med. Klin. Berlin.*, **4**, 817
80. Péan, E.J. (1894). Des moyens prothétiques destinés à obtenir la réparation osseuse. *Gaz. des. Hôp. Paris*, **32**
81. Chlumsky (1896). *Zbl. f. Chir.*, **5**
82. Foedre (1896). *Zbl. f. Chir.*, **5**
83. Jones, R. and Lovett, R.W. (1929). *Orthopaedic Surgery.* (Baltimore, Wm. Wood)
84. Murphy, J.B. (1905). Ankylosis arthroplasty, chemical and experimental. *J. Am. Med. Assoc.*, **44**, 1573
85. Murphy, J.B. (1913). Arthroplasty. *Ann. Surg.*, **57**, 593
86. Lexer, E. (1912). Die Verwertung der Freien Sehnentransplantation. *Arch. f. klim. Chir.*, 818
87. Mankin, H.J. *et al.* (1976). Massive resection and allograft replacement in the treatment of malignant bone tumors. *N. Engl. J. Med.*, **294**, 1247
88. von Baeyer, H. (1932). Translocation of tendons. 49th Report of Progress in Orthopaedic Surgery. *Zbl. f. Chir.*, **58**, 3140
89. Madelung, O. (1878). Die spontane Subluxation der Hand nach Vorne. *Verh. dtsch. Ges. Chir.*, **7**(2), 259
90. Stöffel, A. (1913). Treatment of spastic contractures. *Am. J. Orth. Surg.*, **10**, 611
91. Selig, R. (1914). Die intrapelvine extraperitoneale Resektion des Nervus obturatorius. *Arch. f. klin. Chir.*, **103**, 994
92. Lange, F. (1910). Support for the spondylitic spine by means of buried steel bars attached to the vertebrae. *Am. J. Orth. Surg.*, **8**, 344
93. Lange, F. (1924). Die operative Schienung der Spondylitische Wirbensäule mit Zelluloid-staben. *Ztschr. f. orth. Chir.*, **45**, 492
94. Lange, F. (1900). Über periosteale Sehnenverpflanzung bei Lähmungen. *Münch. med. Wchschr.*, **47**, 486

95. Lange, F. (1930). *Die epidemische Kinderlähmung.* (Munich, Lehmann)
96. (1913). *Allgemeine Orthopädie und Spezielle Orthopädie.* (Munich)
97. Payr, E. (1910). Über die operative Mobilizierung ankylosierte Gelenke. *Münch. med. Wchschr,* **37**
98. Payr, E. (1934). *Gelenksteifen und Gelenkplastik.* (Berlin, Springer)
99. Schanz, A. (1905–7). *Handbuch der orthopädischen Chirurgie.* (Jena)
100. Schanz, A. (1925). Über die nach Schenkelhalsbrüchen zurückbleibended Gehstörungen. *Dtsch. med. Wchschr.,* **51**, 730
101. Gaensslen, F.J. (1935). Schanz subtrochanteric osteotomy for irreducible dislocation of the hip. *J. Bone Jt. Surg.,* **17**, 76
102. Hohmann, G. (1923). Über Hallux valgus und Spreizfuss. *Arch. f. Orth. u. Unfall Chir.,* **21**, 525
103. Hohmann, G. (1934). *Fuss und Bein.* (Munich)
104. Hohmann, G. (1933). Das Wesen und die Behandlung des sogenannten Tennisellenbogen. *Münch. med. Echschr.,* **80**, 250
105. Langenbeck, B. (1878). Zur Resektion des Kniegelenks. *Verh. dtsch. Ges. Chir.,* **7**, 34
106. Langenbeck, B. (1854). Die subkutane Osteotomie. *Dtsch. Klinik.,* **6**, 327
107. König, F. (1891). Osteoplastische Behandlung der kongenitalen Hüftgelenksluxation. *Verh. dtsch. Ges. Chir.,* 75
108. König, F. (1892). Die Gelenkerkrankungen bei Bluten mit besonderer Berücksichtigung der Diagnose. *Klin. Vorträge,* **36**, 233
109. König, F. (1878). *Verh. dtsch. Ges. f. Chir.,* **1**, 93
110. Vulpius, O. (1897). Zur Kasuistik der Sehnentransplantation. *Münch. med. Wchschr.,* **16**
111. Vulpius, O. (1910). *Behandlung der spinale Kinderlähmung.* (Leipzig)
112. Vulpius, O. (1908). Arthrodese der Schultergelenks. *Z. f. orth. Chir.,* **19**
113. Vulpius, O. (1897). Über die Verwendung der Cellulose in der Orthopädie. *Z. f. orth. Chir.,* **5**, 6
114. Schmorl, G. (1932). Über Osteitis deformans Paget. *Virchow's Arch. f. Path. Anat.,* **283**, 694
115. Schmorl, G. (1927). Über die an den Wirbelbandscheiben vorkommenden Ausdehnungs und Zerreissungsvorgänge und die dadurch in ihnen und der Wirbelspongiosa hervorgerufen Veränderungen. *Verh. d. dtsch. path. Ges.,* **22**, 250
116. Schmorl, G. and Junghanns, H. (1932). *Archiv und Atlas der normalen und pathologisch Anatomie in typischen Röntgenbilden.* (Leipzig, Georg Thieme)
117. Strümpell, A. (1884). *Lehrbuch der speziellen Pathologie und Therapie der inneren Krankheiten.* (Leipzig)
118. Erb, W.H. (1877). *Verh. naturh.-med. Ver. Heidelb.,* **1**, 130
119. Virchow, R. (1853). Das normale Knochenwachstum und die rachitische Störung derselben. *Arch. path. Anat. Physiol.,* **5**, 409
120. Virchow, R. (1851). Die Identität von Knochen-, Knorpel- und Bindgewebskörperschen. *Verh. Physikal-medizinische Ges. Würzburg,* **2**, 150
121. Virchow, R. (1872). Arthritis deformans. *Virchow's Arch.,* **2**
122. Virchow, R. (1864). *Die krankhaften Geschwülste.* (Berlin)
123. Röntgen, W. (1896). *Nature,* 53, 274
124. Underwood, E.A. (1944–5). W.C. Röntgen and the early development of radiology. *Proc. Roy. Soc. Med.,* **38**, 27
125. Küntscher, G. (1959). Die Technik des Aufweitens der Markhöhle. *Der Chirurg.,* **30(1)**, 28
126. Böhler, L. (1944). *Technik der Knochenbruchbehandlung im Frieden und im Krieg.* (Vienna)

127. Böhler, L. (1948). *Medullary Nailing of Küntscher.* (London)
128. Heim, H. (1943). Die Marknagelung der langen Röhrenknochen nach Küntscher. *Der Deutsche Militärarzt,* **8(3)**, 137
129. Westerborn, A. (1944). Nailing of the marrow cavity in cases of recent fractures and pseudarthroses. *Acta Chir. Scand.,* **90**, 89
130. Küntscher, G. (1948). Recent advances in the field of medullary nailing. *Ann. Chir. et Gynaec. Fenniae,* **37(2)**
131. Laurence, G. (1944). L'enclouage médullaire des fractures des os longs: méthode Küntscher. *Rev. d'Orth. et de Chir. de l'appareil moteur.,* **30**, 32
132. Chigot, P.L. (1946). A propos des ostéosynthèses diaphysaires intramédullaires. *Presse Méd.,* **54**, 89
133. Watson-Jones, R. *et al.* (1950). Medullary nailing of fractures after 50 years. *J. Bone Jt. Surg.,* **32B**, 694
134. Hey Groves, E.W. (1916). *On modern methods of treating fractures.* (Bristol, John Wright)
135. Rush, L.V. and Rush, H.L. (1939). Technique for longitudinal pin fixation of certain fractures of the ulna and femur. *J. Bone Jt. Surg.,* **21**, 619
136. Lambrinudi, C. (1940). Intramedullary Kirschner wires in the treatment of fractures. *Proc. Roy. Soc. Med.,* **33**, 153
137. de Sahagún, B. (1952). Historia general de las cosas de Neuva España, Mexico 1946. *J. Bone Jt. Surg.,* **34A**, 506
138. Wolffsohn, S. (1796). *Verzeichnis und Beschreibung der neuesten und brauchbarsten Bruchbänder, chyrurgischen Maschinen und Verbandstücke.* (Vienna). Cited by Valentin, B. (1961). In *Die Geschichte der Orthopädie.* (Stuttgart, Georg Thieme)
139. von Breuning, G. (1841). *J.F. Dieffenbach's chirurgische Leistungen in Wien.* (Vienna)
140. Lorinser, F.W. Die Krankheiten der Wirbelsäule. In Pitta-Billroth, *Handbuch der allgemeine und spezielle Chirurgie*
141. Albert, E. (1890). *Zur Theorie der Skoliose.* (Vienna)
142. Albert, E. (1882). *Wien. med. Pr.,* **23**, 725
143. Albert, E. (1871). Über die Struktur der Synovialhäute. In Stricker *Handbuch der Lehre von den Geweben des Menschen und die Tiere.* (Leipzig)
144. Albert, E. (1877). Implantation der Fibula in die Fossa intercondyloidea femoris bei angeborenen Defekt der ganzen Tibia. *Wien. med. Pr.,* **4**
145. Albert, E. (1888). Arthrodese bei einer habituellen Schulterluxation. *Internat. klin. Rundschau,* **9**
146. Lorenz, A. (1886). *Pathologie und Therapie der seitlichen Rückgratsverkrümmungen.* (Vienna)
147. Lorenz, A. (1895). *Pathologie und Therapie der angeborenen Hüftverrenkung auf Grundlage von hundert operativ behandelten Fällen* (Vienna and Liepzig)
148. Lorenz, A. and Reiner, M. (1905). Die angeborene Huftverrenkung. In *Handbuch der Orthopädischen Chirurgische.* (Jena)
149. Lorenz, A. (1920). *Die sogenannte angeborene Hüftverrenkung, ihre Pathologie und Therapie.* (Stuttgart)
150. Lorenz, A. (1896). Über die Stellung der funktionelle Methode der Belastung des eingerenkten Schenkelkopfes mit dem Körpergewicht zu den anderen unblutigen Behandlungsmethoden der angeborenen Hüftverrenkung. *Wien klin. Wchschr.,* **36**
151. Lorenz, A. (1897). *Wien klin. Rundschau,* **21**
152. Nicoladoni, C. (1880). Über Sehnentransplantation. *Versamml. dtsch. Naturforsch. v. Ärzte im Salzburg,* **54**
153. Nicoladoni, C. (1882). Nachtrag zur pes calcaneus und zur Transplantation der peroneal Sehnen. *Arch. klin. Chir.,* **27**, 660

154. Waterman, J.H. (1902). Tendon transplantation, a review. *Med. News*, 54

155. Büdinger, K. (1906). Über Ablösung von Gelenkteilen und Verwandte Prozesse. *Dtsch. Z. Chir.*, **84**, 311

156. Büdinger, K. (1908). Über traumatische Knorpelrisse in Kniegelenk. *Dtsch. Z. Chir.*, **92**, 510

157. Spitzy, H. (1912). *Z. orth. Chir.*, **30**, 221

158. Dieffenbach, J.F. (1846). Neue sichere Heilmethode des Falschen Gelenks oder der Pseudarthrose mittels Durchbohrung der Knochen und Einschlagen von Zapfen. *Wchschr. Ges. Heilk.*, 729

159. Detmold, G.H. (1851). *Nordamerik. Ber. f. Natur- und Heilk. Philadelphia*, **3**, 379

160. Brainard, D. (1854). *Essay on a new method of treating ununited fractures and certain deformities of the osseous system.* (New York)

161. Böhler, L. (1931). Diagnosis, pathology and treatment of fractures of the os calcis. *J. Bone Jt. Surg.*, **13**, 75

162. Bankart, A.S.B. (1942). Fractures of the os calcis. *Lancet*, **ii**, 175

163. Freud, S. (1897). *Die infantile Cerebrallähmung.* 1897

164. Zippel, J. and Meyer-Ralfs, M. (1975). Themistocles Gluck: Wegbereiter der Endoprosthetik. *Z. für Orthop.*, **113**, 134

165. Gluck, T. (1890). Die Invaginationsmethode der Osteo- und Arthroplastik. *Berl. klin. Wschr.*, **32**, 752

166. Gluck, T. (1891). Referat über die durch das moderne chirurgische Experiment gewonnenen positiven Resultaten betreffend die Naht und den Ersatz von Defecten höherer Gewebe: sowie über die Verwertung resorbierbarer und lebendiger Tampons in der Chirurgie. *Arch. klin. Chir.*, **41**, 182 and 239

CHAPTER 4

National Histories – France

The very name 'orthopaedics' was devised in France, in 1741, by Nicolas Andry, Dean of the Paris Faculty. We discuss this later. To go back much earlier, one **Lanfranc** (originally Lanfranchi di Milano), an Italian who moved to Paris via Lyons, became an eminent French surgeon and published his *Chirurgia Magna* in 1296. He was a member of the faculty at the College of St Côme, in later centuries to be in competition with the rising guild of barber-surgeons*. Lanfranc stressed the importance of cleanliness in wounds and believed that exposure to the air, or entry of air, was the cause of suppuration, a view that persisted until John Hunter's time and even later. He was followed by Mondeville (1260–1320) and then by Guy de Chauliac.

De Chauliac (c.1300–1368) was a professor at the University of Montpellier. He wrote a *Chirurgia Magna* or *Inventarium et Collectarium Artis Chirurgicalis Medicinae* and also a *Chirurgia Parva* or *Minor Surgery*. In the former he describes the treatment of femoral fractures with traction by weights and pulleys[1] and stressed the importance of the preparations for fracture treatment: the place, the assistants, bandages steeped in whites of eggs and red oil, splints of willow, iron or leather, rather longer than the limb, 'provided that they do not touch nor injure the joint.' These splints were evidently quite narrow and placed round the limb like barrel-staves at fingerbreadth intervals and bound together by a tightly twisted cord. There was a suspensory cradle and a bed with an aperture for excretion and an overhead rope for the patient to pull himself up. De Chauliac used his traction to soften and redirect the callus when union was progressing badly and did not hesitate to refracture for malunion. Like Hippocrates, he thought that Colles' fracture was a posterior dislocation of the carpus and reduced it. He sutured nerves like Lanfranc before him. **Dalechamps**, of Lyons (b.1513)[2] described spinal caries, as the Greeks had done, but added – two

---

* Both were hierarchially inferior to the physicians of the Faculty of Medicine.

centuries before Pott – that it was sometimes associated with paraplegia. 'These patients are subject to abscesses which are difficult to cure and point in the loins and groins ... When the vertebrae of the neck are displaced, all the parts below lose sensation and movement, but if they are displaced in a rounded form (i.e. not sharply angulated) movement and sensation are little or not at all affected.' He agreed with Galen that the fundamental cause was a 'tuberculum', whatever that might be (it was apparently derived from the nodular appearances of the lungs in the phthisis known to be associated with vertebral caries from the Hippocratic period).

The most famous surgical figure of the 16th century in France (or anywhere else) is that of **Ambroise Paré** (1510–1590), a Renaissance figure but one of the end of the Renaissance, who revolutionized the treatment of war wounds and ushered in the modern age of prostheses and brace-making.

Paré was born at Bourg Hersent, in Maine, and his father and other relatives were barbers or other paramedicals. In 1532 he was apprenticed to a Parisian barber-surgeon and worked for four years at the Hôtel-Dieu in Paris and then as an army surgeon under Henri IV and surgical adviser to a succession of French kings (which is why he was spared by royal decree from the Massacre of St Bartholomew, though a Huguenot). Paré was humane, at a time when humanity was not a marked feature of military surgeons, and was glad to find methods of treatment that lessened suffering.

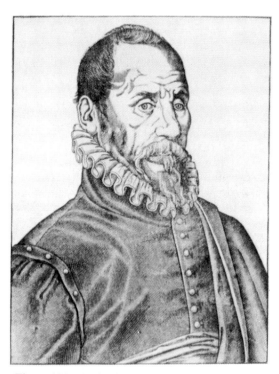

Figure 101   Ambroise Paré (1510–1590) aged 68

He wrote, of the expedition against Turin, in 1537:

'We entered the throng in the City and passed over the dead bodyes, and some which were not yet dead; we heard them cry out under our horses' feet, which made my heart relent to leave them ... I entered into a stable ... where I found foure dead soldiers, and three which were leaning against the wall, their faces wholly disfigured, and neither saw not heard, nor spoke; and their cloathes did yet flame with the gunpowder which had burnt them ... There happened to come in an old souldier, who asked me if there were any possible means to cure them, I told him no; he presently approached them, and gently cut their throats without choler. Seeing this great cruelty, I told him he was a wicked man, he answered that he prayed to God that whensoever he should be in such a case, that he might find someone that would doe as much for him, to the end he might not miserably languish.' (From *The Apologie and Treatise of Ambroise Paré*, trans. Th. Johnson 1643, ed. Keynes G. University of Chicago Press 1952).

In 1564, he published his great treatise, the *Dix Livres de la Chirurgie*, in modern French instead of the conventional medical Latin[3,4]. This encyclopaedic work begins with an excellent section on surgical anatomy. He describes ganglia, which he ruptured after using emollients. There is a careful account of injuries to nerves, joints and ligaments, and Bick stresses that Paré was the first surgeon known to have performed excision of an elbow joint for persistent infection, yet this was not repeated or revived until the late 18th century. Perhaps his greatest contribution was the use of the ligature for the large vessels in amputations. It seems not to be generally appreciated that Paré used a tourniquet in amputation – 'a strong and broad fillet, like that with which women are used to bind up their hair' – and for three purposes: to hold the muscles retracted with the skin so that they might redescend to cover the bone-ends and relieve pain after the operation; to 'prohibit the flux of blood by pressing and occluding the veins and arteries'; and 'to dull the senses of the part by stupefying it, the animal spirits being hindered by tight compression from passing in by the nerves'. The bone was smoothed after being sawn and the vessels drawn down from where they lurked within the muscles with 'crow's-beak' forceps – the haemostats of the time – and tied with a double thread. (This practice lingered on through the Napoleonic Wars and after, the threads being left long and dangling until they came away naturally.) It is sometimes stated that this marked the end of the use of boiling oil or the cautery for amputation stumps, but it was only contributory; Paré had already discovered, fortuitously, that these were not only unnecessary but noxious. Having performed many amputations after a battle, he wrote:

'I was willing to know first, before I applied it, how the other Chirurgions did for the first dressing, which was to apply the said oyle (of elders) the hottest that was possible into the wounds, with tents and setons; insomuch that I tooke courage to doe as they did. At last I wanted oyle and was constrained instead thereof to apply a digestive of yolkes of

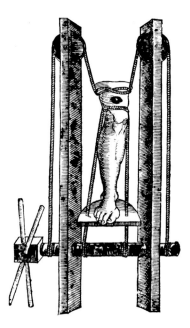

Figure 102   Paré's adaptation of the *glossocomium* of antiquity, ingeniously providing simultaneous traction and countertraction

eggs, oyle of Roses, and Turpentine. In the night I could not sleep in quiet, fearing some default in not cauterizing ... which made me rise very early to visit them, where beyond my expectation I found those to whom I had applyed my digestive medicine to feel little paine and their wounds without inflammation or tumour ... the others to whom was used the sayd burning oyle I found feverish, with great paine and tumour about the edges of their wounds ... And then I resolved with myself never so cruelly to burne poor men.' (From Johnson's translation of the *Apologie*.)

He also noted the cleansing action of maggots in dirty wounds.

Paré used rope and windlass traction for femoral fractures and was able to distinguish hip dislocation from fracture of the femoral neck. He confirmed the cord compression in vertebral fractures that had been recognized by the Egyptians and Hippocrates: 'numbness and palsy of the arms, legs, fundament and bladder ... so that their urine and excrements come from them against their wills and knowledge.' Because death was imminent, 'by reason that their spinal marrow is hurt ... you may make an incision to remove the splinters of the broken vertebrae (in cases where the neural arch has been injured) which, driven in, press on the spinal marrow and the nerves thereof.' This was not a novel idea; it had been suggested and possibly practised, by Paul of Aegina in the 7th century, but Paré seems to have been the first who actually did it.

Paré used appliances and methods rather like those of Hippocrates for reducing hip and shoulder dislocations, and one or two special to himself. He describes displacement of the 'appendices' (i.e. epiphyses) of the long bones, to be restored if deformity is to be avoided, and reduced neck dislocations by manipulation and traction. He designed a wide variety of forceps, instruments and braces of all kinds. His artificial limbs were made of iron, by armourers who were finding that the advent of gunpowder was making their trade obsolete. These limbs were mainly cosmetic, but they also had working catches and springs for hands and fingers. All spinal curvatures he thought to be dislocations in various directions, and he attributed the scolioses of young girls to habitual malposture; some curves were clearly congenital, others ascribed to injury, or idiopathic. He was the first to use a corset, of sheet iron or steel and perforated for lightness: 'Those who are hunchbacked, having a curved spine, to repair and conceal this deformity they are to wear corselets of supple iron which should be perforated so as not to be too heavy, and padded so as not to cause excoriation, and the said corselets should be often changed ... for those who are growing they must be changed every three months, more or less, for otherwise, instead

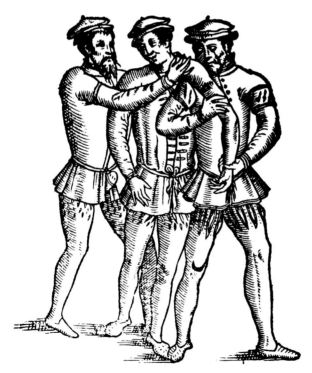

Figure 103 Paré: figure which demonstrates how to reduce a complete dislocation of the left shoulder: the one in the middle is the patient, and the surgeon is the one who reduces the bone into its place, pushing it into its socket with his shoulder. 'And he is to be higher than the patient.' The other is the assistant

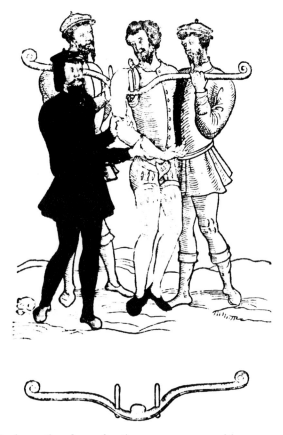

Figure 104   Paré: another figure for the same purpose with a curved stick in the middle of which there is a protuberance to push the bone into its place, and two pegs preventing vacillating here and there

of doing good, one would do harm.' These supports remained popular for well over a century. In 1655, Bartholinus[5] advised that such *instrument ferrea* be worn day and night, and Purmann[6] was still recommending them in Germany in 1705.

'There are,' he wrote, 'three general causes of Luxations: internall, externall and hereditarie.' The internal dislocations were due to humours, often associated with separation of the appendices (i.e. the epiphyses); these were cases of suppurative arthritis. The external displacements were traumatic. He agreed with Hippocrates that dislocation led to atrophy of the limb, 'for the performance of the proper action encreases strength ... but idleness debilitates and makes the part leane.' If dislocation were associated with severe fracture or wound, it was better to accept lameness than to risk damaging the nerves and vessels by heavy traction. His general methods of reduction obviously go back to Hippocrates, but he had some ingenious

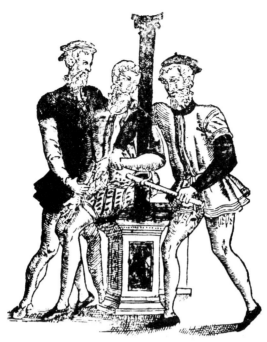

Figure 105   Paré: another figure, which shows how to reduce the bone of the elbow around a pillar with a cord and a stick

devices of his own, such as the *manubrium versatile* or hand-vice to rack out straps attached to the limb. Dislocations occurred more readily in the lean and wasted than in 'fleshie bodies', but were easier to reduce, and bones were more brittle in cold weather and healed faster in the summer.

Paré also invented boots for club-feet, a finger-stall for mallet thumb, and an elongated crutch for leg inequality. He taught the importance of functional positions for splintage: the fingers to be flexed, the shoulder semi-abducted with a pillow in the axilla, the knee and hip straight. He noted that the Achilles tendon could rupture with trivial trauma and 'a crack like a coachman's whip', and could never be so cured as to give complete recovery. He reported the case of a bullet lodged in the spinal cord of the King of Navarre at the siege of Rouen, and located bullets in muscle by reconstructing the position of the limbs and body at the time of injury. He enlarged missile wounds to release exudate and remove all foreign bodies; *débridement* in its true sense of relieving tension, not in the modern bastard sense of removing debris.

Paré also described gout and the other arthritides, and their origin from humours descending from the brain, as Galen had done;* and this concept

---

* Guillaume de Baillou (1538–1616) or Ballonius, 'the father of rheumatism', was the first modern to distinguish gout from rheumatism, in his posthumous *Liber de Rheumatismo* of 1642.

Some Practitioners in stead of this Pulley make use of the hereafter described Instrument, which they terme *Manubrium versatile*, or a Hand-vice. The end therof is fashioned like a Gimblet, and is to be twined into a Poste. Within

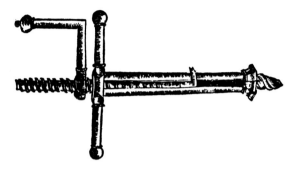

Manubrium versatile, or, *A Hand-vice.*

that handle lyes a screw with a hooked end, whereto the string or ligature must be fastened. Now the screw-rod or male-screw runnes into the female by the twining about of the handle: and thus the ligature is drawne as much as will suffice, for the setting the dislocated bone.

Figure 106   Pare's *manubrium versatile*

of a 'cararrhal' cause for these and other disorders (the very word *pituita* means phlegm) persisted well into the 18th century[7]. He used bandages stiffened with whites of eggs reinforced with additives, directly derived from those of Hippocrates, for the correction of club-feet and other deformities. Club-feet he attributed, if congenital, to such mechanical influences as the mother during pregnancy sitting too long with her legs crossed; or the mother might have had the same defect; or the nurse might hold the child awkwardly, 'pressing the foot against its natural configuration'.

Paré sustained a compound fracture of his own leg in 1561, at the age of 51; both bones were broken four fingers above the ankle. He was carried off with less compunction than Pott under similar circumstances (p. 93), the bearers pulling him this way and that; the pain was severe. However, he instructed his colleagues to treat him and 'not to spare me more than any stranger in his care, that in reducing the fracture he forget the friendship he bore me. Moreover, I admonished him ... to strongly pull the feet straight and that if the wound was not large enough, to open it with his razor to let him easily put the bones in their normal position, and that he carefully search the wound with his fingers ... for the sense of touch is better than any instrument to remove the fragments and pieces of bones that were widely separated.' This tells us a lot about Paré's own practice. It was important to have the foot and heel exactly right; if they were too high it would cause

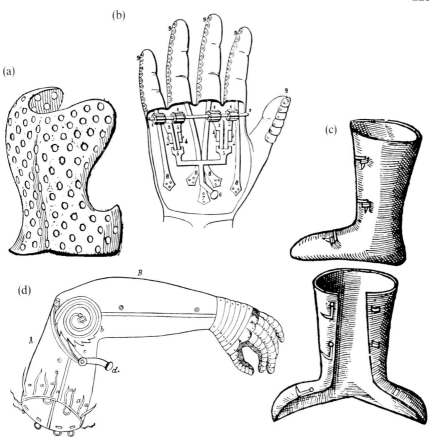

Figure 107 Paré: various devices (a) scoliosis corset; (b) wrist and hand prosthesis; (c) club-foot boot; (d) artificial arm

a concavity at the fracture, if too low a convexity. He suffered an abscess, and some sequestration, but recovered entirely and without any limp; he was lucky.

Paré raised the dignity and status of the barber-surgeons of France to a new level. The Faculty of St Côme had to accept him, and them, after long and stubborn resistance. His originality and initiative exerted an enormous influence on the progress of surgery.

Denis Fournier (d.1683) treated spinal deformity with traction machines inherited from the Hellenistic period, such as the *glossocomium* of Nymphodorus, and other racks of his own devising like the *Polyceste*[8] (all these machines had stylish names like the motorcars of today) and invented the term *apocataostéologie*, meaning 'reestablishment of the bones of the human body'[9].

Jean-Louis Petit (1674–1750)[10] is credited with having invented the inclined plane for the reduction and splintage of leg fractures. For compound tibial fractures he used a wooden 'case', bent at the knee and resembling the

Braun's frame, a precursor of the double inclined plane introduced by Robert Chessher into England in the late 18th century (p. 88). For a fractured tibia he used brandy compresses, bolsters, wood or pasteboard splints, or the limb was enclosed in *joncs*, i.e. bundles of reeds as used by the ancient Hindus and Egyptians, sewn together or strapped overall and including the joints above and below the fracture. Femoral fractures were treated with joncs plus traction by straps extending to the tibial condyles, with countertraction by a sheet between the thighs attached to the bedhead. Some such measures remained in force until the advent of effective traction in the 19th century. Petit also invented a screw-type haemostatic ligature round the limb which he called his *tourniquet* (*tourner* = to turn or twist) and demonstrated to the Academy of Sciences in 1718.

Jacques Croissant de Garengeot (1668–1759) in his *Traité des Instruments les plus utiles* of 1725, refers to the ancient system of classifying operations as synthesis, diaeresis, exeresis and prosthesis.

Jean Méry (1658–1747) of Paris, may have been the first to note that lateral spinal curvatures were accompanied by rotation of the vertebral bodies[11].

We now come to a very important figure in the history of orthopaedics, even though – as we shall see – the importance is somewhat factitious. **Nicholas Andry** (1658–1747), professor of medicine at the University of Paris and Dean of the Faculty of Physick, published in 1741, at the age of 81, a very famous book: *L'Orthopédie, ou l'art de prévenir et de corriger dans les enfants, les difformités du corps, le tout par des moyens a la portée des Pères*

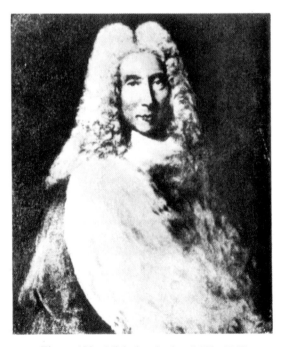

Figure 108   Nicholas Andry (1658–1747)

et des Mères, et de toutes les Personnes qui ont des Enfants a élever (Orthopaedia: or the Art of Correcting and Preventing Deformities in Children: by such Means as may easily be put in practice by Parents themselves and all such as are employed in Educating Children). The English title is that of the translation of 1743 'printed for A. Millar, at Buchanan's Head, opposite to Catharine Street, in the Strand.'

In the preface he says, 'As to the Title, I have formed it of two Greek words, viz. *orthos*, which signifies straight, free from Deformity, and *paidion*, a child. Out of these two words I have compounded that of orthopaedics, to express in one Term the Design I propose, which is to teach the different methods of preventing and correcting the deformities of Children.' 'Orthopaedics' was the term that was to gain acceptance over many others now long discarded. Other names were used before and after Andry. He himself gives credit to two earlier publications. In 1584, Scévole de Sainte-Marthe (Scaevola Sammarthanus 1536–1623) wrote his *Paedotrophia*, a Latin poem on the suckling and rearing of young children, whom, like Andry, he compared to tender plants to be braced against environmental pressures. Sainte-Marthe advised pregnant women to avoid tight clothing, the passions, conjugal embraces and immoderate diet, to have their babies standing up, and how to care for them. The other work, also in Latin, was the *Callipaedia* (or the art of having beautiful children) of 1656, by the Abbe Claude Quillet (1602–1661); and of this we need only note that it relates conception to the constellations, and the sex of the child to the position of the mother and the testicle performing its office, the right for boys and the left for girls, the unwanted one to be temporarily tied off.

For various reasons, partly because of confusion of *paidion* with the Latin *pes* = foot, so that orthopaedists were often confused with chiropodists, many attempts were made to replace Andry's term: Deformities of the human body (Jalade-Lafond 1827)[12], the Orthomorphy of the great Delpech (1828)[13]; the Orthosomatics of Bricheteau (1824)[14]; Deformities of the human frame (W J Little 1853)[15]; Maladies de l'appareil locomoteur (Bouvier 1858[16], Kirmisson 1890[17]); Orthopraxy (Heather Bigg in London, 1862)[18]. The complete expression 'orthopaedic surgery' was perhaps first used by Louis Bauer in America in 1864[19], echoed by St Germain in Paris in 1883 as *Chirurgie Orthopédique*[20].

Andry's chief aim was the prevention of postural defects, symbolized by his famous illustration of a young tree to be supported if it was not to grow crooked. Compelling as this is, every arboriculturist knows that a bent trunk cannot be so straightened, and that the function of the stake is to steady the roots as they develop. A better illustration of orthopaedic technique is given in Diderot's great *Encyclopaedia*: 'In the background a child is engaged in straightening a young tree; this child is the symbol of orthopaedics', for this is straightforward splintage.*

---

* It was this reference to the subject in this great work that did most to establish the term as standard. Just as Celsus was a Roman encyclopaedist whose range happened to include medicine, so the great 18th century French encyclopaedist, Denis Diderot (1713–1780) included surgery and orthopaedics (with some of Andry's illustrations) in his works: *Encyclopédie ou Dictionnaire raisonné des Sciences, des Arts et des Matiers.* (35 vols), Paris 1751–1780.

ORTHOPÆDIA:

Or, the A R T of

CORRECTING and PREVENTING

DEFORMITIES

I N

CHILDREN:

By fuch M E A N S, as may eafily be put in
Practice by P A R E N T S themfelves, and
all fuch as are employed in Educating
C H I L D R E N.

To which is added,

A D E F E N C E of the O R T H O P Æ D I A,
by way of S U P P L E M E N T, by the A U T H O R.

Tranflated from

The *French* of M. *A N D R Y,*

Profeffor of Medicine in the R O Y A L C O L-
L E G E, and Senior Dean of the Faculty of
P H Y S I C K at *Paris.*

I N T W O V O L U M E S.

Illuftrated with C U T S.

V O L. I.

L O N D O N:

Printed for A. M I L L A R, at *Buchanan's Head,* oppo-
fite to *Catharine-ftreet,* in the *Strand.*

M. DCC. XLIII.

Figure 109 Title page of English translation of Andry's *Orthopaedia,* 1743

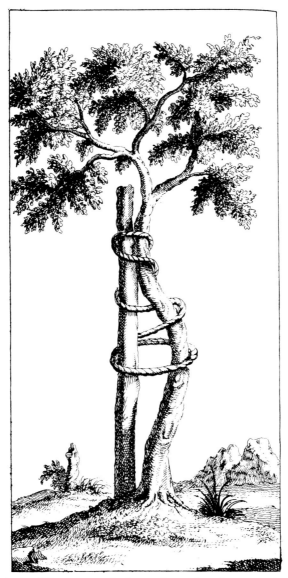

Figure 110 Andry: 'The same method must be used ... for recovering the Shape of the Leg, as is used for making straight the crooked Trunk of a young Tree.'

Andry attributed skeletal deformities to faults of posture and shortness of muscles. Thus, scoliosis was not necesarily due to defects in the spine itself: short muscles could bend it as a tight string bends a bow, and it was the persistence of this myogenetic theory that led to quite extraordinary exertions in unilateral myotomy and tenotomy in France in the early 19th century (see p. 250). Scoliosis was to be treated by rest, suspension, posture (all

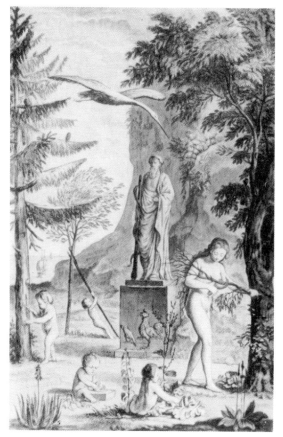

Figure 111   Diderot's *Encyclopédie*, Paris 1763: 'In the background a child is engaged in straightening a young tree; this child is the symbol of orthopaedics.'

everyday activities are carefully analysed), adjustment of desks and chairs, whalebone corsets stuffed over the prominences with the padding increased as these diminished, the corsets to be replaced every three months, a principle directly related to the management of scoliosis by Abbott and others in the USA in the 19th century. Shoes were important, 'Shoes with heels that are too high produce curvature of the trunk in young persons and, for this reason, high heels should not be allowed before the age of 15, especially for girls.' This approach was typical of the Enlightenment (*c.*1740–1830): 'For the layman and doctor of the Enlightenment, prevention was more important than treatment. The concept of prophylaxis is the essential contribution of the study of medicine of the Enlightenment[21].'

Andry seems to have been both underrated and overrated. He did not begin his own medical studies until he was 32, in 1690, was envious and quarrelsome, and seems to have spent much of his life studying diseases caused by worms interspersed with unsuccessful litigation against surgeons who barred his entry to the Paris Faculty, and in polemics, in particular against the *Traité des maladies des os* of Petit in 1723 and against surgeons in general. But for physicians to condescend towards surgeons was the normal posture in the Europe of his age.

Irritating as he may have been, Andry does give a vivid idea of the child's body as a dynamic and *plastic* structure responsive to stress and strain in both the genesis and cure of deformities. And he emphasized the superiority of active over passive exercises, as in torticollis, 'When the Hand is employed to turn the Head of the Child to one side, it is only the Effort of the Hand that does the Affair. But this Force is foreign, and consequently not so effectual, *because it is not seconded by any Effort of the Child.* (My italics, DLV.) It is the Effort of Nature that ought to do all this … when the Hand performs the Motion, the animal Spirits of the Child do not act, neither do the Muscles contract of themselves, but the Motion you give them is quite passive on their part and consequently must be of very little service: for in this Case it ought to come from within.' We are reminded of a remark by a British medical colonel in World War I, 'The factor of volition is vital … a fraction of movement obtained in this way is infinitely more valuable than a greater amount gained by passive methods[22].'

Andry can be forgiven a great deal for having enunciated this absolutely basic principle of all orthopaedic treatment and rehabilitation. He was as assiduous in the fashioning of the human body (usually that of a young woman of fashion) as the great Le Nôtre was later in landscaping the gardens for the King at Versailles. Posture was corrected by loading in the appropriate places, by hard beds; deformities overcorrected by enforcing opposite habits. For rickets, he mentions suspension by a bandage across the chest, under the axillae and crossed under the chin. (This was Glisson's sling of the previous century, but he does not acknowledge Glisson.) He thought that better than any medicine was sprinkling with cold water to excite muscle activity or rubbing with a towel, dry or soaked in white wine, or tickling.

On envy (of sibs) as a cause of wasting: 'For Children have more Cunning than we can well imagine … and indeed in this sense we are frequently their Dupes; for they make it their whole Business to dive into our Thoughts; nay, sometimes they are jealous even before they are weaned. I have seen, says St Augustine, an Infant jealous; he had not yet learned to pronounce a single word, and yet he regarded with a pale Face, and sparkling Eyes, another Child that sucked at the Breast with him.' (It has taken modern psychoanalysts to rediscover this original sin.)

Andry shared the common ideas of his time on prenatal influences as causes of deformity. His treatment for limb and spinal deformities is generally naive and useless, but he shows a marked aesthetic bent in depicting the ideal contours and configurations of parts. For knee angulations he used an iron splint but gives no details.

Andry is often called the Father of Orthopaedics, but this is a serious misnomer. He invented the name, but that is almost all. The reader will look in vain for a rational treatment of even the commonest fractures and orthopaedic disorders. Most of the contents of his book deal with the trivialities of a medical gossip column: complexion, hair, eyes, nails, deportment. He is a beautician rather than a physician. Yet the impression steals through that, in his actual practice, he probably did a fair amount of good. He was interested in the individual, in his or her psychological make-up, and always stressed the importance of self-help in terms of muscular activity. If it is true, as has been said, that in France orthopaedics entered the 20th century clinging to the skirts of paediatrics, this is partly due to the influence of Andry. Perhaps he is better called the Stepfather of Orthopaedics.

Jean-Pierre David (1737–1784) was professor of anatomy and surgery in Rouen at an early age and in 1778 won the prize for an essay set by the Paris Academy of Surgery, 'To explain the effects of motion and of rest, and the indications according to which either should be prescribed in surgical diseases.' David advocated time and rest for joint disease; if it were severe, the aim was ankylosis, in other cases early movement. The diseased part was ready for motion when the inflammation had resolved: natural movement was best and Nature would soon improve on the slightest degree. This exactly corresponds to Hugh Owen Thomas's concept of 'soundness' and 'unsoundness' in joints.

According to Vander Elst, in 1775 the Journal Français de Chirurgie carried a report from one Icart, based on the work of two Toulouse surgeons, Lapoyde and Sicre, on a method of using brass wire for the suture of broken bones, an innovation that aroused fierce opposition. It is certainly true that, at the end of the 18th century, bone surgery became more adventurous in one specific field, that of bone resection, though this was only a continuation of an activity going back to Hippocrates, Celsus, Galen, Paul of Aegina, Guy de Chauliac and Ambroise Paré and many lesser figures. Leopold Ollier (1830–1900) (p. 260) gives the details in his epic *Traité des Resections*[23] and, like his contemporary, Farabeuf (1841–1910), taught that a resection might begin with the soft parts but that it was always necessary to prepare for removal of bone and restoration of bony continuity.

We now come to two surgeons of the Napoleonic Wars: Pierre Percy and Dominique Larrey, both ennobled as barons.

Pierre Percy (1754–1825) was chief surgeon to the revolutionary armies in Flanders and the Rhineland and later an inspector of army medical services. In 1792 he wrote his *Manuel de chirurgie de l'armée*, and his *Journal des campagnes du Baron Percy* was reissued in Paris in 1904.

Dominique Jean Larrey (1766–1842) was trained at the Hôpital St Jean in Toulouse, where he wrote a thesis on spinal caries, and then worked with Bichat at the Hôtel-Dieu in Paris. At 26 he was appointed director of medical services to the Army of the South, was transferred to the Rhine, and in 1797 Napoleon made him organizer of medical services of the army of occupation in Italy, where he founded a medical school in Milan. For the Egyptian campaign he recruited staff from the medical schools of Montpellier and Toulouse and organized a medical centre in Cairo. He then became surgeon to the Imperial Guard and was at Austerlitz and continued in post after the restoration of the monarchy. His own surgical skill was outstanding: he could disarticulate a hip in a few minutes. He had to struggle against administrative inefficiencies, which were associated with a hospital death-rate of around 30 per cent[24].

We may note here that, at Waterloo, on either side, treatment was based on that of previous campaigns, the British on the Peninsular War as managed by James McGrigor, director-general of the Army Medical Department, the French more on the central European struggles, organized by Percy and Larrey and their *ambulances volantes*. Limb surgery offered the major field for surgeons, since wounds of the trunk and head were usually fatal. As often noted in battle, even severe limb injuries such as avulsions sometimes let the victims walk or travel several miles before collapse. The amputation rate was around 12 per cent, 500 in all on the British side. The French were more conservative. Guthrie disarticulated a hip, the first such operation by a British surgeon. Amputations were usually of guillotine type, the soft tissues sewn or taped across, the arteries tied with silk or linen sutures left long for later removal in an attempt to prevent secondary haemorrhage from sepsis. All amputations were very rapid, taking no more than a few minutes or a quarter of an hour. No formal debridement of wounds was done, but there was frequent probing for foreign bodies and dilatation for drainage. The British often did primary wound closure, using sutures or adhesive tape or pins stuck in the skin edges and tied together. Splintage was crude, mainly long straight wooden splints. Death was due to shock, haemorrhage (this included over-enthusiastic venesection), cross-infection and hospital gangrene[25].

Before mentioning further medical figures, it is desirable to stress the importance in France of the *bandagistes*, who were really appliance-makers and mechanics. They were even more important than in England, and it was their close collaboration with the doctors that put new mechanical ideas into practice. The discipline often ran in families, from father to son, and they often engaged in independent treatment. They were also known as *machinistes*, *mécaniciens* or *chirurgiens herniaires*, and it was common for a doctor of orthopaedic bent to have a long and intimate professional relationship with a favoured mechanic.

Thus, we know of a self-styled ingenieur-physician, Alex Magny, who constructed a corset for a Parisian doctor, Augustin Roux, in 1762[26]. There were the Verdiers: Jean Verdier (1735–1820) was the son-in-law of one Tiphaine, known for his management of deformities by methods he kept strictly secret; later, Verdier's son, Jean-Francois Verdier-Heurtin (1767–1823) gave an account of Tiphaine's appliances[27], and a nephew, Pierre-Louis Verdier (b.1780) was the first to introduce rubber surgical appliances into France[28]. A M Delacroix is specifically mentioned in the 1819 *Diction-naire des Sciences Médicales* for the inventions he used in combating deformities, and worked in close collaboration with a physician, Pierre Nicolas Gerdy (1797–1856) who gave Delacroix the utmost credit[29]. It would seem that it was customary for the doctor to provide a general idea of what he wanted and the appliance-maker would flesh it out, a position not much changed until Thomas and others like him began to make their own appliances after the mid-century. Certainly, Delacroix constructed the most elegant and efficient braces for Gerdy, and he also produced artificial extensor tendons for the fingers made of thin elastic metal strips before rubber came into general use.

Just as in England, France had a strong bonesetting tradition, often

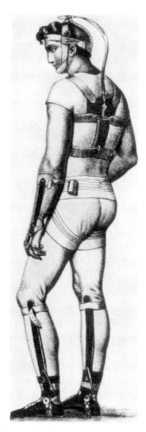

Figure 112   P N Gerdy: *Traité des Bandages et Appareils de Pansement*, Paris 1837–
1839. Appliances to correct lateral inclination of the head and club-foot ('conceived
by M. Delacroix')

handed down in such families as the Bailleuls, who gave their name *bailleul*
to this type of unqualified practitioner, also known as *rabouteurs* or
rhabilleurs. There were also the chiropodists, whose discipline seems to have
originated in France. The most famous of these was one Laforest, surgeon-
pedicurist to Louis XIV, who wrote a standard work on foot care[30]. Their
relevance to orthopaedics is that they gave clear accounts of the nature of
hallux valgus and hammer-toes and their relation to tight footwear in women
and directed the doctors' attention to these conditions.

Nevertheless, the orthopaedists of the second half of the century came to
resent the aspirations of the upstart appliance-makers and lay therapists. St
Germain wrote in 1883 of the negligence of the medical corps, which had
left orthopaedics in the hands of charlatans and empirics, or at least in those
of the appliance-makers, who were, however, useful if kept in their place[31].

Two medical characters worthy of mention are the brothers **Levacher** or
Le Vacher. The elder, François-Guillaume Levacher (1732–1816) was surgeon

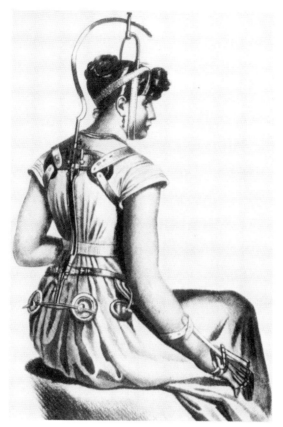

Figure 113 Gerdy: appliance to correct the vertebral column ('invented by M. Delacroix')

to the Court at Parma, and devised a spinal corset incorporating head traction which he showed to the *Académie Royale de Chirurgie* in Paris in 1764. He also developed the 'Minerva' jacket, based on the pelvis and incorporating a 'jury-mast' (jury is a naval term for a temporary aid), though this was not original to him. Thomas Levacher de la Feutrie (1738–1790) was Dean of the Medical Faculty of Paris. He wrote of the treatment of spinal curvature, especially in rickets[32], and devised an apparatus combining an 'extension chair' with lateral pressure. He also constructed an above-knee splint for club-foot.

We now come to a very great man, one of the founding fathers of modern orthopaedics, both in France and in the world in general, one whose name must be linked on equal terms with those of Jean-André Venel in Switzerland and Hugh Owen Thomas in Britain, a man who invented subcutaneous tenotomy and whose practice coincided with the start of the 19th century; **Jacques-Mathieu Delpech** (1777–1832).

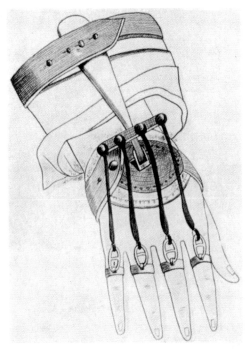

Figure 114 Delacroix: elastic metal replacement of extensor tendons, Paris 1819

Delpech was born in Toulouse on 2nd October 1777 and apprenticed at the age of 12 to a surgeon, Alexis Larrey, who had treated his father, the uncle of the great Dominique Larrey of Napoleon's armies. Perhaps this is why, when only 15, he was enlisted as a surgical dresser in the Army of the South, where he served in the Pyrenees for five years. After short further training and graduation at Montpellier, he studied from 1801 in Paris under Alexis Boyer (1757–1833). Boyer can be seen to have had an influence on Delpech's mature thought, for he wrote, of club-foot, that its cause was 'an inequality in the respective strength of the adductor and abductor muscles of the foot[34].'

In 1812, aged 35, Delpech won a competitive appointment as professor of surgery and chief surgeon as the Hôpital St Eloi in Montpellier. Here he treated the French wounded retreating from Wellington's armies in Spain, aiming at primary healing as he considered the admission of air to wounds to be noxious. Long before Semmelweis, he stressed the importance of transfer of infection by contaminated hands and dressings, and his first major publication was on hospital-acquired wound sepsis, the *pourriture d'hôpital* or hospital gangrene[35].

It was this fear of air-borne wound infection, together with his own and Scarpa's work on club-foot, that underlay his development of subcutaneous tenotomy of the Achilles tendon for paralytic equinus to neutralize the deforming force (open tenotomy had been done long before), first performed

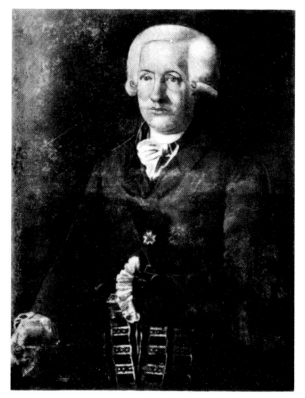

Figure 115   François Guillame Levacher (1732–1816)

on 9th May 1816[36], which influenced, first Stromeyer in Hanover, and then the entire world. But the procedure met with opposition in Paris and he seems to have repeated it only a few times, discouraged by infection and sloughing. Indeed, Delpech is said to have tried to dissuade W J Little from undergoing the operation, eventually performed on the Englishman by Stromeyer, with momentous consequences.

His great book, *De l'Orthomorphie*, with its fine accompanying Atlas, appeared in 1828[37]. This treatise was based on the physiologic concept that the ligaments were only secondary supports of the joints, protected by muscle tone, that the balance between agonists and antagonists together with muscle proprioception regulates posture, and that imbalance leads to deformity, ideas obviously imbibed from Boyer and, at a longer remove, from Andry.

In 1825, he founded his own private institute just outside the city gates on the Toulouse road, one of the first of many such institutes to embellish Europe in the first half of the century. This embraced a grand courtyard, a heated winter gymnasium, an English Garden with an open-air summer gymnasium, a swimming-pool, and an orchard with a wide range of gymnastic appliances used mainly by young women in decorous pantaloons of his own devising. This was essentially a centre for the treatment of postural spinal

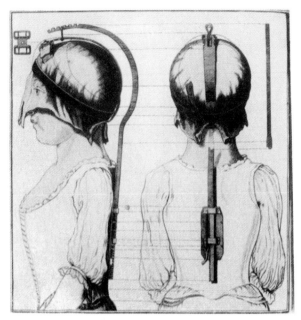

Figure 116   François Guillame Levacher: Minerva jacket with jury-mast suspension
for spinal curvature, Paris 1768

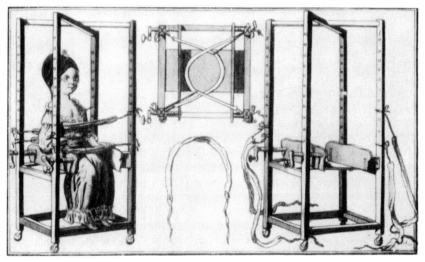

Figure 117   Levacher de la Feutrie: Traité du Rakitis, Paris 1772. Extension chair
for scoliosis with lateral pressure on convexities

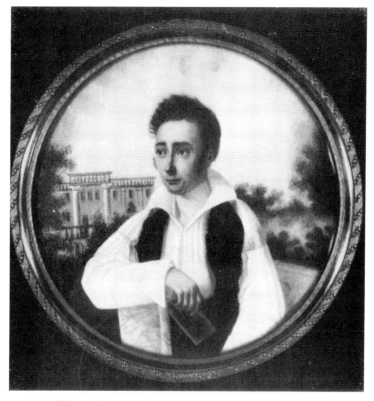

Figure 118 Jacques-Mathieu Delpech (1777–1832)

curves by remedial exercises, which he acknowledged to be much influenced by the scientific concepts of 'the celebrated and clever Dr John Shaw' of London (p. 95). Delpech found it essential to distinguish curvatures due to malposture, poliomyelitis, scoliosis and kyphosis from those due to tuberculosis, and seems to have been the first to insist that the *mal de Pott* should be called *affection tuberculeuse des vertèbres*. 'The tuberculous nature of gibbus spine,' wrote Garrison, 'had been surmised by Hippocrates, confirmed by Galen, revived by Planter, and finally established by Delpech[38].' We must not overlook Dalechamps (p. 221). Delpech determined by suspension whether or not a curve was fixed. His treatment for scoliosis included a hard bed, head traction and pelvic countertraction while supine, and uninterrupted maintenance of correct posture throughout all daily activities, even including piano-playing and carriage drives, using devices which he acknowledged were derived almost entirely from the work of Shaw.

One gets the impression of a driving remedial activist who could direct his energies thus because he was *not* treating caries or other true diseases of the spine, and that this was because his practice was mainly with well-to-do middleclass young women – not that this lessens the achievements and understanding of pathology illustrated in the great *Atlas*.

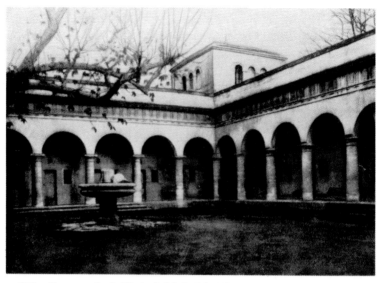

Figure 119   Courtyard of *Hôpital Général* in Montpellier where Delpech initially practised, demolished 1938

On 29th October 1832, driving back to his institute in an open carriage, Delpech (and his coachman) was shot dead by a disgruntled and probably deranged patient on whom he had operated for varicocoele, the bullet traversing the arch of the aorta. The horses left to their own devices, conveyed his body back to the Institute.* There is a good general account of his life in Rochard's *Histoire de la Chirurgie Française au XIXme Siècle* (Paris, Baillière, 1875). The institute was taken over by Victor Trinquier, who had previously directed a similar establishment in Bordeaux and who published some of Delpech's work posthumously[39].

According to Valentin, at about the time of Delpech's death orthopaedics in France began to organize itself in depth under influences emanating from Switzerland and Germany. Elsewhere, we discuss the role of the great precursor, Jean-André Venel, in Switzerland. His nephew, **Louis d'Ivernois** (1789–1844) came to work in Paris around 1813 and was the first there to use Venel's shoe – the *sabot de Venel* – for club-foot. He opened an 'orthomorphic establishment', presumably adopting Delpech's terminology, with **Isidore Bricheteau** (1787–1862) as a partner to propagate the new massage. He also popularized Venel's extension bed. D'Ivernois returned to Orbe in 1830.

At the turn of the 18th–19th centuries, **P F Moreau**, of Bar-le-Duc in north-east France near Nancy, like his contemporary Henry Park in Liverpool, was performing excision of tuberculous joints, intended – or at

---

*Orthopaedic surgeons seem rather vulnerable to execution by dissatisfied patients; for a complete list, see p. 352, 362.

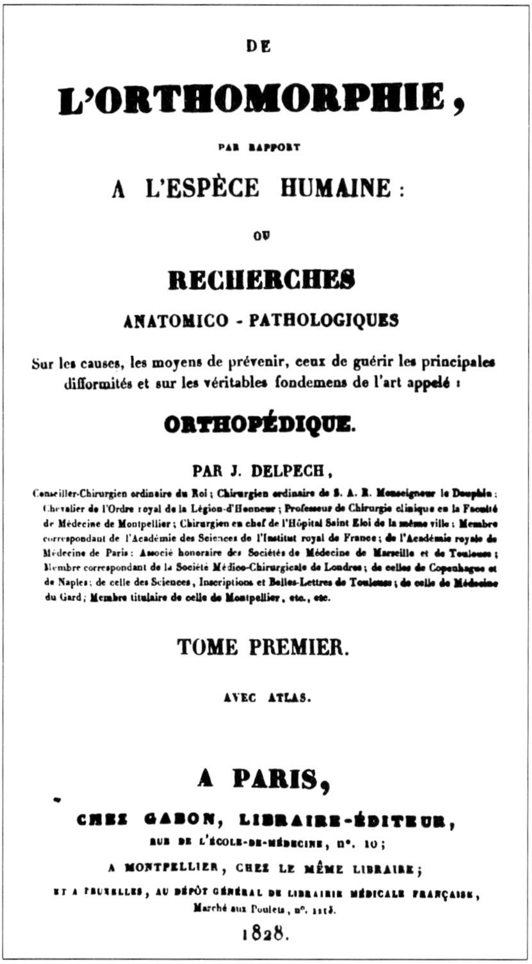

DE

L'ORTHOMORPHIE,

PAR RAPPORT

A L'ESPÈCE HUMAINE :

OU

RECHERCHES

ANATOMICO - PATHOLOGIQUES

Sur les causes, les moyens de prévenir, ceux de guérir les principales
difformités et sur les véritables fondemens de l'art appelé :

ORTHOPÉDIQUE.

PAR J. DELPECH,

Conseiller-Chirurgien ordinaire du Roi ; Chirurgien ordinaire de S. A. R. Monseigneur le Dauphin ;
Chevalier de l'Ordre royal de la Légion-d'Honneur ; Professeur de Chirurgie clinique en la Faculté
de Médecine de Montpellier ; Chirurgien en chef de l'Hôpital Saint Eloi de la même ville ; Membre
correspondant de l'Académie des Sciences de l'Institut royal de France ; de l'Académie royale de
Médecine de Paris ; Associé honoraire des Sociétés de Médecine de Marseille et de Toulouse ;
Membre correspondant de la Société Médico-Chirurgicale de Londres ; de celles de Copenhague et
de Naples ; de celle des Sciences, Inscriptions et Belles-Lettres de Toulouse ; de celle de Médecine
du Gard ; Membre titulaire de celle de Montpellier, etc., etc.

TOME PREMIER.

AVEC ATLAS.

A PARIS,

CHEZ GABON, LIBRAIRE-ÉDITEUR,

RUE DE L'ÉCOLE-DE-MÉDECINE, n°. 10 ;

A MONTPELLIER, CHEZ LE MÊME LIBRAIRE ;

ET A BRUXELLES, AU DÉPÔT GÉNÉRAL DE LIBRAIRIE MÉDICALE FRANÇAISE,
Marché aux Poulets, n°. 1113.

1828.

Figure 120   Delpech: title page of *De l'Orthomorphie*

any rate likely – to result in fusion, for he followed the operation by placing
the bone-ends in contact and immobilizing the limb until consolidation
occurred, much as Paré had done 200 years earlier[40]. This was a difficult
and time-consuming procedure, unpopular with some – particularly military
surgeons – who preferred the rapidity of amputation, which was precisely
why its advocacy was necessary. (As we have seen, Hugh Owen Thomas was
to despise both as unnecessary and inferior to conservatism.) Moreau is also
said to have attempted, unsuccessfully, to wire an ununited fracture of the
humerus as early as 1805. Moreau's son continued the practice of excision
and another Frenchman, P J Roux (not to be confused with the Augustin
Roux of the 18th century) was also active in this field. It is sad to have to
record that the elder Moreau, though he reported his method to the *Académie*

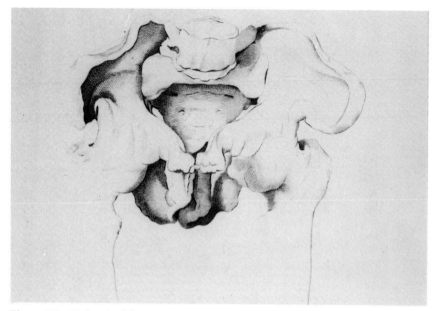

Figure 121   Delpech: rickety pelvis (from the *Atlas* accompanying *De l'Orthomorphie*),

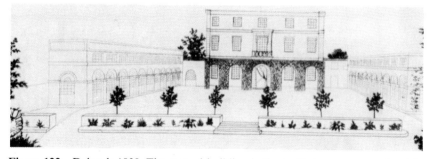

Figure 122   Delpech 1828. The central building is the institute proper; on the right there is a hot-house and on the left the winter gymnasium

de Chirurgie in 1782, and demonstrated it to Percy in 1786, and though he carefully described excision of the elbow, knee and ankle, was virtually ignored. It took another 30 or 40 years for the operation to become respectable in France, where it was reintroduced from England as a 'novelty' by Léon le Fort in 1859, just as Delpech's tenotomy had to be reintroduced, with embellishments, from Germany.

Not far from Bar-le-Duc, at Morley (Meuse), but distant from any university, **Francois Humbert** (1776–1850) founded an *établissement orthopé-*

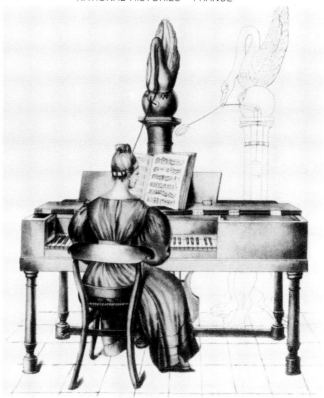

Figure 123 Delpech: 'Column with counterweight, for study of the piano, harp, drawing etc. The idea of this instrument is not our own; we have taken it almost entirely from the work of Dr Shaw.' (1828)

dique in 1817 which he claimed to be the first in France[41]. It certainly predated Delpech's institute at Montpellier and initially resembled it in treating mainly spinal curvatures. He invented an instrument, the 'hybometer', to measure the changes produced by curvatures and was a very capable constructor of extension beds and chairs. Humbert was one of the first to attempt to cure congenital dislocation of the hip by manipulative reduction. In a book published with Jacquier in 1835[42], he asserted that by forcible instrumental extension he had succeeded in replacing the femoral head in its socket in a single 55 minute session in both congenital and pathological dislocations (even in an 11-year-old girl!). Pravaz (see below) argued that this was not a reduction but an anterior transposition, by no means unknown before the era of X-rays and sometimes deliberately aimed at, for it was certainly an improvement. Nevertheless, Pravaz (who was, incidentally, the first to achieve genuine reduction) gave Humbert full credit for his 'bold initiative' in conceiving that reduction might be a possibility and for obtaining a more stable position[43,44], while Gerdy also conceded the originality of the conception, even if unsuccessful[45].

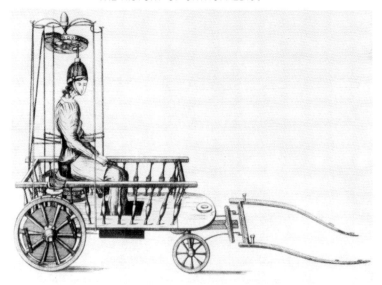

Figure 124   Delpech: 'rotary carriage' (1828)

Charles-Gabriel Pravaz (1791–1853) was a doctor's son who was called on to give orthopaedic advice to schoolgirls, and thus led to found an institute in Paris in 1826, at Passy, where he took Guérin into partnership. Here he devised new types of bed for the traction treatment of scoliosis[46], similar to beds being used by many others in England and the Continent, all of which seem to have dated back to Venel in Switzerland, described in 1789. Pravaz also invented special appliances for gymnastic correction, such as his self-propelled bed and his *balançoire orthopédique*[47], and gave some credence to creeping or crawling exercises. Like Andry, he thought scoliosis due to unequal muscle growth or activity.

In 1834, leaving Guérin to run the Paris institute, he moved to Lyons, where he took a special interest in congenital dislocation of the hip. In that year he reduced a dislocation in an 8-year-old child by traction, abduction and pressure over the trochanter, and by 1847 had treated 19 children with 15 cures, the treatment lasting some 18 months[48]. There can be little doubt of his priority in this field. Later, he enthusiastically adopted Bouvier's subtrochanteric osteotomy for old unreduced cases.

Pravaz is credited with the invention of the hypodermic syringe. This came about because he was interested in curing aneurysms with an electric current and discovered the coagulating effect of iron sesquichloride, and devised a metal syringe with a hollow needle to inject this into the vessels[49].

Jules Guérin (1801–1866), the Parisian orthopaedic surgeon, was a man of extraordinary character, and that often far from amiable since he could be as contentious as Andry or Thomas. He was respected (and feared) by his colleagues and visited by surgeons from the world over, especially from the USA. Like Thomas, he was convinced that he, and only he, knew what orthopaedics was about and that he had personally invented it. However,

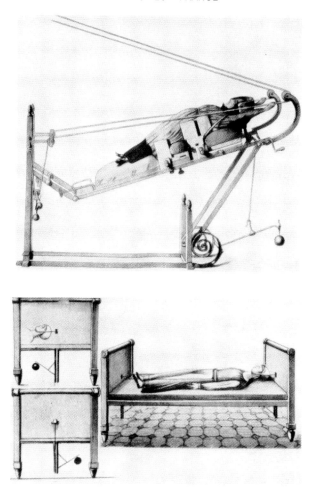

Figure 125 Pravaz: Bed with progressive extension; 'a new method for the treatment of deviations of the vertebral column.' Paris, 1827

his foreign visitors found him courteous and helpful. In 1842, Valentine Mott, from New York, wrote, 'The princely establishment of my excellent friend Dr Jules Guérin in Paris at Passy may be cited as passing all the rest. The ingenious and distinguished founder has done more than all his contemporaries in the practice of myotomy and tenotomy[50].' But then, none of us is altogether unfamiliar with orthopaedic prima donnas who are irritantly clamant of priority on their home ground but bland and welcoming to visitors from abroad.

One problem – and it is still not universally solved – related to the dividing line between the territories of general surgeons and orthopaedists. Guérin was severely criticized for treating patients who did not come within his sphere, so much so that a commission of the Paris Faculty deliberated on

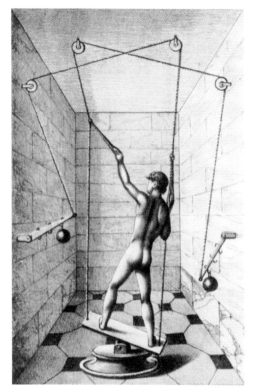

Figure 126   Pravaz: '*Balançoire Orthopédique*', Paris 1827

the matter for three years and could only conclude that it was very difficult to fix the demarcation between orthopaedics and surgery, 'of which it is a subsidiary[51]'.

Guérin's visitors were amazed at his enthusiasm for tenotomy and myotomy for treating scoliosis (p. 537), which, though owing its origin to Delpech, had to be reimported from Germany. Guérin regarded scoliosis (and all other deformities, including club-foot) as due to 'convulsive muscular contraction'. Hence, spinal myotomy was entirely justified and in 1838 he deposited a sealed envelope with the *Académie des Sciences* claiming priority[52]. However, he used the method to such excess, and made such extravagant claims for its results, as to arouse reaction among his colleagues – from Bouvier[53], and from his especial enemy, Malgaigne, who reported to the Academy that he had investigated Guérin's patients and found these girls not only unimproved, but worse or even crippled by the weakness the operation had created[54]. This was entirely confirmed by a special commission[55]. In 1844 the Academy formally endorsed Malgaigne's criticisms and that was the end of spinal myotomy in France. Indeed, we are told that, as a result, Guérin was ousted from his hospital appointments, ironically enough for providing the first purely orthopaedic service in France[56]. Guérin

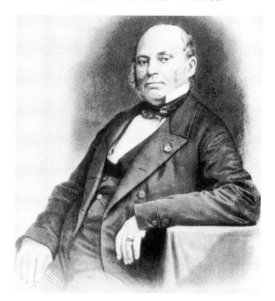

Figure 127   Jules Guérin (1801–1866)

brought a legal action against Malgaigne and Velpeau (a member of the commission) for slander and won his case, but only to further damage himself in public opinion. The situation was ironic because Guérin had previously exposed the fake cures of scoliosis by Hossard (p. 537) and had been sued by Hossard and lost the case. It is only fair to say that Guérin's method found considerable support in Germany and Italy and, remarkably, in very recent times, from such an eminent surgeon as Joseph Trueta.

Guérin also practised subcutaneous tenotomy for torticollis[57] and claimed reduction of congenital dislocation of the hip after multiple myotomies and tenotomies around the joint, sparing scarcely a single muscle[58]. Pravaz pointed out that the weakened muscles were now unable to contain the femoral head in the rudimentary acetabulum. Perhaps because of this, Guérin now went a step further and attempted to enlarge the acetabular roof by scarifying the periosteum above the labrum with a tenotome and asserted that this created a ridge which stabilized the joint. This, too, had to be officially investigated, 'M J Guérin announces that subcutaneous periarticular scarification and later resumption of mechano-gymnastic treatment result in provoking the formation of a cotyloid rim and consolidating the articulation … (he) performs subcutaneous section of the tight muscular band and practises periarticular scarification behind and slightly above the point currently occupied by the femoral head: these scarifications involve the entire thickness of the soft parts down to the bone[59].'

Guérin was one of the first to use a type of plaster bandage for correction of club-foot and also performed tarsal osteotomy for this condition[60,61].

Sauveur-Henri-Victor Bouvier (1799–1877) was a hardworking and sincere physician who inherited an orthopaedic institute in Paris from one Milli, who had been a patient of Heine at Würzburg (p. 181). His 1837 survey of bony deformities earned him a prize from the *Académie des Sciences*[62], and he wrote an encompassing account of the corset in history[63] and a series of lectures on orthopaedic subjects which used the term 'locomotor apparatus' for the first time[64]. He practised at the *Hôpital des Enfants Malades* in Paris and was noted for refusing to speak for two weeks before he was due to address a medical meeting, to spare his voice. He died tragically, after a winter's day in 1877, when, now almost blind, he fell into the icy water of the great basin in the Tuileries gardens.

Bouvier was an enthusiast of the orthopaedic bed that provided traction, often called extension, as introduced by Venel. For scoliosis, he gave his young female patients crutches so long that their feel hardly touched the ground and they had to swing themselves along, as Dieffenbach remarked, like kangaroos[65]. This was in order to unstress the spine; and Delpech noted wrily that if one of these young women happened to break a crutch after months of such locomotion, they were quite unable to make their way indoors, so used were they to not standing on their own feet[66].

Bouvier distinguished between rachitic and postural curves, considering the latter an exaggeration of physiologic deviations. Club-foot accompanying spina bifida was, he thought, due to 'perversion' of muscular activity by a disturbance of nervous activity. It was Bouvier who, 20 years later, in 1836, followed up Delpech's first historic subcutaneous tenotomy of 1816 and reported it a complete and lasting success, describing the organization of a 'tendinous callus' within the tendon sheath[67]. He himself practised the operation and proposed subcutaneous section of the plantar structures for

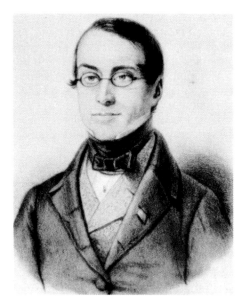

Figure 128   Sauveur-Henri-Victor Bouvier (1799–1877)

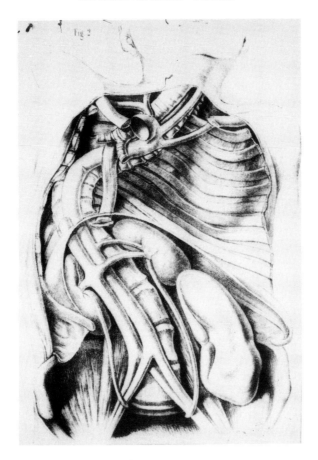

Figure 129 Bouvier: the pathology of scoliosis

the accompanying cavus.

Bouvier would not at first believe that Pravaz had succeeded in reducing a congenital dislocation of the hip by long-continued traction and abduction and never retracted his opposition, despite his own exertions in the field, for he was convinced that the constriction of the joint capsule, rather than shallowness of the socket or muscle contracture, made reposition anatomically impossible[68]. However, he did suggest, in 1835, that late deformity might be corrected by subcutaneous subtrochanteric osteotomy and obtained good results which were copied elsewhere and adapted to older patients:

Orthopaedics was first accepted as an independent speciality in France around 1850, and it may be said that Bouvier was the first 'official' orthopaedist. The early decades of the 19th century were marked by a rash of orthopaedic institutes in France. One such was founded in Paris in 1823 by **Guillaume Jalade-Lafond** (b.1805), deviser of an 'extension chair' and an 'oscillatory bed' with which he even attempted reduction of congenital hip

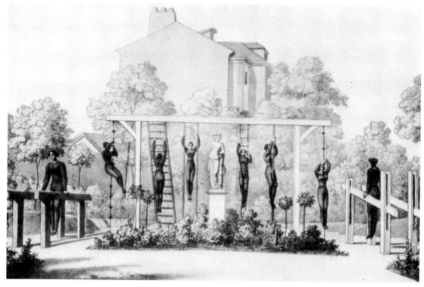

Figure 130   Jalade-Lafond: gymnastic exercises in the garden of his institute, (1827)

dislocation. The gardens of his intitute at Chaillot abounded with elegantly clad maidens engaged in varied gymnastic activities. Lafond took his son-in-law, **Vincent Duval**, into partnership. Duval gained a reputation for his treatment of club-foot,* on which he wrote a treatise[69], and it was this treatise that the novelist Gustave Flaubert consulted when he was planning for his character, Doctor Bovary, to perform an ill-fated section of the Achilles tendon (p. 504). Towards the end of the century, Duval's son Emile produced his own book on the subject[70].

From 1849, the elder Duval edited the *Revue des Spécialités et des Innovations médicales et chirurgicales*, writing a number of orthopaedic articles himself, and in 1825 there appeared a *Journal clinique sur les difformités*, but this lasted only until 1829. One of its editors was **Charles-Amédée Maisonabe** (b.1804), who seems to have written most of the material singlehanded as a step towards his comprehensive 1834 treatise on deformities[71]. At about this time, **Pierre Nicolas Gerdy** (1797–1856) published his treatise on bandaging and appliances[72], his elegant constructions have been mentioned earlier. Gerdy had the courage to speak out against what was rapidly becoming a mania for extension beds, and it was his support that gained the approval of the commission set up to assess Pravaz's efforts with congenitally dislocated hips.

We have referred to Guérin's running battle with **Joseph-François Mal-**

---

* It is indicative of the poor relation status of orthopaedic surgery at this time that Duval's weekly session at the *Hôpital des Enfants Malades* was monitored by a commission of physicians and surgeons who checked his diagnoses and results.

gaigne (1806–1865). Malgaigne was born at Charmes, in the Moselle, began medical studies at Nancy at 15, endured privation in Paris, in 1830 took a hospital unit to help the Poles in their struggle against Russia. He was professor of operative surgery in Paris from 1850 until his death, the first to operate under general anaesthesia in France, in January 1847, less than 3 months after Morton in Boston; but, as sometimes happens, he was not very dextrous himself: a critic described him as having two left hands.* However, Malgaigne was a man of outstanding erudition and application. Notable are his edition of the works of Ambroise Paré in 1840[73], his treatise on fractures and dislocations of 1847–55[74], his study of appliances used in fracture treatment from the time of Hippocrates[75] and his monumental *Leçons*

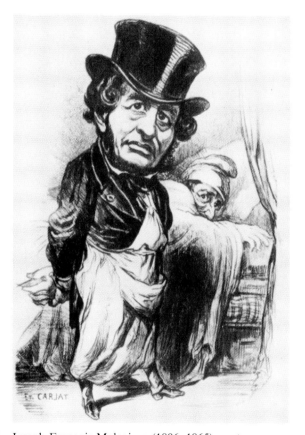

Figure 131   Joseph-François Malgaigne (1806–1865): contemporary caricature

---

* When the present writer, as a medical student at University College Hospital, London, before World War I, was assisting the great philosopher–surgeon, Wilfred Trotter, the latter asked him why he was using his left hand. 'I am trying to become ambidextrous, Sir' met with the crushing retort from the sardonic Trotter: 'Well, you're making progress; you're ambisinistrous already!'

d'Orthopédie of 1862. He died of a cerebral haemorrhage sustained while chairing a meeting of the *Académie de Médecine* in 1865.

In 1845, Malgaigne defined orthopaedics as 'a branch of surgery which has as its aim to render to deviated joints their form and function and to bony levers their natural direction ... placed in the hands of specialists who were empirics and not surgeons, or of surgeons without much talent who had abandoned surgery to devote themselves to this speciality. Orthopaedics remained in obscurity until the last century: it was increasingly limited to the treatment of spinal kyphosis and club-foot.'

Malgaigne added trauma to orthopaedics, revised Boyer's *Leçons sur les maladies des os* of 1803, took an interest in fractures (he described ischaemic forearm contracture due to tight dressings 34 years before Volkmann) and did experimental work in animals which proved the existence of incomplete and longitudinal fractures. He designed the racquet incision for amputation, an advance on the circular incision, and was an enthusiast for the traction treatment of fractures introduced in the USA at the midcentury. We refer elsewhere to his early attempts at external fixation for fracture by pins or prongs, as for fractures of the patella, where the clamps were held by screw-plates allowing compression, and how he applied this to the tibia (p. 557), but there must have been some trouble with sepsis as it fell into disrepute until revived by Ombredanne at the turn of the century. Although Malgaigne was an opponent of Guérin, he did try the latter's method of multiple myotomy for scoliosis, but not for long. In 1840 he founded the *Journal de Chirurgie* and in 1847 became chief editor of the *Revue médico-chirurgicale de Paris*. It was as an editor that he thought it his duty to quarrel with Guérin.

We now step back somewhat to refer to **Baron Guillaume Dupuytren** (1777–1835). Rang tells us that he was the son of a poor lawyer, kidnapped by a rich woman attracted by his looks, rescued and taken to study medicine in Paris (where he was alleged to have used the fat of cadavers to fuel his lamp). He became chief surgeon at the *Hôtel-Dieu* in 1813 at the age of 36 and worked enormously hard, starting at dawn or earlier every day and became known as 'the first of surgeons and the least of men' or the 'brigand' of the Hôtel-Dieu, probably because of his harsh and over-weening habits towards patients and colleagues, remarked on with amazement by American visitors. Peltier says that 'he reigned there as an absolute monarch for twenty years, the greatest French surgeon since Paré[76]. What was more important was that he combined enormous clinical experience and observation with an interest in pathology, far from a common combination for the age. We associate his name with the eponymous contracture of the palmar fascia and a particular ankle fracture, but he wrote on many subjects: congenital dislocation of the hip, the nature of callus formation, subungual exostosis (he operated on 30 cases) and many others[77]. He had his fracture service on the ground floor for ease of transportation and followed Pott and Chessher in treating lower limb fractures with the hip and knee semi-flexed.

In 1826, he wrote at length on 'original' (i.e. congenital) dislocation of the hip[78], asserting that he was the first to do so though clinical descriptions go back to Hippocrates and its tendency to be hereditary had been noted by

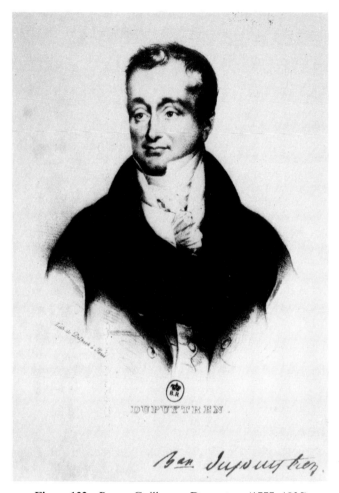

Figure 132   Baron Guillaume Dupuytren (1777–1835)

Paré. He based his remarks on a series of observed cases and post-mortem examinations. It was a triumph of clinical and pathologic observation, at a time when there were no X-rays and when dislocation in children due to suppuration and in adults due to trauma was common. It was, he thought, 'a transposition which exists at birth and appears due to a defect in the depth of the acetabulum rather than to accident or disease'. He describes the shortening and telescoping, the lumbar lordosis, the waddling gait, the Trendelenberg sign (which he does not name). He stigmatizes the cruelty of useless treatment such as blistering, the absence of signs of inflammation, the tendency to be bilateral (which he thought universal) and even stresses that indications of the lesion may be detected at birth if only sought for, yet the diagnosis is usually made only after several years. It was not scrofulous or rachitic. The trochanters might eventually rise as high as the iliac crests and the pelvifemoral muscles became contracted. The femoral head was misshapen, the acetabulum absent or defective, while a secondary superficial socket formed above and behind it. Almost all his cases were in females and he speculates on the flexed position of the hips *in utero* as a cause, the capsular ligament yielding under the strain, a supposition still valid in some cases where hormonal influences are added to genetic dysplasia.

On the basis of his anatomic studies, Dupuytren concluded that treatment was pointless, 'What is the use of traction exerted on the lower limbs? Supposing that by this means one could restore these limbs to their length, is it not obvious that, the femoral head finding no cavity disposed to receive it and capable of retaining it, the limb would lose the length afforded it as soon as it was left to itself[79]?' He said this to save colleagues from unprofitable manoeuvres other than a palliative girdle, and patients from distress. Yet only two years later one of this pupils, Caillard-Bilonière, refers to an 8-year-old girl with bilateral dislocation whom Dupuytren had transferred to the institute of Jalade-Lafond and Duval, where she was treated by continuous traction in the *machine oscillatoire*. 'It was not without great surprise that, after three or four months of continuous extension, Dupuytren saw the greater part of the good effects produced by this means persist after several weeks ... This case is important in itself, and may become even more so because of the consequences it may have[80].'

The effect did not last, and Dupuytren remained absolutely pessimistic. However, Valentin suggests that it was this very pessimism that kept the problem permanently on the agenda, perhaps because it eventually led to the idea that the acetabulum or the femoral head, or both, must be reshaped[81], possibly because, in orthopaedics, juniors are always hoping to prove the 'Old Man' wrong.

There is a well known story of a murdered man being dismembered to make him unrecognizable; the pieces were found in a sack. Dupuytren established a congenital hip dislocation, and the judicial authorities, advised of this defect, striking in life, were able to identify both victim and murderer.

Dupuytren invented, or reinvented, subcutaneous tenotomy of the sterno-mastoid for torticollis, dividing the sternal and clavicular heads of the muscle in a 12-year-old girl in 1822 with a 'Pott's buttoned bistoury' passed behind the tendon. The shoulder was brought down by tying the right hand to the right foot.

In an essay on callus formation, written about 1808, Dupuytren distinguished between provisional and permanent callus. The former was external (periosteal) and medullary, brittle and eventually reabsorbed; the latter was cortical and even stronger than the original bone. Final organization of the permanent callus occupied 8–12 months and was marked by disappearance of the provisional callus and reopening of the medullary canal. His account of the stages of fracture union is detailed, redolent of close observation and well worth reading.

As for the palmar contracture, it had already been clearly described by Henry Cline in 1808[82] and by Astley Cooper[83], in 1808 and in 1822, both of whom advised section of the contracted bands with narrow knife, so it is difficult to see why Dupuytren's accounts in 1832[84] and 1834[85] should have gained priority. He noted that it tended to affect those with occupational pressure on the palm, started at the ulnar side, and was due to contraction of the palmar fascia – 'from its lower portion are given off kinds of cords which pass to the diseased fingers' – while the joints, tendons and ligaments were perfectly normal. Some surgeons proposed section of the tendons, but Dupuytren simply did a fasciotomy through several small incisions and splinted the fingers straight, leaving the wounds open. He distinguished between osteosarcoma (though he did not use the term in its modern sense) and 'spina ventosa', distension of a bone, often in the hand, from a tuberculous or nonmalignant process, and thought that it was not uncommon for the latter to become malignant[86].

Marie Francois Xavier Bichat (1771–1802) was a Paris surgeon who helped to establish the histology and histopathology of joints on a sound basis with his *Traité des Membranes en Général et de Diverses Membranes en Particulier* (Paris 1799–1800). A section of this book is devoted to the synovial membrane. Paracelsus had uses the term synovia for the fluid, which Havers later thought was secreted by the fat pads, acting as glands. Bichat corrected this error: the fat pads were mere mechanical buffers; the fluid did not result from glandular action or transudation from the bone-ends, it was 'exhaled' from the many orifices of a serous membrane analogous to the pleura or peritoneum, i.e. it was a dialysate from the blood, and was returned to the circulation by absorption. Nevertheless, Havers, whom we consider elsewhere (p. 72), was not altogether wrong in regarding the synovial cells as mucin-secreting. Bichat also wrote a *Traité d'Anatomie Humaine* in 1819 in which he stated that the dorsal spine had a normal deviation to the right to accommodate the aorta, and that idiopathic scoliosis was an exaggeration of this curve.

We now come to the important place held in orthopaedics, and especially in both pathology and physiology, by the Lyons school. Here, an orthopaedic precursor was **J P N Nichet** (1803–1847), who confirmed Delpech's rather intuitive recognition of the essential nature of Pott's disease by a careful study of the morbid anatomy in a series of autopsies. 'It is the scrofulous tubercle that constitutes the essence of this grave deterioration of the vertebral column[87].' His treatment was by rest and reclination, with local bleeding and caustics.

Even before Pravaz removed to Lyons from Paris in 1835 there had been an orthopaedic establishment in the city. Subsequent famous names include those of Bonnet, Ollier, Poncet, Leriche and Policard.

Amédée Bonnet (1809–1858) was chief surgeon at the *Hôtel-Dieu* from 1835 and professor at the medical school from 1839. In 1840 he studied the preferential position of inflamed joints by experimental injection of cadaver articulations[88]. Like everyone else he wrote a book on tenotomy, which he applied to squint and stammering as well as club-foot[89]. He elaborated the wire splints for limb fixation introduced by Mayor of Lausanne and added a triangle attached to the foot of the splint to limit painful instability in arthritis of the knee. Bonnet wrote an early *Traité des maladies des articulations* (Paris and Lyons 1845) and a later work in 1860, the *Nouvelles* *méthodes de traitement des maladies articulaires.* Like Malgaigne in Paris and Hilton in London and many others, Bonnet was an apostle of rest for joint disease, fixing the joints proximal and distal to the diseased joint. He insisted on the need for a functional position in ankylosis (though he was one of the first to mobilize a fibrous ankylosis under general anaesthesia) and wrote on every aspect of joint disease, thus orienting the Lyons school towards orthopaedics and its apogee under Ollier, soon to follow.

Louis-Xavier-Edouard-Léopold Ollier (1830–1900) followed Bonnet in the surgical chair. As his name is so closely linked with bone growth, we cannot proceed without looking first at some earlier work in this field.

In 1736, **John Belchier** (1706–1785), a young surgeon recently appointed to Guy's Hospital in London, was given for supper pork from pigs fed on madder-soaked bran by a calico printer. He noted that the bones were stained red and was able to reproduce this by feeding madder to a cock: 'but why the bones only are affected, I shall consider of in the Course of more Experiments[90]' (of which there is no record). Perhaps he became interested because he had been a pupil of William Cheselden (p. 83), who taught that bones grew by the supply of matter via the periosteal vessels[91].

The polymath, Hans Sloane, mentioned Belchier's paper to **Henri-Louis Duhamel** (1700–1782), an amateur scientist and member of the Paris *Académie des Sciences*, who repeated Belchier's experiments during 1739–43[92]. He noted that, when madder was fed during fracture healing, only the newly-deposited bone was stained and that the new bone was mainly periosteal, that the madder was laid down peripherally in layers and could be alternated with unstained layers by intermittently interrupting the supply of madder, and concluded that the periosteum must be osteogenic, a supposition that was to be hotly disputed through the next century, and even in the same century by John Hunter. Duhamel realized that the marrow cavity must enlarge with growth, but could not account for *how* it expanded. Silver markers he inserted in the shaft did not become separated, i.e. longitudinal bone growth had to take place at the bone ends, though he was unable to clarify this.

Duhamel's views on periosteal osteogenesis ran directly counter to those of the famous Swiss–German physiologist, Albrecht Haller (1708–1777) at Göttingen, who, writing before the days of cell histology, believed that minerals were deposited by the arteries and that bone formation was a function of blood-supply. Hunter repeated Belchier's work and showed that long bones were being continuously remodelled, bone being simultaneously deposited externally and absorbed internally (he thought via the lymphatics). This must also occur in the process of sequestration, 'While Nature is busied in getting rid of that part of the bone which is dead, she is laying on additional bone on the outside.' Hunter thought that fracture callus came from the arterioles of the bone-ends or periosteum or other membranes; it was not a mere product of the periosteum.

Marie Jean-Pierre Flourens (b.1794), permanent secretary of the Academy, confirmed this remodelling process but also thought that Duhamel was right, that the periosteum *was* osteogenic and could even reproduce the entire shaft[93].

We may now return to Ollier, a contemporary of Lister, both exemplars of a new type of surgeon relying on observations in experimental physiology and pathology. Ollier studied at Lyons and Montpellier. In 1857–9, working in Paris, he proved in rabbits that periosteal strips, even completely detached and buried under the skin, could and did form bone if the deep layer with the osteoblasts was intact. In 1868, now in Lyons, he wrote his *Traité expérimentale et clinique de la regéneration des os et de la production artificielle du tissue osseux*. Irritation of a bone was osteogenic because the 'corpuscles' multiplied; arterial ligature had no effect; a transplanted bone fragment died and was absorbed; and in fractures the greater part of the callus came from the periosteum, only a little from the marrow, least from the bone itself. If a segment of the shaft were removed subperiosteally, regeneration was complete, from the 'cambium' layer of the membrane. True, the epiphyseal cartilage formed bone, but only *in situ*, never if transplanted. In 1864, Ollier removed the upper half of the humerus subperiosteally for tuberculosis in a girl of five; by age seven it had reformed, though two inches short.

Here, we have an extraordinary historical counterpart to William Macewen of Glasgow (p. 131), who took exactly the opposite view; only the osteoblasts were osteogenic, the periosteum was completely inactive, osteoblasts and osteoclasts acting reciprocally presided over bone growth and remodelling. Bone defects could be reconstituted by inserting bone chips stripped of their covering. In 1878, as if to counter Ollier, he did his famous operation on a boy aged three affected by chronic osteomyelitis of the entire right humerus, in whom excision of the entire shaft save for the epiphyses had left the arm useless. He denied the parents' request for amputation and inserted a series of tibial wedges obtained from corrective osteotomies for rickety knee deformities, devoid of periosteum. At 35 the patient was a workman with a humerus only three inches shorter than the left, i.e. free grafts *could* survive and grow, and if the shaft regrew, it must be from the growth-plates[94]. It does not seem to have occurred to Macewen that he might have removed the dead shaft from within an intact periosteal sleeve. Of course, both the periosteal and the shaft schools of thought were right, though the work of the Swiss school of osteosynthesis has tended to stress the role of the cortex.

Nevertheless, the two schools remained in such bitter, almost theological, opposition, sustained by thousands of experiments, that Sir Arthur Keith concluded that the only explanation must be that the bones of Parisian dogs were constructed on different principles from those of Glasgow and London! Ollier was partly motivated by the idea that joint excision, if it was to leave a mobile pseudarthrosis, must be accompanied by excision of the periosteum, and that if ankylosis were the object the membrane should be left intact. When he aimed at mobility, he used active and passive motion and, in treating fused joints, anticipated arthroplasty by interposing adipose tissue between the bone ends.

It is of great historic interest – and not much known – that as far back as 1877 Ollier suggested that bone-growth might be inhibited by resection of the epiphyseal plate for the correction of certain deformities[95], a method not to be rediscovered or applied until employed by Phemister 56 years later (p. 432).

In 1899, Ollier described dyschondroplasia[96], based on two cases of growth disturbances in young girls in whom the newly discovered X-rays showed translucent masses of cartilage within the shafts. He also described, in 1864, a type of chronic osteomyelitis, reported later by his pupil Antonin Poncet (1845–1913) as 'periostitis albuminosa[97]', which may or may not have been identical with Garré's sclerosing nonsuppurative osteomyelitis. (Poncet also discovered, or invented, a disease called 'tuberculous rheumatism[98]'.)

Ollier was an army surgeon in the Franco-Prussian War of 1870 and is credited with the use of long-term occlusive dressings many years before Winnett Orr and Trueta, a method found in some form in Larrey's memoirs.

Alexandre Rodet (1814–1884) was chief surgeon at the *Hôpital de l'Antiquaille* in Lyons and is known for his work on the experimental production of osteomyelitis in animals by the intravenous injection of staphylococci (or what he called a micrococcus of a yellow–orange colour), in which he noted the remarkably constant localization of the lesions at the subperiosteal zone of the metaphyses and the sparing of the epiphyses[99]. This work exactly anticipated that of Clarence Starr in Toronto in 1922.

Gabriel Nové-Josserand (1868–1949) was a pupil of Ollier, began as a general surgeon, was influenced by congenital deformities to conceive of orthopaedic surgery as a special field – one of the first French surgeons to do so – and was appointed to the first chair of orthopaedics in Lyons in 1921. He devoted his life to crippled children there, save for his work in the civilian reincorporation of soldiers disabled in World War I, and practised the manipulative reduction of congenital dislocation of the hip. He may have

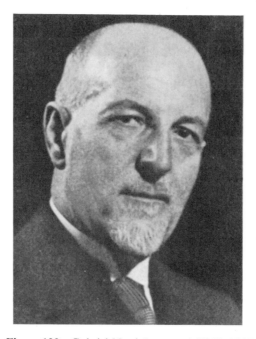

Figure 133   Gabriel Nové-Josserand (1868–1949)

been the first to perform arthrodesis for arthrosis of the hip. He was a wise and reserved man and was associated with the foundation of SICOT (p. 475) and presided over its Second Congress in London in 1933. His successor in the Chair was **Louis Tavernier**, with whom he wrote an account of malignant bone tumours in 1927[100]. Tavernier was interested in knee derangements, publishing *Pathologie des Menisques du Genou* (with Mouchet) in 1927 and becoming known after World War II for his work on denervation of the painful arthritic hip[101].

Two younger members of the Lyons school were **René Leriche** (1879–1955) and **Albert Policard** (1881–1949), both of whom took an interest in the problems of bone growth[102] before passing to the surgery of the vascular/autonomic system. Leriche became world-famous as professor of surgery at Strasbourg from 1925 to 1939, when he moved to the *Collège de France* in Paris. He did fruitful work on the surgery of the vascular system, of pain and of peripheral nerve injuries, much of which has become incorporated into orthopaedic practice. Though a general surgeon, he retained an interest in skeletal disorders.

Also in Lyons, **Jules Froment** (1878–1946), professor of medicine, studied nerve injuries in World War I and in 1915 recorded his *signe de pouce*, the weakness of the flexor pollicis brevis in low ulnar nerve palsy causing inability to prevent flexion of the interphalangeal joint when attempting to press the thumb straight down on a flat surface[103]. To this we may add the name of **Jules Tinel** (1879–1952), of Rouen and Paris, also a neurologist in the first world war, whose eponymous sign of 'formication' elicited below the site of nerve injury when the nerve is percussed, if elicited at progressively distal levels, indicates regeneration of nerve-fibres, and whose absence conveys a gloomy prognosis[104].

It may be relevant to add that France had some primacy in modern endeavours at nerve suture in the 19th century. In 1863, Lengier of Paris made an early attempt at suture of the median nerve at the wrist, and Letiévant of Lyons refers to median suture in an 1873 treatise on nerve section[105]. Nicasse wrote an article on nerve suture in 1885[106], while in 1893 the great neurologist, Brown-Séquard, reported on the features of recovery after suture[107]. In 1886, Assaky proposed and practised *suture à distance*[108], when gaps too wide for end-to-end suture were bridged by sutures to guide fibre regrowth (one imagines that nowadays strips of muscle would be implanted). In 1873, Letiévant dealt with this problem by 'nerve implantation', inserting the central or distal ends of both of the divided nerves into a sound nerve.

Auguste Nélaton (1807–1873) came to the same conclusions as Nichet (p. 259) as to the nature of Pott's disease in a Paris thesis of 1836[109], written at the early age of 29, in which he also described chronic infiltrating tuberculosis of the long bones, or 'tuberculous osteomyelitis'. Nélaton was early convinced of Pravaz's success in reduction of congenital dislocation of the hip, and said so, 'Pravaz has succeeded in obtaining this long-sought reduction. Reduction of congenital luxations of the femur must therefore now be regarded as a general method in which only the indications remain to be specified[110].'

Nélaton's line, connecting the anterior superior spine, tip of the great trochanter and the ischial tuberosity, should really be called the Roser–Nélaton line as Wilhelm Roser described it in 1846 whereas Nélaton did not do so until a year later. Any displacement of the trochanter above this line was thereafter regarded as evidence of disease or fracture of the hip. Nélaton was one of the surgeons called in as a consultant when Garibaldi suffered a gunshot wound of the ankle in the rising of 1862, and reported his observations in the Paris *Gazette des Hôpitaux*. (Garibaldi went to London two years later with the foot in fixed equinus and was treated there by Henry Heather Bigg.)

Nélaton seems to have been the first to coin, or at least to use, the term 'osteomyelitis' for pyogenic or other infection. In 1860 he published a classic monograph on sarcomas and benign tumours of bone, which recognized the giant-cell lesions[111]. Before this, even experienced pathologists like Virchow had regarded sarcomata as forms of metastatic carcinoma[112], Dupuytren had been one of the first to differentiate true tumours from expanding intraosseous tuberculosis (spina ventosa).

To digress only slightly, in 1882 **Philippe C E Gaucher** (1854–1918) gave the first description of his eponymous 'primary epithelioma of the spleen: splenic hypertrophy without leukaemia[113].' He thought it a neoplasm and was unaware of possible bone involvement, which was pointed out in the 1920s by Cushing[114], Pick[115] and others. It was apt that, in 1927–9, a Leningrad military surgeon, M I Arinkin, introduced sternal puncture as 'an intravital method of examining the bone marrow[116]. Others had suggested that, if peripheral blood examination was unhelpful in diagnosing obscure haematopoietic disorders, the sternum could be trephined through an open incision. Arinkin decided to puncture the manubrium instead with a heavy needle, and this was adapted later (but not by him) to the diagnosis of metastases and to transfusion.

A very famous figure in the orthopaedic world in Paris before and after the turn of the century was **Edouard Kirmisson** (1848–1927), whom Sir Harry Platt has called the acknowledged doyen of French orthopaedics in his time. Kirmisson was the first chief of paediatric and orthopaedic surgery at the *Hôpital des Enfants Malades*, and professor of paediatric surgery from 1901 to 1919 with a reputation for the staged reduction of congenital dislocation of the hip. He wrote, in 1898, on the surgery of congenital deformities[117] and, in 1890, on disorders of the locomotor system[118], while a text on acquired deformities in 1902[119] became the standard work for a generation. Kirmisson popularized (though he did not invent) osteotomy for irreducible congenital hip dislocation and made the connection between slipped upper femoral epiphysis and hypopituitary obesity. In 1890, he founded the *Revue d'Orthopédie* and this was continued as the *Revue de Chirurgie Réparatrice de l'Appareil Moteur*, the official organ of the French Society of Orthopaedic Surgery and Traumatology when that body was founded by himself, Broca, Ombredanne, Nové-Josserand, Mouchet and Froelich in 1918 with Kirmisson as first president.

After Kirmisson, the chair at the *Enfants Malades* was occupied by **Louis**

Ombredanne (1871–1956) from 1921 to 1942. During World War I he had initiated base hospitals in the castles of the Loire, where he practised reconstructive surgery and worked on improved prostheses; but long before that, as early as 1904, he had been using cross-leg skin-flaps and in 1907 devised a simple safe apparatus for ether anaesthesia which was almost the only one in use in France for many years. He is known for his interest in arthrodesis of the paralysed foot[120], spinal fusion in scoliosis (sometimes using the vertebral border of the scapula as a graft), and for shelf operations in congenital dislocation of the hip. Later, he became more interested in adult orthopaedics and was instrumental in creating, in 1932, the first chair in this subject, held by P Mathieu, with whom he wrote an orthopaedic textbook[121]. Before 1932, the only teaching on adult orthopaedics was given by Mauclaire of the Paris Faculty.

In 1930, Ombredanne was one of the founders of SICOT (p. 475), whose first congress was held in Paris in 1933. He published his ideas in his *Clinical and Operative Summary of Paediatric Surgery* in 1923. In 1913, he modified Codivilla's technique of femoral lengthening by performing an oblique osteotomy and applying skeletal traction with a screw device for daily extension[122].

Ombredanne was succeeded, in 1942, by **Jacques Leveuf** (1886–1948), who had been an assistant to Pierre Delbet in the early attempts to nail the fractured neck of femur under X-ray control. At the *Enfants Malades* he was professor of 'Infantile and Orthopaedic Surgery', a combination which was

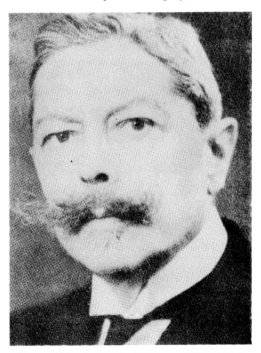

Figure 134   Louis Ombredanne (1871–1956)

the cornerstone of Parisian orthopaedics and typified the paediatric/orthopaedic link in France. It meant the practice, by the same surgeon, of orthopaedic and plastic surgery, neurosurgery and the management of trauma. He established in Brittany, where the condition was common, a centre for congenital dislocation of the hip and performed arthrography on the newborn to detect soft-tissue obstacles to reduction, in his view an indication for operation.

Special mention is due to the work on bone and joint tuberculosis carried on for many years, in the second half of the 19th century and before World War I in particular, at the hospital on the Normandy coast founded by **Victor Ménard**. Ménard remained at the Berck-Plage institution throughout his career, whereas some of his successors came from Paris only on secondment. His work on the tuberculous spine and hip attracted visitors from the world over; the hospital became a long-term institute analogous to similar centres such as the Oswestry Hospital in Britain. Ménard's *Orthopédie et Tuberculose Chirurgicale* of 1914 is a classic. The work was continued by **Etienne Sorrel** and **Madame Déjérine-Sorrel**. Etienne was the surgical side of this marital partnership and wrote on, among other subjects, extra-articular fusion of the hip[123] while his wife wrote a classic monograph on Pott's paraplegia during their ten-year stay at Berck after World War I, before Sorrel was appointed to the *Hôpital Trousseau* in Paris. He was a co-founder of SICOT.

It was at Berck that **Jean-François Calot** (1861–1944) had his own semi-

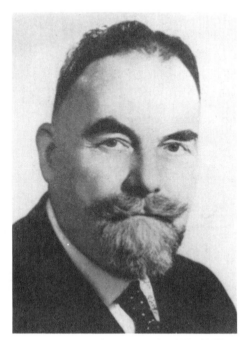

Figure 135   Etienne Sorrel (1882–1965)

independent fiefdom and practised his *redressement brusque* for the kyphosis of Pott's disease[124], so exactly reminiscent of methods of vigorous correction of spinal deformity down the ages from the time of Hippocrates. (Valentin points out that John Shaw (1792–1827) had warned against attempting this procedure – 'If it were possible to push them in or out, the operation would certainly be fatal to the patient[125]' – and comments that, if Calot had been aware of this passage, many patients might have been spared their sad fate.)

It is possible that Calot anticipated Hibbs in performing (or suggesting) spinal fusion in Pott's disease by turning up periosteal flaps from the spinous processes. He injected tuberculous joints and sinuses with antiseptics such as iodoform suspended in oil[126], and it is interesting that he described his manipulative reduction of congenital dislocation of the hip[127] at about the same time as Lorenz, but was completely overshadowed by the latter. Calot believed that congenital hip dysplasia underlay subsequent disorders, such as Perthes' disease and arthrosis, and in this he was, of course, partly correct. The 'Calot jacket' or cast was a plaster jacket for scoliosis incorporating pressure pads over the convexities. His textbook of 'indispensable orthopaedics' was popular in its time and went into nine editions[128].

One of Ménard's pupils and a subsequent assistant surgeon at Berck was **Jacques Calvé** (1875–1954), whom we think of in connection with Legg of Boston and Perthes of Tübingen, all of whom described the hip disease now

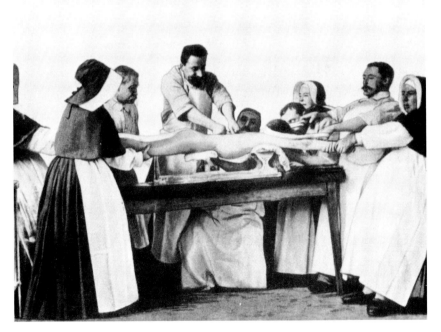

Figure 136   Jean-François Calot and his *redressement brusque* for the kyphosis of Pott's disease, 1896

accorded the name of the last, and in the same year of 1910.*

Calvé and the X-ray arrived at Berck almost simultaneously, at a time when the widening application of radiography was revealing a group of osteochondritides in growing children. This led to the discovery that some of the 'tuberculous' hips were really cases of coxa plana. These were rare cases of hip irritability, suggestive of tuberculosis but with motion retained and X-ray evidence of coxa vara, hypertrophy of the femoral head, increased density, fragmentation and flattening of the epiphysis, but *not* by total destruction or osteoporosis, of short clinical duration, recovering with full movement except full abduction, and without adenopathy or abscess and never relapsing. 'We have described a type of hip which does not correspond to any previously described, and which until now has been considered to be coxotuberculosis[129].' (We need only add Girdlestone's warning that tuberculosis of the hip could present very much in this way, a veritable wolf in sheep's clothing, if the disease chanced to produce vascular occlusion at the outset.)

However, Calvé did have undisputed priority in describing vertebral osteochondritis with collapse, given at length in his contribution to the *Robert Jones Birthday Volume* in 1928 (p. 658). His quite original accounts in 1925[130] were of cases presenting with a painful dorsal kyphosis, sharply angulated, diagnosed and treated as tuberculous but distinguished by complete recovery, negative tuberculin tests and X-ray evidence of sclerotic involvement and collapse of a single vertebral body without involvement of the discs. 'It is impossible not to recognize ... some connection between these two cases and coxa plana ... the affection I have just submitted to you is, I believe, to the spinal column what coxa plana is to the hip and Koehler's disease is to the foot.' Calvé attributed the condition to vascular changes subsequent to trauma, but eosinophil granuloma is now commonly incriminated. (Earlier, in 1922, applying the X-ray to the masses of clinical material at Berck, Calvé had discovered calcification of the intervertebral disc, another condition simulating Pott's disease[131].)

Calvé practised the delicate art of aspirating the intraspinal abscess of Pott's disease to relieve paraplegia, without great success, but his studies of the pathology and mechanics of the disease were masterly. He was not over-enthusiastic over the role of fusion; he did foresee the introduction of ischiofemoral arthrodesis of the hip. He was busy with casualties in the first world war, married the daughter of an American officer, became the director of the Franco-American Foundation at Berck until his retirement in 1945, and spent his last years in the USA.

It is a pleasant duty to call attention to the work of a neglected and obscure Frenchman, **Pierre Le Damany** (1870–1963) in the early detection and treatment of congenital dislocation of the hip which far antedates that

---

* Legg's paper noted 'an obscure affection of the hip joint which clinically and radiologically simulated tuberculosis but did not pursue the usual destructive course.' Perthes called it 'arthritis deformans juvenilis'. It was Waldenström, in 1920, who first called it coxa plana (and claimed to have discovered it in 1909).

of much better known workers[132]. His theories on pathogenesis may have been fanciful (it was 'anthropologic' or 'teratologic' or due to the effect on the human foetus of increased leg-length or brain size); but in and after 1910, 50 or more years before von Rosen[133] or Barlow[134] and 20 years before Ortolani[135], he began large-scale routine examination of the hips of the newborn at the Rennes maternity hospital (hip dysplasia is endemic in Brittany) and described a test essentially similar to the one we use today, 'The operator produces a displacement of the femoral head in the opposite direction to the foregoing. The pulp of the middle finger pushes the trochanter from without inwards at the same time as the thigh is brought suddenly into abduction. With this manoeuvre, the head re-enters the cavity over the posterior rim and this re-entry is accompanied by a jerk ... sometimes sufficiently marked to be audible. The double movement which subluxates the head and then returns it to the acetabulum may be repeated as often as may be desired for careful monitoring.' His work was confirmed by a Parisian colleague, Sauget at the *Maternité de Paris*, in 1500 cases. Le Damany distinguished between those hips that rapidly stabilized and those that remained unstable and sometimes proceeded to complete placement. His treatment was by simple abduction and flexion, maintained by a thigh bandage fastened to a bodice, but he treated only those hips still unstable after six months. The older child was managed by traction, manipulation and plaster[136–138].

Just Lucas-Championnière (1843–1913) was a Parisian surgeon directly opposed to the orthodox management of fractures by rest, who emphasized the importance of early movement and mineral splintage[139]. Noting the excellent function obtained in some untreated cases, he deliberately advocated abandoning splintage for movement on the grounds that the irritation encouraged callus formation, prevented muscle atrophy and was particularly valuable for fractures involving joints. Ultimately, he came to use splints only for femoral and tibial fractures. His methods were not adopted to any extent by the French Army in World War I, except for some articular injuries, though the campaign of the Belgian, Willems, for early movement after infected penetrating joint wounds did gain some acceptance (but not by the patients).

Championnière was also very radical in the surgery of club-foot, not hesitating to excise the talus or even all the tarsal bones[140]. His views on fracture management were of course directly opposed to Hugh Owen Thomas's 'rest, uninterrupted and prolonged' and were a reaction against the stiffness often resulting from long immobilization. Though, like all enthusiasts, he overstated his case, it contained an essential truth, the value of mobilization at the earliest safe opportunity, which gained force with Robert Jones in England in World War I and with Watson-Jones in World War II, and is now part of orthopaedic practice everywhere.

Mention of the world wars reminds us of the part played by **Alexis Carrel** (1873–1944), a Lyons doctor of an experimental frame of mind whose many endeavours had an enormous influence on orthopaedic surgery though he was not an orthopaedic surgeon himself. He early developed the technique of arterial suture and its role in organ transplantation[141], which laid the foundations of modern organ transfer, including the pedicled bone-graft. He received the Nobel Prize in 1912, and his work in World War I in connection with wound treatment with hypochlorite irrigation by means of the Carrel–Dakin method and the technique of serial culture to ascertain the best moment for secondary wound suture is referred to elsewhere (p. 646).

It is commonly accepted that the introduction of formal synovectomy into orthopaedic surgery was due to **Mignon**, when he reported a case of synovectomy of the knee, chronically swollen after injury, to the *Société de Chirurgie de Paris* in 1900[142]. This was done through two lateral incisions; the operation was complicated by the formation of new bone at the lateral femoral condyle, requiring excision after three months. The result at six months was fair, with 70° flexion, and the patient able to kneel and run. However, Volkmann of Leipzig, bolstered by Listerian antiseptics, had done partial synovectomies, mainly for synovial tuberculosis without caries, during the 1870s; Schüller reported four cases of total synovectomy for rheumatoid arthritis in 1887[143]; Müller, also German, reported in 1894 on a very successful end-result four years after total synovectomy for rheumatoid disease[144]; Albertin, in 1895, reported two successful operations for the sequelae of penetrating wounds[145]; and during the discussion of Mignon's paper, Lucas-Championnière said that he had done this operation for various indications with good results. It may be noted that both Schüller and Müller routinely divided the cruciate and one or both collateral ligaments to gain access.

Jean-Martin Charcot (1825–1893), the first professor of neurology anywhere in the world, spent his professional life at the Salpetrière in Paris, where he wrote the first thesis distinguishing between gout and rheumatoid arthritis; as well as between chronic joint disease arising primarily in the synovial membrane ('progressive symmetrical arthritis' or rheumatoid arthritis) and degeneration of the articular cartilage (osteoarthritis)[146,147]. However, his main claim on our attention lies in the original description[148] of the arthropathy known by his name, 'the arthropathy of ataxic patients', which he ascribed, without actually mentioning syphilis (the spirochaete had yet to be discovered), to lesions of the spinal cord as seen in Pott's paraplegia, acute myelitis, and injury of the cord (quoting Weir Mitchell's observations in the American Civil War). 'Behind the disease of the joint there is a disease far more important in nature, which in reality dominates the situation – sclerosis of the posterior columns.' Charcot found these joints in the spine as well as the limbs. (Bick says that the first account of destructive joint disease of central nervous origin was by John K Mitchell of Philadelphia in 1831.)

We must also recall that, in 1869 with Joffray, Charcot described certain cases of progressive muscular atrophy, now known as amyotrophic lateral sclerosis[149], and in 1886, with Marie[150], the peroneal atrophy described independently in the same year by Tooth in England[151].

Pierre Marie (1853–1940), like Charcot, to whom he was an intern and subsequent associate and whom he succeeded in the Chair of Neurology at the Salpetrière, was primarily a neurologist whose interests inevitably overlapped into orthopaedics since the two fields are so closely related.

Marie was the first to describe acromegaly as associated with pituitary tumour, in 1886; he also described hypertrophic pulmonary osteoarthropathy in 1890[152], but he had been anticipated there by Bamberger[153], and of course clubbing of the fingers in chronic lung disease was familiar to Hippocrates and his successors. In 1898, with Sainton, he published the first account of craniocleidal dysostosis, based on his own cases, marked by increased skull diameter, failure of ossification at the fontanelles, disordered dentition and partial aplasia of the clavicles, but with remarkably little impairment of function[154].

In 1898, Marie gave a description of ankylosing spondylitis (which he called *spondylose rhizomélique*, though this was not altogether unknown*, 'a particular characteristic of which is the occurrence of complete fusion of the spine together with a more or less pronounced ankylosis of the joints at the bases of the limbs, while the small joints remain unaffected[155]. He noted that the kyphosis was mainly cervicodorsal, that the spinal joints were fused down to the sacrum, that the limb joints truly fixed were the hips and that in flexion, that there was marked flattening of the pelvis and thorax, and that respiratory excursion of the ribs was almost eliminated. Despite the pain, there was never any evidence of an acute arthritis in the sense of swelling and inflammation. 'The tendency to ankylosis with deformity is predominant and unavoidable.' All Marie's patients were males, and the rigidity was such 'that the spine would fracture rather than allow the slightest movement in it.' In ambulation, 'the patients look like wooden dolls, in which the leg movements occur about one transverse axis through both knees.'

Delpech had, however, already described the condition in 1828, as had Paget in 1877, describing it as a condition somewhat similar to osteitis deformans, 'a rare form of what I suppose to be general chronic rheumatoid arthritis of the spine involving its articulations with the ribs. The spine droops and is stiff, the chest is narrow, the ribs scarcely move[156].' Similarly, in 1695, a Dr Bernard Connor, described as an Englishman by Golding and an Irishman by Rang, who was physician to the King of Poland, described 'an extraordinary human skeleton, whose vertebrae of the back, the ribs and several bones down to the os sacrum, were all firmly united into one solid bone, without jointing or cartilage[157].

In 1913, with Foix, Marie described the autopsy finding of median nerve compression in the carpal tunnel in a case with bilateral thenar atrophy.

André Léri (1875–1930) was a polymath, much influenced by Charcot, who combined neurology with psychiatry and orthopaedics (as an orthopaedic physician). In 1922 he described, and it was a truly original observation, 'a flowing hyperostosis along the entire length of a limb' which he called melorheostosis because the dense thickening seemed in the X-rays to drip like candle-wax along the bones on one side only of the limb[159]. He reported further cases in 1928[160] and found the bone like ivory at biopsy of a metacarpal[161].

Also from the Salpetrière came the first account, in 1912[162], of the syndrome named after **Maurice Klippel** (1858–1942) and his interne **André**

---

* It had been described in Germany by Strümpell and by Bechterew.

Feil (b.1884), both of whom were neurologists. This related to a tailor aged 46, 'who appeared to have no neck, the head seeming to rest on the trunk.' The clinical and radiographic examination revealed a thoracic cage reaching to the base of the skull, with a fused cervicodorsal mass. But Bick, to read whose *Source Book* is always humbling, states that the first report of this condition was by Hutchinson in England in 1894.

To finish with the Salpetrière, another neurologist there, Jules Déjérine, married a woman medical student from San Francisco, **Auguste Klumpke** (1859–1927) an early woman doctor who described her eponymous brachial palsy in 1885[163] as a lesion of the lower trunks of the plexus to be distinguished from Erb's palsy, giving an accurate description of the ocular manifestations elsewhere defined by Horner, 'characterised by myosis, narrowing of the palpebral fissure, and, in some cases, by the eyeball retracting and becoming smaller.' (For completeness, we may add that Wilhelm Heinrich Erb (1840–1921) was a Heidelberg neurologist who described his own palsy in 1877, though only one of his five cases was obstetric in origin, the others due to injury or spondylosis or Pancoast's tumour[164]).

We should also mention **Guillaume Armand Duchenne** (1806–1875), of Boulogne, noted for the first account, in 1868, of the weakness and connective tissue hyperplasia in pseudohypertrophic muscular atrophy, the first group of the muscular dystrophies to be characterized[165]. He had already briefly noted this in this *Eléctrisation localisée* of 1861 (2nd edition), which describes his use of a faradic stimulator to study the function of normal and abnormal muscle. He originally thought the condition a paralysis, but the name was later changed to dystrophy.

Jules Emile Péan (1830–1898) was a leading Parisian general surgeon at the Hôpital St Louis whose interest here lies in his early attempts at metal joint prostheses. In 1894 he wrote on the use of such prostheses to replace bone components[166]. Others, like Gluck (p. 201), had tried ivory or animal bone with unsatisfactory results. Péan used metal, particularly platinum, which did not corrode like iron or steel. He reports an operation, amazingly advanced for the period, in which he removed the upper shaft and head of a humerus grossly affected by tuberculosis and inserted a platinum and rubber prosthesis which gave an excellent functional result despite extensive preceding suppuration. He concluded that major parts of the skeleton, including joints, could be replaced, that the prosthesis should be nonabsorbable and was well-tolerated and preserved movement, and that for grossly infected lesions this was an alternative to disarticulation. But he was not, at that time, advocating replacement operations for tumours or arthrosis.

Between the two world wars, French orthopaedics had made advances in separating itself from paediatric surgery. Fracture and rehabilitation services were built up. This progress was brought to a halt by the second world war. French surgeons found themselves isolated from their colleagues and lacking the most elementary equipment. After the liberation, their renewed contact with Anglo-American colleagues and techniques led to a remarkable resurgence. Of the leading personalities since that time we shall mention only one.

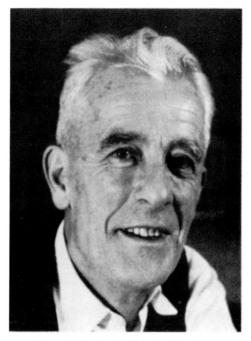

Figure 137   Robert Merle d'Aubigné

Robert Merle d'Aubigné, successor to Mathieu, was a leading figure in the orthopaedic scene in Paris, at the *Hôpital Cochin*, in France and the entire world, for many years. He has reviewed the recent history of French orthopaedics in relation to his own career[167]. His contributions include being the first, after Walter Mercer in Edinburgh, to perform transperitoneal fusion for spondylolisthesis; the addition of a long intramedullary stem to the Judet hip prosthesis; his widely adopted grading for functional assessment of the hip; his series of cases of idiopathic necrosis of the femoral head, presented at the Watson-Jones Lecture in London in 1959, at a time when this condition was hardly recognized in the UK; his massive block resections of bone tumours, supplemented by grafting, plating or medullary nailing; and his bone shortenings or lengthenings by transposition of femoral segments and medullary nailing.

REFERENCES

1. Neuburger, M. (1911). *Die Geschichte der Medizin.* (Stuttgart)
2. Dalechamps, J. (1570). *Traité de Chirurgie.* (Lyons)
3. Paré, A. (1586). *Les Oeuvres d'Ambroise Paré, Conseiller et Premier Chirurgien du Roy.* (4th edn.) (Paris)
4. Malgaigne, J-F. (1840). *Oeuvres Complètes d'Ambroise Paré.* (Paris)

5. Bartholinus, T. (1663–7). De gibbositate virginis nobilissimae. In *Epistolarum Medicinalium*.

6. Purmann, M.G. (1705). *Lorbeer-Krantz oder Wund-Artzney*. 2nd edn. (Frankfort and Leipzig)

7. Du Port, F. (1694). *La Décade de Médecine*. (trans. Le Vay, D.) (Springer-Verlag, Heidelberg and Berlin, 1988)

8. Fournier, D. (1668). *Explication des Bandages*. (Paris)

9. Fournier, D. (1671). *L'oeconomie chirurgicale, pour le r'habillement des os du corps humain. Contenant l'ostéologie, le nosostéologie, l'apocataostéologie et le traité des bandages*. (Paris)

10. Petit, J.L. (1723). *Traité des maladies des os*. (Paris)

11. Méry, J. (1707). Observations faites sur un sequelet d'une jeune femme agée de 16 ans, morte a l'Hôtel-Dieu de Paris, le 22 février 1706. *Hist. Acad. Roy. Sci.*, Paris

12. Jalade-Lafond, G. (1827). *Recherches pratiques sur les principales difformites du corps humain et sur les moyens d'y remedier*. (Paris)

13. Delpech, J.-M. (1828). *De l'Orthomorphie*. (Paris)

14. Bricheteau, I. and d'Ivernois, L. (1824). In *Encyclopédie Méthodique de Médecine*. (Paris)

15. Little, W.J. (1853). *On the nature and treatment of the deformities of the human frame*. (London)

16. Bouvier, H. (1858). *Leçons cliniques sur les maladies chroniques de l'appareil locomoteur*. (Paris)

17. Kirmisson, E. (1890). *Leçons cliniques sur les maladies de l'appareil locomoteur*. (Paris)

18. Bigg, H.H. (1862). *Orthopraxy: the mechanical treatment of deformities*. 2nd edn. (London)

19. Bauer, L. (1864). *Lectures on orthopaedic surgery*. (Philadelphia)

20. St Germain, L.-A. (1883). *Chirurgie Orthopédique*. (Paris)

21. Ackerknecht, E.H. (1957). Medizin und Aufklärung. *Schweiz. med. Wchschr.*, **20**

22. Deane, H.E. (1918). *Gymnastic Treatment for Joint and Muscle Treatment*. (Oxford)

23. Ollier, L.X.E. (1885). *Traité des resections et des opérations conservatrices qu'on peut pratiquer sur le système osseux*. (Paris)

24. Larrey, D. (1812–16). *Mémoires de chirurgie militaire et campagnes d'Amérique, d'Italie, d'Espagne et de Russie*. (5 vols.) (Paris)

25. Crumplin, M.K.H. (1988). Surgery at Waterloo. *J. Roy. Soc. Med.*, **81**, 38

26. Roux, A. (1762). Utrum deformitatis a Rachitide oriundae, dum ipsa Rachitis curatur, Thoracibus, Ochreis et aliis machinamentis corrigi debeant. *Thesis submitted to the Paris Faculty 18 March 1762*

27. Verdier, J.F. (undated). *Discours sur un nouvel art de développer la belle nature, et de guérir les difformités au moyen d'exercises, aidé par les machines mobiles de M. Tiphaine*. (Paris)

28. Verdier, P.-L. (1822). *Rapport et notes sur les bandages et appareils inventés*. (Paris)

29. Gerdy, P.N. (1839). *Traité des bandages et appareils de pansement*. 2nd edn. (Paris)

30. Laforest (1781). *L'art de soigner les pieds*. (Paris)

31. Saint-Germain, L.A. (1883). *Chirurgie Orthopédique*. (Paris)

32. Le Vacher, F.-G. (1768). Nouveau moyen de prévenir et de guérir la courbure de l'épine. *Mém. Acad. Chir.*, **4**, 596

33. Levacher de la Feutrie, T. (1772). *Traité du Rakitis*. (Paris)

34. Boyer, A. (1803). *Leçons sur les maladies des os*. (Paris)

35. Delpech, J.-M. (1815). *Mémoire sur la complication des plaies et des ulcères connue sous le nom de pourriture d'hôpital.* (Paris)
36. Delpech, J.-M. (1823). Ténotomie du tendon d'Achille. *Chir. Clin.*, **1**, 184
37. Delpech, J.-M. (1828). *De l'Orthomorphie par rapport a l'espèce humaine.* (Paris)
38. Garrison, F. (1929). *History of Medicine.* 4th edn. (Philadelphia and London, Saunders)
39. Delpech, J.-M. and Trinquier, V. (1833). *Observations cliniques sur les différences de la taille et des membres.* (Paris and Montpellier)
40. Moreau, P.F. (1803). Observations pratiques relatives à la resection des articulations affectées de carie. Thesis, Paris Faculty, 1803
41. Humbert, F. (1834). *Notice sur les appareils et machines inventés par F. Humbert.* (Bar-le-Duc)
42. Humbert, F. and Jacquier, N. (1835). *Essai et observations sur la manière de réduire les luxations spontanées ou symptomatiques de l'articulation iliofémorale.* (Bar-le-Duc and Paris)
43. Pravaz, C.-G. (1838). Rapport sur l'ouvrage de M. Humbert, présenté a la *Société de Médecine de Lyon le 22 janvier*
44. Pravaz, C.-G. (1871). *Traité théorique et pratique des luxations congénitales du fémur.* (Lyon and Paris)
45. Gerdy, N. (1838–40). Rapport sur deux mémoires du docteur Pravaz relatifs a l'etiologie, au causes et au traitement des luxations congénitales du fémur. *Bull. Acad. Méd.*, **6**, 121, 160
46. Pravaz, C.-G. (1845). *Mémoire sur la réalité de l'art orthopédique et ses rélations nécessaires avec l'Organoplastie.* (Lyon)
47. Pravaz, C.-G. (1827). *Methode nouvelle pour le traitement des déviations de la colonne vertébrale.* (Paris)
48. Pravaz, C.-G. (1847). *Traite théorique et pratique des luxations congénitales du fémur.* (Lyon and Paris)
49. Pravaz, C.-G. (1835). Sur un nouveau moyen d'opérer la coagulation du sang dans les artères, applicable à la guerison des anevrismes. *Compt. Rend. Acad. Sci.*, **36**, 88
50. Mott, V. (1842). *Travels in Europe and the East.* (New York and London)
51. Rapport sur les traitements orthopédiques de M. le Docteur Jules Guérin. 1848. (Paris)
52. Guérin, J. (1839). Traité des déviations latérales de l'épine par myotomie rachidienne. *Gaz. Méd.*
53. Bouvier, S.-H.-V. (1841). Appréciation de la myotomie appliquée au traitement des déviations rachidiennes. *Ann. Chir. Franc. Etrang.*, **7**, 108
54. Malgaigne, J.-F. (1845). *De la valeur réelle de l'orthopédie et spécialement de la ténotomie rachidienne dans le traitement des déviations latérales de l'épine.* (Paris)
55. Report of Commission on Guérin's tenotomies for scoliosis (1844–45). *Bull. Acad. Roy. Méd.*, **10**, 188 and 279
56. Chigot, P.L. and Moinet, P. (1972). *Clin. Orthop.*, **82**, 268
57. Guérin, J. (1838). Mémoire sur une nouvelle methode de traitement du torticollis ancien. *Gaz. Med.*, **14** and **17**
58. Guérin, J. (1841). *Recherches sur les luxations congénitales.* (Paris)
59. Rapport sur les traitements orthopédiques de M. Jules Guérin. Paris 1848
60. Guérin, J. (1838). *Mémoire sur l'étiologie générale des pieds bots congénitaux.* (Paris)
61. Guérin, J. (1962). Note sur l'ostéotomie et la tarsotomie dans le traitement du pied bot congénital. *Bull. Acad. Med. Paris*, **37**
62. Bouvier, S.-H.-V. (1837). Sur les difformités du système osseux. *Comptes rendus. Acad. Sci. Paris*, **5**, 253

63. Bouvier, S.-H.-V. (1853). *Etudes historiques et médicales sur l'usage des corsets.* (Paris)
64. Bouvier, S.-H.-V. (1858). *Leçons cliniques sur les maladies chroniques de l'appareil locomoteur.* (Paris)
65. Dieffenbach, J.F. (1838). Einige Bemerkungen über die Orthopädie in Frankreich. *Z. Ges. Med.,* **8,** 57
66. Delpech, J.-M. (1828). In *De l'Orthomorphie.* (Paris)
67. Bouvier, S.-H.-V. (1838). Mémoire sur la section du tendon d'Achille dans le traitement des pieds-bots. *Mém. Acad. Roy. Méd.,* **7,** 411
68. Bouvier, S.-H.-V. (1838). *Mémoire sur la reduction des luxations congénitales du fémur.* (Paris)
69. Duval, V. (1839). *Traité pratique du pied-bot.* (Paris)
70. Duval, E. (1890). *Traité pratique et philosophique du pied-bot.* (Paris)
71. Maisonabe, C.A. (1834). *Orthopédie. Clinique sur les difformités dans l'espèce humaine.* (Paris)
72. Gerdy, P.N. (1826). *Traité des bandages et appareils de pansement.* (Paris)
73. Malgaigne, J.-F. (1840). *Oeuvres complètes d'Ambroise Paré.* (Paris)
74. Malgaigne, J.-F. (1847–55). *Traité des Fractures et des Luxations.* (Paris)
75. Malgaigne, J.-F. (1841). *Recherches historiques et pratiques sur les appareils employés dans le traitement des fractures en général depuis Hippocrate jusqu'à nos jours.* (Paris)
76. Peltier, L.F. (1958). Guillaume Dupuytren and Dupuytren's fracture. *Surgery,* **43,** 868
77. Dupuytren, G. (1847). *Injuries and diseases of bones* (trans. Le Gros Clark) (London, New Sydenham Society)
78. Dupuytren, G. (1832–4). Original or congenital displacement of the heads of the thigh-bones, from *Leçons orales de clinique chirurgicale faites a l'Hotel-Dieu de Paris.* (Paris, Germer-Baillière) (trans. Le Gros Clark as above)
79. Dupuytren, G. (1826). Mémoire sur un déplacement original ou congénitale de la tête des fémurs. *Repert. Gén. Anat. Physiol. Path. Clin. Chir.,* **2,** 82
80. Caillard-Bilonière, A.J. (1828). *Sur les luxations originelles ou congénitales des fémurs.* Thesis, Paris Faculty, 1828
81. Poggi (1880). Contributio alla cura cruenta della lussazione congenita coxofemorale unilaterale. *Arch. di Ortop.,* **7,** 105
82. Windsor, J. (1834). *Lancet,* **ii,** 501
83. Cooper, A. (1822). *A treatise on dislocations and fractures of the joints.* p. 524. (London)
84. Dupuytren, G. (1832). De la rétraction des doigts per suite d'une affection de l'aponeurose palmaire. *J. Univ. Hebd. Med. Chir. Prat.,* **5,** 348
85. Dupuytren, G. (1834). *Lancet,* **ii,** 222
86. Dupuytren, G. (1847). On osteosarcoma, spina ventosa and tubercles in bone. In *Injuries and Diseases of Bones.* (trans. Le Gros Clark, London, New Sydenham Society)
87. Nichet, J.P.N. (1835, 40). Mémoire sur la nature et le traitement du mal vertébral de Pott. *Gaz. méd.*
88. Bonnet, A. (1840). Mémoire sur la position des membres dans les maladies articulaires, considerées sous le rapport de leurs applications thérapeutiques. *Gaz. méd.,* **14** and **21**
89. Bonnet, A. (1841). *Traité des sections tendineuses et musculaires.* (Paris and Lyons)
90. Belchier, J. (1736). *Phil. Trans.,* **39,** 287
91. Cheselden, A. (1741). *The Anatomy of the Human Body.* (London)
92. Duhamel, H.-L. (1742). Sur le développement et la crue des os des animaux.

Hist. Mém. l'Acad. Inscriptions Belles-Lettres, **2**, 481

93. Flourens, M.J.P. (1842). *Recherches sur le développement des os et des dents.* (Paris)

94. Macewen, W. (1912). *The growth of bone; observations on osteogenesis.* (Glasgow)

95. Ollier, L. (1877). De l'excision des cartilages de conjugation pour arrêter l'accroissement des os et a rémédier à certaines difformités du squelette. *Rev. Mens. Med. Chir.*

96. Ollier, L. (1900). *Lyon méd.*, **93**, 23

97. Poncet, M.A. (1874). De la periostite albumineuse. *Gaz. Hebd. Méd.*, **11**, 133 and 179

98. Poncet, M.A. (1897). *Gaz. Hôp. Paris*, **79**, 1219

99. Rodet, A. (1884). Etude expérimentale sur l'ostéomyélite infectieuse. *Comptes Rend. Acad. Sci.*, **89**, 569

100. Nové-Josserand, G. and Tavernier, L. (1927). *Tumeurs des os.* (Paris)

101. Tavernier, L. and Godinto, C. (1945). *Traitement chirurgical de l'arthrite sèche de la hanche.* (Paris, Masson)

102. Leriche, R. and Policard, A. (1926). *Les problèmes de la physiologie normale et pathologique des os.* (Paris)

103. Froment, J. (1915). *Presse Méd.*, **23**, 409

104. Tinel, J. (1917). *Nerve wounds.* (trans. Rothwell). (London, Baillière)

105. Letiévant, J.J.E. (1873). *Traité des sections nerveuses.* (Paris)

106. Nicasse (1885). Sur la suture des nerfs. *Rev. Chir.*, **7**

107. Brown-Séquard, C.E. (1893). Faits tendants à montrer le retour de la sensibilité et du mouvement apres la suture des nerfs. *Bull. Acad. Med. Paris*, **20**

108. Assaky, G. (1886). De la suture des nerfs à distance. *Arch. Gen. Méd.*, **2**, 529

109. Nélaton, A. (1836). *Recherches sur l'affection tuberculeuse des os.* Thesis, Paris Faculty, 1836, No 376

110. Nélaton, A. (1847). *Elements de pathologie chirurgicale.* Vol. 2, p. 510. (Paris)

111. Nélaton, A. (1860). *Tumeurs benignes des os, tumeurs à myéloplaxes.* (Paris)

112. Virchow, R. (1864–5). *Die krankhaften Geschwülste.* (Berlin)

113. Gaucher, P.C.E. (1882). *De l'epithéliome primitif de la rate: hypertrophie de la rate sans leucémie.* Thesis, Paris Faculty, 1882

114. Cushing, E.H. and Stout, A.P. (1926). Gaucher's disease with report of a case showing bone disintegration and joint involvement. *Arch. Surg.*, **12**, 539

115. Pick, L. (1927). Die skelettform (ossuäre form) des morbus Gaucher. In *Kriegs- und Konstitutionspathologie.* (Jena)

116. Arinkin, M.I. (1927). *Vestn. Khir.*, **30**, 57

117. Kirmisson, E. (1898). *Traité des maladies chirurgicales d'origine congénitale.* (Paris)

118. Kirmisson, E. (1890). *Leçons cliniques sur les maladies d l'appareil locomoteur.* (Paris)

119. Kirmisson, E. (1902). *Les difformités acquises de l'appareil locomoteur pendant l'enfance et l'adolescence.* (Paris)

120. Ombredanne, L. (1921). L'arthrodèse du pied. *Ann. Soc. Franc. Orth.*, **5 Oct**

121. Ombredanne, L. and Mathieu, P. (1937). *Traité de chirurgie orthopédique.* (Paris, Masson)

122. Ombredanne, L. (1913). Allongement d'un fémur sur un membre trop court. *Bull. Mém. Soc. Chir.*, **39**, 1177

123. Sorrel, E. (1930). Arthrodèse extra-articulaire pour coxalgie chez un adulte. *Bull. Mem. Soc. Nat. Chir.*, **56**, 101

124. Calot, J.-F. (1896). Des moyens de guérir la bosse du mal de Pott. *France Med.*, **52**

125. Shaw, J. (1823). *On the nature and treatment of the distortions to which the spine and the bones of the chest are subject.* (London). Cited by Valentin, B. (1967).

Die Geschichte der Orthopädie. (Stuttgart)
126. Calot, J.-F. (1896). Du traitement des tumeurs blanches par les injections intra-articulaires. *French Surgical Congress, Paris 1896*
127. Calot, J.-F. (1903). La technique du traitement non-sanglant de la luxation congénitale de la hanche. *Ann. Chir. Orth.,* **12**
128. Calot, J.-F. (1923). *L'orthopédie indispensable aux praticiens.* 8th Edn. (Paris)
129. Calvé, J. (1910). Sur une forme particulière de pseudo-coxalgie greffée sur des déformations caracteristiques de l'extremité supérieure du fémur. *Rev. Chir.,* **30**, 54
130. Calvé, J. (1925). Sur une affection particulière de la colonne vertébrale chez l'enfant simulante le mal de Pott: ostéochondrite vertébrale infantile. *J. Radiol. Electrol.,* **9**, 22; also *J. Bone Jt. Surg.,* **7**, 41
131. Calvé, J. and Galland, M. (1922). Sur une affection particuliere de la colonne vertebrale simulante le mal de Pott (calcification du nucleus pulposus). *J. Radiol. Electrol.,* **6**, 21
132. Dickson, J.W. (1969). Pierre Le Damany on congenital dysplasia of the hip. *Proc. Roy. Soc. Med.,* **62**, 575
133. von Rosen, S. (1957). *Acta Orthop. Scand.,* **26**, 136
134. Barlow, T.G. (1962). *J. Bone Joint Surg.,* **44B**, 292
135. Ortolani, M. (1937). *Pediatria (Napoli),* 45, 129
136. Le Damany, P. (1908). *Z. Orthop. Chir.,* **21**, 129
137. Le Damany, P. and Sauget, J. (1910). *Rev. Chir. (Paris),* 45, 512
138. Le Damany, P. (1912). *La luxation congénitale de la hanche.* (Paris)
139. Lucas-Championnière, J. (1899). *Le massage et la mobilisation dans le traitement des fractures.* (Paris)
140. Lucas-Championnière, J. (1900). Traitement des formes graves du pied-bot par l'ablation de la totalité des os du tarse. *13th International Medical Congress,* Paris
141. Carrel, A. (1902). La technique opératoire des anastomoses vasculaires et la transplantation des viscères. *Lyon Med.,* **98**
142. Mignon, M.A. (1899–1900). Synovectomie du genou. *Bull. Mém. Soc. Chir., Paris,* **26**, 1113
143. Schüller, M. (1887). *Die Pathologie und Therapie der Gelenkentzüundungen.* (Vienna)
144. Müller, W. (1894). Zur Frage der operativen Behandlung der Arthritis deformans und des chronischen Gelenkrheumatismus. *Atch. f. klin. Chir.,* **47**, 1
145. Albertin (1896). De la synovectomie et de l'arthrectomie dans les arthrites infectieuses aiguës du genou consécutives aux plaies pénétrantes de cette articulation. *Prov. med.,* **10**, 195
146. Charcot, J.-M. (1867). Caractères anatomiques de l'arthrite rheumatismale chronique. *Gaz. des Hôpitaux*
147. Charcot, J.-M. (1868). Sur quelques arthropathies. *Arch. Physiol.,* **161**
148. Charcot, J.-M. (1872–87). *Leçons sur les maladies du système nerveux faites à la Salpetrière.* (Paris)
149. Charcot, J.-M. and Joffray, A. (1869). Deux cas d'atrophie musculaire progressive avec lésions de la substance grise et des faisceaux antéro-latéraux de la moelle épinière. *Arch. Physiol. Norm. Path.,* **2**, 744
150. Charcot, J.-M. and Marie, P. (1886). Sur une forme particulière d'atrophie musculaire progressive souvent familiale. *Rev. Med.,* **6**, 97
151. Tooth, H.H. (1886). The peroneal type of muscular atrophy. *Cambridge doctoral dissertation.* (London, HK Lewis)
152. Marie, P. (1890). De l'ostéo-arthropathie hypertrophiante pneumique. *Rev. Méd.,* **10**, 1

153. Bamberger, E. (1889). Über Knochenveränderungen bei chronischer Lungen- und Herzkrankheiten. *Wien. klin. Wchschr.*, **2**, 226

154. Marie, P. and Sainton, P. (1898). Sur la dysostose héréditaire cleidocranienne. *Rev. Neurol.*, **6**, 835

155. Marie, P. (1898). *Rev. Méd.*, **18**, 285

156. Paget, J. (1877). On a form of chronic inflammation of bones (osteitis deformans). *Med. Chir. Trans.*, **60**, 37

157. Connor, B. (1695). *Phil. Trans.*, **19**, 21

158. Marie, P. and Foix, C. (1913). *Rev. Neurol.*, **26**, 647

159. Léri, A. and Joanny (1922). *Bull. Soc. Méd. Hôp. Paris*, **46**, 1141

160. Léri, A. and Lièvre, J.A. (1928). *Presse Méd.*, **36**, 801

161. Léri, A., Loiseleur and Lièvre (1934). *Bull. Soc. Méd. Hôp. Paris*, **54**, 1210

162. Klippel, M. and Feil, A. (1912). Un cas d'absence des vertèbres cervicales avec cage thoracique remontant jusqu'à la base du crâne. *Nouv. Iconogr. Salpetrière*, **25**, 223

163. Klumpke-Déjérine, A. (1885). *Rev. Méd.*, **5**, 591 and 739

164. Erb, W.H. (1877). *Verh. naturh.-med. Ver.*, **1**, 130

165. Duchenne, G.B.A. (1868). Recherches sur la paralysie musculaire pseudohyper- trophique ou paralysie myosclérosique. *Arch. Gen. Méd.*, **1**, 5

166. Péan, E.J. (1894). Des moyens prothétiques destinés à obtenir la réparation des parties osseuses. *Gaz. Hôp. Paris*, **67**, 291

167. d'Aubigné, R.M. (1982). Surfing the wave: 50 years in the growth of French orthopaedics. *Clin. Orthop.*, **171**, 3

CHAPTER 5

National Histories – Italy

It was fortunate that **Leonardo da Vinci** (1452–1519) lived at a time when dissection had ceased to be illegal in Italy and when the Renaissance was being marked by a burst of scientific endeavour. His motives in studying the human body, particularly its muscles, may have been primarily artistic, but they yielded results valuable to orthopaedics, for he analysed muscle structure in relation to function, the principles of leverage and synergistic action, and this meant taking an engineering look at the skeleton. Anticipating Vesalius (1514–1564), he was one of the midwives at the birth of modern anatomy; but because his main interest lay in function, he was also a precursor in physiology, and particularly in myology and the analysis of movement.

This is cognate with the work of **Aloysio Luigi Galvani** (1737–1798) of Bologna, because of the latter's seminal studies on the electrical stimulation of muscle. His *De Viribus Electricitatis in Motu Commentarius* (The effects of artificial electricity on muscular motion) was published in a Bologna scientific journal in 1791, and later that year in book form, but it was not translated into Italian until the bicentennial of his birth in 1937 and there was no English translation at all until 1953. 'I wish to bring to a degree of usefulness those facts which came to be revealed about nerves and muscles through many experiments involving considerable endeavour, whereby their hidden properties may possibly be revealed and we may be able to treat their ailments with more safety.' The story is familiar. It was an accidental discovery. He had dissected a frog, there was an electrical machine in the same room; whenever his scalpel touched one of the crural nerves at the same time that a spark was produced, and at no other time, the leg muscles went into violent spasms. Also, the finger had to touch the metal of the blade; holding a bone handle did not work, nor could the scalpel be replaced by a glass rod. But it did work if the experimenter substituted for himself an iron wire of sufficient length, and whether the frog were near or far from the spark machine. The intensity of the spasm was proportional to the strength of the spark. A *conductor* was essential and could be applied to either the muscles or to their nerve.

Later, Galvani obtained similar results without a machine, simply by applying dissimilar metals to the spinal cord and muscles and bringing them together to complete the circuit, or by placing the cord and muscles on sheets of different metals or in different solutions and bridging them with a single curved metal strip. It was thought by some that this was a new and mysterious form of 'animal electricity'. **Alessandro Volta** (1745–1827), of Pavia, showed that this was not so, and that the discharge from his simple pile could cause continuous contraction. Volta's experiment also showed (though he did not fully appreciate it) the distinction between efferent and afferent nerves. Stimulating the former caused contraction of the muscles to which they were attached, whereas stimulation of the latter, unconnected to any muscle, still caused contraction by relay through the central nervous system. It was an outcome of this work that some, including Benjamin Franklin, himself an electrical experimenter in the intervals between bouts of American diplomacy, thought that electricity might be useful in treating paralysis. In the late 18th century, static machines were in use at various of the London hospitals, including St Thomas's; and there is a remote but historical connection between this development (and this hospital in particular) and the much later development of electrical methods for treating nonunion of fractures (p. 581).

Domenico Cotugno (Cotunnius) (1736–1822) must have been a remarkable figure since he was appointed professor of surgery at the Naples Hospital for Incurables at the age of 30 and remained there until his death at the age of 86. His researches related to the cerebrospinal fluid – 'it seems beyond doubt that this fluid ... oozes out from the extremities of the small arteries and is again absorbed by the small inhaling veins, so as to be in a continual state of renovation' – the aqueducts of the inner ear, the coagulable proteinuria of nephritis, and sciatica. As to the last, he distinguished between localized 'arthritic' sciatica, evidently due to hip disease, and the true nervous sciatica which ran down to the foot. He thought it clear that the cause was an affection of the sciatic nerve, due to an excess of fluid in its sheath, observed the paresis that might result, and compared the condition to brachial (or cubital) neuralgia[1,2].

Geronimo Mercuriali (1530–1606) produced the first illustrated book on sports medicine: *Artis gymnasticae apud antiquos celeberrimae, nostris temporibus ignoratae* (Venice 1569), which dealt mainly with the health habits, sports and exercises of Greek and Roman antiquity and went into six editions. He also wrote works on dermatology, paediatrics and ear disease.

Perhaps the first true clinical orthopaedist in Italy was **Antonio Scarpa** (1752–1832), who was an anatomist (Scarpa's fascia) and general surgeon who published an important study of club-foot in 1803[3]. This is discussed elsewhere (p. 491), and we need only recall here that Scarpa clearly saw that there was a talonavicular dislocation, and that the position and shape of the talus remained normal. For its treatment, he adapted Venel's splint by incorporating spring correction which he had stolen (it is the only word) from Typhesne in Paris. He also wrote on osteomyelitis, though that term itself had not yet been invented.

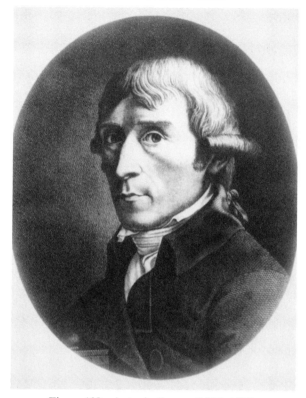

Figure 138 Antonio Scarpa (1752–1832)

Another surgeon-anatomist, **Giovanni Palletta** (1748–1832), of Milan, gave a very clear account of the morbid anatomy of congenital dislocation of the hip based on an autopsy of a 15-day-old boy with bilateral lesions[4]. Many years later, he gave a detailed description of the changes in the shape of the head and socket and in the capsule in neglected cases[5], and he was a very early practitioner of deliberate subtrochanteric osteotomy to correct the flexion-adduction deformity in such cases.

Bartolommeo Borella (1784–1854) was the first Italian to devote himself exclusively to orthopaedics (and, incidentally, to use this name habitually for this discipline), and it was he who founded, in 1823, the first orthopaedic institute in Italy, the *Regio Stabilimento Ortopedico*[6], on the hills of Moncalieri at the town of San Donato, an institute run after his death by his son-in-law, Giovanni Fistono, which survived until after the mid-century. Borella described himself as surgeon and hernial specialist to the army and royal family and had travelled in Europe, mainly to study the management of club-foot in Rome and Paris. His chief publication, *Cenni d'Ortopedia*, appeared in the Proceedings of the Royal Academy of Sciences of Turin in 1821[7], and has an elegant frontispiece incorporating his appliances, reminiscent of the *hoplomochlion* of Aquapendente of 1647 (p. 56), though John Shaw of London thought it merely 'a good proof of the mania for complicated machinery.'

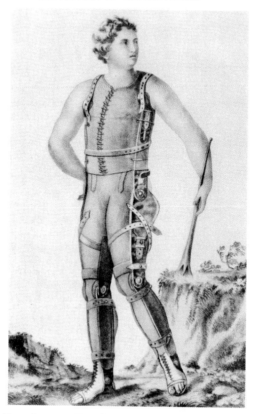

Figure 139   Bartolommeo Borella: *Cenni d'Ortopedia* (frontispiece, 1821)

Lorenzo Bruni founded the second orthopaedic institute in Italy, in Naples, in 1838 at Posilippo, mainly for the treatment of scoliosis and club-foot. He also ran an orthopaedic department at the Ospedale de Santa Maria di Loreto, where he was professor of clinical orthopaedics from 1840[8]. He was an enthusiast for the physical education of the young. He was also joint publisher of the *Giornale di Ortopedia* from 1839, but this does not seem to have lasted very long; and he produced an excellent atlas of deformities in 1845[9]. Bruni vigorously refuted the claims made by Rogier and Carbonai for myotomy in scoliosis as advocated in Paris by Guérin[10].

Ferdinando Carbonai (19805–1855), with his brother Angelo, founded an institute emphasizing gymnastics and hydrotherapy in Florence in 1840, the *Imperiale e Reale Istituto Ortopedico Toscano*[11], originally within the city but later transferred to the delectable rural surroundings of the nearby village of San Giusto, and was professor of practical and clinical orthopaedics in the local medical school from 1841 until the chair lapsed in 1849. Carbonai had travelled to visit, among others, Little in London and Guérin and Pravaz in France, acquiring from Guérin the enthusiasm for myotomy in scoliosis which Bruni had so deplored. This enthusiasm was shared by **Catullo Rogier**,

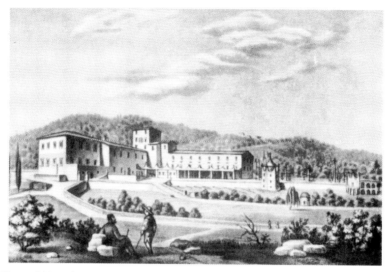

Figure 140   The Carbonai Institute near Florence, from a prospectus of 1850

the remarkable Baron de Beaufort di Modena, author of the first Italian treatise on orthopaedics in 1845[12], a work totally devoted to Guérin's methods and attributing most orthopaedic disorders, not to mention squint and stammer, to Guérin's 'convulsive muscular contraction'.

Carbonai's nephew, **Paolo Cresci Carbonai** (1839–1882) founded a further institute in Florence in 1860, the *Regio Stabilimento Ortopedico e Idroterapico*, and wrote on spinal curvature[13].

Giovanni Battista Monteggia (1762–1815) was a Milanese pathologist who acquired syphilis by cutting himself at an autopsy (an unusual explanation) and became a surgeon and professor at Milan. In 1814, he described his eponymous fracture in a girl with a fracture of the shaft of the ulna accompanied by an anterior dislocation of the radial head which could not be replaced[14].

The first tenotomy for club-foot in Italy was performed by Sperino in Turin in 1838, followed by Sani[15], Sillani[16] and others.

If we have to assign a particular name and place to the true beginnings of Italian orthopaedics, these must be those of Rizzoli and Bologna, for **Francesco Rizzoli** (1809–1880) was responsible for creating the world-famous institute that bears his name and was later to be directed by the great Putti[17]. The institute, however, was a posthumous creation, for, though Rizzoli was professor of surgery and obstetrics in Bologna and left his entire estate for the foundation of an orthopaedic institute, purchasing the site of the San Michele monastery, wonderfully perched on Mount Oliveto above the city, the actual building did not materialize until 1896, 16 years after his death.

Rizzoli was an enthusiast for osteotomy and practised it extensively. He was also attracted by the challenge of inequality of leg-length and began by exploiting an accidental fracture of the femur on the sound side, allowing union with overlap to compensate for shortening of the opposite limb[18]. He

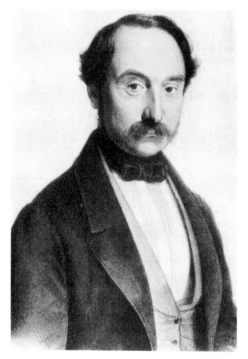

Figure 141   Francesco Rizzoli (1809–1880)

then proceeded deliberately to fracture the sound femur to compensate for shortening, of whatever origin, an undertaking that a German contemporary, Ernst Julius Gurlt (1825–1899) considered to be in no way deserving of imitation and not to be recommended with a clear conscience[19]. To produce the fracture, Rizzoli devised an osteoclast, one of the first of its kind, which had an iron ring on either side of the intended fracture site, connected by a bar traversed by a screw device allowing pressure to be exerted on a metal bow. He later incorporated a dynamometer to measure the pressure accurately, and began to extend the procedure: thus his pupil, Antonio Giovanini, used it to correct ankylosis of the knee in flexion[20]. He also tackled the problem surgically. Fearing to injure the nerves and vessels of the short limb by operative lengthening, he decided to shorten the sound limb by resecting part of the femur, and first did so in 1847, a method later developed by his successor, Codivilla, who also applied it to the tibia and fibula.

The institute proper was directed for its first three years by Rizzoli's pupil, **Pietro Panzeri** (1849–1901), who had directed a provisional establishment before this date, and who simultaneously directed the Milan *Istituto dei Rachitici*, founded in 1881 and originally devoted to the orthopaedics of children. By the end of the 19th century, Italian orthopaedics was dominated by these two great institutes.

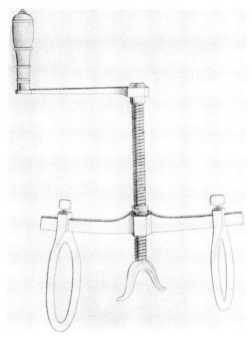

Figure 142 Rizzoli's *macchinetta ossifraga* or osteoclast of 1849

From 1899, the Rizzoli was directed by **Alessandro Codivilla** (1861–1912). During his short tenure, Panzeri had adhered to classical patterns of management. Codivilla changed all this to usher in the modern era in his short life-span, becoming a world figure in orthopaedics at the turn of the century.

He was an activist, and in 1899 wrote a classic paper on tendon transplantation[21], a topic then very much in the air but still rather novel in Italy, having been introduced, or reintroduced, by Nicoladoni in nearby Innsbruck in the Tyrol in 1880. This was directly linked to his interest in the surgery of the after-effects of poliomyelitis, on which he wrote a paper in 1900[22]. He reported 30 operations, laying down the principles of redistribution of muscle power around the joint. Each case had to be individually analysed and planned for, and the tendon transfer might have to be combined with release of contractures or arthrodesis or osteoclasis to correct deformity. If the transferred tendon was too short, it could be lengthened by fascial strips (Lange was using silk strands). He described transfer of the tibialis posterior through the interosseous membrane and also used tenodesis, especially as a check to foot-drop.

He also described an operation to compensate for loss of opposition of the thumb by transfer of the superficial flexor of the little finger which completely anticipated that of Sterling Bunnell 40 years later, in 1938. He recognized that spastic paralysis presented quite different problems and that tendon lengthening, with or without transfers, had much to offer here.

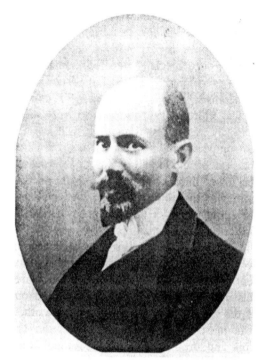

Figure 143   Alessandro Codivilla (1861–1912)

Elsewhere, he advocated the avoidance of disabling peritendinous adhesions and preservation of the gliding mechanism by utilizing the sheath of the tendon of the paralysed muscle, a technique that influenced Fritz Lange in Munich and, through him, Leo Mayer (p. 429). In 1905, he reported on methods of leg lengthening[23]; he had already introduced skeletal traction by means of a pin transfixing the os calcis and now used this to distract the tibia and fibula after osteotomy, gaining increases of 3 to 8 cm in 22 cases, work that greatly influenced the similar endeavours of Magnusson and Freiberg in America, Ombredanne in France, and Codivilla's own successor, Vittorio Putti. As early as 1901, he conceived, but did not perform, excision of a hemivertebra for congenital scoliosis[24], but this was considered too risky until performed by Royle in Australia 27 years later.

Bick rightly says that Codivilla was one of the greatest creative minds that was ever devoted to orthopaedic surgery, and refers to the brilliance, variety and soundness of the methods which became source material for modern techniques. He preferred to write in his native Italian journals and his name was therefore less well-known abroad to readers of the French, German and English language literature than that of his successor.

Surely Bick's encomium applies even more fittingly to Codivilla's successor, **Vittorio Putti** (1800–1940), whom Valentin calls 'a noble man endowed by Nature with extraordinary gifts of body and spirit'. Putti was indeed noble in character and achievement (and modesty) and, as Harry Platt writes,

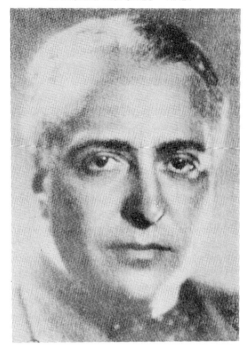

Figure 144   Vittorio Putti (1880–1940)

destined to outshine his master. Born of a Bolognese surgeon and a poetess, a multilingual scholar in an ancient university city, he became director of the Rizzoli Institute in 1911 at the age of 31 and made it famous during the first world war as a centre for reconstructive surgery and rehabilitation. At the end of the war, when he was still only 40, Putti had done work on peripheral nerve injuries, cineplastic amputation[25,26]* and knee-joint arthroplasty that set him squarely in the front rank of European orthopaedists.

Under his guidance between the wars, the Institute was enlarged and given a fine library, aided from his own pocket, and became a Mecca where young men were trained to work throughout Italy (and also in South America). Like Wren, Putti touched nothing that he did not adorn. He wrote of his extensive local resections for bone tumours for which others would have considered amputation inevitable; of lumbar spondylosis as a cause of low back pain and sciatica; in his last year of a compression screw for fractures of the neck of the femur. However, he is best known for his work on congenital dislocation of the hip, particularly important in northern Italy where the condition was endemic, providing major contributions to our knowledge of its morbid anatomy[27] and on preventive measures. He

---

* These had originally been conceived by another Italian, Vanghetti, after experience in the 2nd Italo-Abyssinian War (see p. 484).

promoted an intensive educational programme among general practitioners and the lay public to obtain early diagnosis and used a simple triangular cushion to maintain reduction in young children. Over 3600 cases were treated by manipulative reduction beween 1899 and 1938. Writing in 1950, Platt said that the years between the world wars were a golden age for orthopaedic surgery, and that the heroes of this age were surely Robert Jones and Vittorio Putti. No-one can dispute this.

Putti was also a great medical historian, particularly on the history of artificial limbs, describing such famous museum specimens as the iron hands of Goetz von Berlichingen and the devices of Paré. In 1910, he described congenital platyspondyly[28]. He contributed significantly to the literature on bone tumours[29]. At about the same time as McMurray in Liverpool, in 1937, he practised transverse intertrochanteric osteotomy for ununited hip fractures[30]. He improved on Codivilla's technique and results in femoral lengthening, obtaining up to four inches increase by means of a Z osteotomy and a distraction apparatus incorporating two transfixion pins, with controlling springs and screws[31,32]. This he called an osteoton; but it did not always efficiently control angulation and alignment until Leroy C Abbot, of St Louis, used two pins in each fragment. Putti began his career at a time when plaster had still to compete against the older splints and braces, and paid full homage to Mathysen for his invention of the plaster bandage[33]. Soon after World War II he was writing of the cerclage of fractures with metal bands[34]. He made advances in arthroplasty[35]; like Willis Campbell, he designed bone-block operations not amounting to arthrodesis to control paralytic equinus and calcaneus. For major procedures on the knee he made a U incision, dividing the patellar ligament and reflecting the patella upwards[37], not the happiest of procedures unless intended for arthrodesis.

Putti was active in organizing societies for the aid and rehabilitation of crippled children and adults. One very important service was his active fostering of the development of orthopaedic surgery in Latin America, particularly Argentina with its huge Italian population, and arranging scholarships for young men at the Rizzoli Institute. Finally, though anyone who has reason to consult his bibliography will be reluctant ever to use that word, in 1917 he founded the journal *Chirurgia degli Organi di Muovimento* and edited it until his death. Before this, there had been only the ephemeral *Giornale di Ortopedia* of Bruni and, in 1884, the appearance of the *Archivio di Ortopedia* issued by Panzeri and Fedele Margary in Turin.

Fedele Margary was a very active and surgically-minded orthopaedist at the turn of the century and is referred to elsewhere (p. 631). He is said to have performed the first subcutaneous osteotomy in Italy, in 1879, and certainly removed a medial meniscus in 1882[38]. The names of Italian orthopaedists crop up frequently in any discussion of congenital dislocation of the hip because of its high incidence in their country: Palletta, Poggi, Paci, Ortolani all made important contributions.

Alfonso Poggi (1848–1930) realised that it might be necessary to deepen the acetabulum and remodel the femoral head if stable reduction were to be achieved. He was chief of surgery at Bologna when, in 1880, he wrote his historic paper[39], the first known in the literature to describe acetabular reconstruction, the essential complement to Dupuytren's observation of half a century earlier that the joint components were incongruous and the forerunner of all subsequent procedures for late cases. It related to a previously untreated girl of 12 with unilateral dislocation. 'I had decided in my own mind ... to replace the femoral head in its natural position, deepening or reconstructing the acetabulum, even adjusting the femoral head if it were altered in shape.' He exposed the misshapen head on the ilium, divided the capsular constriction, found a shallow filled acetabulum, remodelled the joint components to obtain good congruous reduction and excised the redundant capsule. Had he used this capsule for interposition, we would have had the essence of Colonna's capsular arthroplasty[40] 56 years beforehand. The follow-up at one year was excellent.

Agostino Paci (1845–1902) was a Pisan surgeon who, in 1889, recommended adapting to the treatment of congenital dislocation the manoeuvre of levering the head over the posterior acetabular rim as used for traumatic dislocations (by Bigelow, among others)[41]. This was a move away from reduction by gradual traction and a resuscitation of the single-stage manipulation of Humbert and Jacquier in France earlier in the century (p. 247). However, in the period before X-rays, it was always uncertain whether true reduction, rather than an improved position, had been obtained. Paci became over-keen on claiming priority in a dispute with Lorenz; however, Bick claims him as an outstanding orthopaedist of 19th century Italy and his series of papers on closed reduction as epoch-making. Paci really does seem to have the priority, as Lorenz did not report his 'bloodless' method until 1895, after stating publicly, only the year before, that Paci's manipulative reduction was impossible! Such sudden conversions are not infrequent in orthopaedics: Whitman denounced astragalectomy before proceeding to perform many thousands (p. 503).

We refer elsewhere to Ortolani's advocacy of early recognition of congenital dislocation of the hip in 1937 (and how this had been long anticipated by Le Damany in France). **Marino Ortolani** was a professor of paediatrics at Ferrara and described his sign in 1937[42], and later in a book on congenital dislocation in 1948[43]. It was just the same as that Le Damany had described a quarter of a century before, and the same as the snapping heard and felt during reduction by the Paci–Lorenz manoeuvre as the femoral head jerked over the labrum and posterior acetabular rim. But – and Le Damany had also emphasized this – it was essential for the child to be relaxed, preferably by a swig at the nipple.

Between the two world wars, the Milan *Istituto dei Rachitici* became a famed European centre under the direction, over 35 years, of **Ricardo Galeazzi** (1866–1952), known for his enormous experience with congenital dislocation of the hip (he reviewed 12 000 cases), for his work with structural scoliosis, begun as far back as 1913. He used a method very much like that of Abbott, produced by forced correction in traction but with the lateral pressure produced by leverage in a machine, and with similar tedium and disadvantages, but not altogether unrewarding[44]. In 1934, he complemented the description by another Milanese, Monteggia, of his eponymous forearm fracture by reporting on ulnar shaft fracture accompanied by disruption of

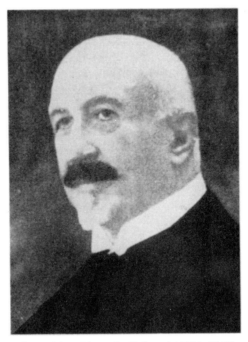

Figure 145   Riccardo Galeazzi (1886–1952)

the inferior radio-ulnar joint, analogous to Monteggia's lesion but much commoner[45]. Galeazzi also advanced procedure in cineplastic amputation[46]. At one time, in 1910, he thought it might be possible to correct the anteversion of CDH by powerful manual external derotation of the shaft, the femoral head being held in position, so as to produce a sort of stress or greenstick fracture, but this did not last long[47].

Carlo Marino-Zuco (1893–1965) was a Roman who became professor and head of the department of orthopaedic surgery and traumatology at the medical school of the University of Rome, which became a world centre. He was especially renowned for his work on the pathogenesis and treatment of scoliosis, the treatment of paralysis in poliomyelitis, and femoral lengthening. He helped found the Italian Society for Rehabilitation of the Disabled.

Raffaele Zanoli (1897–1971) became Putti's assistant at the Rizzoli institute in 1924 and assistant professor of orthopaedics in 1929. From the latter year he worked in Genoa, eventually as professor, and in the latter year succeeded Delitalia as Director of the Rizzoli. He was editor of the *Chirurgia degli Organi di Muovimento* and author of over 200 papers on every aspect of orthopaedic surgery.

More recently, we must just mention the names of Scaglietti, in Florence and of Dalla Vedova, who assumed charge of the new University Orthopaedic Clinic in Rome in the 1930s.

REFERENCES

1. Cotugno, D. (1764). *De Ischiade Nervosa Commentarius*. (Naples)
2. Cotugno, D. (1775). *A Treatise on the Nervous Sciatica*. (London)
3. Scarpa, A. (1803). *Memorie chirurgica sui piedi congeniti dei fanciulli e sua maniere di corregere questa difformita*. (Pavia)
4. Palletta, G.B. (1803). *Adversaria chirurgica prima*. (Milan)
5. Palletta, G.B. (1820). *Exercitationes pathologicae*. (Milan)
6. Borella, B. (1826). *Osservazione critiche sui modo du curare varie storpiature delle ossa e particolarmente il gobbo. Con un succinto raguaglio delle cure vantagiosamente intraprese nel Regio Stabilimento Ortopedico*. (Turin)
7. Borella, B. (1821). Cenni d'Ortopedia. *Mem. Acc. Sci.*, **26**, 163
8. Bruni, L. (1841). *Risultamenti clinici ottenuti nella sala ortopedica nell'ospedale di Santa Maria di Loreto in tutto l'anno dei 1841*. (Naples)
9. Bruni, L. (1845). *Atlante ripristinante nel loro stato naturale le varie deformita*. (Naples)
10. Bruni, L. (1840). *Sulla inefficacia della tenotomia dorso-lombare nella cura delle deviazioni della colonna vertebrale*. (Naples)
11. Carbonai, F. (1840). *Primo Istituto Ortopedico in Toscana creato e diretto dal Dott. Carbonai*. (Florence)
12. Rogier, C. (1845). *Trattato completo di Ortopedia umana teorico-pratico*. (Rome)
13. Carbonai, P.C. (1867). *Sopra le deviazoni della colonna vertebrale*. (Florence)
14. Monteggia, G.B. (1814). *Istituzioni Chirurgiche*. (Milan)
15. Sani, F. (1844). *Alcune operazione di tenotomia e miotomia*. (Rome)
16. Sillani, S. (1844). *Cenno storico sull'ortopedia, e di due casi di piedi torti da lui operati con tenotomia e sezione da tendini*. (Macerata)
17. Putti, V. (1939). Francesco Rizzoli. *Chir. Organi Mov.*, **25**, 149
18. Rizzoli, F. (1849). Nuovo metodo per togliere la claudicazione dell'accavallamento e reciproca union dei frammenti del femore. *Nov. Comm. Acad. Sci. Inst. Bononiensis.*, **10**, 245
19. Gurlt, E.J. (1862). *Handbuch der Lehre von den Knochenbrüchen*. (Hamm)
20. Giovanini, A. (1871). Trattamiento di alcune achilosi del ginocchio, mediante un nuovo meccanismo. *Boll. Sci. Med. Bologna*, **2**, 161
21. Codivilla, A. (1899). Sur trapianti tendinei nella pratica ortopedica. *Arch. Ortop.*, **16**, 225
22. Codivilla, A. (1900). Il trattamiento chirurgico moderni della paralysi infantile spinale. *Policlinico*, **7**, 110
23. Codivilla, A. (1905). Means of lengthening, in the lower limbs, the muscles and tissues which are shortened by deformity. *Am. J. Orth. Surg.*, **2**, 353
24. Codivilla, A. (1901). Sulla scoliosi congenita. *Arch. di Ortop.*, **18**, 65
25. Putti, V. (1917). Plastische e protesi cinematiche. *Chir. Org. Muov.*, **1**, 5
26. Putti, V. (1818). Utilization of muscles of a stump to activate artificial limbs. *Brit. Med. J.*, **10**, 7
27. Putti, V. (1935). *Anatomia della lussazione congenita dell'ancha*. (Bologna)
28. Putti, V. (1910). Die angeborenen Deformitäten der Wirbelsäule. *Fortschr. a. d. Ge. d. Roentgenstr.*, **15**, 70
29. Putti, V. (1929). Malignant bone tumours. *Surg. Gyn. Obstet.*, **48**, 324
30. Putti, V. (1937). L'ostéotomie intertrochanterienne dans le traitement des pseudarthroses du col du fémur. *Presse méd.*, **45**, 1841
31. Putti, V. (1918). La trazione per doppia infissore e l'allungamento operative dell'arto inferiore. *Chir. Org. Muov.*, **2**, 421
32. Putti, V. (1921). Operative lengthening of the femur. *J. Am. Med. Assoc.*, **77**, 934
33. Putti, V. (1938). Antonius Mathijsen. *Chir. Org. Muov.*, **24**, 1

34. Putti, V. (1921). L'encerclage ou ruban dans le traitement sanglant des fractures. *Lyon Chir.*, **18**, 133
35. Putti, V. (1917). Le mobilizzazione chirurgica della anchylosi del ginocchio. *Chir. Org. Muov.*, **1**, 1
36. Putti, V. (1921). Arthroplasty. *Am. J. Orth. Surg.*, **3**, 421
37. Putti, V. (1921). Technica dell'arthrotomia del ginocchio. *Chir. Org. Muov.*, **5**, 1
38. Margary, F. (1882). Estirpazione della cartilagine semilunare interne del ginocchio sinistro. *Gior. Roy. Acad. Med.*
39. Poggi, A. (1880). Contributio alla cura cruenta della luzzazione congenita coxofemorale unilaterale. *Arch. di Ortop.*, **7**, 105
40. Colonna, P.C. (1936). An arthroplastic operation for congenital dislocation of the hip – a two-stage procedure. *Surg. Gyn. Obstet.*, **63**, 777
41. Paci, A. (1885). *Studie ed osservazione sulla lussazione iliaca comune e sua cura razionale.* (Genoa)
42. Ortolani, M. (1937). *Paediatria*, **45**, 129
43. Ortolani, M. (1948). *La lussazione congenita dell'anca.* (Bologna)
44. Galeazzi, R. (1929). Treatment of scoliosis. *J. Bone Jt. Surg.*, **11**, 81
45. Galeazzi, R. (1934). *Arch. Orthop. Unfallchir.*, **35**, 557
46. Galeazzi, R. (1911). Sulla protesi cinematici. *9th Congr. Soc. Ortop. Ital.*
47. Galeazzi, R. (1910). Über die Torsion des verrenkten oberen Femurendes und ihre Beseitung. *Verh. d. dtsch. Ges. f. orth. Chir.*, 334

CHAPTER 6

National Histories – Switzerland

Jean-André Venel (1740–1791), a Genevese physician, was a late developer who went to Montpellier for a year at the age of 39 to study dissection and then, in 1780, established the first orthopaedic institute in the world at Orbe, in Canton Waadt.

There had been homes for crippled children before, but this was the first

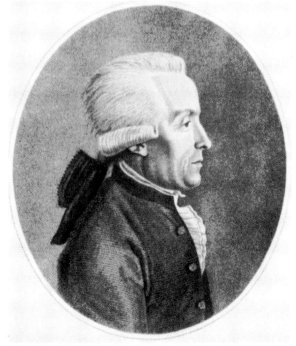

Figure 146   Jean-André Venel (1740–1791)

true hospital, for it established the essentials of orthopaedic management: segregation of patients in one centre under medical control, unalloyed by other disciplines; braces and appliances made in its workshops by individual fitting; education for children and vocational training for adolescents. Venel was also the first true orthopaedist, for he recorded and published his methods, unlike Deventer at the beginning of the century who had kept his methods secret (p. 309).

Valentin quotes Bouvier as calling Venel 'the father of orthopaedics'[1] but the inverted commas are not necessary; the description is a true one. Venel and his institute served as the model for all the many institutes that developed on the continent of Europe after 1800; and these, in turn, anticipated all the organized services for cripples and the academic establishments that now exist the world over.

Most of Venel's patients were children; some were adolescents, especially young girls, but this was not like the later institutes that were often mainly for teaching deportment. It treated real diseases; club-foot, tuberculosis, scoliosis. Venel was well aware of the benefits of sunlight and stressed, in 1776, that lack of exposure of the body was particularly noxious in young girls, that its benefits were well known to the ancients and ought not to be neglected[2].

Venel kept a visual record of his cases, sometimes by drawings, but also by plaster casts made on admission, partly to facilitate the construction of the requisite appliance, partly for graphic contrast with a cast made after correction. These casts were stored in a special room.

Where spinal disease was concerned, he was convinced of the importance

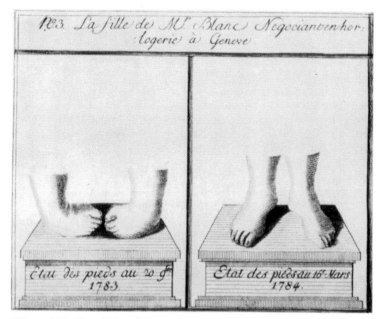

Figure 147   Venel: drawings to show status before and after treatment

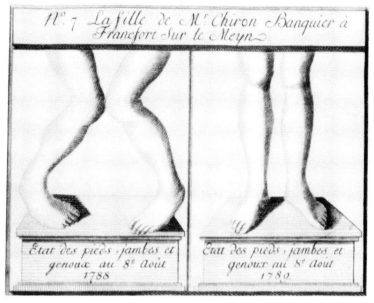

Figure 148   Venel: drawings to show status before and after treatment

of long recumbency and of maintained traction (often then called extension). His 'daytime appliance' for spinal curvature may not have been particularly original; but he also believed that, logically, traction should continue through the night and designed a 'night appliance' which was truly novel and was copied and modified in many countries. He argued that traction was more effective in the relaxed warmth of the bed with the spine relieved of body-weight. It was exerted via the head and axillae, with counter-traction by straps from a pelvic girdle fastened to the foot of the bed. Not a particularly vain man, even Venel could not shrug off the usual orthopaedist's mania for priority, 'I now turn to this appliance, which is exclusively my own and which is the basis of my special method.'

Also his own was the famous *sabot de Venel*, a club-foot appliance, a mechanical triumph unlike any previous splint which utilized leverage by a sole-plate connected to a metal rod on the outer side of the calf, with an encircling strap below the knee. This principle was the basis of many subsequent appliances, right up to and including the Denis Browne splint of our own times. Placide Nicod (1876–1953) reported that Venel's shoe was still in use in his hospital in Lausanne in 1908, and a modification was still in use by his son and successor Louis Nicod at the *Hospice Orthopédique de la Suisse Romande*, in 1955[4]. It was applied after manipulation and relaxing baths and the treatment was gradual, so that the child had to stay in hospital throughout treatment. No publications on the method ever appeared, as he died soon after drawing up the heads of a work to be entitled *Nouveaux moyens de prévenir et de corriger dans l'enfance les déjettements, courbures et difformités des pieds, des jambes et des genoux, même de ceux de naissance* (New methods of preventing and correcting in infancy the twists, curvatures

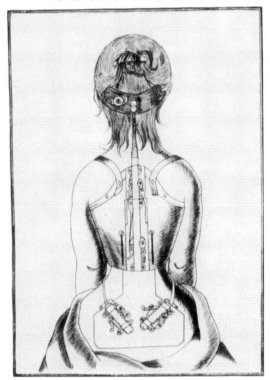

Figure 149   Venel's 'daytime appliance' for spinal curvature, 1789

and deformities of the feet, legs and knees, even those present at birth). Venel died early, at the age of 51, in 1791, of phthisis. For a time the institute was carried on by his brother and his nephew, Pierre-Frédéric Jaccard (1768–1820), but in 1820 Jaccard's son-in-law, Antoine-Paul Martin transferred it to Aubonne. His son, Henri Martin Crinsoz (1842–1914) founded the Hospice mentioned above in Lausanne. His successor was Placide Nicod (1876–1953) in 1927, and Placide was followed by his son, Louis.

To stay with institutes, there were few in Switzerland compared with other countries. One, in Zürich, for ophthalmic and orthopaedic cases, was founded by Joseph Konrad Heinrich Giesker (1808–1858), who had been Langenbeck's assistant at Göttingen, but he later became an obstetrician. During the 1850s, Jakob Frey (d.1883) became enthused by Swedish remedial gymnastics and set up a centre for this, also in Zürich[5], and after his death a new institute was founded by August Lüning (1853–1925) and **Wilhelm Schulthess** (1855–1917), who were the authors of a popular *Atlas and Outline of Orthopaedic Surgery* at the turn of the century[6]. Schulthess also wrote on scoliosis[7], and in 1907 opened the Balgrist Institute or Swiss Remedial and Educational Institute for Crippled Children, directed for many years by **Richard Scherb** (1880-1955), the first such in the country. Scherb was one of the very few exclusively orthopaedic surgeons in Switzerland of his time and unusual also in holding a chair in the subject. Karl Streckeisen (1811–1868), paediatrician

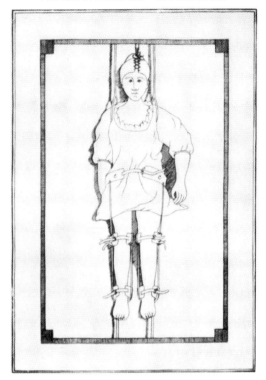

Figure 150 Venel's extension bed, ('lit à extension,' 1789)

at Basel, reviewed the subject of club-foot in 1869[8]. We recall that wire splints were the invention of the Lausanne surgeon, Mathias Louis Mayor (1775–1847), who also used steel wire and cotton in surgery[9].

H von Meyer, of Zürich, described the screw-home locking mechanism of the knee in 1873[10], and this impressed Goodsir in Edinburgh[11], who thought the menisci helped to ensure this good fit. In 1867, von Meyer published a paper on the architecture of spongy bone[12] which led, indirectly, to Julius Wolff's historic studies of the relation between form and function. In 1866 he published a treatise on spinal deformities, postulating mechanical imbalance as the cause of scoliosis[13].

Theodor Kocher (1841–1917) graduated in Berne in 1865, studied widely abroad, and became professor of surgery in Berne in 1872. He was also an anatomist who developed many useful surgical incisions and approaches; his posterolateral or 'southern' exposure of the hip is still regarded by many as the best[14]. His chief interest was in thyroid surgery, yet he is now best known for his method of reducing shoulder dislocation[15], which some have claimed goes back to ancient Egypt (p. 10). It was Kocher who was one of the first to designate slipped upper femoral epiphysis as adolescent coxa vara[16], and he was an early reporter of disc prolapse compressing the cord[17].

Kocher was succeeded in the chair of general surgery in Berne by **Fritz de Quervain** (1868–1940). Rang[18] quotes a note by Grey Turner, relating to

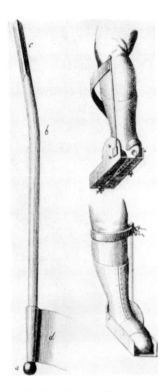

Figure 151   Venel's club-foot appliance, the *sabot de Venel*

a visit in 1908, which gives de Quervain some priority in medullary nailing; for, experiencing difficulty with a fractured femur, 'he sent for an old-fashioned vulcanite pessary. This he heated and moulded into a sort of angulated peg which fitted into the medullary cavities of the bones and served to give stability to the fragments.' He is best known for his 1895 description[19] of the eponymous tendon sheath thickening at the radial styloid, one of the very few orthopaedic conditions in which one can guarantee an immediate cure for a disabling condition. One wonders how it escaped notice before, and what was the natural history of the untreated condition. According to Girdlestone[20], de Quervain was using the spine of the scapula to graft fracture-dislocations of the spine in 1911 and later used this for Pott's disease, possibly even antedating Hibbs. He certainly wrote on the subject in 1917[21].

César Roux (1857–1934), originally from Lausanne but a Berne graduate in 1880, studied in Vienna, Prague and Halle and became Kocher's assistant in 1883, when he began surgical practice in Laussane. In 1890 he became extraordinary professor and in 1893 ordinary professor of surgery. Despite making advances in orthopaedics, such as his operation for recurrent

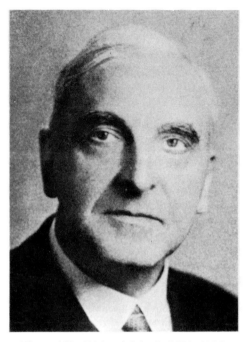

Figure 152   Richard Scherb (1880–1955)

dislocation of the patella by lateral release, medial reefing and medial shift of the patellar tendon[22], he was always a general surgeon.

Fritz Steinmann (1872–1932), also of Berne, gave an enormous impetus to the technique of fracture management in 1907, when he described nail transfixion of bone for the application of skeletal traction[23]. He had been impressed by the bad results shown by the newly invented X-rays and by the waste and disability revealed by national insurance schemes. Traction offered a compromise between total immobilization and the active method of Lucas-Championnière (p. 269), but adhesive strapping was difficult to manage and could cause sores and gangrene. He used two nails for the lower femur, one inserted from each side but not transfixing the opposite cortex, inserted under local or general anaesthesia, or none. This permitted easy access to and observation of the fractured limb, especially if compound, and controlled rotation. A single nail could also be used above the malleoli, through the lower humerus, across a dislocated acromioclavicular joint or in the great trochanter. It was a painless method, allowed early movement, tolerated more loading than strapping and avoided vascular complications; and its rapid acceptance at a time when iatrogenic infection of bone was an ever-present fear is a tribute to its value. We must remember, however, that Codivilla was using os calcis pins two years earlier in connection with his leg-lengthening operations (p. 288), and that the Kirschner wire was introduced at about the same time.

Switzerland has two special claims to our interest. One of these relates to its special place in the treatment of tuberculosis – of the skeleton as of the lungs – in its mountain sanatoria in the pre-streptomycin days. One thinks of Rollier at Leysin. The other, more recent, is the compression method of osteosynthesis of fractures, the AO method that began as a working-party on problems of internal fixation in the early 1950s and in 1958 became the official policy of a group of Swiss surgeons[24] who developed special powered tools, implants, screws, etc., a method that has gained worldwide popularity among the mechanically minded but appeals rather less to those who see the role of the orthopaedic surgeon as aiding, rather than supplanting, biological process. It may be unkind to quip that this beautifully efficient and precise technique was what one might expect from a nation of watch-makers (the equipment was originally manufactured in a disused watch factory) but older surgeons will recall Hugh Owen Thomas's bitter remark about 'practitioners too prone to look upon bones as mere machines, possessed of no automatic repairing quality.'

We ought to mention **Hans Debrunner** (1889–1974), a Zürich graduate influenced by working with Hermann Gocht in Berlin in 1915–24. In Zürich he set up an orthopaedic clinic at the University Hospital, helped found the Swiss Orthopaedic Society in 1941, and was President in 1952–5. In 1948 he became professor of orthopaedic surgery in Basel. He is known for his work on club-foot. Also, **Eugen Bircher** was using ivory as a transplant or insert in 1886[25], and was a pioneer of arthroscopy of the knee joint around 1918–19, when he carried out the first experimental endoscopies in cadavers, developing this field almost simultaneously with the Japanese[26]. The subject is dealt with more fully at p. 575.

REFERENCES

1. Valentin, B. (1956). Jean-André Venel, der 'Vater der Orthopädie'. *Sudhoffs Arch. Gesch. Med.*, **40**, 305
2. Venel, J.-A. (1776). *Essai sur la santé et sur l'éducation médicinale des filles, destinées au mariage.* (Yverdon)
3. Venel, J.-A. (1789). Description de plusieurs nouveaux moyens mécaniques propres à prévenir, borner et même corriger, dans certains cas, les courbures latérales et la torsion de l'épine du dos. *Hist. et Mém. Soc. Phys.*, **2**, 66 (Note Venel's use of the word *torsion.*)
4. Valentin, B. (1961). *Die Geschichte der Orthopädie*, p. 69. (Stuttgart, Thieme)
5. Frey, J.J. (1860). *Die Behandlung der Lähmungen und Verkrümmungen.* (Zürich)
6. Lüning, A. and Schulthess, W. (1901). *Atlas und Grundriss der orthopädischen Chirurgie.* (Munich)
7. Schulthess, W. (1905–7). *Die Pathologie und Therapie der Rückgratsverkrüm-mungen.* In *Handbuch der orthopädische Chirurgie.* (Jena)
8. Streckeisen, K. (1869). Notizen über Bau und Behandlung des Klumpfusses. *Jahrb. Kinderheilk.*, **2**, 49
9. Mayer, M.-L. (1836). *Sur le dessin linéaire en relief, et l'usage en chirurgie du fil de fer et du coton.* (Paris)
10. von Meyer, H. (1873). *Die Mechanik und Statik der Gelenke.*
11. Goodsir, J. (1868). *Anatomical Memoirs* (edited Wm. Turner). (Edinburgh)
12. von Meyer, H. (1867). Die Architektur der Spongiosa. *Reichert u. Dubois-*

Reymonds Arch., 615

13. von Meyer, H. (1866). Die Mechanik der Skoliose. *Virch. Arch.*, **35**, 125
14. Kocher, T. (1894). *Chirurgische Operationslehre.*
15. Kocher, T. (1870). *Berlin klin. Wschr.*, **7**, 101
16. Kocher, T. (1894). Ueber coxa vara. *Dtsch. Z. f. Chir.*, **38**, 521
17. Kocher, T. (1896). Die Verletzungen der Wirbelsäule zugleich als Beitrag zur Physiologie des menschlichen Rückenmarke. *Mitt. a.d. Grenzgeb. d. Med. u. Chir.*, **1**, 415
18. Rang, M. (1968). *Anthology of Orthopaedics*, p. 115. (Edinburgh, Livingstone)
19. De Quervain, F. (1895). *Korresp. Bl. Schweiz. Arz.*, **25**, 389 (letter)
20. Girdlestone, G.R. (1923). The place of operations for spinal fixation in the treatment of Pott's disease. *Brit. J. Surg.*, **10**, 372
21. De Quervain, F. and Hoessly, H. (1917). Operative immobilization of the cervical spine. *Surg. Gyn. Obstet.*, **24**, 428
22. Roux, C. (1888). Luxation habituelle de la rotule: traitement opératoire. *Rev. Chir.*, **8**, 682
23. Steinmann, F. (1907). Eine neue Extensmethode in der Frakturen Behandlung. *Zbl. f. Chir.*, **34**, 938
24. Müller, M.E., Allgöwer, M. and Willinegger, H. (1965) *Techniques of Internal Fixation of Fractures.* (Springer-Verlag, Berlin)
25. Bircher, E. (1886). Eine neue Methode unmittelbare Retention bei Frakturen der Rohrenknochen. *Verh. d. dtsch. Ges. f. Chir.*, **15**, 130
26. Bircher, E. (1921). Die Arthroendoskopie. *Zbl. Chir.*, **48**, 1460

CHAPTER 7

National Histories – The Netherlands

Many orthopaedic advances originated in the Netherlands during the 150 years from the mid 17th century to around 1800, yet little of note emerged after that period even though the 19th century saw the flowering of orthopaedics in Europe generally.

In 1652, Isaac Minnius, a surgeon with some reputation for operating for congenital torticollis, was consulted by one Tulp or Tulpius, presumably, an instance of the old relationship between surgeon and physician, for the cure of a 12-year-old boy. Tulp describes how Minnius began by making an eschar over the muscle with caustic and then divided the muscle over the clavicle with a knife 'from the ear towards the throat[1]'. Minnius was the first, or rather the first we have absolute knowledge of, to do this operation and, as Dieffenbach remarked, secured immortality merely by thinking of this unconventional procedure, though he added that by placing a skin scar over the muscle Minnius did everything likely to bring about a recurrence[2].

We then have Daniel Florianus, whose operation for neck correction is described by Job van Meekren (1611–1666), a pupil of Tulp, in his posthumous *Heel- en Geneeskonstige Aanmerkingen* (Amsterdam 1668). Meekren, 'widely renowned surgeon of the City, Admiralty and Hospital of Amsterdam', persuaded Florianus to operate on a 14-year-old boy, tied to a chair and held down while the tendon, but adroitly, 'gave such a snap ... as if one had plucked the string of a musical instrument.' Meekren gives the first known illustration of torticollis.

In 1668, **Hendrik van Roonhuyse** (d.1672) divided the muscle in a 23-year-old patient, 'and it was our great good fortune that our little knife was rather broad and blunt at the back, for otherwise we might easily have damaged the windpipe and the artery, which were most plainly to be seen the following day, from which it may be sufficiently deduced how dangerous and destructive it would be to use caustic and corrosive agents as the above-mentioned Tulp asserted, and how cautiously the knife must be used and everything kept ready for a severe haemorrhage, which could so easily follow[3].' Roonhuyse did a similar operation in 1670 on a 16-year-old, but this time he divided

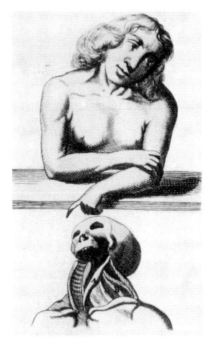

Figure 153   Job van Meekren: pathology of torticollis, Amsterdam 1668

the muscle from within outwards with a sickle-shaped knife which he passed
under the tendon after raising the skin fold, which sounds very much like
the first subcutaneous tenotomy.

None of these surgeons describe deliberate postoperative overcorrection.
Moreover, at much the same time, Antonius Nuck (of the nuciform sac) used
a head suspension appliance called the *torques*, though he admitted a place
for operation[4].

It should be added that it seems very probable that operations had long
been performed for torticollis (and other deformities) by charlatans, quacks
and mountebanks (French *saltimbanques*, Italian *saltimbanci*, German *Bänkel-
sänger*), i.e. those who jumped on a bench to shout their wares, before doctors
dared overcome their fears that convulsions and other disasters might follow
division of the sinews they had never clearly distinguished from nerves.
(Hippocrates had warned of the dire consequences of division of the Achilles
tendon.) The accounts given above stress the anxiety of the operators,
Valentin refers to an account, in the diary of an English cleric, the Reverend
John Ward[5], for 1648–79, of how a quack divided three tendons in a child's
neck, making a small incision with a lancet and elevating the tendon for fear
of wounding the jugular vein and inserting a knife to divide the tendon
'upwards' (presumably outwards) with a loud snap. The skin wound was
trivial and hardly bled. This practitioner did overcorrect, by means of a cap
bandaged to the opposite armpit.

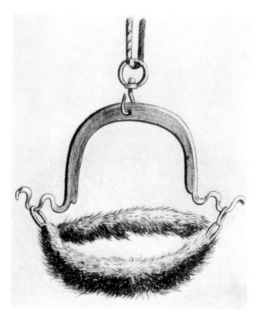

Figure 154   Antonius Nuck: the *torques* to be applied to the neck for head suspension, Leiden 1696

Another Dutchman, the famous anatomist **Theodor Kerckring** (1640–1693) reports how his 6-year-old great-niece was treated for congenital dislocation of the hip by a bonesetter, but in vain[6].

Hendrik Ulhoorn (1692–1749) is known for his extension chair, used in the treatment of spinal curvatures; this had an iron post with a hook over the head and traction was over pulleys. He describes this in his translation into Dutch of Heister's *Institutiones Chirurgicae* (Amsterdam 1741). Heister (p. 54) was one of the early great German surgeons.

A prominent 17th century figure was **Hendrik van Deventer** (1651–1724), who was born in Leiden and apprenticed as a goldsmith at the Hague and somehow acquired an interest in appliances for deformities. He studied pharmacy in Germany, returned to Holland at Wiewerd in Friesland, and practised mainly in obstetrics, in which field the complications of the narrow pelvis led to an interest in skeletal disorders, particularly scoliosis, which he treated by suspension from axillary slings. This led to an invitation to Copenhagen to treat the two children of King Christian V for rickety deformities, and he spent several periods there during 1689–91 and was decorated for his orthopaedic appliances[7]. As he was unqualified and successful, the Danish doctors cordially detested him, and when he did graduate at Groningen he had to be examined in Dutch as he knew no Latin. Even when he wanted to move to the Hague, the profession there would not recognize his diploma and he had to settle at nearby Boorburg, where he built an orthopaedic institute that attracted many patients from at home and abroad, and where he lived from 1709 to his death in 1724.

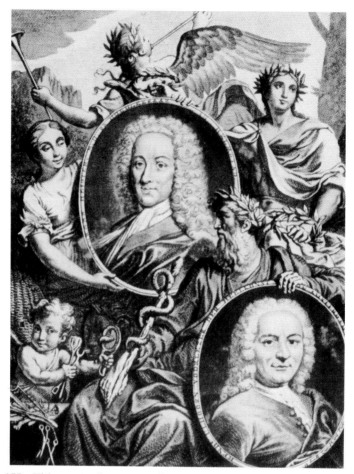

Figure 155 Title page of Hendrik Ulhoorn's translation into Dutch of Lorenz
Heister's *Institutiones Chirurgicae* (Amsterdam, 1755). Heister is the central figure,
Ulhoorn below

Most of Deventer's writings were on obstetrics. A purely orthopaedic text
was published posthumously, in 1739, which translates as 'An account of the
disorders of bones, and especially of rickets, or the English disease[8].' Valentin,
to whom most of this information is due, says that it is doubtful whether
Deventer actually wrote the text himself; it was handed down by his heirs,
polished by others, and remained a valuable literary property until 1765.
But an earlier work, the *Novum Lumen* of 1701, alludes to his superior
orthopaedic prowess in such terms as, 'If anyone has one or more vertebrae
displaced, and ... the lower part of the body is so paralysed that he is unable
to move either limb, and if the upper part is hunched and misshapen, I
reduce the vertebrae and by restoring to the nervous fluid its freedom of
circulation I also restore the ability to walk.'

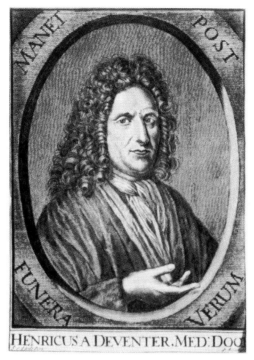

Figure 156   Hendrik van Deventer (1651–1724)

He was canny as well as self-important, stipulating prior payment for treatment of a wide range of conditions including wry-neck, scoliosis, dislocated hip, club-feet, knock-knee and bow-legs. Like many skilled practitioners of the day, he also wanted to keep it all in the family, 'I keep secret for my own children ... the knowledge of certain chemical preparations, as well as of manipulations to eliminate all kinds of physical malformities, *reliably, without risk, gradually* and *rapidly.*' He is careful to stress that the appliances must be bent to fit the knees and ankles, must apply pressure where needful and nowhere else, that the pressure should be adjustable and not excessive, and that treatment must be uninterrupted until the limb is straight. Deventer was probably as skilful as he claims, and one aspect of this is that he made plaster casts of his patients' limbs before and after treatment to demonstrate his success, a form of visual record in the days before photography in which he was a precursor of Venel. There ought to have been no doubt that he was the founder of scientific orthopaedics in Holland; but this was not the case because he left few records or publications, kept his methods secret and founded no school. Even the Dutch literature of the late 19th century makes little reference to him.

Pieter Camper (1722–1789) was professor of medicine in Amsterdam, an anthropologist and anatomist who described his eponymous fascia and, probably, the olecranon bursa, and wrote a famous dissertation on shoe-induced deformities in 1781[9]. The first paragraph reads as if written by Swift,

'This little treatise originated in a jest ... I wished to prove to my pupils ... that the most trifling matter, were it but a *shoe*, might become interesting if discussed by one able to speak with entire knowledge of both causes and results.' In this work, which made static foot deformities a fit and respectable subject for doctors to discuss and rescued them from the chiropodists, he refers to his dissections of club-feet, which had convinced him of the impossibility of complete correction, and blamed 'lack of room in the womb' for this deformity, one of many who were to take this view. He regarded deformation of the calcaneus and talus as primary, resulting in the forefoot being drawn in by the tibialis anterior and posterior, with loss of power in the peronei, 'so that the talus is even more twisted and turned outwards; but this is not all, for the calcaneum itself becomes crooked and is bent completely by the small flexor muscle and the abductor muscle of the great toe, and the Achilles tendon likewise loses its action.' Camper also made a contribution to geographic pathology when he noted that congenital dislocation of the hip was particularly common in certain parts of Holland, especially in young girls and irrespective of social status, 'so that this affliction cannot be ascribed to lack of either care or remedies.'

In 1851, **Antonius Mathysen** (1805–1878), a Dutch military surgeon* invented the plaster of Paris bandage, which, after heated debate for and against, was to transform orthopaedic practice. This is discussed at length elsewhere (p. 568).

The Netherlands Orthopaedic Association was founded in Amsterdam in 1898. Platt says that the story of Dutch orthopaedics in the first 30 years of the 20th century is simply that of **Murk Jansen** (1867–1935), an inspiring multilingual polymath who fought for the recognition of the discipline. His views of certain errors in embryogenesis as the cause of congenital deformities are not now accepted, but he did valuable work on bone growth and form and paved the way to the reputation of the Anna Kliniek and the Wilhelmina Hospital Clinic in Amsterdam as orthopaedic centres of excellence.

Another pioneer was **Guillaume Franciscus Joseph Marie Bär** (1905–1968), who trained as a general surgeon but was invited in 1935 to build and direct the St Maartenskliniek in Nijmegen for the treatment of the handicapped, this at a time when there was no Dutch university with a chair or even a separate department for orthopaedics, and when there was little or no training. This was then only the second such institute in the country. Nor must we forget **Cornelius Pieter Van Nes** (1897–1965), head of the Annakliniek from 1935 to 1952, who specialized in traumatology and reconstructive surgery, and whose expertise in osteosynthesis brought him patients from all over Europe. His 'turn-up plasty' for lower limb tumours was a *tour de force*.

Jan Derk Mulder (1907–1968) directed the Annakliniek at Leiden from

---

* Mathysen is variously described as Dutch or Belgian; but he was actually born in Budel in the Netherlands before the emergence of Belgium as an independent country, and his birthplace remained in Holland. Though he worked across the frontiers, and may perhaps best be described as Flemish, he was technically a Dutch citizen.

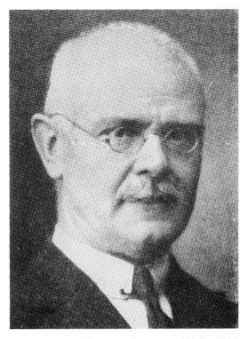

Figure 157   Willem Murk Jansen (1867–1935)

1952, becoming professor there in 1967, largely responsible for the development of orthopaedic surgery at a difficult time for this discipline in Holland. He was President of the Dutch Association in 1949–52.

REFERENCES

1. Tulpius, N. (1652) *Observationes medicae*. (Amsterdam)
2. Dieffenbach, J.F. (1841). *Über die Durchschneidung der Sehnen und Muskeln*. (Berlin)
3. van Roonhuyse, J. (1672). *Genees- en Heelkonstige Aanmerkingen*. (Amsterdam)
4. Nuckius, A. (1696). *Operationes et experimenta chirurgica*. (Leiden)
5. Severn, C. (1839). *Diary of the Rev. John Ward*. (London). The MS was discovered in the library of the Medical Society of London.
6. Kerckring, T. (1670). *Spicilegium anatomicum*. (Amsterdam)
7. Lamers, A.J.M. (1946). *Hendrik van Deventer, Med. Doct. Leven en werken*. (Assen)
8. van Deventer, H. (1739). *Beschryving van de Ziektens der Beenderen. En inzonderheyd, van de Rachitis of engelsche Ziekte*. (Leiden)
9. Camper, P. (1789). *Ober den besten Shoen*. (Amsterdam)

CHAPTER 8

National Histories – Belgium*

Belgian orthopaedics displays two influences. As in France, it was to some extent traditionally associated with paediatrics and paediatric surgery, the chair in which was held by **Jules Lorthioir** (1864–1931) at the Saint Pierre Hospital in Brussels. Thus, in 1911 he reported eight cases of pantalar fusion for paralysis by removing, denuding and replacing the bone[1]. Lorthioir's son, Paul, played an important part in the affairs of SICOT and his father's successor, Adolphe Maffei (1872–1945), also prominent in SICOT, died in Belsen during the occupation. On the other hand, there was a vigorous school interested in fracture management, which will be discussed later.

We should perhaps begin with the Professor **Baron Seutin**[2] (1793–1865). Growing up at Nivelles in a country under Napoleonic domination, he opted for medical studies to avoid conscription and was attached to the Hôpital Saint Pierre, but was eventually designated as a military surgeon after examination by Baron Larrey, cared for the wounded at Dresden and Leipzig, was taken prisoner, returned to the military hospital in Brussels in 1814 and organized several of the ambulance services for the wounded at Waterloo. In 1822, he founded the *Société des Sciences Médicales et Naturelles* of Brussels, to which he devoted much time and money and which endured for over a century. In 1824, he became director of the St Pierre and instructor in operative surgery and obstetrics, renouncing private practice after usefully marrying an heiress. He was active surgically in the 1830 Revolution and became medical director of the Belgian Army and attended the siege of Antwerp.

Seutin's claim to fame lies in his introduction, in 1835, of a method of treating fractures inspired by chance. He found a goat with a broken leg next to the establishment of a woman who starched linen; and it occurred

---

*I am greatly indebted to Professor Maurice Hinsenkamp and the late Dr Vander Elst for much of this material.

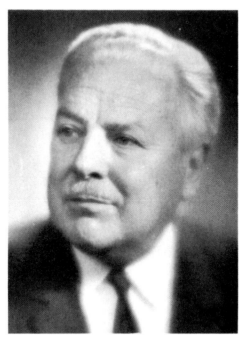

Figure 158   Paul Lorthioir

to him (as it had occurred to others for 2000 years) to use starch-paste to impregnate his bandage, so creating the *méthode amovo-inamovible* (removable-irremovable), i.e. a stiff bandage which could be incised to expose the fracture the next day and yet have its rigidity restored to allow crutch ambulation. This he claimed as original; admirers spoke of genius; yet we have seen that similar bandages go back to Larrey, Cheselden, even Hippocrates. In 1840, he published a book on his method, followed by a second volume with 114 figures describing the invention as 'a great victory for the whole of humanity', and made a grand tour to promote its advantages, taking him, via Langenbeck in Berlin, to Poland and Petrograd, thence to the Army of the Caucasus engaged in the Crimean War (did he influence Pirogoff towards closed methods?) and home by Turkey, Greece, Italy and France. In Brussels, at a medical banquet, he was awarded a medal with his portrait on one side, and on the other, 'To the author of the *méthode amovo–inamovible*, from Medicine and Humanity'. A second celebrity tour followed through France, Portugal, Spain and North Africa, from which he returned to become a baron in his own country and holder of a clutch of honours from most of Europe. It is always convenient when personal vanity coincides with the honour of one's country.

Seutin boasted that his method required only starch and bandages, no egg-white or whalebone like that of Larrey and others. It provided gentle uniform splintage and compression, immobilized the fracture and prevented oedema, and could be removed and reapplied like no bandage before, saving

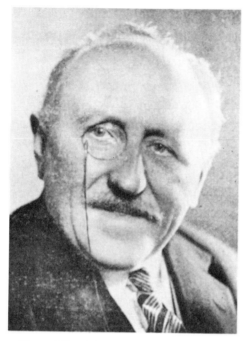

Figure 159 Adolphe Maffei (1872–1945)

many limbs from amputation. Velpeau may have made counterclaims; but his bandage was a mere counterfeit and published later, and anyway he used dextrin. Velpeau's graceful retraction in no way mollified Seutin, who also polemicized against Malgaigne.

Vain as he was, Seutin was nevertheless a perfectionist in matters of hospital hygiene and treatment and the virtues of his method cannot be refuted. Moreover – a hit at Lister – there was no need 'to saturate the air with so-called disinfectants under the pretext of destroying microscopic organisms fashionably attributed with a noxious influence that was certainly contestable.' This more than a decade after Pasteur's discoveries! Still, he promoted conservation over amputation, practised subperiosteal resections and excised the fractured femoral head. He became a member of the Senate, organized homes for the sick, and left his money to hospitals and bursaries and his heart to his birthplace. Even so, Seutin is now almost entirely forgotten. If we resurrect him here at length, it is to show that surgical hype is not a new phenomenon, and because it seems probable that he helped to foster the closed treatment of wounds and the evolution of the plaster bandage.

We now come to an undeniably very great figure, that of **Albin Lambotte** (1866–1955)[3,4]. Lambotte was influenced by his father, who was professor of comparative anatomy in Brussels, but more by his brother Elie, who was chief of surgery at the Schaerbeek Hospital in the Brussels suburbs. Elie was an indisputable genius, the first to operate for gastric ulcer, the second to

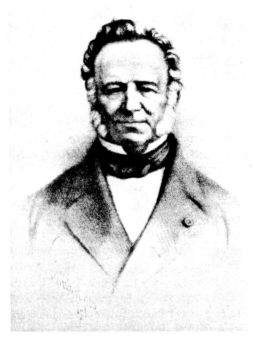

Figure 160   Baron Seutin (1793–1865)

perform cholecystectomy, and Albin was an intern in his department. Elie died at 32, but had already operated on leg fractures. Albin soon became head of surgery at Antwerp, where, in 1894, he began his series of gastric resections, laminectomies, posterior root sections and craniotomies; the date indicates how formidable this undertaking was. He was, however, destined to shine most brightly in bone surgery, which he attacked with immense energy from around 1900, reporting in 1907 on the operative treatment of 185 fractures. In 1907 he wrote, 'My aim is primarily to study bony suture, or to be more precise, osteosynthesis[5].' It was Lambotte who created the name, the technique and the instruments for this procedure. He reinvented the external fixator and devised bone-clamps, rugines, metal prostheses and a great variety of plates and screws. These he modelled in wood and sent to the surgical workshops in Paris (he also constructed the most beautiful violins and cellos). He (and Delbet in Paris) screwed the fractured femoral neck in 1899 and in 1908 presented 35 operated femoral fractures completely recovered. In 1928 he described the operative management of the injured hand; the pinning of Bennett's fracture, cerclage for phalangeal fractures and medullary nailing of phalangeal fractures through the articular cartilage of the head[6]. These procedures all illustrated at pp. 592 and 593.

In the early days (as now), infection was the great hazard of bone operations. Lambotte succeeded by an absolute no-touch technique, never using an instrument more than once without resterilization, never soiling his immaculate white gloves with a drop of blood. The source of infection, he

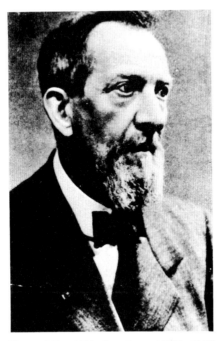

Figure 161   Albin Lambotte (1866–1955)

wrote, was an operation poorly and infrequently performed by a hesitant surgeon groping in the depths of the wound. Asepsis meant making an operation a short and mathematically conceived procedure. No surgeon should operate without special training, proper technique and equipment, in purpose-designed institutions to which the patients were admitted from the time of injury.

Despite violent opposition, he gained disciples – Tuffier in Paris, Arbuthnot Lane in England; and in 1913–14 he operated in Paris and Lyons for the benefit of the International Surgical Congress. His 70th birthday in Antwerp was attended by Leriche, Sauerbruch, Albee, Hey Groves, Putti, Tavernier and many others, and Leriche recalled how, as a young assistant at Lyons in 1913, he had been overcome by Lambotte's skill. 'They'd saved a difficult leg for you, in seven or eight fragments. You were on a strange ground, surrounded by experienced surgeons more given to criticism than admiration. Calmly, without apparent effort, without in the least soiling your white gloves, you magnificently assembled the diaphyseal jig-saw.' Leriche had then mentioned to Poncet that Lambotte was about to operate again, on an even more difficult case. 'How very unwise,' said Poncet, 'When one has once brought off a difficult feat in public, it's wiser not to start again,' and declined to watch. Leriche duly reported that the second operation had been even more successful. 'Well then,' replied Poncet, 'this Lambotte is more than skilful, he's lucky!' Perhaps the best tribute a surgeon can receive. Now, in 1935, Leriche, himself a professor, was to say to his face, 'I wonder whether Monsieur Lambotte, so modest and reserved, has ever fully appreciated the profound influence he has exerted on the surgeons who were young around 1910.'

Another sign of a good clinician was his hatred of administrators. When admonished to economy, he sewed up his private patients with the string they used to fasten their documents. He was a rounded, civilized man, an inspiration to his juniors, founder-member and first president of the Belgian Orthopaedic Society. Far from being rivals, he and Lane share the renown for introducing the operative fixation of fractures: Lane's *Operative Treatment of Fractures* appeared in 1905 and Lambotte's *L'intervention opératoire dans les fractures* in 1907, but both had been working steadily on the subject since the 1890s.

Lambotte's pupil, **Jean Verbrugge** (1896–1964), a Brussels graduate of 1921, held a Mayo Clinic fellowship in 1922–3 and spent 1925 with Putti in Bologna and Leriche in Strasbourg. He then settled in Antwerp with Lambotte, perfecting his techniques and applying them to paediatric ortho-paedics. He was interested for a time in the use of the magnesium alloys[7]. In 1946 he became *Professor Ordinaire en Orthopédie et Physiotherapie* at Ghent, thought he still lived and worked in Antwerp. He maintained a link with London's Royal National Orthopaedic Hospital for the training of junior surgeons from Europe. Vander Elst has left an exquisite personal portrait of this delightful man[8].

Robert Danis (1880–1962) was born in Tournai and qualified in 1904[9]. He at once attacked the then formidable problems of thoracic and vascular surgery and cancer of the breast. He was a prolific innovator in many fields: vascular, thoracic, portocaval surgery, spinal anaesthesia. In 1921 he became professor of surgery in Brussels. Dissatisfied with the available instruments and techniques, he invented his own, studied the metallurgical aspects of internal fixation, and enunciated two main principles; axial compression and the primary healing of fractures without external or internal callus. His great work, *Théorie et Pratique de l'Ostéosynthèse*, appeared in Paris (Libraires de l'Académie de Médecine) in 1949. In all this, of course, he was a disciple of Lambotte, whose work he desired to emulate, aiming to combine biology with mechanics, to develop atraumatic surgery and the 'primary suture' of bone, so as to allow immediate movement of adjacent joints, complete anatomic restoration and direct union without visible callus. 'If the adjacent joints are immobilized with a cast following internal fixation, the main benefit of the operation is lost', an opinion vigorously endorsed by George Perkins later in London. He even advocated internal fixation for fractures without separation if a cast would otherwise be necessary. There was no place for external callus in fractures so treated by *soudure autogène* (internal welding), for such callus should be regarded as essentially pathological, could hamper forearm rotation and was to be eliminated by osteosynthesis. The material used had to be biochemically and electrically inert; internal fixation must maintain absolute rigidity of the fragments and compress them along their main axes. To secure this he invented wire-guides, tighteners, saws, screws,

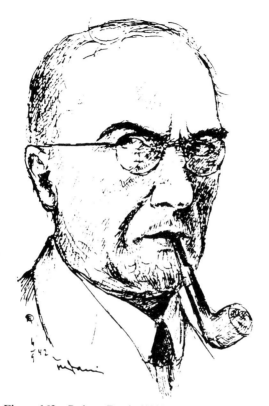

Figure 162 Robert Danis (1880–1962): self portrait

extractors, the single and double coaptor. The initiation of the AO movement in Switzerland in 1958 was largely due to the impression created by Danis.

An endearing man, he used to say to his pupils, 'Son, you can spit in the peritoneum, it will get better with drainage. Irrigate and clean a cranial wound and it will recover. As for bones, don't touch them; you're too young.' He taught them to treat ankle fractures by immediate splintage with reduction the next day; but when he himself fell in the street and crawled to his department and was given this timid advice, his response was: 'You're mad! Haven't you ever heard of Lucas-Championnière? Put on a Velpeau bandage.' He organized a bone-bank at a time when this was illegal in Belgium and used his retirement for painting and musical composition and performance.

Pierre Lacroix (1910–1971), of Louvain, was chief of orthopaedic surgery at the St Pierre University Hospital in that city and engaged in a long programme of research, summed up in his book, *The Organisation of Bone*, of 1949, which reviews the microphysiology of normal, diseased and ageing bone.

In 1943, **Robert Soeur**, despite war difficulties, inserted the first medullary

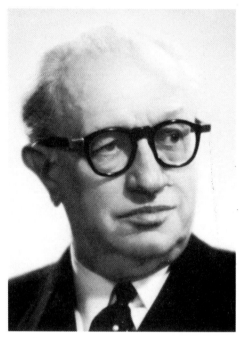

Figure 163   Jean Delchef (1882–1962)

nail to be used in Belgium and was able to report 74 cases in 1946[10,11].
After World War II, **Edouard Vander Elst** was a valiant orthopaedic historian
and edited the proceedings of SICOT for many years, as well as the history
of SICOT itself[12]. **Jean Delchef** was a father figure in Belgian orthopaedics,
a great teacher (though he held no academic post), a founder of the Belgian
Orthopaedic Society in 1920, and the first Secretary-General of SICOT,
which he nursed for its first 25 years.

REFERENCES

1. Lorthioir, J. (1911). Huit cas d'arthrodèse du pied avec extirpation temporaire d'astragale. *Ann. Soc. Belge. Chir.*, 6–7
2. Colard, A. (1983). Sur le Professeur Baron Seutin et sa méthode amovo-inamovible. *Rev. Méd. Brux.*, **4**, 39
3. de Marneffe, R. (1982). *Rev. Méd. Brux.*, **3**, 493
4. Vander Elst, E. (1964). Souvenirs sur Albin Lambotte. *Rev. Méd. Normande*, **6**, 473
5. Lambotte, A. (1907). *L'intervention opératoire dans les fractures récentes et anciennes envisagée particulièrement du point de vue de l'ostéosynthèse avec la description des plusieurs techniques nouvelles.* (Paris)
6. Lambotte, A. (1928). *Arch. France Belges Chir.*, **31**, 759
7. Verbrugge, J. (1937). L'utilization de magnésium dans le traitement chirurgical des fractures. *Acad. Chir. Mém. Paris.*, **63**, 813

8. Vander Elst, E. (1946). Jean Verbrugge. *Acta Orthop. Belg.*, **30**, 599
9. Vander Elst, E. (1962). *Ortho-Scop.*, **7**, 9
10. Soeur, R. (1946). *L'ostéosynthèse au clou.* (Paris, Masson)
11. Soeur, R. (1946). Intramedullary pinning of diaphyseal fractures. *J. Bone Jt. Surg.*, **28**, 309
12. Vander Elst, E. (ed.) (1978). *Société Internationale de Chirurgie Orthopédique et de Traumatologie.* (Springer)

CHAPTER 9

National Histories – Scandinavia

'The lame can ride a horse as well as any man, the handless can drive a herd'. These lines were written a thousand years ago in Iceland when in southern Europe the handicapped were abandoned to the wolves[1]. The handicapped were even given their chance in war. There is a figure of a double arm amputee springing from a boat to invade Britain. Bertelsen and Snorrason[2] tell us of Ivar the Boneless, who evidently had osteogenesis imperfecta, for he had blue eyes and brittle bones; yet he was carried into battle on a shield when, in the 9th century, he campaigned against the English in Northumberland, and drew a bow easily 'though he had only gristle in his limbs where other men had bones'. (When he caught King Ella, he made an 'eagle' of his back, dividing the ribs near the sternum and bending the chest-wall back on either side to make a pair of wings. This was also a Roman atrocity.)

'King Inge, who later ruled the southern part of Norway, suffered from ill-health as long as he lived; his back was severely curved, one leg was shorter than the other, and it had wasted so much that he walked with difficulty.' This was evidently poliomyelitis, as he also had a prominence on his loin and another on the chest, evidence of a paralytic scoliosis. Sometimes a nickname gives the diagnosis: Torolf Bent-Foot, Torstein Ox-Foot or Torbjørn Horn-Hoof, all presumably cases of congenital club-foot. Names such as Catback, Prow-Chest and Crooked-Leg suggest rickety deformities.

There was also tuberculosis, as evidenced by findings in early skeletons, though this was very late in reaching Iceland. Leprosy came to the Nordic countries with the Vikings and is often mentioned in the Icelandic sagas. Exposure of defective infants was acceptable as late as the 13th century, though under the influence of Christianity the indications became restricted to monsters.

Feet and legs were lost in war, from leprosy or ergotism, or as punishment. A sword might be called Foot-Biter. Survivors were nicknamed Wood-Leg, Wood-Foot or Beech-Foot, evidence of the existence of artificial limbs from

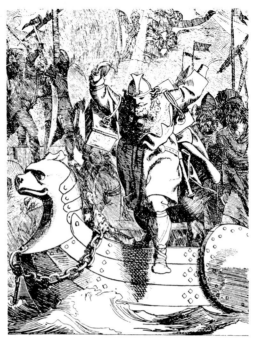

Figure 164   Olav Trygvason springing out of boat, ready for battle despite two amputated arms (Bertelsen, A. and Snorrason, M. D. [1972]. *Clinical Orthopaedics and Related Research*, **89**, 23)

at least the 9th century AD. Wounds were sutured with silk or catgut unless they were irreparable, as when an axe split a man in two. The Eyrbegga Saga tells of Torodd Torbrandson, wounded in the nape of the neck with an arrow through to the tongue; the arrow-head was removed but he was never able to bend his head again[3]. The sagas abound with such stories; as in the Iliad, the writings show that army leaders were also expected to act as surgeons.

For most of this historical material we are indebted to the late Arne Bertelsen (1910–1971), professor and orthopaedic surgeon at the Copenhagen Rigshospitalet. Bertelsen wrote a fascinating paper with Norman Capener, of Exeter, England on *Fingers, Compensation and King Canute*[4]. Canute, King of England, Denmark and Norway, established a code of mediaeval Latin/Anglo-Saxon laws which included a table of compensation for injuries, reckoned in schillings or solidos. The maximum compensation, 100 schillings, was for death or a broken neck with tetraplegia. Of digital amputations, a thumb was worth 30, the index (*demonstrarius*) 15, the middle finger (*impudicus*, for reasons not to be discussed here) 12, the ring finger (*annularis*) 18 and the little finger (*auricularis*, the ear-picker) 9. There is an extraordinary equivalence here to modern British pension scales for war injuries. These had been adopted almost verbatim from Alfred the Great (848–900), and by

Alfred from Aethelbert, first Anglo-Danish king of Kent (d.616), and *he* had them from the Salic Franks, his mother having been a Merovingian. At 507–511 a hand or foot was reckoned at 100 shillings and an index (now *sagittarius*) at 35. Incidentally, Montaigne[5] tells us that, in Roman times, a man might attempt to avoid military service by cutting off a thumb; hence the word *poltroon* (*pollex truncus*) for a coward. Vanquished enemies might have their thumbs amputated to make them incapable of handling oars or weapons.

Let us come to modern times.

SWEDEN

In 1827, **Nils Åkerman** (1777–1850) opened an orthopaedic institute in Stockholm called the Josephinska Orthopaediska Institutet after the Crown Princess and later wrote its history[6]. It was Åkerman who really introduced systematic orthopaedics into Sweden. In 1847 he transferred his institute to **Carl Herman Sätherberg** (1812–1897), who concentrated on remedial gymnastics[7], a field which flourished at this time in Sweden, under the influence of the school founded by **Pehr Henrik Ling** (1776–1839)[8]. Ling, of Lund University, started as a teacher of fencing and gymnastics and then applied these to therapy; he was not a doctor, and not popular with the doctors, but persuaded the authorities to allow him to found an institute, the Royal Central Institute of Gymnastics, in 1813. Ling developed what Valentin calls a rational science of calisthenics based on ancient Greek methods that had a worldwide influence[9].

In the mid century the institute was directed by **Lars Gabriel Branting** (1779–1881) and a centennial report appeared in 1913[10]. The strict Swedish system prescribed only free exercises, sometimes resisted by other gymnasts or apparatus, and seems to have had almost a masonic flavour, for there was a secret numerical code or gymnastic formula known only to adepts. The system was introduced into other countries, notably Germany, America and England and, like bonesetting, its management became the preserve of certain families: the Cyriaxes, of German origin, and the Kellgrens, originally Swedish but later transferred to England[11]. Some of the descendants of these families acquired a reputation for what has been termed (by themselves) 'medical orthopaedics'.

One gains the impression that Swedish gymnastics was a self-perpetuating, closed and comprehensive system like Marxism or psychoanalysis in which heterodoxy was not tolerated. Like the latter, the exercises were conducted on a one-to-one basis with a physician or instructor and only one patient could be treated at a time. So it was an advance when **Jonas Zander** (1835–1920) in Stockholm constructed batteries of appliances activated either by the patients themselves or by electric motors to allow passive and resisted exercises, focussed on individual muscles or muscle groups. Such machines were much used for rehabilitation of the wounded in World War I[12], but were in no way as useful as purposeful active movements. These medico-mechanical institutes became fashionable, if only as a way of losing weight;

they provided the equivalent of modern weight-training.

The pattern of orthopaedic services in Sweden was pioneered by **Patrik Haglund** (1870–1937), who had been a pupil of Hoffa in Berlin (p. 192) and became the first professor of orthopaedics in Sweden in 1913, with a clinical base at the Karolinska Institute. For a long time he was the only academic teacher of orthopaedics in the country. Perhaps this was why, initially, Scandinavian orthopaedics developed along German lines, with institutions for the care and training of cripples and the supply of appliances and artificial limbs. Like too many orthopaedic pioneers, Haglund achieved his ambition of a new and specialized orthopaedic unit only when he was due to retire, at the age of 65 in 1935. He wrote, in German, *The Principles of Orthopaedics* and for many years worked virtually singlehanded, in dismal premises. Certainly, most cases of congenital dislocation of the hip in the country were referred to him, and this led to the expertise manifested in this field by his pupil, **Erik Severin**. In 1941, Severin analysed 454 hips treated over 20 years and showed that, while the functional results might be better than the X-ray appearances suggested, late deterioration was common[13].

Henning Waldenström (1877–1972) succeeded Haglund in the chair in 1936, but ran the new institute for only a short time, until 1942, for reasons of age. It seems clear that he had recognized juvenile osteochondritis of the hip independently of Legg, Calvé and Perthes, and at almost exactly the same time in 1909; nevertheless, he did not describe it under the name of

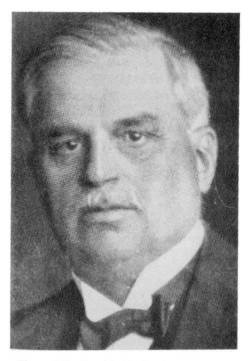

Figure 165 Patrick Haglund (1870–1937)

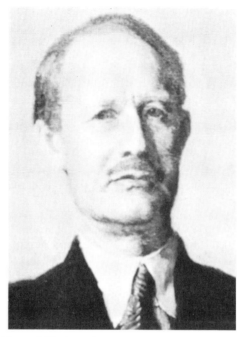

Figure 166   Henning Waldenström (1877–1971)

coxa plana until 1920[14]. He was more surgically oriented than Haglund and urged use of the term 'orthopaedic surgery' rather than plain 'orthopaedics' – a change not officially accepted for many years – and visited military hospitals in England and France in World War I to gain experience.

In 1922, **Sven Johansson** (1880–1959) in Stockholm described osteochondritis of the patella[15], as he thought for the first time; but, as usual with such claims, he was wrong, for the Norwegian, Sinding-Larsen (1866–1930) had given an account in the previous year[16]. In 1932 Johansson, who was interested in the metallurgical aspects of fracture fixation, did very nearly bring off a first when he described blind nailing of the femoral neck with the three-flanged nail that Smith-Petersen had been inserting under direct vision since 1925 and first reported in 1931. Johansson placed it over a guide-wire under X-ray control[17]. It was not quite a first because Westcott in Virginia had made a preliminary report of the same technique earlier in that same year[18].

Carl Hirsch (1913–1973) graduated at the Karolinska in 1944 and became head of orthopaedics at Uppsala in 1957 and professor there in 1957. In 1960 he moved to the orthopaedic chair at Göteborg and in 1969 to that at the Karolinska. He had studied under Langenskiöld in Helsinki in 1946, and with Seddon and Trueta in Oxford in 1948 and with Joseph Barr in Boston in the same year. He had a special interest in the biomechanics of the hip and spine and had his own laboratory. He published over 200 papers and presided over the Scandinavian Orthopaedic Association from 1963 to 1966.

In the 1930s, **Svante Orell** made a series of studies on autogenous bone grafts, interesting then but not of much current importance, which are described at p. 550. He was also interested in recurrent dislocation of the shoulder[19].

Ivar Palmer (b.1897), a Stockholm graduate of 1923, was a resident at the Serafimer Hospital, then part of the Karolinska, and, after service elsewhere in Sweden, became senior staff member of the surgical division of the Sabbatsberg Hospital in Stockholm, where he wrote his famous thesis[20] on knee ligament injuries. From 1939 to 1942 he was chief of trauma and military surgery in the newly reopened Karolinska, until 1947 he was chief of surgery at the Sabbatsberg Hospital, and was then chief at the new Southern Hospital of Stockholm until retirement in 1962.

His book[21] discusses injuries of the menisci and of the cruciate and other ligaments and their repair (including meniscus resuture). He devised instruments for cruciate repair and methods of dealing with torn collateral ligaments. He vigorously contested the idea, current in 1938, that few surgeons knew much about anterior cruciate injuries, how to diagnose or repair them; he was right. Galen had described the ligament[22]. In England, Battle in 1898[23] and Mayo Robson in 1900[24] had described satisfactory repair of the anterior or both cruciate ligaments, and Hey Groves in Bristol had reported similarly in 1917[25] and 1919[26]. Groves had detached a fascial strip from the iliotibial band and directed it through a tunnel in the lateral femoral condyle through the old course of the damaged ligament. Alwyn Smith reported a similar procedure in the British Journal of Surgery in 1918[27], while in 1936 and 1939 Willis Campbell in Tennessee described the triad of torn medial meniscus, tibial collateral ligament and anterior cruciate and their repair[28,29].

In 1948, **Knut Lindblom**, at the Karolinska, reported his technique of direct injection of the lumbar intervertebral discs with radio-opaque dye which both reproduced the symptoms if done at the lesional level and showed the nature of the rupture[30]. The fact that this could be done fairly simply made it possible for others to proceed to chymopapain injection later.

In the 1950s and 60s, Severin continued his thoughtful work on congenital hip dislocation, illuminating its pathology by arthrography and showing that soft tissue obstructions to concentric reduction in the depths of the acetabulum could be worn down by splintage and activity.

We should also refer to the work of Göran Bauer on radioactive isotopes, of Bo Nilsson on bone metabolism, of Alf Nachemson on low back pain and of Bertil Stener on orthopaedic oncology. The first thesis on osteogenesis imperfecta was published in 1788 by a Swedish army surgeon, Olaus Jacob Ekman, who called it 'congenital osteomalacia' and traced it as a hereditary condition through three generations[31]. Ekman expressed definite eugenic views, 'Since there is no reason to believe that the girl just mentioned will ever marry, let us hope that this family of poor wretches will die with her!' The condition was also described, as 'osteopsathyrosis', by Lobstein, professor of pathological anatomy at Strasbourg, 50 years later[32].

Finally, Swedes made important contributions to our understanding of poliomyelitis which will be dealt with a little later.

NORWAY

An orthopaedic institute was opened in Lillehammer by a **Gunder Kjoelstad** (1794–1860) in 1836, transferred to Christiana (Oslo) in 1844 and to Eidsvold in 1857. His assistant, August Tidemand, founded his own establishment in the capital in 1837. But the real founding father of orthopaedics was **Ivar Alvik** (1905–1971). He began as a general surgeon (there were no others), spent World War II in Sweden, and returned to Norway as initially the *only* orthopaedic surgeon in the country and worked in tuberculosis hospitals. He then trained in orthopaedic surgery in England and New York and became professor at Sophies Minde, the institute for crippled children founded by Queen Sophie (of Norway and Sweden). This he turned into a modern orthopaedic hospital, with workshops, bioengineering laboratories, prosthetic departments and physiotherapy. This led a drive to stimulate the formation of orthopaedic departments in general hospitals. Alvik was a founder of the Nordic Orthopaedic Association (*q.v.*)

We have mentioned **Sinding Larsen**, who was director of a long-stay seaside hospital treating mainly skeletal tuberculosis at Frederiksven and became director of the Rikshospitalet in Oslo in 1911. The name of **Bülow-Hansen** (1861–1938) is linked with the treatment of congenital hip dislocation and poliomyelitis.

DENMARK

In the 17th century, **Niels Stensen**, or Nicolaus Steno (1638–1686), of Copenhagen, pondered on the contraction of muscles, criticizing the conventional view that this was due to an influx of animal spirits and showing that contraction could occur in isolated muscle tissue by stimulating either its nerve or the muscle directly. He recognized that each muscle unit had a certain potential contractility, and that the power of muscle was the sum of the action of its fibrils[33,34]. Stensen died at 38, after quitting science for the Church. In the18th century, a celebrated anatomist, **Jakob Benignus Winslow** (1669–1760) published in 1733 his great *Exposition anatomique de la structure du corps humain*, which was a standard anatomical text for a century. He described the bursae, subscribed to the glandular theory of synovial function and wrote widely on matters of orthopaedic interest.

As in Sweden, early developments in modern times rested on the shoulders of a very few individuals. These included **Poul Guildal** (1882–1950), a key figure, closely involved in the development of Danish orthopaedics, who organized the Copenhagen Orthopaedic Hospital, with his pupil, **Sven Kiaer**, and **P G K Bentzon** at Aarhus, succeeded by **Thomasen**. Guildal was a pupil of Herman Slomann who founded a private orthopaedic clinic in Copenhagen in 1901, the first true clinic in Scandinavia. There had been 'institutes' before this. In 1834, Johannes Peter Langgaard, a layman, had founded one at Store Tuborg near the capital which will be found in Hoffa's list of the more important centres of the first half of the century (p. 193). **Johann Christian August Bock** (1813–1879) was a regular doctor who studied with Dieffenbach in Berlin and started his own centre in Copenhagen in 1847; he translated Dieffenbach's *Operative Surgery* into Danish and became a professor and Court physician, but later lapsed into trade and politics.

Knud Jansen (1913–1983) was essentially a team man, favouring collaboration between every discipline for the benefit of the disabled. He was chairman of the Danish Orthopaedic Association and the Danish Society for Orthopaedic Surgery, Secretary-General of the Scandinavian Orthopaedic Association, editor of *Acta Orthopaedica Scandinavica* from 1968, a prominent member of SICOT (*q.v.*) and of World Orthopaedic Concern, and founder of the International Society for Prosthetics and Orthotics, and its President from 1970 to 1977.

Arne Bertelsen (1910–1971) occupied the first chair of orthopaedic surgery in Denmark in Copenhagen in 1957. He had graduated in 1935 and became an anatomist and pathologist at Aarhus. He then moved to Copenhagen for surgical training, and in 1945 became chief of the University Hospital Polyclinic. In 1945–7 he made an orthopaedic study tour of Sweden, the UK, USA and Canada, and in 1952 became chief of one of the two departments at the Orthopaedic Hospital in Copenhagen (the other was first under Sven Kiaer and then Hjalmar Larsen). In 1968 he moved to the University Hospital. He urged and achieved the building of country-wide orthopaedic and accident units, pursued plastic and hand surgery, was president of the Danish Orthopaedic Association in 1954–6, and was involved in the care of cripples, nationally and internationally.

Holger Werfel Scheuermann (1877–1960) was interested in both orthopaedics and radiology, but eventually became chief of radiology at the Copenhagen Cripples' Hospital and the leading Danish radiologist. He described adolescent kyphosis in 1921 as a pubertal lesion much commoner in males, due to epiphyseal lesions as part of an osteochondritis, totally unamenable to treatment[35]. The first major clinical and experimental study of fluorosis of bones and ligaments was published in 1932 by Møller and Gudjonsson from the radiology department of the Copenhagen State Hospital[36]. This was an accidental discovery in cryolite workers being examined for silicosis. In 1949, **Seedorf** published a massive study of osteogenesis imperfecta, its clinical features and heredity, based on 55 families comprising 180 affected members[37]. Fairly recent Copenhagen orthopaedic surgeons known personally to the present writer include **Arne Bertelsen**, now deceased, **Hjalmar Larsen** and **Johannes Mortens**. These, with others, also undertook the periodic supervision of orthopaedic services in Greenland.

As in other fields, it was convenient for the small populations of the Nordic countries to act together in orthopaedics. In 1919 there were only some 25 orthopaedic surgeons for the whole of Scandinavia with a population of 18 million, and in that year there was founded in Göteborg the Nordisk Ortopedisk Förening (Nordic Orthopaedic Association) for the social care of cripples under the impetus of Slomann from Denmark and with Haglund as first president and Johansson as first secretary. Gradually, the orthopaedists took over fracture care from the general surgeons. The association was inactive in World War II, but grew rapidly thereafter and at its 50th anniversary in 1959 had 232 members. At first, orthopaedic papers were published by the Scandinavian Surgical Society, but in 1930, at a meeting of eleven Scandinavian orthopaedists, Haglund of Stockholm and Bentzon of Denmark (Aarhus) proposed a new publication, the *Acta Orthopaedica Scandinavica*, privately financed by the eleven founders. In 1947 the chief editor was Professor Sten Friberg, succeeded by Knud Jansen and then by Gorän Bauer.

The Swedish Orthopaedic Association was founded in 1944 on the stimulus of Sophus von Rosen, of Malmö, with 23 original members, now many hundreds. The original Nordic Association now has around 1000 members.

A Danish pioneer in rehabilitation was the Rev. Hans Knudsen, who founded the Society and Home for the Disabled in 1872. This was matched by the Sophies Minde in Norway, the Finnish Invalid Foundation, and by Swedish centres in Stockholm, Göteborg and Halsingborg.

SCANDINAVIA AND POLIOMYELITIS

The association between Scandinavia and poliomyelitis is not, on reflection, so very odd. In those countries of the Third World and around the Mediterranean where the disease was endemic, and immunity often gained in childhood, severe epidemics were unusual even though, in sum, there may have been – and still is in some African countries, like Malawi – a lot of individual disease. The really severe epidemics were reserved for countries where this pool of infection did not exist, where high standards of hygiene paradoxically increased vulnerability, the countries of north-west Europe, North America and Australia.

We have referred elsewhere (p. 186) to the work of Jacob Heine, of Cannstatt, in establishing the identity of the disease, previously fragmented into individual local paralyses, and in establishing its natural history and the principles of management. That it existed in ancient Egypt is evidenced by the stele shown at p. 9 and other findings; however, epidemics in the Old and New Worlds were not reported until around 1800, but they could hardly have escaped mention if they had occurred. Each informant thought he was describing a new disease. A good clinical description was given by the London physician, Michael Underwood, in the second edition of his *Treatise of the Diseases of Children* of 1789 under the heading 'Debility of the Lower Extremities', 'When both lower extremities have been paralysed, nothing has seemed to do any good but irons for the legs, to support the limbs and enable the patient to walk.' Underwood recognized it as occurring between the first and fifth years and as associated with disorders of the alimentary tract, but found it puzzling because previously undescribed. Monteggia has been credited with a prior account, but this differs little from Underwood's and is certainly much later. John Shaw (1792–1827), the renowned London orthopaedist, said very little of the disease, but what he did say no one had said before, 'Certain paralytic affections of the muscles are sometimes so instantaneous that we must consider them as depending on a change which has suddenly taken place in the brain, or spinal marrow, or in the nerves which supply the affected parts[38].'

Heine briefly reported some cases in 1838[39] and elaborated on this in a monograph two years later[40] and produced a much larger treatise in 1860[41], attributing the disorder to spinal cord lesions, differentiating it from spastic paralysis and noting the epidemic nature of the disease, its effect on growth, the contractures and their treatment by tenotomies. The term 'acute anterior poliomyelitis'* originated with Adolf Kussmaul (1822–1902). The localization of the lesion to the anterior horn cells of the cord is often ascribed to workers in Charcot's service in Paris around 1865, but it seems that Duchenne discovered this ten years earlier.

Recurrent small epidemics occurred in Scandinavia in the 19th century and were first documented by Cronberg and Øberg in Sweden in 1801 and 1807. The first large epidemic documented in the literature was Scandinavian, described by Bergenholz, in 1855. We owe the first detailed study of an epidemic, that in Stockholm in 1887, to the Swedish physician, Oscar Medin, who read a paper to the paediatric section of the International Medical Congress in Berlin in 1890[42]. This had been a typical summer epidemic with maximum incidence in August–September, affecting 44 children, with three deaths; none were over six years of age. Medin noted every aspect of the disease: that the victims were usually children in good health, that – unlike other infections – it did not select the poorest, the deceptive latent phase after onset and the existence of polioencephalitis, supported by histologic observations of acute inflammation in the anterior horns and secondary tract degeneration. Medin's service was to clearly establish the infective nature of the condition. For very many years it was known as the Heine–Medin disease.

Christian Leegaard, in 1909, described over 1000 cases from an epidemic in Norway in 1905, pointing out that the many nonparalytic or abortive cases which would not have been noted under other circumstances were, he believed, responsible for the spread of the disease. Between 1911 and 1913 there were several large epidemics in Sweden, described by Otto Wickman in 1917 – over 6000 cases; it was a disease that had previously gained his attention. He noted that in rural areas recurrence was unusual within five years, because of immunity gained by the local population, whereas annual epidemics might occur in cities. The lowest mortality was in the 0–5 year age-group; it rose with age and only 15 per cent of patients were over 15 years old. Early physiotherapy was important to prevent contracture.

We now come to the great Copenhagen epidemic of 1952, a monument to human courage[43]. In 1952, Copenhagen had about a million inhabitants. There had been epidemics in the two previous years and the Blegdams Hospital for infectious diseases, under its director, Professor Lassen, was expecting a further intake. But it was not prepared for a very large number and had no respirators, it seems because of unsatisfactory results in previous epidemics. The epidemic began at the end of July and the last cases were seen in January of the following year. During these six months, 1289 paralytic and 1631 nonparalytic cases were recorded in central Copenhagen; 110 died.

---

* Greek *polios* = grey.

The Blegdams Hospital was the only one covering this area and admitted 2727 patients, though some came from as far away as Bornholm or even Greenland. The epidemic peaked around 15th September, when 50 patients were admitted daily. All admissions went through the Blegdam; the most serious (respiratory) cases were retained, but many of the others went to other hospitals or temporary premises. Forty-three per cent of those admitted were paralysed, but many of these could be transferred fairly rapidly to treatment centres, some of these set up in renovated hotels.

Nearly 10 per cent of cases had respiratory paralysis. There were not nearly enough respirators, whether of cuirass of iron lung type. Some were obtained from Norway and Sweden, but of 31 patients with severe paralysis admitted up to 27th August, 27 died. The situation was not under control. In 1948, tracheotomies had been performed in Sweden, but with a 70 per cent mortality, death being due to anoxia and carbon dioxide narcosis. A new approach was vitally needed. Lassen called on an anaesthetist, Bjørn Ibsen, for assistance. A 12-year-old girl with total paralysis was chosen for testing; she was both hyperpyrexic and cyanosed. She was tracheotomized and a tube inserted. She lost consciousness, developed lung collapse, stopped breathing. Only manual ventilation with a balloon for weeks saved her life. It became clear that ventilation countered the anoxia and CO_2 accumulation and reduced brain damage. As a result, oral intubation was done at the earliest sign of breathing difficulties and tracheotomy as indicated. Most patients required manual ventilation, and this called for an immense programme in which doctors, nurses, medical, dental and veterinary students, porters, even volunteers from the street, were called on for ventilation round the clock. They knew there was a risk of contracting the disease, and some did, but there is no evidence that any patient died for lack of a volunteer to continue the manual ventilation.

Of 345 patients with life-threatening poliomyelitis, 270 had tracheotomies and 277 were ventilated. One hundred and forty-four died in the acute phase. Apart from very numerous quadriplegics, frequent complications included shock, ileus, hyperpyrexia, pulmonary oedema and uraemia. Pulmonary physiotherapy was of the first importance. Many of the survivors were permanent respiratory cripples, but they were all cared for and enabled to lead remarkably satisfactory lives by a combination of voluntary and state aid. The last patient was discharged from the Blegdam in 1959.

The essentially novel feature of this epidemic was the institution of intratracheal positive-pressure ventilation at the earliest sign of respiratory failure and its manual continuation over as long a period as required. Eventually, a mechanical respirator was developed to do this, but the human presence could not be substituted and the bulk of the work depended on the hands of individuals. All this gave an impetus to the development of intermittent positive pressure ventilation systems now familiar in intensive care units for the care of traumatic, coronary and postoperative cases, accompanied by the routine estimation of blood-gases which was also used in Copenhagen. Indeed, the whole concept of the intensive care unit, often under the direction of an anaesthetist, was furthered by the Copenhagen experience. This also stimulated the use of physiotherapy for emptying the lungs and retraining the respiratory or ancillary muscles.

No convalescent serum or vaccine was used during the epidemic. The Salk vaccine arrived in 1955 and prevention is now assured where it is used, but there is still no treatment and, if immunization levels fall too far or the supply of vaccine is ever interrupted, new epidemics will occur as in the past for, unlike smallpox, the virus still exists in quantity in many parts of the world and could emerge again, like Aids from Africa or from elsewhere in the tropics.

REFERENCES

1. Miller, D.S. and Davies, E.H. (1972). *Clin. Orthop.*, **89**, 76
2. Bertelsen, A. and Snorrason, E. (1972). Orthopaedics in West Scandinavia during the Middle Ages. *Clin. Orthop.*, **89**, 23
3. Jonsson, F. (1912). *Laegekunsten i den nordiske oldtid.* (Copenhagen)
4. Bertelsen, A. and Capener, N. (1960). Fingers, Compensation and King Canute. *J. Bone Jt. Surg.*, **42B**, 390
5. Montaigne, M. de: Des Pouces. *Oeuvres complètes*, p. 670. (Paris, Gallimard)
6. Åkerman, N. (1840). Utdrag of Josephinska Orthopediska Institutets Journal från dess stiftelse den 9 October 1827 til October 1840. *Svenska Laek. Saellsk.*
7. Sätherberg, C.H. (1894). *Gymnastik-ortopediska Institutets Historia.* (Stockholm)
8. Cyriax, R.J. (1914). A short history of mechano-therapeutics in Europe until the time of Ling. *Janus*, **19**, 178
9. Ling, P.H. (1836). *Reglement foer gymnastik.* (Stockholm)
10. *Kungl. Gymnastika Centralinstitutets Historia 1813-1913* (1913). (Stockholm)
11. Cyriax, E.F. (1871). *Elements of Kellgren's Manual Treatment.* (London)
12. Hemingway, E. (1955). In Another Country. In *Men Without Women.* (Penguin)
13. Severin, E. (1941). Contribution to the knowledge of congenital dislocation of the hip joint. *Acta Chir. Scand.*, **84** (Suppl.), 63
14. Waldenström, H. (1920). Coxa plana, osteochondritis deformans coxae, Calvé–Perthessche Krankheit, Legg's disease. *Zbl. f. Chir.*, **47**, 539
15. Johansson, S. (1922). En fornt icke beskriven sjukdom i Patella. *Hygeia*, **34**, 161
16. Larsen, S. (1921). En hittel ukjendt sygdom i patella. *Norsk. Mag. f. Laegevidensk*, **82**, 856
17. Johansson, S. (1932). *Acta Orth. Scand.*, **3**, 262
18. Westcott, H.H. (1932). Preliminary report of a method of internal fixation of transcervical fractures of the neck of the femur in the aged. *Virginia Med. Monthly*, **59**, 197
19. Orell, S. (1940). Surgical treatment of recurrent dislocation of the shoulder joint. *Surg. Gyn. Obst.*, **70**, 945
20. Palmer, I. (1938). On the injuries to the ligaments of the knee joint. *Acta. Chir. Scand.*, (Suppl.), 53
21. Palmer, I. (1962). *Oppen Behandling av Frakturer och Ledskador.* (Stockholm, Almquist and Wiksell)
22. Galen, C. *On the usefulness of the parts of the body* (trans: May, M.T., 1968). (Cornell University Press)
23. Battle, W.H. (1900). A case after open section of the knee joint for irreducible traumatic dislocation. *Trans. Clin. Soc. Lond.*, **32**, 232
24. Mayo Robson, A.W. (1903). Ruptured crucial ligaments and their repair by operation. *Ann. Surg.*, **37**, 716
25. Hey Groves, E.W. (1917). Operation for the repair of the crucial ligaments.

Lancet, **2**, 274

26. Hey Groves, E.W. (1919). The crucial ligaments of the knee joint: their function, rupture and the operative treatment of the same. *Brit. J. Surg.*, **7**, 505

27. Alwyn Smith, S. (1918). The diagnosis and treatment of injuries to the crucial ligaments. *Brit. J. Surg.*, **6**, 176

28. Campbell, W.C. (1936). Repair of the ligaments of the knee. *Surg. Gyn. Obst.*, **62**, 964

29. Campbell, W.C. (1939). Reconstruction of the ligaments of the knee. *Amer. J. Surg.*, **43**, 473

30. Lindblom, K. (1948). Diagnostic puncture of the intervertebral discs in sciatica. *Acta Orthop. Scand.*, **17**, 231

31. Ekman, O.J. (1783). Dissertatio medica descriptionem et casus aliquot osteomalaciae sistens. *Thesis*, University of Uppsala, 10 May 1783

32. Lobstein, J.F.G.C.M. (1833). De la fragilité des os, ou de l'ostéopsathyrose. In *Traite d'Anatomie Pathologique*. (Paris)

33. Stensen, N. (1664). *De musculis et glandulis observationum specimen*. (Copenhagen)

34. Stensen, N. (1662). *Observationes anatomicae*. (Leyden)

35. Scheuermann, H.W. (1921). Kyphosis dorsalis juvenilis. *Z. Orth. Chir.*, **51**, 305

36. Møller, P.F. and Gudjonsson, S.V. (1932). Massive fluorosis of bone and ligaments. *Acta Radiol. Scand.*, **13**, 269

37. Seedorf, K.S. (1949). Osteogenesis imperfecta: a study of clinical features and heredity based on 55 Danish families comprising 180 affected members. *Opera ex Domo Biologiae Hereditaraiae Humanae Universitatis Hafniensis*, **20**. 1

38. Shaw, J. (1823). *On the nature and treatment of the distortions to which the spine and the bones of the chest are subject*. (London)

39. Heine, J. (1838). Proceedings of the *Versammlung deutscher Naturforscher und Ärzte*. (Freiburg)

40. Heine, J. (1840). *Beobachtungen über Lähmungszustande der untern Extremitäten und deren Behandlung*. (Stuttgart)

41. Heine, J. (1860). *Spinale Kinderlähmung*. (Stuttgart)

42. Medin, O. *En epidemi af infantil paralysi*

43. Lassen, H.C.A. (1956). *Management of Life-Threatening Poliomyelitis: Copenhagen 1952–1956*. (Edinburgh and London, Livingstone)

CHAPTER 10

National Histories – Ireland

In the pre-Christian era, one Liancecht was a medical deity, or at least a human physician, of around 480 BC. Assisted by Creidne, a famous silversmith, he made an articulated silver hand to replace that lost by King Nuadhat at the Battle of Magh Tuireadh between Tuatha de Danann and the Firbolgs, a loss that had excluded him from office for seven years – hence 'Nuadhat of the Silver Hand', one of the first western European references to artificial limbs.

The Barber-Surgeons' Guild controlled surgery in Ireland until the foundation of the Royal College of Surgeons in Ireland in 1784, at much the same time as similar separations in France and England.

Abraham Colles (1773–1843), born in Kilkenny of humble origins, was professor of surgery at the College of Surgeons in Dublin from the age of 29 for 32 years. He was the first to tie the right subclavian artery. He was the first, in 1814, to describe the eponymous* fracture an inch or so above the lower end of the radius and its typical deformity, often previously mistaken for a sprain or dislocation[1]. He showed that the late result was often one with full painless movement, even if treatment were defective, and used two tin splints after reduction, as did Robert Jones, and my own chief, Paul Jenner Verrall, at the Royal Free Hospital in London up to World War II. 'I should consider this by far the most common injury to which the wrist or carpal extremities of the radius and ulna are exposed ... one consolation only remains, that the limb at some remote period will again enjoy perfect freedom in all its motions and be completely exempt from pain;

---

*Let us, however, always bear in mind Ravitch's caustic comment on eponyms, 'Given an eponym, one may be sure (1) that the man so honoured was not the first to describe the disease, the operation or the instrument, or (2) that he misunderstood the situation, or (3) that he is generally misquoted, or (4) that (1), (2) and (3) are all simultaneously true[2].'

the deformity, however, will remain undiminished throughout life.' Colles made no dissection observations on his fractures; these were made, and Colles' name attached, later by Robert Smith (see below).

Colles' fracture had, of course, been considered earlier by Hippocrates and many others, as a dislocation of the wrist or inferior radio-ulnar joint. In 1783, Claude Pouteau (1725–1775)[3], of the Hôtel-Dieu at Lyons, described fractures of the distal radius, some with crepitus, some impacted, some with diastasis, though Colles was unaware of this at the time of his own publication. (We may complete this historical aspect by adding that Dupuytren, in 1847[4], stated that fractures of the distal radius were extremely common, 'I have always found that these supposed dislocations of the wrist prove to be fractures; and I have never met with or heard of a single well-authenticated and convincing case of the dislocation in question.' The pathology was clarified by Jean-Gaspar-Blaise Goyrand (1803–1866)[5] of Aix-en-Provence, who distinguished epiphyseal separations from fractures, and by Nélaton (1807–1873) in 1844[6], who produced these fractures experimentally in cadavers by transmitted force. It was Velpeau (1795–1866) who coined the term *talon de fourchette* (dinner-fork deformity).

The discovery of X-rays led to some rethinking, as fractures of the distal radius were among the first to be thoroughly studied; there was an X-ray report of Colles' fracture as early as 1897[7]. Finally, there is Barton's description, in 1838, of *his* eponymous injury of the wrist[8], a subluxation associated with a dorsal or palmar marginal fracture of the end of the radius.

Colles wrote a book on surgical anatomy in 1811 and a paper on congenital talipes equinovarus in 1818[9].

Robert William Smith (1807–1873) was one of the most distinguished Irish anatomists and surgeons. He founded the Dublin Pathological Society with Colles, Graves, Corrigan and Stokes (there's eponymy for you!) and became professor of surgery at Trinity College. He conducted the autopsy on Colles. In 1849, he published in Dublin *A Treatise on the Pathology, Diagnosis and Treatment of Neuroma*, with excellent clinical illustrations, which described neurofibromatosis long before von Recklinghausen did so in 1882. His classic work, *A Treatise on Fractures in the Vicinity of the Joints, and on certain forms of Accidents and Congenital Dislocations* in 1847, with 200 excellent illustrations, included an account of the fracture of the radius known by his name, and also of Madelung's deformity before Madelung described it[10].

Robert Lafayette Swan, sometime President of the College of Surgeons in Dublin, graduated in 1863 and was one of the first modern Irish orthopaedic surgeons, founding the Dublin Orthopaedic Hospital at his home at 11, Ushers' Island (later transferred to Upper Merrion Street). His successors included such men as Sir William De Courcy Wheeler, who began bone-grafting for Pott's disease at Mercers' Hospital in 1922, and Arthur Chance; but neither he nor they ever confined themselves to orthopaedic surgery.

Edward Hallaran Bennett (1837–1907) succeeded Smith as professor of surgery at Trinity College in 1873 and was later President of the College of Surgeons. He was famous as a bone pathologist, described the well-known fracture at the base of the thumb metacarpal[11], introduced antisepsis to Dublin and did many osteotomies for rickets.

Robert M'Donnell, President of the College in 1877, is said to have given the first blood transfusion in Ireland, in 1865. He operated for an unstable fracture–dislocation at the dorsolumbar junction of the spine with cord damage, 37 days after the injury and in the presence of Brown-Séquard, who was visiting Dublin at the time. Despite considerable sensorimotor recovery, death ensued after 17 days; the autopsy showed the cord to have been damaged by a slice fracture of the body of L1. 'But unsuccessful cases are often more instructive to the practical surgeon than those which terminate favourably ... it must be admitted that ... the judiciousness of trephining the spine, with a view to remove pressure from the spinal marrow, is one of the nicest which can be presented to the surgeon.' It was, in fact, very controversial, and M'Donnell gives a surprisingly long list of operated cases going back as far as 1827 (see also p. 422 for experience in the American Civil War). The problems were the risk to life of the operation, the risk of creating a compound fracture of the spine, and the stability of the spine after laminectomy; but we now know the answers to these. Oddly, M'Donnell himself felt certain that even very severe cord injuries were capable of recovery, 'I have often more or less completely cut the cord and have often seen the animals operated upon almost completely recover from the paralysis[12].'

The only Irish surgeon known to have specialized entirely in orthopaedic surgery at an early date was **Grattan**, of Cork, known for his invention of an osteoclast (see p. 618).

We should also mention **Peter Redfern** (1820–1912), born in Derbyshire, a Fellow of the Royal College of Surgeons in England in 1851, who moved via Aberdeen to become lecturer in pathology in Belfast for 33 years, and was described by Keith as 'the founder of our knowledge concerning the microscopic structure of cartilage and discoverer of the process by which its wounds are repaired[13].' Experimental breaches either remained open or healed by fibrous tissue, but were never repaired by the same substance.

In southern Ireland, those general surgeons with orthopaedic interests included De Courcy Wheeler, Somerville-Large and others, particularly perhaps **Arthur Chance** (1889–1980), son of the Sir Arthur Chance already mentioned, on the staff of Dr Steevens' Hospital in Dublin from 1916 to 1966, a general surgeon who came to devote himself to orthopaedics and was professor of surgery at the College of Surgeons.

Other Dublin figures of the early post-World War II period include **John Sugars** and **John Cherry**. At Cork for many years, the regional orthopaedic centre was directed by **St John O'Connell**, a former assistant to E P Brockman in London, with M A Connail and F H Moore. Other regional centres have been developed in recent decades.

In northern Ireland, the first purely orthopaedic surgeon was **Robert James Wilson Withers** (1909–1965), energetic and a great teacher, who initiated the Irish Orthopaedic Club, commemorated by the Withers Orthopaedic Unit at Musgrave Park. The first whole-time orthopaedic surgeon appointed in Belfast was Piggott, in 1940, and there is now a regional clinic system run by a number of surgeons.

Robert Adams was a Dublin physician, who was the first, in 1857, to distinguish between osteoarthritis and rheumatoid arthritis in *A Treatise on Rheumatic Gout, or Chronic Rheumatic Arthritis of all the Joints*. He invented the term *malum coxae senilis* for nonarticular arthrosis of the hip. And it was an Irishman, Bernard Connor, who published in Rheims in 1691 an excellent, and what must surely have been the first, account of ankylosing spondylitis[14]

REFERENCES

1. Colles, A. (1814). *Edinb. Med. J.*, **10**, 181
2. Ravitch (1979). Dupuytren's invention of the Mickulicz enterotome, with a note on eponyms. *Perspect. Biol. Med.*, **22**, 170
3. Pierres, Ph.-D. (1783). *Oeuvres posthumes de M. Pouteau: Mémoire contenant quelques réflexions sur quelques fractures de l'avant-bras, sur les luxations incomplètes du poignet et sur le diastasis.* (Paris)
4. Dupuytren, G. (1847). *On the injuries and diseases of bones, being selections from the collected edition of the clinical lectures of Baron Dupuytren* (Trans. Le Gros Clark, F., London, Sydenham Society)
5. Goyrand, G. (1832). Mémoires sur les fractures de l'extremité inférieure du radius, qui simulent les luxations du poignet. *Gaz. Méd.*, **3**, 664
6. Nélaton, A. (1844). *Éléments de Pathologie Chirurgicale.* (Paris)
7. Beck, C. (1898). Colles' fracture and the Roentgen-rays. *Med. News*, **72**, 230
8. Barton, J.R. (1838). Views and treatment of an important injury of the wrist associated with marginal fracture of the dorsal or palmar aspect of the end of the radius. *Med. Examiner*, **1**, 365
9. Jones, A.R. (1950). *J. Bone Jt. Surg.*, **32B**, 126
10. Peltier, L.F. (1959). *Surgery*, **45**, 1035
11. Bennett, E.H. (1882). Fractures of the metacarpal bones. *Dublin J. Med. Sci.*, **2**, 73
12. M'Donnell, R. Case of fracture of the spine in which the operation of trephining was performed, with observations. (Dublin, HMSO)
13. Keith, A. (1919). *Menders of the Maimed.* (London)
14. Connor, B. (1695). *Phil. Trans.*, **19**, 21–7

Dr Patrick Heraghty of Sligo tells us in his book on Inishmurray, an island off the Sligo coast, now abandoned, that in the early years of this century the island's 'doctor', one Crimley, used a 'plaster' made of comfrey leaves pounded with stones, which dried into a pliable and resilient cast for fractures. He also applied green freshwater algae to burns to give a firm occlusive coating of alginate equivalent to tannic acid. (Heraghty, P. [1982]. *Inishmurray*. Dublin, O'Brien Press)

CHAPTER 11

National Histories – Australia

Australia was a late developer in the orthopaedic field and resembles other late developers, of originally colonial origin and of vast geographic extent, in certain aspects; an initial professional dependence on the 'mother country', in this case Britain, or on other European countries, and a largely isolated regional development by states until the growth of air transport made communication in person relatively easy. Nearly all the growth of orthopaedics took place after 1900; the earlier work being that of two early pioneers, Hamilton Russell and Sir Charles Clubbe. Young Australian orthopaedists might make the 'grand tour' of European centres once and then find themselves too busy as their practices grew to repeat it, though this too has changed in recent years. Orthopaedic development was both facilitated and hampered by a closer initial association with paediatric surgery than existed in England, and was definitely hindered by the reluctance of general surgeons to recognize orthopaedics as an independent discipline. To be fair, there was a reluctance of some orthopaedists to abandon general surgery.

In such a foreshortened story, history must come closer to the present day, and include more details of individuals, than is usually desirable in books of this nature. And – at least to home-bound parochials in the old country – these individuals often seem to have led lives of enviable freedom and eccentricity. The best source of information is Hugh Barry's fine book, *Orthopaedics in Australia*[1], together with an article by H Jackson Burrows[2]. Barry classes Australian orthopaedists and allied practitioners into three groups: immigrants, natives and renegades. The renegades or expatriates include Sir Grafton Elliot Smith (1871–1943), anatomist and anthropologist, E T C Milligan, pioneer of wound excision in World War I, William Gissane, linked with the Birmingham Accident Hospital in England, Hubert Sissons, who built up the department of bone pathology at the Royal National Orthopaedic Hospital in London, Campbell Golding, of the radiology department at London's Middlesex Hospital, Howard Florey, to whom we owe the practical application of penicillin. All these are discussed at the appropriate places.

PIONEERS

Robert Hamilton Russell (1860–1933) graduated at King's College Hospital in London, was a dresser and house-surgeon to Lister, emigrated to Australia in 1889 and became surgeon to the Children's Hospital in Melbourne in 1892 and to the Alfred Hospital in 1901. He was a general surgeon with orthopaedic interests and is known for his traction for femoral fractures and hip disorders to eliminate muscle spasm[3]. In 1908 he resected an osteocla-stoma of the lower ulna and substituted a cadaveric graft, possibly for the first time. A gentle handsome man, he was a founder-member of the Royal Australasian College of Surgeons.

    Sir Colin MacKenzie (1877–1938) was a Melbourne graduate of 1898, initially an anatomist, who worked with Vulpius at Heidelberg and visited Robert Jones in Liverpool. He advanced the treatment of poliomyelitis, a recurrent scourge in Australia, with the principle of muscle rest and coined the term 'reeducation'. He stated the most important principle in such reeducation, 'An ounce of scientifically directed volitional effort is worth pounds of passive movement', important at a time when passive mechanical motion was much in vogue. He was the first to describe the shoulder abduction splint. During World War I he worked with Arthur Keith at the Royal College of Surgeons in London and with Robert Jones at the

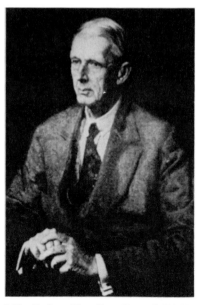

Figure 167   Robert Hamilton Russell (1860–1933)

Shepherd's Bush Military Hospital and there set up a department of muscle retraining, a world first. He wrote *The Action of Muscles, including Muscle Rest and Reeducation.*

Frederick Wood Jones (1879–1954) was a London Hospital graduate, an anatomist, who worked on nerve injuries at Shepherd's Bush (the importance of this London military hospital as a training ground for young orthopaedists from the old British Empire, and elsewhere, during the first world war cannot be overemphasized). He rotated between professorial chairs in anatomy in England and Australia after the war, restored the Hunterian Museum after its partial destruction in World War II, and wrote *The Principles of Anatomy as seen in the Hand*, a classic, and a corresponding book on the foot.

Max Herz (1876–1948) was the only man trained as an orthopaedic surgeon and practising solely in this field in Australia before the first world war. A Munich graduate, he worked with Schanz in Dresden and Lorenz in Vienna and studied club-foot and Pott's disease. In 1902, Herz assisted Hoffa in Berlin in an operation on a patient from New Zealand, who persuaded Herz to go back to New Zealand with him, where he worked in Christchurch and Auckland. In 1910, he moved to Sydney, became a figure in Australian surgery, wrote on the surgery of poliomyelitis, and in 1911 reported to the Sydney Australian Medical Congress a successful nailing of an ununited fracture of the neck of the femur with a five inch silver nail. In 1911 he became Honorary Orthopaedic Surgeon at St Vincent's Hospital, Sydney. (The term 'Honorary' is equivalent to 'Attending' in the USA; it has dropped out in Britain since the advent of the National Health Service there.) He was treated badly in World War I, interned for six years and then banned by professional bodies and hospitals, and had to set up his own hospital in 1921. He was shunned by many Sydney surgeons, the local British Medical Association tried to get him deported, and he was never elected to the Australian Orthopaedic Association.

Hugh Compson Trumble (1894–1962) was a general surgeon with orthopaedic interests, best remembered as a neurosurgeon at the Alfred Hospital who eventually confined himself to neurosurgery. He did develop a method of extra-articular bone-graft arthrodesis of the hip joint in 1932[4] which was later developed by Brittain[5] in Norwich, England and by Bosworth[6] in New York.

In World War I, Sir Neville House, Director-General of the Australian Army Medical Services, foresaw the orthopaedic problems of ex-soldiers and sent several officers to train at the Alder Hey military hospital at Liverpool set up by Robert Jones, under T P McMurray and others. These included Denis Glissan from Sydney, A V Meehan from Brisbane and Alex Juett from Perth. This marked the beginning of a continuing pilgrimage of Australian would-be orthopaedists to Britain for training, so that by the second world war orthopaedics had become a fully-fledged speciality. For long, Liverpool had more influence than London – it granted an orthopaedic diploma, the MCh Orth, which London did not – though at the present time both are perhaps being ousted by the USA.

Norman Royle (1888–1944) had an interesting life. A Sydney graduate with a lifelong interest in muscles and physical culture, partly an anatomist,

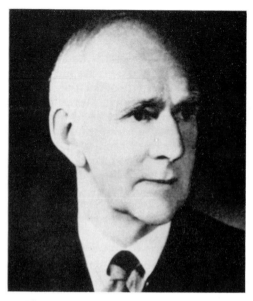

Figure 168   Hugh Trumble (1894–1962)

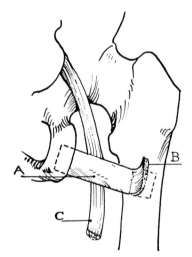

Figure 169   Sketch of Trumble's ischio-femoral arthrodesis

he collaborated with John Irvine Hunter, a young professor of anatomy, in experimental work on the sympathetic supply to muscle which convinced him that the spasticity of a number of disorders – wounds of the central nervous system, stroke, cerebral palsy – was due to sympathetic overaction. He began publishing work on sympathetic ramisection in 1924 (later ganglionectomy[7-9]) and applied this to cerebral palsy. This was partly based on Foerster's section of the posterior nerve roots for spasticity in 1908[10], but Royle became an enthusiast, always to be deplored in new and unproved surgical fields. He travelled, operated and orated in Britain and the USA and met with general acclaim; but his results were not reproducible and his later life, ironically, was clouded by Parkinson's disease. He was perhaps the first to excise a congenital hemivertebra for kyphoscoliosis[11]. To some extent, he may have paved the way to those, like Leriche, who used operations on the sympathetic for vascular disease – though these, too, have fallen into desuetude.

Let us now consider the various States separately.

NEW SOUTH WALES

This State, and the city of Sydney, has always been dominant in Australian orthopaedics. The first specialist group in the country was the orthopaedic section of the New South Wales branch of the British Medical Association, founded in 1923, while the Australian Orthopaedic Association was founded in 1936 in Sydney, its permanent headquarters. This State has the greatest share of membership and the first chairs of orthopaedic surgery in Australia were at the University of Sydney and that of New South Wales.

Early orthopaedic work was associated with the *Royal Alexandra Hospital for Children* (founded 1880), though there was no department as such until 1935. It was originally the Sydney Hospital for Sick Children at Glebe, but changed its name after moving to Camperdown in 1904. It is associated with some famous early personalities. **Sir Charles Clubbe** (1854–1932), who emigrated from England in 1882 and pursued the French tradition of orthopaedics as part of paediatric surgery. His operations for club-feet, including astragalectomy, and subcutaneous tibial osteotomies for curvatures were, Barry suggests, among the earliest orthopaedic procedures in Sydney. **Sir Robert Wade** (1874–1954), though chief general surgeon also at the Royal Alexandra Hospital from 1913, was a leading Sydney orthopaedic surgeon and was Director of Army Orthopaedics in World War I, based at Randwick Military Hospital. **Sir Norman Gregg**, in 1941, discovered the relationship of pregnancy rubella to congenital deformity. **Gerald Keith Smith** (1886–1963) became an eminence in the orthopaedic department. Wilfred Vickers Laurence Macdonald, Gordon Colvin and R W D Middleton were successive heads of the department, all with a basic feeling for physiotherapy and muscular reeducation that has always been a feature of Australian orthopaedics.

The Royal Prince Alfred Hospital, Sydney, founded in 1882, the largest and most influential hospital in New South Wales since World War II, was the training ground for many young orthopaedists. The new orthopaedic unit of 1920 was placed under **Lennox Teece** (1889–1959), who had been with Robert Jones at Shepherd's Bush in 1916–18 and was therefore largely an operator on knee menisci and feet. Teece was the first Australian-born surgeon to specialize in the field in Australia, a charismatic, larger-than-life figure with a large medicolegal practice, fond of gambling, skiing and horse-

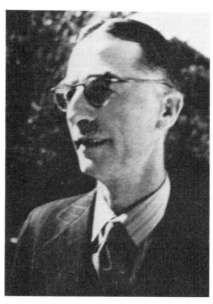

Figure 170   Lennox Teece (1889–1959): orthopaedic surgeon, Royal Prince Albert
Hospital, Sydney

racing. He had an enormous private practice and described a sign for
meniscus tears which some consider better than the McMurray sign. His
assistant and successor at the Prince Alfred was **F H McClements Callow**
(b.1908), originally a general practitioner, who towards the end of World
War II toured Britain, America and Canada as part of a study team with
Bryan Keon-Cohen and John Jens investigating developments in amputations
and prostheses. He was secretary to the AOA and its president in 1962.

The Australian Orthopaedic Association was founded in 1936 at a Sydney
meeting of ten orthopaedic surgeons: E B M Vance (1885–1939), Alex
Hamilton (b.1899), J W R Hoets (1885–1961), Norman Royle (1888–1944),
Dennis Glissan (1889–1958), Laurence Macdonald (1900–1986), F H McC
Callow (b.1908), S H Scougall (1889–1965), A L Webb (1898–1969) and
Harold Sweetapple (1898–1947). Other foundation members co-opted later
were Lennox Teece (1889–1959), L O Betts (1886–1943), Roy Grantham
(1889–1950), A V Meehan (1890–1955) and L W N Gibbon (1899–1937).
The first president was Vance (who was also the first Australian to gain the
Liverpool MCh Orth and was always a Liverpool adherent) and Hamilton
the first secretary. Earlier in 1936, Hamilton had consulted E P Brockman
in London, then secretary of the British Orthopaedic Association, as to
whether the proposed Australian Association should be exclusive. Brockman
replied that it would be unwise to exclude men who combined orthopaedic
and general surgery, or to restrict membership to members of the British
Medical Association. In a later letter he added that, when the AOA was
strong enough, *then* it should be restricted to purely orthopaedic practitioners.
In the event, those who were not offered foundation membership included

Robert Wade, Tom King and J B Colquhoun of Melbourne, Juett and McKellar-Hall of Perth. And, says Barry, 'Max Herz was never seriously considered at any time.'

Alexander Robert Hamilton (b.1899), a Sydney graduate of 1923 and for some years a general practitioner, was persuaded by Vance to go to Liverpool and took his diploma there in 1931. He was a partner in Vance's Sydney practice in Macquarie Street and took over the practice when Vance died in 1939. He became senior orthopaedic surgeon at the Balmain District Hospital and Royal North Shore Hospital and helped design the Margaret Reid Orthopaedic Hospital at St Ives.

William Lawrence Macdonald (b.1900) also took the route from Sydney to Liverpool, was asked by Robert Jones to help out at Oswestry for three months and stayed five years. (Oswestry always had and retains a strong Australian association. Macdonald's tenure came between those of Douglas Parker and Bryan Keon-Cohen. The present Director is an Australian.) He designed the hospital at St Ives on the same lines as Oswestry, was on the staff of many Sydney hospitals, and the editorial secretary of the AOA and on the editorial board of the Journal of Bone and Joint Surgery (B) for many years.

Harold Algar Sweetapple (1898–1947) was another Sydney graduate (1921) persuaded by Vance to take the Liverpool trail. It has tended to be customary for such pilgrims to return with both the MCh Orth and a Fellowship of one of the Royal Colleges of Surgeons; Sweetapple did so and returned to work at St Vincent's and as Teece's assistant at the Prince Alfred. He died young of a malignant melanoma.

Allan Frederick Dwyer (1920–1975), a Sydney graduate of 1942, trained at home, and moved from general practice to orthopaedics to become known in three fields: arthrodesis of the hip using internal fixation with an iliofemoral medullary nail*, the anterior approach for scoliosis[12] with removal of the discs and use of a cable threaded through cannulated screws, and electrical stimulation of spinal fusion. In the latter part of his career he moved to the USA.

St Vincent's Hospital, Sydney is linked particularly with **Denis Joseph Glissan** (1889–1958). After service in the first world war, he was sent, with Juett and Meehan, by the Australian Army Medical Corps to Alder Hey and returned to St Vincent's to form the first orthopaedic department. Greatly influenced by McMurray, he naturally disliked internal fixation or any use of metal in the body, and is described by Barry as meticulous, demanding and a tedious operator.

Stuart Scougall (1889–1964), originally a Queenslander, graduated at Sydney in 1920, toured the orthopaedic centres of Europe, Britain and the USA in 1929 and became a full-time orthopaedic surgeon. He was on the staff at the *Royal North Shore Hospital* during 1921–38, where he founded (and resigned from) the orthopaedic department. He developed open reduction and

---

*To see a patient who has been so operated walking and going home a few days later is one of the great experiences of orthopaedic surgery.

Kirschner wiring for the edentulous mandible. Barty describes him as a lonely complex man, interested in aboriginal culture.

The first chair of orthopaedic surgery in Sydney University was based at the Royal North Shore in 1970 and held by **T K F Taylor**, a Sydney graduate of 1955, trained at the Wingfield-Morris Orthopaedic Hospital at Oxford under Trueta and later in Seattle.

At the *Sydney Hospital*, a department was formed in 1923 under C Nigel Smith, succeeded in 1932 by **John William van Rees Hoets** (1885–1961), who had initially been an anaesthetist and so acted for Royle's animal experiments. He assumed orthopaedic practice in 1920 and was eventually senior orthopaedic surgeon at the Lewisham and Sydney Hospitals with an extensive private practice. He was an early enthusiast for cup arthroplasty. The department expanded rapidly in 1958 when it moves out to the Prince of Wales Annexe. **Roy Vescys Graham** (1889–1948) was a general surgeon at the Sydney and Lewisham hospitals, but took up orthopaedics, practised with Royle and accompanied Hunter and Royle in 1924 on their US tour. He habitually removed the medial meniscus by turning up a flap of the tibial collateral ligament including the meniscus, refixing the ligament with a screw of bone, the patient walking next day. He was the first Australian orthopaedic surgeon to enlist in World War II and served throughout.

Thomas Barry McMurray (1917–1964), son of Liverpool's T P McMurray, had been a parachute medical officer in World War II, sustained a cervical fracture–dislocation treated by his father, emigrated first to Cape Town and then to Australia in 1961. In Sydney he became director of orthopaedic surgery at New South Wales University, based on the Prince Henry and Prince of Wales Hospitals but never felt at home in the country and died prematurely.

Ronald Lawrie Huckstep (b.1926), after service in Africa, was appointed professor of orthopaedic surgery at the University of Sydney in 1973 (he was originally a Londoner, graduating at the Middlesex Hospital there in 1952). His work in Kampala, Uganda, gave him enormous experience in poliomyelitis, osteomyelitis, tuberculosis and the relevant appliances. His *Poliomyelitis: A Guide for Developing Countries including Appliances and Rehabilitation* has been a bible for many working in the Third World.

In 1973 he founded World Orthopaedic Concern, which fosters such work. He is known for his interest in biomedical engineering and ingenious methods of fracture fixation, sometimes enabling salvage of the limb with high femoral metastases.

William Anderson Hugh Smith (1901–1981) was a Sydney graduate of 1933 whose life was interrupted by two world wars: in the first he served as a naval rating and in the second as a surgeon in New Guinea. Then, after the obligatory stay in Liverpool, he became senior orthopaedic surgeon at the Mater and St Vincent's Hospitals between 1951 and 1961, president of the AOA in 1964 and very influential in the Association. He personally endowed the first chair of orthopaedic surgery in Australia at the Royal North Shore Hospital in 1970 and a second chair at the University of New South Wales in 1972. He also established the Hugh Smith Orthopaedic Research Department in 1979.

Edmund Bruce Mortimer Vance (1885–1939), a charming diffident man, graduated at Sydney in 1911, served in World War I, and was the first Australian to take the MCh Orth course (and get it – Barry says that he was the *only* student at the first course in 1923). He was associated with Oswestry and became friendly with Robert Jones, who wanted him to stay on, but returned to Australia with Jones's recommendation as an orthopaedic surgeon, started a department at St George's Hospital in 1927 but soon resigned, and found his main hospital interest at the Royal South Sydney Hospital. His pervasive influence on the training of generations of young Australians has been indicated. He is not to be confused with his son, R A B ('Dick') Vance, first orthopaedic surgeon in Canberra.

Hugh Collis Barry (b.1912) moved from early medical studies in Sydney to a Rhodes Scholarship at Oxford, researched with Florey and completed the medical course at the London Hospital. After war service he specialized in orthopaedics and was appointed to the Royal Prince Alfred in 1947, becoming chief of orthopaedics from 1964 to 1970. He wrote a monograph on Paget's disease in 1969[13].

The New South Wales Society for Crippled Children originated in 1929 and developed the Margaret Reid Home at St Ives on Sydney's North Shore in 1937; this became an orthopaedic hospital on the pattern of the Robert Jones and Agnes Hunt Hospital at Oswestry in North Wales. Its original complement of patients suffered mainly from poliomyelitis, rickets, osteomyelitis, skeletal tuberculosis (now largely vanished), spina bifida and muscular dystrophy. There was education and vocational training; peripheral clinics were maintained. Though a good centre for training and paediatric surgery, the changing clinical pattern had greatly reduced the demand for longterm orthopaedic beds and liaison with other institutions was poor; it closed in 1981. The Spastic Centre of New South Wales, started in 1945, is now at three sub-centres: Mosman, Allambie Heights and Newcastle.

VICTORIA

Developments in this State were centred on Melbourne. In 1929, a 40 bed orthopaedic unit was attached to the Royal Children's Hospital at Frankston, by the sea, the first purely orthopaedic hospital in Australia. The first medical superintendent was **John Colquhoun**, who had arrived from Scotland via Oswestry and the Massachusetts General Hospital; nevertheless, the board would not agree a designated orthopaedic appointment. His successor in 1934 was a paediatrician, Douglas Galbraith (the hospital was closed in 1970 as longstay beds were no longer required). Colquhoun had had an honourable career in Britain. Born in 1899, he served as a soldier in World War I, graduated at Edinburgh in 1925, came to Australia in 1929 and commanded the First Australian Orthopaedic Unit in the Middle East in World War II. He was president of the AOA in 1958. It was sad that, even after some years as superintendent at Frankston, his elevation to Honorary Surgeon had to be in general surgery; he was not formally recognized as an orthopaedic surgeon until 1946, and that at the parent Royal Children's Hospital. Of his successors we mention only **Malcolm Menelaus** (b.1930), a Melbourne graduate of 1954, trained partly in England at Pyrford and the Birmingham Accident Hospital (evidently, the Liverpool influence was on the wane), who became chief of orthopaedic surgery at the Royal and gained a reputation in the surgery of spina bifida. He wrote, in 1971, *The Orthopaedic Management of Spina Bifida Cystica.*

In 1933, the Royal Melbourne Hospital set up an orthopaedic unit and appointed as its first director **Charles Littlejohn** (1889–1960). Littlejohn was a New Zealander by birth, educated in Melbourne and graduating at St Bartholomew's Hospital in London in 1914. He served and was decorated in both world wars (the reader will have observed by now just how cardinal such service was in the lives of Australians) and delayed his orthopaedic advancement by insisting on continuing with some general surgery. This kept him out of the AOA. In World War II he commanded the surgical division of the Australian General Hospital at the siege of Tobruk and invented the Tobruk splint, a combination of the Thomas splint with plaster-of-Paris which facilitated evacuation of soldiers with femoral fractures. Later, he became consultant orthopaedic surgeon to the Australian Army, and the only general surgeon to be elected an honorary member (but never a full member) of the AOA.

Bryan Tobyn Keon-Cohen (1903–1974), a Melbourne graduate of 1927, was to become a leading figure in both the AOA and the Royal Australasian College of Surgeons, an unusual pattern. Originally a resident to Sir Allan Newton at the Royal Melbourne Hospital, his chief advised him to take up orthopaedics and he went to England to obtain his surgical fellowship and to work under Harry Platt, McMurray and Naughton Dunn at Oswestry. He returned to Melbourne in 1938 as assistant to Littlejohn, served as an orthopaedic surgeon overseas in World War II, and then succeeded Littlejohn as chief of orthopaedic surgery at the Royal Melbourne in 1947, retiring in 1963. He was well-known, thoughtful and well-spoken, and an international-ist, with links to bodies in Britain, Canada and the United States.

In 1934, St Vincent's Hospital in Melbourne appointed **Tom King** (1899–1973) to run a new orthopaedic clinic as the first purely orthopaedic surgeon in Victoria. Hugh Barry says, 'He received no help from his general surgical colleagues', i.e. here as elsewhere orthopaedic surgery developed in spite of and not because of general surgery. King had graduated at St Vincent's Clinical School in 1923, travelled widely, obtained his English surgical fellowship, and was greatly influenced by Böhler in Vienna. Though not himself greatly concerned with trauma, he was a pioneer of internal fixation of the fractured neck of femur; in 1934, independently of Sven Johannson (p. 327), he devised a centrally cannulated modification of the Smith–Petersen pin for closed insertion over a guide-wire under X-ray control[14], whereas its originator had been using an open operation. He also advocated compression as an aid to fracture union[15], devised a nail-plate for internal fixation after McMurray's osteotomy and excised the medial humeral epicondyle for ulnar neuritis, a useful procedure which has never gained popularity. Both his sons became surgeons.

Henry Vernon ('Harry') Crock succeeded King at St Vincent's in 1961.

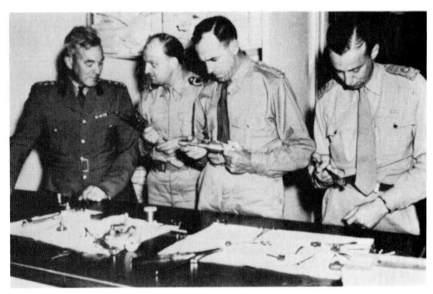

Figure 171   Colonel R I Harris, Lt-Commander John Jens, Major C Callow and Major B T Keon-Cohen

His training included a period with Trueta at Oxford. His main interest has been in spinal disorders and his injection studies of the spine are beautiful as well as informative[16] and gained him the Wood Jones medal when it was first created in Australia. He is a founder-member of the International Society for the Study of the Lumbar Spine.

QUEENSLAND

Various factors accelerated orthopaedic developments in Queensland. In 1935, the British Medical Association report on fractures stimulated the transfer of fracture managment at the Royal Brisbane Hospital from general surgeons to a special orthopaedic service. In 1937, in Queensland, honorary specialists were replaced by paid staff – totally unlike in the rest of Australia – and this was made the opportunity for the creation of an orthopaedic department. Simultaneously, hospital treatment for accident cases became free in the State; as general surgeons no longer had a financial interest, the orthopaedists were able to take over without rancour. Finally, Sister Kenny (see below) was given beds at the Brisbane Children's Hospital for exploitation of her ideas on the treatment of poliomyelitis and, though this gave rise to controversy, it also gave useful publicity to orthopaedics as a discipline.

Here, a pioneer was **Arthur Vincent Meehan** (1890–1955), a Sydney graduate of 1914 who served in France in World War I, suffered amputation of a foot and several reoperations. He worked at Alder Hey with Robert Jones. He was orthopaedic surgeon to Brisbane Children's Hospital from

1922 until 1928 and later ran a clinic at the Mater Children's Hospital in a fine combination with J R S Lahz (see below).

John Rudolph Sergius Lahz (1900–1959) suffered a severe fracture of the femur at the age of 15, operated in Sydney, which may, as so often, have influenced his choice of career. After graduation in Sydney in 1924 he joined Meehan in Brisbane. His own operation had been by plate fixation and left him with recurrent infection (26 operations in 20 years) and an inch of shortening.

George Alexander Clarence Douglas (1890–1966), a 1912 Edinburgh graduate, moved to Australia and was a Medical Officer there in World War I. After study in England, he became Senior Orthopaedic Surgeon at the Brisbane General Hospital and did the first open reductions and internal fixation of fractures there. He was a prime mover in founding the Montrose Home for Crippled Children.

L W Norman Gibson (1899–1937) was honorary orthopaedic surgeon at the Children's Hospital, where he had to deal with a large epidemic of poliomyelitis. He was largely responsible for the report of a royal commission on this disease, which, incidentally, found against Sister Kenny.

Harold Crawford (1894–1959) moved to orthopaedics from general surgery and became senior orthopaedic surgeon at the Children's hospital in 1938. In 1941 he had repeated clashes with Sister Kenny when she was given beds at the hospital.

Arthur Russell Murray (1910–1955) was a Tasmanian who had lost a leg in childhood, trained at Edinburgh and returned to take an interest in hand surgery in Brisbane, and in the training of social workers and occupational therapists.

It is no coincidence that both Meehan and Murray died in 1955, before their natural term. A migrant, Karl Kast, had been refused certification for incapacity due to backache by several orthopaedic surgeons, including Meehan, Lahz, Michael Gallagher and Andrew Murray, who said that he was exaggerating his symptoms. He decided to kill them all. Conveniently for him, they all practised in sets of rooms in downtown Brisbane, at Wickham House or Ballow Chambers nearby. On 1st December 1955 he visited these with a revolver and a suitcase of bombs. At Wickham House he severely wounded Gallagher, who later recovered. At Ballow Chambers he shot and killed Meehan and Murray. He then confronted Lahz, who managed to escape, but suffered a heart-attack a few hours later. Kast then blew up Lahz's office and shot himself.*

This may be a convenient place to write of **Sister Elizabeth Kenny** (1880–1952). An Australian Army nurse in World War I, though never properly trained, she opened a clinic for poliomyelitis in Townsville, Queensland in 1928. She abandoned splintage in favour of hot packs and early passive (and very painful) movements and was given hospital beds for this purpose. This

---

*This must be regarded as a little intemperate, much as one sympathizes with the 'Let's kill all the lawyers' attitude at times. We recall the assassination of Delpech (p. 244) and the attempt on Moll in South Africa (p. 362).

was based on a concept of 'spasm'[17], but in 1935 a royal commission found against her method. However, she found popular and medical support in the USA[18] and went to work there, though she died in Australia. It is now agreed that there was no scientific basis for her policies, and it is a fact that the type of early treatment has little or no effect on the extent of the residual paralysis[19]; nevertheless, her enthusiasm in rehabilitation was valuable.

Before immunization, poliomyelitis was much feared in Australia and it is interesting to compare Kenny with another remarkable woman, **Dame Jean MacNamara** (1899–1968), a Melbourne graduate of 1922 and a lifelong student of poliomyelitis and other viral disorders. Between 1933 and 1937 she engaged in the full-time treatment of poliomyelitis and spastic paralysis at the Royal Children's Hospital in Melbourne, was very conservative in management, and espoused treatment with convalescent serum – not now thought of any value – in a world tour. She was largely responsible for introducing myxomatosis for rabbit control.

Three other women doctors deserve mention. **E E ('Betty') McComas** (1906–1962) was the first resident surgeon in the orthopaedic division of the Melbourne Children's Hospital annexe at Frankston and in 1936 became the first woman to gain the MCh Orth at Liverpool. Much of her subsequent life was devoted to treatment of the after-effects of poliomyelitis. In 1937 she was appointed to the Queen Victoria Hospital for Women and Children and became a member at the first meeting of the AOA.

Claudia Burton-Bradley (1910–1967), a childhood diabetic and a Sydney graduate of 1943, was the first director of the New South Wales Spastic Centre from 1945 for 17 years.

A fifth woman, **Marion Radcliffe-Taylor** (b. 1894) was a New Zealand graduate of 1922 who took an Edinburgh surgical fellowship, was an intern at Oswestry, and returned to New Zealand as assistant to Renfrew White at Dunedin for two years. She then moved to Perth, where she became acting or assistant orthopaedic surgeon to the Children's and Perth Hospitals, doing early work on hip forage for arthrosis. She later gave up clinical practice in favour of administrative governmental duties.

SOUTH AUSTRALIA

This state was a late starter in orthopaedics.

Lionel Oxborrow Betts (1886–1943), born and brought up in the state and an Adelaide graduate of 1907, became the first purely orthopaedic surgeon there after a period as a general practitioner and invaliding in the first world war. In 1927 he was the second entrant for the MCh Orth diploma at Liverpool (Vance had been the first), won the Gold Medal and acted as locum for Robert Jones for some months. Back in Australia he became attached to the Adelaide Children's Hospital and was the second president of the AOA. He is known for his clarification of the cause of Morton's metatarsalgia[20] and for showing that incisions in the sole of the foot are benign. His son, William James Betts, followed him as president of the AOA in 1975.

Norman Stannus Gunning (1895–1964) was a colleague of Betts, took the Edinburgh surgical fellowship and the MCh Orth in 1933, and became orthopaedic surgeon to the Adelaide Children's Hospital and the Royal Adelaide Hospital. In 1942 he commanded a field ambulance in New Guinea. His career was marred by the usual troubles with general surgeons, who were appointed his nominal superiors even though he did the actual orthopaedic work.

Lansdale Bonnin (1918–1966) was an Adelaide graduate of 1941 who, typically, served in the second world war and then obtained his surgical fellowship and MCh Orth in England and worked for two years at Oswestry. He then became honorary orthopaedic surgeon to the Adelaide Children's Hospital and medical adviser to the Crippled Children's Association of South Australia. He died early, at 48, and was succeeded by **(Sir) Dennis Paterson** as director of orthopaedics at the hospital, knighted for his services in 1976.

John Russell Barbour (1910–1976), an Adelaide graduate of 1934, was a registrar at the London Hospital when the second world war began and served with the Australians in the Middle East and New Guinea. He then practised in Adelaide as an anatomist and orthopaedist and became senior orthopaedic surgeon to the Royal Adelaide Hospital in 1956. In 1962 he started a paraplegic unit but continued with some general surgery privately and so was never admitted to the AOA. This had its advantages; Barry tells us that on one occasion, faced with a patient with haematemesis in whom spinal deformity from ankylosing spondylitis made gastric surgery impossible, Barbour did a spinal osteotomy and a gastrectomy two weeks later with great success, and this while his chief, Alan Lendon, was convalescing from a laminectomy performed by Barbour, his junior! One feels one would have liked to meet Barbour.

WESTERN AUSTRALIA

In 1923 there were two orthopaedic clinics in Perth, one at the Children's Hospital (later the Princess Margaret Hospital for Children) and one at the Perth Hospital (later the Royal Perth). Both were run by **Alexander Juett** (1886–1953), born in Adelaide, educated in Perth, a 1905 Rhodes Scholar at Oxford and a graduate of London's Middlesex Hospital in 1913. He returned to Western Australia as a general practitioner, was gassed in World War I, worked with casualties in England and introduced orthopaedics in Perth afterwards. Juett did not travel or go to meetings. This was done by his partner, **Reginald McKeller-Hall**, a Melbourne graduate of 1922 who had higher surgical training in Britain and then teamed up with Juett at the hospitals mentioned above. He was honorary orthopaedic surgeon to the Children's Hospital for 27 years, from 1926 to 1953. Before following Juett in that position he took a year for postgraduate study in Liverpool and Leiden, with the Judets in Paris, with Putti and Galeazzi in Italy. In 1936, Hall became impressed with Sister Kenny and adopted her treatment in the severe poliomyelitis epidemic of 1948 in Western Australia. Other epidemics followed, in 1954 and 1956; these spurred physiotherapy and rehabilitation services in Western Australia, where Hall became medical adviser to the regional branch of the Crippled Children's Society, formed in 1935.

Perth has a special association with **Sir George Bedbrook** and spinal injuries. Bedbrook was a Melbourne graduate of 1944, who had postgraduate orthopaedic experience in England in 1950, especially at Stoke Mandeville. Back in Australia by 1953, he partnered McKellar-Hall after Juett's death. The Royal Perth Hospital established a paraplegia unit under his direction, now one of the best in the world. He became a national and international adviser on paraplegia and was knighted in 1978. He became deeply involved in the organization of rehabilitation for the handicapped nationally and in the Western Pacific and Indonesia, with an interest in the Paraplegic Games. He was also President of the AOA and helped promote a chair in orthopaedic surgery at the University of Western Australia. His interests were many, since he pursued the role of orthopaedics in mental retardation, genetic conditions, orthotics and prostheses and was involved in political negotiations to facilitate the rehabilitation of disabled workers. The new chair at Perth was filled by **Sydney M L Nade** (b.1939) from 1978. We may note that Allan Dwyer was senior lecturer in orthopaedic surgery in Perth from 1976 to 1980 before moving to Little Rock, Arkansas.

TASMANIA

Here, the prime mover was **Sir Douglas Parker** (b.1900), a Sydney graduate of 1923 who did some postgraduate study in Britain, obtained a surgical fellowship at Edinburgh and returned to Australia as a general practitioner. In 1928 he returned to England, took his MCh Orth and spent two years at Oswestry, where he was one of the last house surgeons to Robert Jones. In 1933 he moved to Hobart, first as a general practitioner, then as orthopaedic and general surgeon to the Royal Hobart Hospital. After war service he became director of orthopaedic services in Tasmania and organized a system on the Oswestry basis. He did much for orthopaedic training and was knighted in 1954.

REFERENCES

1. Barry, H. (1983). *Orthopaedics in Australia.* (Sydney, Australian Orthopaedic Association)
2. Burrows, H.J. (1980). Australian orthopaedics in the last 50 years. *J. Bone Jt. Surg.,* **32B**, 601
3. Russell, R.H. (1924). Fracture of the femur: a clinical study. *Brit. J. Surg.,* **11**, 491
4. Trumble, H.C. (1931). A method of fixation of the hip joint by means of an extra-articular bone graft. *Austral. N.Z.J. Surg.,* **1**, 413
5. Brittain, H.A. (1941). Ischiofemoral arthrodesis. *Brit. J. Surg.,* **29**, 93
6. Bosworth, D.M. (1942). Femoro-ischial transplantation. *J. Bone Jt. Surg.,* **24**, 38
7. Royle, N.D. (1924). Operation of sympathetic ramisection. *Med. J. Austral.,* **1**, 587
8. Royle, N.D. (1927). Treatment of spastic paralysis by sympathetic ramisection.

Proc. Roy. Soc. Med., **20**, 63

9. Royle, N.D. (1937). Surgical treatment of spastic paralysis. *Med. J. Austral.,* **24**, 979
10. Foerster, O. (1908). Über eine neue operative Methode der Behandlung spastische Lähmungen mittels Resektion hintere Rückenmarkswurzeln. *Z. f. Orth. Chir.,* **22**, 203
11. Royle, N.D. (1928). The operative removal of an accessory vertebra. *Med. J. Austral.,* **1**, 467
12. Dwyer, A.F., Newton, N.C. and Sherwood, A.A. (1969). An anterior approach to scoliosis. *Clin. Orthop.,* **62**, 192
13. Barry, H.C. (1969). Paget's Disease of Bone. (Edinburgh, Livingstone)
14. King, T. (1934). *Med. J. Austral.,* **1**, 5
15. King, T. (1957). Compression of bone ends as an aid to union in fractures. *J. Bone Jt. Surg.,* **39A**, 1238
16. Crock, H.V. and Yoshizawa, H. (1977). *The Blood Supply of the Vertebral Column and Spinal Cord in Man.* (New York, Springer)
17. Kenny, E. (1941). *The treatment of infantile paralysis in the acute stage.* (Minneapolis, Bruce Publications)
18. Pohl, J.F. and Kenny, E. (1943). *The Kenny concept of infantile paralysis and its treatment.* (St. Paul, Bruce Publications)
19. McCarroll, H.R. and Crego, C.H. (1941). An evaluation of physiotherapy in the early treatment of anterior poliomyelitis. *J. Bone Jt. Surg.,* **23**, 851
20. Betts, L.O. (1940). Morton's metatarsalgia: neuritis of the fourth digital nerve. *Med. J. Austral.,* **1**, 514

CHAPTER 12

National Histories – New Zealand

New Zealand is a country with a small population living under generally healthy conditions. The 85 per cent who are of Caucasian origin are mainly of British ancestry and their incidence of orthopaedic disease is virtually that in the UK. In the Polynesian 15 per cent, there is a very high incidence of certain orthopaedic conditions. Most postgraduate orthopaedic training has traditionally been in Britain, though there is evidence of recent change, and this was the last English-speaking country to establish a national orthopaedic association. Orthopaedic surgery was not practised as such before the end of World War I.

Well-known surgical emigrés of the past have included the famous plastic surgeons, Sir Harold Gillies, Sir Archibald McIndoe and Rainsford Mowlem. Their work necessarily overlapped on orthopaedics at many points, and Mowlem is of some particular interest because of his work on cancellous grafting as part of plastic reconstruction in World War II. More recently, JS Batchelor of Guy's Hospital in London and Karl Nissen of the Royal National Orthopaedic Hospital who were both born in New Zealand had their entire training and careers in England. W Bremner Highet, a brilliant young man who worked on peripheral nerve injuries at the Wingfield-Morris Orthopaedic Hospital at Oxford in the second world war, was drowned at sea in that conflict. The late Murray Falconer, who joined the staffs at the Maudsley and Guy's Hospitals in London, was entirely a neurosurgeon, but his interest in the neurologic problems of cervical spondylosis inevitably led to collaboration with his orthopaedic colleagues. During World War I, a number of New Zealand army surgeons were trained in orthopaedics in the British forcing-houses directed by Robert Jones at Shepherd's Bush in London, Alder Hey at Liverpool, and Oswestry in North Wales. In England, Colonel D S Wylie became head of the first New Zealand Army Orthopaedic Unit at No 1 N.Z. General Hospital at Brockenhurst and Colonel Mill was similarly situated at the No 2 Hospital at Walton-on-Thames. Others were Renfrew White, Wallis, Mill, Ulrich and Gower. All returned home in 1918.

Provision was then necessary for the treatment of returned servicemen. Wylie established a department at Christchurch Hospital in late 1918 and Mill became established at the new King George V Hospital at Rotorua (subsequently known as the Queen Elizabeth) and in the Military Annexe at the Auckland Civil Hospital. Renfrew White was at the Dunedin and Ulrich at Timaru. In 1920, W S Wallis became superintendent and orthopaedic surgeon at King George V and initiated a general trend by turning it into a centre for civilian orthopaedic surgery and a general hospital.

James Renfrew White (1888–1961) is usually considered the doyen of orthopaedic surgery in New Zealand. An Otago graduate of 1912, he returned home after war service and orthopaedic training in England (at the Royal National Orthopaedic Hospital and elsewhere) and in 1920 became clinical instructor in orthopaedics at the Otago Medical School and surgeon-in-charge of the first department of orthopaedic and traumatic surgery at the Dunedin Public Hospital. As we have so often noted in other contexts, this was combined for a time with general surgical duties, that is, he was officially considered a general surgeon with orthopaedic interests, but he eventually devoted himself entirely to orthopaedics, became senior surgeon to the orthopaedic department in 1936, handed over his fracture work to others, spent a year in the USA where he became FACS, and retired in 1949. He had a great influence on generations of students, wrote *Orthopaedic Physical Signs and Bandaging*, set up a system of peripheral clinics, was Director of the New Zealand School of Physiotherapy and a Founding Fellow of the Royal Australasian College of Surgeons. He has been described as a genius with a touch of eccentricity: scholarly, erudite and musical.

Between the World Wars, **Alexander Gillies**, trained in England, worked in Wellington from 1929, was a major influence in developing the New Zealand Crippled Children's Society and organized mobile preventive ortho-paedic clinics for children. The Society was formed in 1935 with the aid of private charity and the Nuffield Fund and became a national organization collaborating with the Department of Health. Other figures of the inter-war period included Keith Stuart Mackie, who trained in England after the first world war and arrived in Auckland in 1921, Cuthbert McCaw with a similar history (both were native New Zealanders) who joined Mackie in 1926, Morris Axford who succeeded after Mackie's death in 1936, Selwyn Morris who joined the Auckland staff in 1936 as the first purely orthopaedic surgeon, Allan McDonald, also in Auckland, and Walter Robertson in Wellington.

In World War II there were three New Zealand military hospitals in the Middle East, each headed by an orthopaedic surgeon from civil life, and there was a corresponding expansion in orthopaedic services at home, especially stimulated by exposure to American field hospitals in the country at that time. Later, the treatment of returned servicemen led to developments in rehabilitation, physiotherapy, occupational therapy and vocational train-ing for civilian patients, and by 1950 there were orthopaedic departments in many small towns as well as the great cities. The Auckland General Hospital had three senior and three assistant orthopaedic surgeons. Many young graduates trained in the United Kingdom.

Earlier, professional standards had been related to the Royal Australasian

College of Surgeons and to local hospital requirements, usually in a context of general surgery and bearing in mind that poliomyelitis and osteomyelitis were considerable problems in the first half of the century. Now there was to be a change. 1948 saw the appearance of the British Volume of the *Journal of Bone and Joint Surgery* and this, as in the case of South Africa, implied the desirability of a national orthopaedic association for editorial parity.

It seems fair to say that the New Zealand Orthopaedic Association owed its origin to the patronage of Renfrew White and the driving force of Alexander Gillies. The two men discussed the possibilities in Dunedin in that year and, through the good offices of the New Zealand branch of the British Medical Association, a meeting was held at the Wellington Hospital on 17th February 1950; those present included Gillies, Jennings, Fitzgerald, Blunden, Elliott, Cunningham and Lennane. Despite the tendency of a minority to cling to the skirts of the Australasian College or the British Medical Association, it was decided to form an independent association based on the 16 surgeons then exclusively practising orthopaedics in New Zealand. The first President was Gillies, the first Secretary Kennedy Elliott and Renfrew White was Patron.

The first scientific meeting was in Christchurch in 1950 and meetings followed annually. The 1951 meeting was the visit of Sir Reginald Watson-Jones as Sims Travelling Commonwealth Professor. By 1980, the membership was over 100. The Association has proved a great success. It may have taken some courage and initiative to escape the embrace of the Australians, but New Zealanders have always been noted for these qualities!

George William Gower (1887–1974) was a link with the earliest days of orthopaedic surgery in New Zealand. In World War I, he was in a group of young medical officers selected for training under Robert Jones. In 1919 he moved to Christchurch Military Hospital, then became superintendent at Waikato Hospital, spent nine years in private orthopaedic practice in Hamilton, and was back with the New Zealand Medical Corps in the Middle East and Italy in World War II.

Walter Sneddon Robertson (1889–1968) founded the orthopaedic department at Wellington Hospital. Qualifying in Dunedin in 1912, he served as a medical officer in the first world war and in 1919 received postgraduate training in hydrotherapy and electrotherapeutics in England. Returning to New Zealand, he served at the Trentham Military Hospital for a short period before joining staff at the Wellington Hospital in 1922. The following year he took charge of the fractures and inaugurated the orthopaedic department. He became full-time orthopaedic surgeon to the hospital in 1939 and Director of Orthopaedic Services in 1947. In 1935 he had been appointed a consultant to the newly formed Crippled Children's Society. His services during the poliomyelitis epidemic of 1925 were particularly valuable.

Keith Stuart Mackie (1890–1936) served as a medical officer in World War I and had some postgraduate training under Robert Jones in Liverpool subsequently. In 1921 he was appointed to the Auckland Hospital in charge of the Physiotherapy Department, and this remained his nominal appointment even when he became the first orthopaedic surgeon at the Auckland Hospital and in the Auckland region. He had a short but brilliant career as an orthopaedic surgeon of the highest repute.

James Leslie Will (1894–1968), known as 'Snowy', was the first orthopaedic surgeon at the Christchurch Hospital. A medical student at the outbreak of World War I, he initially served in the ranks but was returned home to be pushed through the medical course and rejoin the Army as a medical officer. After the war he trained in Liverpool and Edinburgh before taking up his post at Christchurch. He had a particular interest in the Crippled Children's Society in the North Canterbury Region.

Morris Axford (1901–1968) was an Otago graduate of 1924, a postgraduate trainee in England, who became senior visiting orthopaedic surgeon to the Auckland Hospital, promoted the Crippled Children's Society, was an early President of the NZOA and retired in 1967.

Selwyn Bentham Morris (1905–1956) was the first orthopaedic surgeon to be trained as such and to devote his entire career wholly to the discipline. After training in London and Vienna, he returned to New Zealand and became an orthopaedic surgeon at the Auckland Hospital in 1936, where he worked until his death. Not only was he a brilliant surgeon and teacher, but his opinion was widely sought and he was a figure in local medical politics.

James Kennedy Elliott (1908–1968) was a Wellingtonian and Edinburgh graduate who eventually became senior orthopaedic surgeon at Wellington Hospital. He made a special study of rehabilitation and limb-fitting in Britain and the USA. In World War II he was surgeon-administrator of the New Zealand forces in the Middle East and Italy. He was a Founding Fellow of the NZOA and on the editorial board of the British volume of the *Journal of Bone and Joint Surgery*.

Richard Henry Dawson (1915–1967) was an Otago graduate of 1939 who served overseas in the war, acquired the MCh Orth diploma, and returned home in 1949 to introduce orthopaedic services into North Auckland. He built up a system of peripheral clinics and moved to Palmerston North in 1952 to do as much there. He was interested in problems of unequal leg-length and osteotomy for coxa vara, and died while in office as President of the Association.

John Bentham Morris (1933–1970) was the son of Selwyn B Morris. Graduating in Otago in 1956, he trained in England, was an Exchange Fellow under the ABC system in 1962 and became visiting orthopaedic surgeon at the Middlemore and Mater Misericordiae Hospitals, with an interest in hip surgery and spina bifida. His premature death was tragic.

Graeme Ballantyne Smaill (1928–1972), also short-lived, was a Dunedin graduate of 1954 who spent two years in England, mainly at Pyrford, became orthopaedic surgeon to the Wellington Hospital in 1963, and established a unit at the Hutt Hospital in 1967. He is known for his promotion of the early diagnosis of congenital dislocation of the hip.

CHAPTER 13

National Histories – South Africa

The first operation under ether in South Africa – an above-knee amputation – was done by a Dr William Atherstone at Grahamstown on 16th June 1847. (Morton's first case in Boston had been done eight months earlier.)

The Boer War of 1899–1902 saw the first use of X-rays on the battlefield, though Roentgen's discovery was as recent as 1895; the British sent out two machines to the Pietermaritzburg Military Hospital which revealed bullets and other metal in wounds. Both sides were served by volunteers in Red Cross units and field ambulances. Serving on the British side was C T Möller senior, a South African who had been studying at Edinburgh and who was to become Superintendent of the General Hospital at Germiston, where he later gave the young Fouché (see below) the beds and facilities denied him by the Johannesburg General Hospital. On the Boer side was a German, Dr E S Sthamer (1873–1957), a general practitioner who had been trained in orthopaedics by Sauerbruch in Berlin, and who stayed on after the war to become the first orthopaedist in the Transvaal before Fouché's start in Johannesburg in 1925. He worked in Pretoria from 1915 as a general surgeon with orthopaedic interests, and then as a purely orthopaedic surgeon at the General Hospital from 1930 to 1943.

As it happens, South Africa's first orthopaedic surgeon was also a German, **Dr Ernst Simon** (1868–1943), who arrived in 1898, having been persuaded to emigrate to the Cape by Albert Hoffa, himself South African born but later professor of orthopaedic surgery at Würzburg and Berlin (p. 192). Simon practised in a private nursing home and was interested in the correction of club-feet. He had to return to Germany in 1914, but resumed practice at the Cape after the war. He retired to Munich in 1931 but finally returned to South Africa in 1938.

To retain the German connection for a moment, **Pieter de Villiers Moll** (1889–1934), though South African born, went to Heidelberg to study under Oscar Vulpius from 1909 to 1914. His stay was prolonged by the war, but he began practice in 1919 and in 1927 became the first ever orthopaedic surgeon at a public hospital as a staff member at the New Somerset Hospital; but he had no beds until 1937, and then only two, a common experience for orthopaedic surgeons everywhere at that period (see under Mather Cleveland, p. 441, and Blundell Bankart, p. 155). He was not appointed a lecturer until 1931. He organized crippled child care for all races and is commemorated in the Pieter Moll and Nuffield Chair of Orthopaedic Surgery at Cape Town University. As has happened with other orthopaedic surgeons (see pp. 244 and 352), a patient dissatisfied with a compensation report tried to shoot him, but Moll overcame him. He ensured his succession by Peter Roux in 1932. Roux (1900–1942) therefore followed Moll at the Somerset Hospital and as Head of Orthopaedics at Cape Town in 1934.

Other forerunners included **Professor Charles M Saint** (1888–1973), who became head of the department of surgery at Cape Town University in 1919, a brilliant surgeon and teacher, author of a famous *Manual* with Rutherford Morison.

In 1925, **F P Fouché** (1886–1962) began specialist practice in Johannesburg and in 1927 was appointed to the General Hospital there, as 'assistant surgeon in charge of orthopaedic cases', later as Honorary Orthopaedic Surgeon as such, and in 1935 as head of the department. (Other prominent staff members later included Sidney Sacks, G T Du Toit and W T Ross.) Fouché created the first orthopaedic unit in the Transvaal at Germiston General Hospital. Fouché's history is interesting, and not untypical. A 'stormy, restless character', he had been born in the Karoo and graduated at Edinburgh as there was then no medical school in South Africa. He returned to work as a general practitioner in the Orange Free State, took his MD at Edinburgh in 1921, decided to take up orthopaedic surgery and worked under Trethowan (p. 150) at Guy's Hospital in London for several years. He also assisted Lambrinudi and coinvented (some say he was the prime mover) the latter's famous eponymous operation for drop-foot. In 1925 he was back in the Transvaal as the first orthopaedic surgeon in Johannesburg and became orthopaedic surgeon and lecturer at the General Hospital until retirement in 1946. It was because the general surgeons were hostile to change that his first appointment was as a general surgeon, albeit in charge of orthopaedic cases; only in 1935 was a specialized department recognized at the General and Children's Hospitals.

We should refer to a rather extraordinary 'orthopaedic physician', **Dr Emilia Krause** (1891–1972), who set up a free service for crippled children at Bloemfontein, Fouché operated on her patients in Johannesburg and returned them to her for aftercare.

Even by 1937, there were only seven orthopaedic surgeons in the entire country, and recognition of orthopaedics as a speciality was very grudging. 'It took many years to break down the resistance of general surgeons, who at one time [the 1920s] included orthopaedic work in their activities,' writes Edelstein.

The early surgeons, once they began to treat non-whites, found themselves faced with immense problems of skeletal tuberculosis, osteomyelitis, poliomyelitis and rickets. All were influenced, in whole or part, by British clinical methods and by British administrative and charitable policies. Thus, the

Education Act of 1917 made education and treatment compulsory for children with long-term illness. Various schemes developed. The Lady Michaelis Orthopaedic Home opened at Plumstead in 1926, with Moll as honorary surgeon, for children of all races, and became a training centre for Stellenbosch University. The Princess Alice Home of Recovery at Retreat, the Cape, opened in 1932 and became the Princess Alice Orthopaedic Hospital and a training centre for Cape Town University. There were the Maitland Cottage Homes founded by the Invalid Children's Aid Fund at the Cape in 1930; in 1946, A J Helfet became their visiting orthopaedic surgeon and in 1952 they became a formal long-stay orthopaedic hospital. Groote Schuur Hospital opened in Cape Town in 1938, but had no initial provision for orthopaedic surgery, which developed there only against the usual difficulties.

In Johannesburg, the Hope Convalescent Home, started in 1915, provided vocational training and became the Hope Training Home for Crippled Children in 1936. Also, in and around Johannesburg, services were provided by the mining industry, such as the Chamber of Mines Hospital at Cottesloe in 1939, the first purely accident hospital in southern Africa and probably in the southern hemisphere.

In Pretoria, orthopaedics was recognized by the Faculty of Medicine in 1943, but as a subdivision of general surgery, with Johann Du Toit in charge from 1945. An orthopaedic hospital was opened in 1947 with the aid of the Nuffield Trust. Other centres for treatment and care of cripples were at East London, Durban and Cape Province. Before World War II there were four main long-stay centres for children with orthopaedic disease; at Cape Town, Johannesburg, East London and Bloemfontein. Durban was less developed. Each area has its Society in Aid of the Crippled Child, which together merged as the National Council for the Care of Cripples in South Africa in 1939.

A tremendous impetus to orthopaedic developments in South Africa was provided by the Nuffield Fund in 1937. Lord Nuffield, the British millionaire motor car manufacturer (then Sir William Morris) was influenced by G R Girdlestone, who was named as one of the Trustees, the two having worked together in the same roles of benefactor and adviser at Oxford. Nuffield had already made great contributions in Britain, Australia and New Zealand and was later to aid many other states of the British Commonwealth. Also, a South African surgeon, Richard Hartley Rose-Innes, had been an intimate friend of Morris while at Oxford, Girdlestone went out to South Africa in 1937 for a month to plan the service. (G T Du Toit, then working in Johannesburg, had been his house-surgeon at Oxford.) The essence of his plans for early detection, efficient treatment and aftercare, was based on a central hospital with peripheral clinics, as at Oswestry and Oxford. Nuffield gave £100 000, which provided funds for many facets of the work; lectureships at Cape Town and Johannesburg, postgraduate training, the subsidy of orthopaedic surgeons to settle in the smaller towns and rural areas, the training orthopaedic technicians and nurses.

We must mention some more individuals.

Hamilton Bell (b.1906) was a Belfast man, an early holder of the Liverpool MCh Orth Diploma, who was persuaded by Roux to join him in Cape

Town. In 1935 he was appointed to the New Somerset Hospital and in 1938 Bell and Roux set up a fracture clinic in the basement of the then new Groote Schuur Hospital. (Bell had been advised by McMurray not to fight the general surgeons, simply to treat fractures better than they did; Roux had set up a clinic at Somerset in opposition to Saint and was soon treating all the fractures.) By 1942, Bell was Senior Surgeon and Lecturer at Groote Schuur, and in 1971 became Professor of Orthopaedic Surgery at the University of Stellenbosch until 1972, having been appointed senior orthopaedic surgeon at the new Stellenbosch University Medical School and Hospital in 1956.

Guillaume Tom Du Toit (b.1909), the first President of the South African Orthopaedic Association, was an original planner in implementing Girdlestone's draft scheme. After having worked in Johannesburg under Fouché, from 1965 to 1971 he was professor of orthopaedic surgery and head of department at Pretoria Medical School, and in 1972 became Honorary Professor at the University of the Witwatersrand.

It was probably Du Toit who was mainly responsible for initiating the Orthopaedic Surgeons' Group (at Girdlestone's instigation) at a meeting in Cape Town on 17th September 1942. The founder members (who were all the orthopaedic surgeons in the country) were Fouché, Du Toit, Hamilton Bell, J M Edelstein, C T Möller, A D Polonsky, J Oberzimmer, A LewerAllen and, as an Honorary Member who happened to be serving in the British Royal Army Medical Corps in the area at the time, Arthur EyreBrook of Bristol (p. 168). There had been a preliminary meeting in July in Johannesburg, convened by Du Toit with only five of these present. The Group had to fight 'the battle of the fractures' against the general surgeons and to lay their claim to the management of all locomotor disorders, not just backache and painful feet. Most national orthopaedic associations seem to have begun in this semi-conspiratorial manner, blended with adventure: we think of Shaffer and the New York meeting that founded the American Orthopaedic Association in 1887, and the dinner at the Café Royal in London in 1917 that led to the British counterpart. The problems and pains of such new directions are not birth-pangs, rather the storms of adolescent separation from an over-clinging parent.

The original Orthopaedic Surgeons' Group was in essence a Transvaal group and an affiliate of the South African Medical Association. The formation of a truly national South African Orthopaedic Association was due to a suggestion by Sir Reginald Watson-Jones, to put it on a par with the Associations of America, Britain, Canada, Australia and New Zealand around the time of the establishment of the British Volume of the *Journal of Bone and Joint Surgery*, so as to allow representation on the editorial board.

The second President of the SAOA was **Joseph Melvin Edelstein** (1896–1966), who went to graduate at Edinburgh and returned to Britain in 1931 to obtain the FRCSE and MCh Orth qualifications in 1933. He started practice in Johannesburg in 1934 and succeeded Fouché in 1947 as Honorary Orthopaedic Surgeon at the General Hospital. He became Lecturer at the Witwatersrand and assumed the newly created Chair of Orthopaedic Surgery there in 1962.

The rather short stay of Thomas Barry McMurray (1917–1964) in Cape Town, short but intense and fruitful, before his further migration to Australia is set out at p. 348.

Carl Theodorus Möller (b.1911) began his career in Johannesburg under the aegis of Fouché, just as Fouché has been aided in his own early days by Möller's father. One of the founding 'Group of Five', he became the third President of the SAOA.

Johann G Du Toit (b.1918), a Cape Town graduate of 1940, trained under Hamilton Bell and Pieter Roux and was chief of orthopaedic surgery at Pretoria University and the Verwoerd Hospital from 1945 to 1964.

Two eminent South African orthopaedic surgeons later emigrated to New York. These were **Sidney Sacks**, senior surgeon at the Johannesburg General and Witwatersrand University between 1947 and 1978, and **Arthur Jacob Helfet**, (b.1907) a Liverpool graduate who became an orthopaedic surgeon in Cape Town after World War II and senior orthopaedic surgeon at Groote Schuur and the fourth President of the Association.

George Dall, a Cape Town graduate of 1944, became professor there in 1976. Martin Singer, a fellow-graduate of that year, became surgeon in charge of hand surgery at Groote Schuur in 1966.

Louis Solomon (b.1928) became professor of orthopaedic surgery and head of the clinical department at Johannesburg in 1967, and soon proved himself a brilliant researcher and team-leader – notable, among many other things, for his studies of primary necrosis of the femoral head in Africans. He is currently (1990) professor at the University of Bristol in England.

There are, at the time of writing, chairs of orthopaedic surgery at Cape Town, Witwatersrand (Johannesburg), Pretoria, Stellenbosch, Natal (Durban), the Orange Free State and the Medical University of Southern Africa (MEDUNSA).

There are many other excellent orthopaedic surgeons working in South Africa whom we cannot mention because their story is too recent, or without making a rather dry and uninformative catalogue. Details of these are available from the invaluable record by G F Dommisse, *To Benefit the Maimed*, published by the South African Orthopaedic Association in 1982 to coincide with the Combined Meeting of the Orthopaedic Associations of the English-speaking World at Cape Town in that year. Virtually all the material in this section has been gathered from this work.

It is satisfactory to reflect that the relations of South African orthopaedic surgeons with their colleagues round the world have not been affected by the prejudices that have bedevilled cooperation in other disciplines. South African orthopaedics is second to none in quality and South African orthopaedic hospitality is outstanding.

CHAPTER 14

National Histories – Canada

Here, orthopaedic development was conditioned by the vastness of the country, historic affiliations to England on the one hand and France on the other, and proximity to and resultant interchange with the USA. As in other young countries, cases now regarded as exclusively orthopaedic were treated by general surgeons, and, when orthopaedics did develop, it was often as a part of paediatrics. World War I gave the greatest stimulus to establishing orthopaedic surgery as a speciality in Canada. There were no organized services in Toronto before 1925.

ONTARIO

In Toronto, orthopaedic surgery originated in a concern for congenital deformities and deforming childhood diseases at the Hospital for Sick Children under **Clarence Leslie Starr** (1867–1920). The greatest problem was skeletal tuberculosis, and Starr was worried about the management of cold abscesses and the prevention of secondary infection, always a nuisance, often a disaster. He was also interested in pyogenic osteomyelitis, stressing the importance of early drainage by incising the periosteum and drilling the cortex, provided this did not increase necrosis[1]. Starr led the Canadian orthopaedic services overseas in the first world war.

W E Gallie (1882–1959) was a man of many parts, with a particular interest in the transplantation of bone, fascia and other materials. His needle for the fascial repair of hernia is universally known. Stimulated by Albee's work, he studied the process of bone repair and thought he had confirmed Macewen's view of the cardinal role of the osteoblast, though he could not repeat the filling of defects with autogenous bone chips, which he thought were not viable and served only as scaffolding for repair and replacement by invasion from the living bone of the host. His work, often with D E Robertson[2-4], formed the basis of teaching regarding the principles of bone

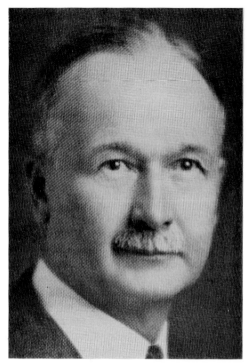

Figure 172   Clarence Leslie Starr (1867–1920)

surgery in the Toronto school and led directly to later work in 1945–6 at the Combined Services Orthopaedic Unit on cancellous grafts for infected bone defects relevant to war injuries[5]. In 1916, he was much engaged with tenodesis procedures to correct deformities in poliomyelitis, especially for calcaneus, but these did not meet with lasting success over the years[6].

Gallie was always interested in the use of autogenous deep fascia as a 'living suture'[7], an interest deriving directly from the work of Lexer in Germany (p. 200). With Le Mesurier[8], he performed animal experiments and used fascial strips to treat ligamentous injuries, mainly cruciate, at the knee[9], ununited fractures of the patella[10], recurrent dislocation of the patella[11] and shoulder[12]. He developed skeletal traction, employing ice-tongs, wiring and grafting for cervical fracture-dislocations[13,14]. He studied stabilization of the paralytic foot and designed a fusion of the subtalar joint by means of a bone graft inserted through a posterior approach and also applied this to fractures of the os calcis[15]. He used a diamond inlay graft for ununited fractures. In 1941, having studied 2500 World War I amputees over 20 years, he advised the Syme amputation whenever low ablation was possible[16], but it was Starr in 1915 who had made this study possible by advising the government on its own artificial limb factory, and the importance of following up amputees. This led to R I Harris, also of Toronto, stating in 1944, when he was Director-General of Canadian Army Medical Services; 'This is the most useful of all amputations of the lower extremity because of the perfection of its weight-bearing properties[17],' a view that influenced policy in the United States. Gallie also favoured the end-bearing Gritti–Stokes procedure for amputations around the knee.

Robert Inkerman Harris (1885–1966), a Torontoan from birth to death, is regarded as the great pioneer of orthopaedic surgery in Canada. He was a very great man, a man of presence, with a wide influence on younger men in Canada, the USA and Australia. Initially appointed as a general surgeon to the Toronto General Hospital in 1930, he became head of the new orthopaedic division in 1940 and was a founder-member of the Canadian Orthopaedic Association. If one were to seek to compare him with any colleague in terms of eminence and respect, it must be with Philip Wilson in New York. His early clinical problems were with skeletal tuberculosis and poliomyelitis. The visit of Royle and Hunter to North America in 1925 to advocate sympathectomy for spastic paralysis, though it proved fallacious, led Harris to study sympathectomy for short legs in poliomyelitis, and he found that it lessened the shortening[18]. He had a special interest in spondylolisthesis. Under him, the orthopaedic service of the hospital, which included Dewar and McIntosh, formed a travelling team visiting clinics throughout Ontario up to a distance of 500 miles in association with the Ontario Society for Crippled Children, patients being brought in to the centre for treatment as required[19].

Harris was orthopaedic consultant to the Canadian army in the Second World War and subsequently helped organize the ABC Exchange Travelling

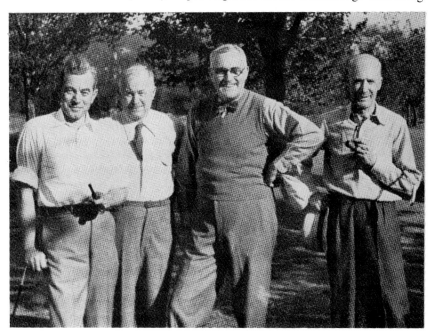

Figure 173　R I Harris, D E Robertson, W E Gallie and A B Le Mesurier

Fellowships of young orthopaedic surgeons between America, Britain and Canada which began in 1948. He was succeeded as chief of service by **Frederick P Dewar**, professor of orthopaedic surgery at Toronto University. Another Toronto figure was **George Frederik Pennal** (1913–1976), trained in the Liverpool school, who became chief surgeon at St Joseph's Hospital, associate professor and responsible for training programmes.

In western Ontario, periodic visits to orthopaedic patients in the early days were made by B E MacKenzie, a general surgeon with orthopaedic interests, and his pupil, Stewart Wright, of the Western Hospital, Toronto. **Hadley Williams** (1864–1932), graduate of the University of Western Ontario in 1888, trained in England and was professor of surgery at his university from 1909 to his death. All three of these remained general surgeons.

Sir Frederick Banting (1891–1941) is usually known only for his work on insulin, but he was in fact the first surgeon in Western Ontario to devote himself exclusively to orthopaedics. He came to London, Ontario from the Hospital for Sick Children in Toronto in 1920, but did not settle and after a year his physiological interests took him back to Toronto.

1922 saw the opening of the War Memorial Children's Hospital at London, promoted by **George Ramsay**, who had trained in surgery in Chicago before World War I and with Robert Jones in Liverpool afterwards. Ramsay became increasingly interested in orthopaedics and helped develop the

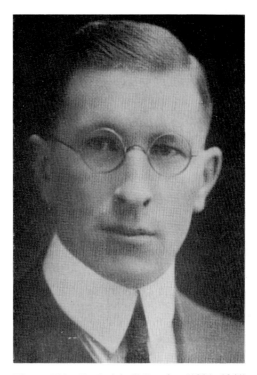

Figure 174   Frederick G Banting (1891–1941)

Western Ontario section of the Society for Crippled Children, centred on London but with outlying clinics.

MONTREAL

Here, the 'father' of orthopaedic surgery was **W G Turner**, a McGill graduate of 1900 who was appointed in charge of orthopaedics *within* the department of general surgery and became clinical professor of orthopaedic surgery at McGill University and head of the local Shriners' Hospital. **Archibald Mackenzie Forbes** (1874–1929) did orthopaedic work at the Montreal General Hospital, helped found the Children's Memorial Hospital and was sometime president of the Canadian Orthopaedic Association. He was succeeded at the General Hospital by Norman T Williamson (1893–1947) who died prematurely.

Around 1934 there developed an informal group of some ten men, engaged exclusively in orthopaedic practice, for informal discussions; with added members from Quebec and Ottawa, these formed the Montreal Orthopaedic Association. This was, of course, bilingual in French and English and one of this group, **J Édouard Samson**, who was a graduate of Laval University in Quebec and had moved to Montreal in 1930, studied with Hibbs and Albee in New York and with Nové-Josserand in Lyons (p. 262). Samson is well known for his fascial interposition arthroplasty of the knee. Samson suggested the formation of a Canadian Orthopaedic Association, which came into being in 1945. At about this time, when the Royal College of Physicians

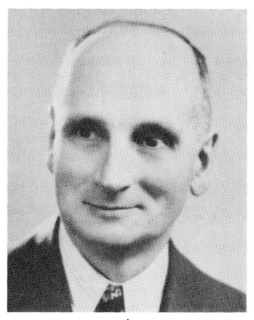

Figure 175 J Édouard Samson

and Surgeons of Canada began to certify specialists, the number of orthopaedic surgeons was just under 50.

WESTERN CANADA

In Western Canada, the pioneer was **H P H Galloway** (1886–1939). He
came from Toronto to Winnipeg in 1905 and began lecturing and practising
in orthopaedic surgery at Winnipeg General Hospital in 1907. He was
president of the American Orthopaedic Association in 1919. In 1939 a
fracture service was developed at the General Hospital modelled on Platt's
service in Manchester, England. After this, orthopaedists multiplied in
Western Canada and acquired closer relations with colleagues in the US
than with those of eastern Canada.

BRITISH COLUMBIA

Here, the initial pattern of linked general and orthopaedic surgery was
perpetuated by **Peter A McLennan**, a McGill graduate of 1898 who moved
to Vancouver in 1905. The first chief of surgery at the Vancouver General
Hospital from 1930, he developed a fracture service there. **Frank Patterson**
(1876–1938) a McGill graduate of the same vintage, was the first purely
orthopaedic surgeon in British Columbia. Initially a general practitioner
who acquired an Edinburgh surgical fellowship in 1900, he worked with
Starr in Toronto after World War I and went to Vancouver in 1919 as an
orthopaedic surgeon. He was the first chief of orthopaedic surgery at the
Vancouver General and St Paul's Hospitals.

EASTERN CANADA

In the Maritime Provinces and Newfoundland, all orthopaedic developments
were after World War I, a few Canadian Army surgeons having been
provided by Robert Jones with orthopaedic training in England before
returning home. **Tom B Acker**, a Dalhousie graduate, worked in MacAusland's clinic in Boston in 1921 and with Whitman and Hibbs in New York,
and began exclusive orthopaedic practice in Halifax in 1923. In 1924,
Dalhousie University created the first orthopaedic clinic and the first
academic posts. At this time, Tom B Acker was appointed (as an associate)
at the Halifax Children's Hospital and, unusually for the period, allotted a
dozen orthopaedic beds. His brother, John Acker, also trained with MacAusland and the two brothers worked with the Canadian Red Cross to construct
a system of peripheral clinics with most of the treatment centred on Halifax.
In the new Victoria General Hospital in Halifax in 1949, the orthopaedic
service was run by the Ackers with B F Miller, who had recently acquired
the MCh Orth, thus expanding the teaching facilities in the subject at
Dalhousie. From as early as 1923, Tom Acker had made regular but

infrequent visits to St John's, Newfoundland. In 1937 a junior surgeon at St John's, Louis Conroy, decided to train in orthopaedic surgery at Steindler's clinic in Iowa and with Willis Campbell in Tennessee and returned to apply his experience at the St John's General Hospital. Others, like E W Ewart, followed this example.

ALBERTA

We must recall that there were no Alberta medical graduates before 1925. Before World War I, orthopaedics were carried out by general surgeons. In 1913 a McGill graduate of 1881, **F H Mewburn**, moved to Calgary as a surgeon and in the first world war was chief of surgery at the Canadian Hospital, Taplow, England. (This survived to become a famous centre for, among other subjects, the management of severe rheumatoid disease in children.) Mewburn became professor of surgery in Calgary and encouraged an integral orthopaedic department with its own head. The first purely orthopaedic surgeons were **Reginald Deane**, who had worked with Mewburn prewar and studied orthopaedics in England later, and Mewburn's son, **F H H Mewburn** (1888–1954). The latter studied in Boston and eventually became clinical professor of orthopaedics at the University of Alberta in 1931. The Alberta Orthopaedic Association was formed in 1948.

We have briefly referred to the founding of the Canadian Orthopaedic Association in 1945. The initiative came from the Montreal Orthopaedic Society in 1943, from its then President, J Edouard Samson and from J Appleton Nutter, who had founded the Society in 1934[20]. These two coopted Andrew P MacKinnon of Winnipeg and R I Harris and a founding committee was formed consisting of all the past presidents of the Montreal Society. Nutter became the first president of the new Association, the vice presidents were Harris, MacKinnon and Samson and the secretary was J Calixte Favreau. The first annual meeting, in Montreal on 11–12th June 1945, was under the aegis of the Canadian Medical Association. The two bodies soon separated but for a time the orthopaedic gatherings continued to be held in Montreal, just before or after the annual meetings of the CMA. Later, there were changes of venue. The initial membership in 1945 was 25; by 1968 it had risen to 300. The second combined meeting of the American and British Orthopaedic Associations (the first had been in 1929) took place in Quebec in 1948 with the Canadian body as a joint participant, and the success of this meeting led to the ABC Exchange Programme of young Fellows of the three countries that has continued since. These combined meetings of the orthopaedic associations of the English-speaking world, which came to include the other members of the British Commonwealth, have since been repeated every few years at different places: London 1952, Washington 1958, Vancouver 1964, Sydney 1970 and Cape Town 1982.

REFERENCES

1. Starr, C.L. (1922). Acute haematogenous osteomyelitis. *Arch. Surg.*, **4**, 567
2. Gallie, W.E. and Robertson, D.E. (1918). Transplantation of bone. *J. Am. Med. Assn.*, **70**, 1134

3. Gallie, W.E. and Robertson, D.E. (1920). The repair of bone. *Brit. J. Surg.*, **7**, 211

4. Gallie, W.E. (1931). The transplantation of bone. *Brit. Med. J.*, **2**, 840

5. Coleman, H.M. *et al.* (1946). Cancellous bone grafts for infected bone defects. *Surg. Gyn. Obst.*, **83**, 392

6. Gallie, W.E. (1916). Tendon fixation in infantile paralysis – a review of 150 operations. *Am. J. Orthop. Surg.*, **14**, 18

7. Gallie, W.E. (1921). The use of living sutures in operative surgery. *Canad. Med. Assn. J.*, **11**, 504

8. Gallie, W.E. and Le Mesurier, A.B. (1922). A clinical and experimental study of the free transplantation of fascia and tendon. *J. Bone Jt. Surg.*, **6**, 600

9. Gallie, W.E. and Le Mesurier, A.B. (1927). The repair of injuries to the posterior crucial ligaments of the knee joint. *Ann. Surg.*, **85**, 592

10. Gallie, W.E. and Le Mesurier, A.B. (1927). The late repair of fractures of the patella and of ruptures of the ligamentum patellae and quadriceps tendon. *J. Bone Jt. Surg.*, **9**, 47

11. Gallie, W.E. and Le Mesurier, A.B. (1924). Habitual dislocation of the patella. *J. Bone Jt. Surg.*, **6**, 575

12. Gallie, W.E. and Le Mesurier, A.B. (1927). An operation for the relief of recurring dislocation of the shoulder. *Trans. Am. Surg. Ass.*, **45**, 392

13. Gallie, W.E. (1936). Fractures and dislocations of the cervical spine. *Am. J. Surg.*, **46**, 495

14. Gallie, W.E. (1937). Skeletal traction in the treatment of fractures and dislocations of the cervical spine. *Ann. Surg.*, **106**, 770

15. Gallie, W.E. (1943). Subastragalar arthodesis in fractures of the os calcis. *J. Bone Jt. Surg.*, **25**, 731

16. Gallie, W.E. (1941). The experience of the Canadian Army and Pensions Board with amputations of the lower extremity. *Ann. Surg.*, **113**, 925

17. Harris, R.I. (1944). Amputations. *J. Bone Jt. Surg.*, **26**, 626

18. Harris, R.I. (1930). The effect of lumbar sympathectomy on the growth of legs shortened after anterior poliomyelitis. A preliminary report. *J. Bone Jt. Surg.*, **12**, 589

19. Harris, R.I. and Coulthard, H.S. (1942). Prognosis in bone and joint tuberculosis. *J. Bone Jt. Surg.*, **24**, 382

20. Hazlett, J.W.L. (1970). The Canadian Orthopaedic Association: A historical review. *Canad. J. Surg.*, **13**, 1

CHAPTER 15

National Histories –
The United States

If we spend what may seem an undue amount of time in detailing the development and achievements of orthopaedic surgery in the United States, this must be because the rate and pace of change in that country, the enormous investment of energy and money and plain humanity, the concentration on innovations in technique as well as on principles, the conviction that almost any problem ought to be capable of solution: all served to transform orthopaedics as it had developed in the Old World. This is not to say that present-day orthopaedics would have been better or worse if America had never been discovered; but it would certainly have been utterly different.

Is it unfair to add that the ideas came mainly from Europe and that the Americans applied them? Provided with a new concept, as so often in other medical fields – one thinks of antibiotics and joint replacement – the Americans developed it with the utmost energy and an almost Teutonic thoroughness and application (after all, over a million German immigrants passed through Ellis Island in the second half of the 19th century.) We also have the ability to survey the entirety of the development of orthopaedics in this new country, so difficult to do in the Old World. Also, as the American Surgical Society was not founded until 1880, and the American Orthopaedic Association was founded as soon after as 1887, orthopaedic surgery as a special discipline was less bound to general surgery by years of tradition and was freer to develop independently, a matter of competition rather than dominance.

At the time of the Revolution, most of the medical men were concentrated in the northern British colonies; and even at the end of colonial rule there were still only two medical colleges, that in Philadelphia, founded in 1765, and that in New York, founded in 1767. (The Harvard medical school was not founded as such until 1783.) Less than fifty medical degrees had been granted before the Revolution; apart from those immigrants already qualified, most doctors learned by apprenticeship or by training in Europe[1]. There, they enjoyed the equivalent of the 18th century Grand Tour; the great figures to be visited included Guérin, Bouvier and Dupuytren in France (some of the visitors were revolted by the way Dupuytren impatiently abused and even struck his patients), Stromeyer in Germany and Little in England.

This tradition was to last right through the 19th century and beyond; in its last quarter a number of Americans from the Atlantic seaboard, notably John Ridlon from New York, were much influenced by the practice of Hugh Owen Thomas in Liverpool. But the flow was quite rapidly to be reversed; for, despite this inevitably late start, as it were at second hand, the actual growth of orthopaedic surgery as an independent discipline proved faster in the USA than in Europe and subsequent generations no longer really needed to travel: so much so that the great Lorenz wrote: 'At that time (around 1883) orthopaedics, in Europe at least, still remained in its infancy, whereas in America it was zealously cultivated[2].' The orthopaedic association of the United States was formed well before that of any European state.

Even before the Revolution, there were plenty of wars – with the Indians, the French – to foster the growth of military surgery. In Philadelphia, in 1775, there was published the *Plain, Concise, Practical Remarks on the Treatment of Wounds and Fractures* by John Jones, professor of surgery at King's College, New York. Jones had studied under Hunter and had served as a surgeon in the French and Indian wars of 1753–63. This was the first American book on military surgery, the first surgical text of any kind, and one much relied on by the surgeons of the Continental Army; there were further editions in 1776 and 1795. It recommended dry lint for wounds, sticking-plaster and bandaging for incised wounds, suture of transverse wounds (that the gaping transverse wound must be sutured goes back to medieval times). Tendons were not to be sutured, but to be held in place by positioning. Balls and bullets were to be removed gently if not too deep, after enlarging the wound, followed by bleeding, purges, opium, bark (as a local astringent with the hope of 'laudable pus' by the fourth day. For severe compound fractures immediate amputation was best, and this was certainly the opinion of the French. Hatchet and club wounds were to be expected from the Indian allies of either side. John Ranby of that time advised, in words almost identical with those used by Paré two centuries earlier, 'to act in all respects as if you are entirely unaffected by their groans and complaints, but at the same time behave with such caution as not to proceed rashly or cruelly, and be particularly careful to avoid unnecessary pain.' In the war of 1812, Baron Percy for the French incised for bullet wounds, evacuated pus and removed deep-seated foreign bodies. A B Bouer, also French, wrote a book which appeared in translation in New York in 1815 as *A Treatise on Surgical Diseases*, and which states, 'When muscles are covered by aponeuroses they should be crossed by incision so as to prevent strangulation when the limb becomes swollen' – a fasciotomy which is the essence of *débridement* before that term became bastardized in modern times. In 1816 an American, John Mann, wrote *Medical Sketches of the Campaigns of 1812, 13, 14* (published at Dedham, Massachusetts), advising early amputation to make wound care easier and treatment more definitive. In Philadelphia, in

1835, W Gibson published *The Institutes and Practice of Surgery*, based on the Indian War of 1830, also advising the incision of skin and fascia to prevent swelling and gangrene.

Philip Syng Physick(1768–1837) of Philadelphia, 'the father of American surgery', was born in America as the son of an English immigrant and apprenticed to a Dr Kuhn, a pupil of Linnaeus. He travelled to London in 1788 and became a pupil of John Hunter in Leicester Fields and was Hunter's close assistant in animal experiments. He spent most of 1790 as house surgeon to Hunter at St George's Hospital but declined an invitation to remain in London and passed a year in Edinburgh, where he graduated, returning to Philadelphia in 1792 at the age of 24. In 1794 he joined the staff of the Pennsylvania Hospital and became professor of surgery at the University of Pennsylvania Medical School in 1805. In 1816, when professor of anatomy, he discovered the absorbability of ligatures made from animal tissues. He applied Hunter's principles of rest for joint disease and of stimulation (by seton) for ununited fractures and acquired some fame when, in January 1822, he successfully treated an ununited fracture of the humerus by the passage of a seton, the 'American' method, not subsequently always successful and sometimes complicated by infection. He also carried the lateral hip splint up to the axilla.

A later professor of surgery, at New York University Medical College, was **Valentine Mott** (1785–1865), a great ligator of the major arteries, including the innominate, perhaps because he had been influenced by spending six months as Astley Cooper's pupil at Guy's Hospital in London in 1807. Mott also performed what may have been the first total excision of the clavicle (for malignant disease) in 1828. He spent the decade of 1831–41 in Europe for health reasons and wrote about his travels on his return[3]. He

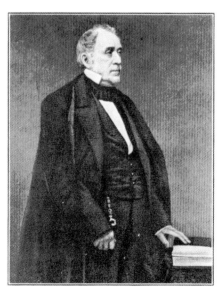

Figure 176   Valentine Mott (1785–1865)

visited Jules Guérin at his 'princely establishment' in Passy, in Paris, and was enthused by seeing Guérin do 50 tenotomies and myotomies on 43 muscles in a scoliotic patient at a single session. Mott found himself happy to have witnessed 'the dawning as well as the meridian splendour of...that beautiful and exact science limitedly denominated orthopaedic surgery' and seems, according to Valentin, to have been the first to use the conjoined term 'orthopaedic surgery' as such. Like many another returning enthusiast, he yearned to diffuse the principles learned in Europe throughout his native land. A site was selected, prospectuses printed, and influence solicited for the founding of an orthopaedic institute at Bloomingdale, New York, for the treatment of spinal curvature, club-foot and so on, but the doctors were against it, 'he yielded to medical ostracism, and the project died with him.' As we shall now see, Boston was to provide a more favourable climate for the new discipline. However, Mott had a *protégé*, James Knight, whom he did persuade to specialize in orthopaedics and who is discussed below.

American orthopaedics, as a separate speciality, began in Boston with **John Ball Brown** (1784–1862) and his son, **Buckminster Brown** (1819–1891), though it was a close-run thing for there were foreign immigrants on the same

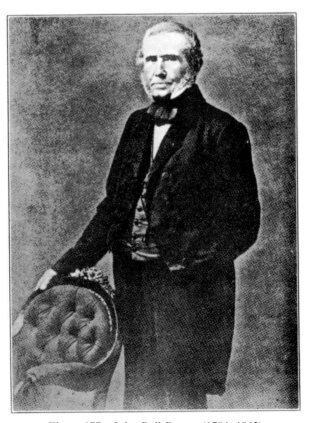

Figure 177   John Ball Brown (1784–1862)

path. John Ball Brown, son of a physician in Wilmington, Massachusetts, and a graduate at Brown University in 1806, moved to Boston in 1812 and five years later was appointed consultant surgeon to the Massachusetts General Hospital. It was not until 1837, at the age of 54, that he decided to restrict his practice to orthopaedics, because of a general concern for the hitherto largely neglected field of the crippled and deformed – it is noteworthy that in Europe the care of cripples as a social duty was a late and secondary adjunct to orthopaedics in historical perspective, whereas in America the two were more or less contemporaneous – and probably because of the havoc skeletal tuberculosis had wreaked in his own family. His son, Buckminster, had Pott's disease and was bedridden for eight years and had a permanent kyphoscoliosis; his elder brother had died from the disease in 1837. John Ball wrote, 'Having lost my eldest son by inflammation of the great spinal cord, and having my second son confined to his bed by a lateral curvature of the spine, my attention has been forcibly drawn to the study and treatment of spinal diseases generally and to the correction of other deformities of the human body[4].'

In 1838 John Ball, joined later by his son, opened what was originally called the 'Orthopedique Infirmary', two blocks from the Massachusetts General Hospital; later it was known as the Boston Orthopaedic Institution. In an early annual report from this centre he wrote, presciently:

> The practice of orthopaedy is a distinct branch of surgery...and should be practised exclusively. It certainly requires all of any one man's mind to treat these deformities judiciously. It would be better for the profession and for the public at large if the duties of the profession were more divided and subdivided...deformities of the human frame cannot be conveniently and judiciously treated except in a hospital or institution expressly devoted to this subject[5].

He therefore resisted the treatment of orthopaedic patients at the General Hospital but seems to have retained his popularity with his colleagues there. He claimed to have been the first to perform subcutaneous tenotomy of the Achilles tendon for club-foot in New England, on 21st February 1839, not long after Stromeyer's first report of his cases at Hanover in 1831[6]. His tenotomies extended to the correction of torticollis, scoliosis and limb deformities. 'The art of Orthopedy is not of recent origin, it was practised a hundred years ago – in the eighteenth century – but the discovery (of recent date) that the tendon could be divided with impunity gave new life to the most useful, but which had become an obsolete, art[6].' (The first Achilles tenotomy in America, an open section, appears to have been done by David L Rogers in 1834, in New York City[7], and Dickson, of North Carolina, operated in the same year. In 1837, in New York, the German immigrant William Ludwig Detmold, a pupil of Stromeyer's, began a series of such operations[8], and we know that in 1830 there appeared in Philadelphia a book in which the author, Thomas Dent Mütter (1811–1859) reported on 28 cases of club-foot treated by tenotomy[9].) Initially, of course, John Ball Brown operated without the benefits of anaesthesia until the arrival of ether in 1846.

Buckminster Brown (1819–1891) obtained his Harvard doctorate in 1844 and spent the years of 1845 and 1846 in Europe studying orthopaedics with Guérin, Bouvier, Stromeyer and Little[10]. When he returned to the States he practised orthopaedics exclusively, the first native American ever to do so from the start of a surgical career. He was initially with his father at the Boston Orthopaedic Institution, or Hospital for the Cure of Deformities of the Human Frame, and then, in 1861, opened a small private hospital of 24 beds, the House of the Good Samaritan, mainly for children, so that he is regarded as the father of children's orthopaedics in America. He was a skilled operator on the foot, knee and hip, and possibly the first to cure bilateral congenital dislocation of the hip, in a girl of four years, whom he treated for two years in double leg traction with counter-traction from a pelvic band fixed to the bedhead.

In 1883, he founded the second chair of orthopaedic surgery in America, the John Ball and Buckminster Brown Professorship at Harvard; the first had been established in 1861, in New York, by Lewis A Sayre at the Bellevue Hospital. In 1868 he published a book containing eight sheets on which were stuck prints from photographic plates, stating that 'the figures in the accompanying Plates are photographic representations of the cases described in the preceding pages. They are copied with an accuracy only attainable by that wonderful art which permits the subject to stamp its own image[11].'

However, despite his operative ability, his treatment was mainly mechanical, by braces, traction and manipulation, and in 1858 he produced a spinal brace rather like that later known as Taylor's brace. With his father, he published the first American textbook of orthopaedics. He was a founder-member of the American Orthopaedic Association in 1887. Edward H Bradford, who was to play such an important part in the later history of

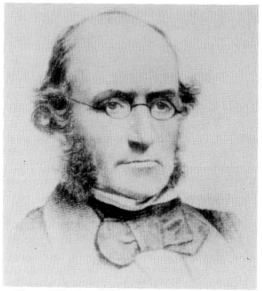

Figure 178   Buckminster Brown (1819–1891)

orthopaedics in Massachusetts, studied under Buckminster Brown and followed him as visiting physician at the orthopaedic division of the House of the Good Samaritan, the only such service then in Boston.

John Rhea Barton (1794–1871) was an assistant to Physick, graduating at the University of Pennsylvania in 1818 and elected to the surgical staff of the Pennsylvania Hospital at the age of 29. He was an innovative and aggressive, but thoughtful, surgeon of great manual dexterity (he was ambidextrous). He did a laminectomy for a fracture spine with paraplegia in 1824, used a 'bran box' for compound fractures of the femur and described his exponymous fracture in 'Views and treatment of an important fracture of the wrist' in the *Medical Examiner* of 1835[12]. He is best known for his work on both arthroplasty and corrective osteotomy for ankylosed joints, an odd instance of a surgeon simultaneously developing two quite differing lines of management for the same problem.

It was an orthopaedic landmark when Barton, on 22nd November 1826, did a deliberate subtrochanteric osteotomy of the femur for a severe flexion–adduction deformity of the right hip, aiming at a pseudarthrosis to be induced by early postoperative movement, analogous to a natural post-fracture pseudarthrosis. The patient was a sailor of 21, John Coyle, injured in a fall at sea and seen by Barton seven months later, when the hip was deformed and stiff after a year in hospital (it was probably an ankylosed tuberculous joint) and not responding to traction.

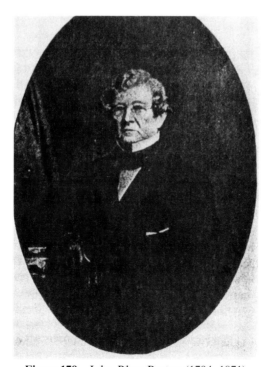

Figure 179   John Rhea Barton (1794–1871)

Barton was well acquainted with the pathology of pseudoarthrosis and hoped for this outcome here, especially 'as in the joint to be formed (by section through the trochanter) the *will* alone must influence the movements, since nearly all of the muscles which exercised their control over the original joint would be carefully preserved by a mere transfer of the point of articulation and resistance from the head of the bone of the acetabulum to the upper end of the shaft of the femur. Although I did not think it essential to the melioration of my patient's condition that the ends of the bone should at its section undergo any change, further than by the absorption of the asperities, I did believe that nature would not passively witness my labours to effect what she herself has so often endeavoured, unaided by art, to accomplish; but that she would be ready to cooperate with me, and to extend to completion that which human art alone would be incapable of in the formation of a new and useful joint.' This was a prophetic statement of the principles underlying joint excision aimed at preserving movement to be further developed in the later 19th century (others used excision with the aim of inducing ankylosis.)

The operation took seven minutes, using a keyhole saw. Movement was begun after six weeks and the patient was walking and weight-bearing at 60 days, walked 150 feet with crutches at 70 days and 100 yards at 78 days, regaining nearly full voluntary hip movement despite some suppuration and transient erysipelas.

'I hope I will not be understood,' wrote Barton, 'as entertaining the belief that this treatment will be applicable to and judicious in every case of an anchylosis...the operation would be justifiable *only*...when the patient's general health is good...where the rigidity is not confined to the soft parts but is actually occasioned by a consolidation of the joint, where all the muscles and tendons essential to the ordinary movements of the former are sound.' The principle, he thought, might be applicable to the hip, knee, shoulder, hallux and finger joints, but only if the muscles were still capable – an idea that has persisted, even though experience has shown that total hip replacement can succeed even in cases of very old ankylosis, where the muscles might be expected to have long wasted. 'If they have been lost,' said Barton, 'it would be palpably wrong to form a joint[13].' Coyle enjoyed the use of his artificial joint for six years, after which ankylosis recurred at the osteotomy site but without recurrence of deformity.

As we note elsewhere, Barton was not the first to aim at deliberate restoration of movement after ankylosis, though some did so by excision of the former joint, some by adjacent osteotomy. Thus, Charles White, of Manchester, England, a student of John Hunter, in 1768, excised several inches of the upper shaft of an osteomyelitic humerus in a boy of 14 instead of doing the conventional amputation, with an excellent result. He reported the case to the Royal Society in 1769 and at this time proposed excision of the femoral head and neck. In 1783, Henry Park (p. 100), surgeon to the Liverpool Infirmary, suggested that excision of diseased joints might sometimes replace amputation – though he was aiming at arthrodesis – while Moreau, in France, was actually doing this at about this time. In 1822, Anthony White, of the Westminster Hospital in London, excised the hip in

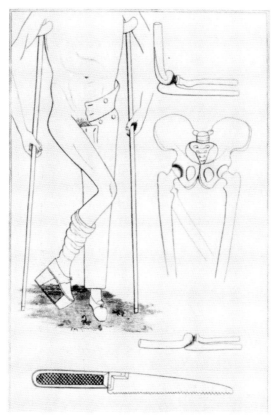

Figure 180   John Rhea Barton: on the treatment of anchylosis by the formation of artificial joints (*North American Medical and Surgical Journal*, **3**, 279 [1827])

a boy of 11, probably tuberculous with secondary infection, sinuses, dislocation and severe adduction deformity. He divided the bone two inches below the greater trochanter and removed the upper femur; there was rapid healing, the leg was straight and the new joint moved well for five years before the patient died of phthisis. The autopsy showed fibrous ankylosis[14]. Thus, by over a century, White anticipated Girdlestone's procedure for this condition. In 1825, James Syme of Edinburgh began his great contributions to excision with the tuberculous shoulder of a woman of 38 and in his 1831 *Treatise on the Excision of Diseased Joints* referred to 14 elbow resections*.

On a contrary course, on 27th May 1835, Barton did a supracondylar wedge osteotomy of the femur for bony ankylosis of the knee at a right angle

---

*We must always recall that, when Hodges wrote his book on *The Excision of Joints* in Boston in 1861, the mortality of hip disarticulation was almost 100 per cent and that of hip excision 50 per cent.

in a doctor, an operation taking only five minutes, correcting the deformity by gradual changes of splintage (he was concerned for the popliteal vessels). There was complete success despite minor infection and extrusion of some small sequestra. The patient was allowed up after four months and resumed his practice, writing to Barton two years later, 'When I think of what I was, and what I am, and that to your firmness, judgment and skill I am indebted for the happy change, I want words to express adequately all that I feel[15].' (In 1845, Gurdon Buck (1807–77) of New York treated a similar case by osteotomy through the former knee joint.)

In 1834, Barton wired a fractured patella, but the patient died of sepsis. However, Bick states that the first published report of this procedure was by E S Cooper of San Francisco, in 1861[16].

The flood of German immigrants in the early 19th century brought two pupils of Stromeyer who became early orthopaedic surgeons in the USA.

William Ludwig Detmold (1808–1894), self-styled Ludwig Wilhelm in his doctoral dissertation at Göttingen in 1830[17], was born at Hanover, the son of the Court physician and was himself surgeon to the Royal Hanoverian Guards. He had acquired a basic training in orthopaedics at Stromeyer's institute in Hanover and emigrated to New York in 1837 at the age of 29 and was thus the first orthopaedic surgeon in that city. An apostle for Stromeyer in the USA, he performed what may have been the first subcutaneous tenotomy in America on 6th September 1837, and by 1840 was able to report on a series of 167 cases, including operations on many

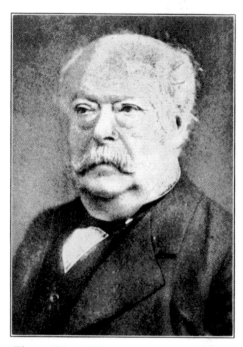

Figure 181   William Detmold (1808–1894)

tendons other than at the heel. In 1841 he established a public clinic for the treatment of crippled children, the first such clinic to be instituted in New York; some authorities state that this was at the Bellevue Hospital[18], others that it was at the College of Physicians and Surgeons[16]; perhaps it was a combined post but in any case he continued it up to 1861. He became a surgeon to the Union Forces in the Civil War and was often called on in advance of impending battles to plan treatment of the wounded and himself worked on many Virginia battlefields. The day after the first Battle of Bull Run he performed 75 amputations in a morning. He devised the Detmold knife, which combined a fork, for one-armed veterans. In 1862 he became Professor of Military Surgery and Hygiene at the College of Physicians and Surgeons.

Although he regarded himself as a Stromeyerian missionary in America, he was not an indiscriminate enthusiast of tenotomy and preferred conservative management if possible; he always followed up the operation with gradual correction in an appliance. In 1842 he gave six lectures to the College, introduced by these remarks, 'Orthopaedic surgery presents to you unequalled and peculiar attractions, for I may safely assert that in every case a satisfactory result may be anticipated and promised, that is, if both patient and surgeon do their best.' That 'unequalled and peculiar attraction'! What good orthopaedic surgeon has not felt like this, and what bad one has? In these lectures, he described a turnbuckle appliance to straighten the flexed knee, not very different from its medieval counterpart. He operated for Dupuytren's contracture, not naming it as such though Dupuytren had described it in 1834[19], he operated for torticollis, and, in 1850, was possibly the first to deal with a cerebral abscess, opening the lateral ventricle[20]. He was on the staff of the Bellevue and Presbyterian Hospitals, a charter member of the New York Academy of Medicine, a founder-member of the New York County Medical Society and its first President. When the American Orthopaedic Association was founded in 1887, Detmold was 79 and was made an honorary member in 1892. He was solitary, a dandy, and rode in the park every day.

Was Detmold the first pioneer of orthopaedic surgery in the USA? He arrived in 1837, but at that time John Ball Brown was already New England's first orthopaedic surgeon and was to establish his Boston institute the following year. Perhaps the two should share the glory. There has been a continuing dispute as to who did the first tenotomies in the US, but Detmold himself never asserted any priority and always acknowledged the work of Dickson in North Carolina in 1835 and of Smith of Baltimore in 1836. Perhaps the best tribute to him is Bick's, 'He was the first of a new breed in American medicine, the trained and self-declared orthopaedic surgeon, who had started practice as such, and who, by publication, teaching and lecturing inspired other physicians to practice the specialty and medical institutions to accept it[16].'

The second of Stromeyer's pupils to arrive was **Louis Bauer** (1814–1898). Carl August Ludgwig Bauer was born in Stettin. A stormy and combative individual, a natural dissident, he was sentenced to 10 months' prison in 1848 for political activities and emigrated to England in the following year. There, as a Stromeyerian, he was welcomed by Little. While in England he

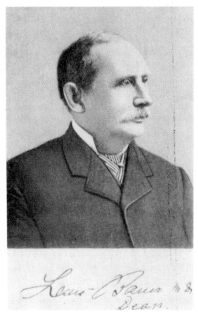

Figure 182   Louis Bauer (1814–1898)

translated into German an English book, *Untersuchungen über das Wesen und die Behandlung der Deformitäten des menschliches Körpers* (Studies on the nature and treatment of deformities of the human frame) by J Bishop (Stettin 1853), and in this he described himself as 'Director of the Royal Orthopaedic Institution in Manchester', though there is no record that such an institution ever existed or that Bauer ever worked in that city, a claim he was to repeat later. We do know that he was listed as a member of the Royal College of Surgeons for 1853.

In that year at the age of 39 he emigrated to New York and, in 1854, founded the 'Orthopaedic Institute of Brooklyn' with Richard Bartelmess and lectured at 'Long Island College Hospital'. This had derived from the German General Dispensary he helped to found and later became the Downstate Medical Center of the State University of New York. His institute was the first of its kind in the city and was modelled on the European pattern, with appliances, a gymnasium, baths and a garden. It therefore resembled John Ball Brown's institute in Boston, but had an outpatient clinic and 50 beds; it eventually became the orthopaedic department of Long Island College of Medicine, chartered in 1858.

In 1861, Bauer gave a series of lectures on orthopaedic surgery at the Brooklyn Surgical and Medical Institute. These were published in 1862 in the Philadelphia Medical and Surgical Reporter and, after editing, as a book entitled *Lectures in Orthopaedic Surgery* in 1864, with a second edition in 1868. This, after the small volume of Buckminster Brown, was the first true orthopaedic textbook in the US, and won the praise of Sir Arthur Keith in

England half a century later[21]. The book stressed the importance of rest and immobilization of the spine. 'No mechanical apparatus, however handsomely constructed...can satisfy this most stringest requirement as long as the patient is permitted the upright position. The doctor must insist on the necessity for the horizontal supine position...*so long as the slightest trace of local disorder is demonstrable, the first therapeutic axiom* in the treatment of joint diseases is *absolute and unconditional rest*, and the next is a functional position of the diseased joint.' These teachings were re-emphasized in a series of lectures given at McGill University Medical College in Montreal and published as *Lectures on Causes, Pathology and Treatment of Joint Disease* in New York in 1868 by William Wood. (Though it is odd that in 1885 he was to state that patients with Pott's disease should be anaesthetized from time to time and the deformity corrected by manual pressure.)

These views on the importance of rest in a functional position were exactly those being preached by Hugh Owen Thomas, 20 years his junior, in Liverpool at much the same time, and it is interesting that both men were entirely dogmatic, convinced they were right – unlike their colleagues – pugnacious and self-isolated and correspondingly somewhat paranoid. Each managed to produce a degree of ostracism. It is not surprising that Thomas called Bauer 'the best exponent of American orthopaedics', adding that 'to the treatment of posterior curvature of the spine I can contribute but little. The mechanical treatment adopted by me is that form of posterior support which my friend, Dr Bauer of St Louis, USA, had introduced into practice[22].' Bauer and Ridlon were the only Americans to whom Thomas felt akin; all three men were cantankerous perfectionists.

Bauer became a critical and prickly colleague of native New York orthopaedists – Sayre, Taylor and Davis – and became a centre of strife, to the degree that, according to John Ridlon, 'he was persecuted out of New York City' by these gentry. But then, Ridlon was a man of similar temperament and, as we shall see, had his own troubles and also had to leave the city. Thus, in his second book, Bauer, referring to Rhea Barton's hip osteotomy, said that *he* did not do it because an artificial joint could never give adequate support, that it excited suppuration, and that, in Sayre's hands, the patient died of pyaemia after a few months without autopsy evidence of neoarthrosis. (Sayre disputed this and quoted witnesses of the autopsy to confirm that there *was* a false joint[23].)

He likewise criticized Taylor's brace: because it was inefficient and had been patented and should – if any good – have been made freely available, and because it was premade without respect for the shape of the patient and assumed, fallaciously, that Pott's disease could be straightened by splintage alone. 'Dr Taylor...need not have gone to the expense of a patent, because it...is not likely to be employed by anyone else.'

H G Davis had devised an extension splint for the lower limb in which a patient with hip disease could get about, a splint improved by Sayre, 'but this apparatus as well as the others above mentioned are all defective in a very essential point: they neither fix the diseased joint nor do they prevent adduction of the limb.' In an article of 1889 on 'Orthopaedic surgery in England and the United States[24]' he wrote, 'Dr Sayre has not given birth to a single original idea but has propagated... the intellectual fruit of his superiors... What revenue would (Dr Taylor) derive from his orthopaedic practice if he relinquished the manufacture of his very glittering, complicated, costly and withal useless instrument?' And, as to Dr Davis's famous appliance, so commended by others, 'this excessive tribute to so indifferent a contrivance did more than anything else to consign it to the mausoleum of the past'.

Bauer, like Thomas, did not hide his light under a bushel. In the same article he wrote, 'The history of orthopaedic surgery in the United States is intimately interwoven with the name of the writer of these pages, and either ignorance or injustice ignores him. This is no empty boast... upon our advent to this country in 1853 there was no specialty as now understood by the term 'orthopaedic surgery': even its name had to be found and cast by us.' This was quite untrue. Detmold had already been 16 years in New York when Bauer arrived; there were Sayre, Knight, Mott and others in the city, John Ball Brown in Boston. If it had been true, why was Bauer not a founder member of the American Orthopaedic Association in 1887, or elected an honorary member as were Detmold, Sayre, Davis and Taylor, if it were not that resentment of his criticisms still rankled?

These criticisms probably provided the impetus for him to leave his Brooklyn workshop in 1869 and settle in St Louis, where he became the first 'Professor of Orthopaedic Surgery' at the College of Physicians and Surgeons of St Louis, founded in 1879, chiefly on his own initiative (the College closed in 1910). It was the first such clinic in the midwest; there was a large German–American community in the city and his reputation had preceded him. He was followed by Ridlon, another self-exile, in Chicago in 1887 and by Steindler in Iowa City. It was no doubt Bauer's influence that secured for Thomas, in 1890, the honorary MD of the University of St Louis as one of the two most distinguished doctors of the year.

A contemporary of John Ball Brown was **Henry Jacob Bigelow** (1818–1890), son of an eminent Boston physician, Jacob Bigelow (1787–1879). He studied medicine at Harvard but then developed lung disease, wintered in Cuba 1839–40 and was then in Europe until 1844. His book, *A Manual of Orthopedic Surgery* (Boston 1845) is sometimes regarded as the first American text on the subject, but this claim has been made so often on behalf of other publications that scepticism is indicated. As he was then still only 27, it is not surprising that the work consists mainly of an account of his experience with Guérin and others in Europe, and the current enthusiasm for tenotomy in all its forms is reflected in his first two chapters, dealing with tenotomy for the cure of squint and stammer. Delpech of Montpellier, Dupuytren and Stromeyer were also among his pantheon, so it is not surprising that he gained the Boylston Prize in 1844 for an essay, 'In what cases and to what extent is the division of muscles, tendons and other parts proper for the relief of deformity or lameness?' He noted that hamstring tenotomy for fixed knee flexion was likely to subluxate the tibia backwards and adopted Little's 'machine' for displacing the tibia forwards during the procedure. For torticollis, he divided if necessary not only the sternomastoid but also the platysma and trapezius, using a brace extending to the pelvis. In 1852 he performed the first excision of the hip joint, though again one must always

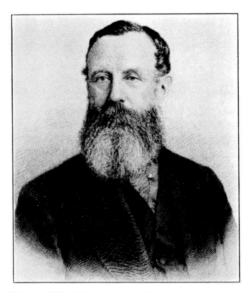

Figure 183   Henry Jacob Bigelow (1818–1890)

be cautious in claiming priority in any of these matters. He also described the correction of flexion–adduction deformity of the hip by subcutaneous section of the adductors, rectus, femoris, sartorius, pectineus, psoas and iliacus, introducing the tenotome three inches below the anterior superior iliac spine parallel to the inguinal ligament as far as the femoral artery. 'Profuse haemorrhage followed but was controlled by compression.'

Bigelow's main claims to fame relate to his contributions to hip surgery and to the introduction of ether anaesthesia. In the former, he stressed the role of the Y–shaped iliofemoral ligament and its use as a fulcrum in reduction of hip dislocations, and his well known method of reducing a traumatic dislocation was based on careful dissections and mechanical studies, described in a book, *The mechanism of dislocation and fracture of the hip* (Philadelphia 1869). This helped to found the subsequent treatment of congenital dislocation by manipulation (Lorenz's 'bloodless method') and open operation (Hoffa). Writing in 1966, Jesse T Nicholson, celebrating the world fame of the Massachusetts General Hospital in hip surgery, refers to the custom, 'whereby, each Wednesday, soon after dawn, the patients are placed beneath Bigelow's bust while members of the orthopedic staff offer petitions which they believe will bring a blessed result.'

Above all, it was Bigelow who was responsible for the first employment of ether for general anaesthesia in surgery at the Massachusetts General Hospital, on 16th October 1846, the Ether Day. He had heard that Dr W T G Morton was extracting teeth painlessly under ether, went to see for himself, and persuaded Dr John C Warren, chief of surgery at the hospital, to allow Morton to administer ether for an operation by Warren himself. Bigelow made known the success of this to the world in a paper published a few weeks later[25], and this only a few years after the great Velpeau in

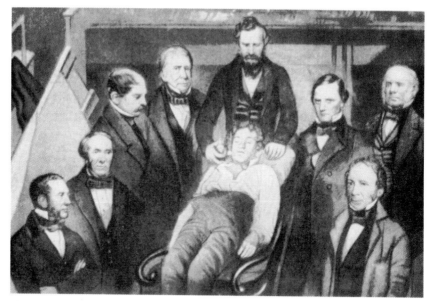

Figure 184   The first public demonstration of ether anaesthesia at the Massachusetts General Hospital on 16th October 1846. Bigelow is the figure below on the left

Paris had asserted that 'the elimination of pain in operations is a chimera which it is not permissible to pursue today[26].' It is fascinating that such *ex cathedra* pronouncements, stressing not only the impossibility but also almost the impiety of a great step forward, recur in the history of medicine and science and usually prove to be presages of such advances. The present writer recalls the great British orthopaedic surgeon, Sir James Seddon, speaking of the 'arrogance' of those who thought that poliomyelitis might be treated or prevented, and this at the very time when Salk was perfecting his vaccine.

Bigelow also constructed an operating chair which the Emperor of Brazil saw at the hospital in 1867 and recommended to the German Empress; Bigelow sent a drawing to Berlin and was rewarded with a copy of von Esmarch's new book, *A Manual of Military Surgical Technique*.

It ought to be added that, several years before the appearance of Bigelow's monograph on the hip, **Murray Carnochan** (1817–1887), professor of surgery at New York College, had published a treatise on congenital dislocation of the hip which was the first comprehensive review of this subject in America[27].

Gurdon Buck (1807–1877), at the New York Hospital, devised in the 1850s 'An improved method of treating fractures of the femur' by adhesive strapping traction in place of Chessher's double inclined plane or the long Liston splint[28]. This was very much as used today, with two side-straps, a spreader and a pulley at the end of the bed, but with countertraction by strap or rubber tubing at the perineum and also with lateral coaptation splints. It had been suggested by Josiah Crosby of New Hampshire[29] and he had also seen his colleague, Henry Gassett Davis, using it for hip disease. Buck demonstrated it to the New York Academy of Medicine in the spring of 1861, and shortly after it became as popular in the Civil War as closed plaster had been in the hands of Pirigoff in the Crimean War. One hesitates to ascribe any priority, since Guy de Chauliac had been using pulley traction at Montpellier in the 14th century, while Josse of Amiens had so treated fractured femurs in 1836 by tying the foot to the raised bed-end. Also, John Haddy James (1788–1869) of Exeter in England in 1839 used continuous weight and pulley traction from a wooden splint in which the leg was bandaged[30].

James Knight (1810–1887), a Baltimore graduate of 1832, practised in New York City from 1835, apparently as a sort of clinical assistant at various centres with a special interest in orthopaedics. He exhibited exceptional ability in designing trusses and braces and from his early days devoted himself to 'displacements of parts of the human system requiring the use of bandages, such as trusses, spring bandages for females ... and suspensory bandages.' (Note the wide range of application of the word 'bandage' in earlier times, and hence the versatility of the 'bandagist'.) He founded the New York Surgeons' Bandage Institute in the late 1830s, 'to be exclusively kept for the reception and sale of the most improved bandages and the treatment of diseases requiring their use', and realized at an early stage the need for a special institution for the crippled poor; but this was not to materialize for over twenty years.

His activities drew the attention of Valentine Mott, who induced him to specialize in orthopaedics, and in 1863 he did what Mott had been unable to do, giving the use of his own home as a hospital for the New York Society for the Relief of the Ruptured and Crippled, prior to the establishment of that Society's own hospital seven years later, with Knight as resident

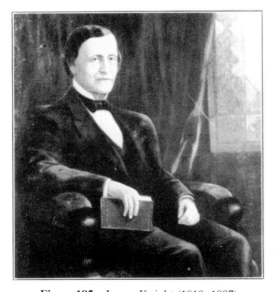

Figure 185   James Knight (1819–1887)

superintendent–physician. The original staff included Mott, William K van Beuren and John M Carnochan. This is the oldest orthopaedic hospital in the US that has been in continuous operation since its foundation, albeit with a change in name. It had 200 beds and only children between the ages of four and 14 with curable diseases were treated.

Knight spoke of himself as a 'surgico-mechanic', dealing only with conditions capable of relief by bandaging and bracing, and absolutely rejected major operations. He refused to have an operating theatre in the hospital and even rejected the plaster bandage invented by the Dutchman, Mathysen, in 1851. Other New York contemporaries, such as Sayre, relied heavily on plaster, especially for suspension jackets for scoliosis and Pott's disease. Knight thought it wrong to compress the respiratory organs or the limbs, 'All such adventurous treatment is avoided in this hospital.' And, in fact, plaster was not used there until after his death, by his successor Virgil Gibney, who also installed the first operating theatre[31]. Hernia was treated there because the orthopaedic appliance-makers also made the trusses, but no skilled mechanics were ever employed since Knight felt that a surgeon ought to be able to fit any brace himself.

Knight was a great autocrat and allowed only treatment of which he approved, and this led to difficulties with his staff. But he did establish the first considerable programme of residency training in orthopaedics in the US, his first assistant being Newton M Shaffer from 1863 to 1868, and his second Virgil P Gibney. His intolerance led to a break with Gibney in 1884, when the latter wrote a book, *The Hip and its Diseases*, which conceded a place for traction or even resection of the tuberculous joint; these were anathema to Knight, who demanded and obtained Gibney's resignation. His later return as head of the hospital seems a piece of poetic justice.

In 1868, Knight published *The Improvement of the Health of Children and Adults by Natural Means*, dealing largely with the diet and the value of electrotherapy, and, in 1874, *Orthopaedia, or a Practical Treatise on the Aberrations of the Human Form*, with Gibney's help. The text was mainly classical, dealing with braces, frames and casts; the only operations mentioned were tenotomies and there was an emphasis on the benefits of electrotherapy with the static machine for chronic ulcers and rheumatism. A second edition ten years later was based on experience with 5000 inpatients and 26 000 outpatients.

Knight was one of the last 'strap and buckle' pioneers in orthopaedics, before and during the expansion of operative methods, and before the foundation of the American Orthopaedic Association in 1887. This, appropriately, was also the year of his death, the end of an epoch, for he was one of the last conservatives at a time when orthopaedic surgeons were struggling desperately to free themselves from the stigma of being 'mere bandagists' and to justify their existence as a separate discipline from general surgery. Of course, Sayre and his colleagues thought him far too conservative, which exemplified the great divide between the non-operators who relied on rest and appliances and the surgically minded, a gap not yet altogether bridged. He practised the 'constitutional' treatment as advocated by Hugh Owen Thomas, and as opposed to what Thomas and Royal Whitman called 'methods of adventure'. Essentially, this relates to the divide between the classical and the romantic in surgery. From ancient times orthopaedics was, and had to be, classical in approach, but when anaesthesia and antisepsis gave the great impetus to operative methods – especially in abdominal surgery, *par excellence* a romantic field – orthopaedists were inevitably not to be left behind. It was precisely the fear that they might now be relegated to being mere 'bandagists' that spurred them on. However, the struggle was never easy. 'There never was a time,' wrote Phelps in 1894, 'when they, the orthopaedic and the general surgeon, could lie peacefully together in the same bed, excepting like the lion and the lamb – one inside the other, and the poor orthopede was always inside.'

What Knight did that had not been done, or not properly done before, was to conceive and establish the ongoing treatment and education and vocational training of the crippled child and adolescent as a unity under his own eye and in his own wards. Though a firm advocate of rest, he placed an emphasis on rehabilitation that had previously been lacking. He really felt for the disabled poor, and that is something without which mere surgical technique is vanity.

We now come to consider a group of men active in New York in the latter half of the century, well grouped as follows by Alfred Rives Shands, to whose historical researches we owe so much[32]. Henry Gassett Davis (1807–1896), 'the greatest mind of the early period', known for the elastic treatment of deformities; Lewis Albert Sayre (1820–1900), 'foremost American orthopedist of all times and probably our first professor'; Edward Hickling Bradford (1848–1926), founder of the modern Boston school of orthopedics and a champion of crippled child care; Charles Fayette Taylor (1827–1899), founder of the New York Orthopedic Dispensary and Hospital, and Newton M Shaffer (1846–1928) who succeeded Taylor (these two, with Knight, relied on mechanical methods and were against operative measures); Virgil Pendleton Gibney (1847–1927), who developed the training programme at the Hospital for the Ruptured and Crippled at the turn of the century; and De Forest Willard (1846–1910), pioneer of orthopaedic surgery in Philadelphia and first professor in the subject at the University of Pennsylvania.

Lewis Albert Sayre (1820–1900) was born in New Jersey, graduated in New York, and was appointed surgeon to Bellevue Hospital in 1853. There he started an orthopaedic dispensary in 1861 and held this clinical appointment until 1898, when he was succeeded by his son, Reginald Hall Sayre. He became the first professor of orthopaedic surgery at Bellevue Medical College (the first at any US medical school), later part of the university of the City of New York. Originally, this was concerned mainly with fractures and dislocations; later it was extended to clinical surgery.

In 1854 he performed the second successful resection of a tuberculous hip in the US[33]; Bigelow had done the first two years before. (Of course, tuberculosis was not then recognized as the cause of 'coxitis'; there was a vague concept of 'strumous diathesis'; Sayre thought it of traumatic origin.) During the next 30 years he excised over 70 hips, though he acknowledged that the operation would eventually be obviated by advances in diagnosis and treatment (it was still being done, and very radically, including the

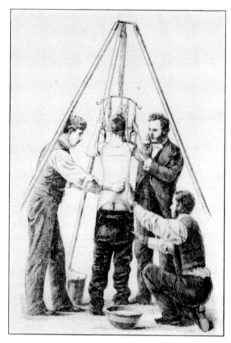

Figure 186   Lewis A Sayre applying a plaster jacket

acetabulum, by Bankart at the Middlesex Hospital in London in the 1930s).
He demonstrated the operation to the International Medical Congress in
Philadelphia in 1876, attended by Lister, who said that this alone would
have been sufficient reward for crossing the Atlantic. He was a great
enthusiast of the plaster bandage, and perhaps his greatest contribution to
orthopaedics was the suspension plaster jacket, the 'Sayre jacket', originally
for Pott's disease[34], his first case being a boy of four with partial paraplegia.
It was later applied to scoliosis[35], sometimes associated with tenotomy of
the latissimus dorsi. For cervical and high thoracic curves the jacket
incorporated a 'jury mast' extending above the head to allow constant head
traction, a forerunner of halo traction. The head was suspended by a sling
from a tripod and lateral pressure was applied to the curve convexities by
canvas bands while the jacket was moulded.

It seems clear from various commissions of enquiry (dubious mid-century
claims in Europe for certain treatments had established the need for objective
assessment) and from the X-ray evidence, when this arrived, that very
complete correction could be obtained; but there was a tendency to recurrence
when the jackets were removed and Sayre himself later came to believe that
the apparent correction was due to the development of compensatory curves.
In 1877, as a delegate from the American Medical Association to the British
Medical Association, he demonstrated his method for spinal diseases at
various centres in England and Ireland (where he complained that the
dampness hindered the setting of his plasters). The tone of these demon-

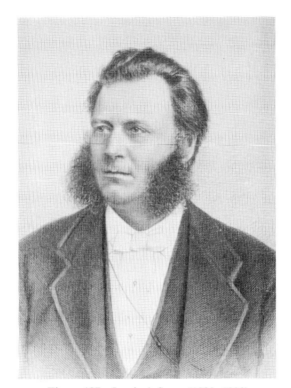

Figure 187   Lewis A Sayre (1820–1900)

strations, and a clue to the temperament of Sayre himself, is sufficiently indicated in a comment by Robert Bigg, who attended one at University College Hospital, 'With a personal and dramatic presumption of supreme superiority...he made a virulent and satirical attack upon all previous treatments. After vilifying these as absolutely worthless, he disclosed...that he himself had...a new and perfect plan of treatment which ought to be adopted to the exclusion of all others, both in cases of spinal caries and in cases of lateral curvature[36].' His book, *Spinal Disease and Spinal Curvature: their treatment by suspension and the use of the plaster of Paris bandage*, (Lippincott, Philadelphia 1877) was actually written during this visit and dedicated to the British medical profession in gratitude for their welcome.

Sayre insisted on the early incision of suppurating joints, but in this, as with all his operations and for spinal injuries, practised careful and prolonged immobilization in casts, nor did his operative enthusiasm prevent him from being an expert brace designer. In tenotomies, he followed Little in delaying correction after operation to prevent air entering the wound. He did many hip osteotomies, aiming, like Barton, at a neoarthrosis[37]. He devised a club-foot shoe, advocated routine examination of all newborn children, and insisted that treatment be instituted from the moment of birth, 'the more frequent the manipulation, the more benefit to be derived.' He also repaired hare-lip and meningocoele immediately. He introduced an inflatable rubber tourniquet and an adhesive strapping method for fracture of the clavicle. His *Practical Manual of the Treatment of Club Foot* (Appleton, New York 1869) was reissued in 1874, 1875 and 1894 and translated into many languages. In 1876, his *Lectures on Orthopedic Surgery and Diseases of the Joints* (Appleton, New York) won wide acclaim as the best American textbook of its time, superseding that of Bauer; it was only the fourth American orthopaedic text ever written. He was an early exponent of bone-lengthening procedures.

Sayre acquired a reputation in Europe as the greatest living practitioner in his field, partly because he was decorated for treating a member of the Swedish royal family. He was a brusque, forceful and therefore controversial personality, an eloquent public speaker, a founder-member of the American Medical Association in 1847 and its President in 1880 – the first orthopaedic surgeon to be so. He prompted the creation of the Journal of the Association in 1882. He was therefore a major force in the development of orthopaedic surgery, raising it from a state of neglect, even contempt. As Bradford wrote in 1889, 'The surgeon no longer looks upon the treatment of orthopaedic cases as a forlorn hope of despairing surgical duty, or as a matter to be relegated to the commercial interests of the maker of the trusses[38].' 'Few men,' said the *British Medical Journal*, 'in this generation accomplished so much for the relief of humanity.'

Because Sayre helped convert orthopaedics from a matter of manipulations and braces into a fully-fledged surgical speciality, it is interesting that he originally opposed the creation of the American Orthopedic Association in 1887 (though he was made an honorary member in 1889) and instead urged his orthopaedic colleagues to join the American Surgical Association. We should add that, from 1861 to 1866, Sayre was appointed Resident Physician of New York City, a sort of Medical Officer of Health, under four mayors. He was an enthusiast of vaccination, improved sewage disposal, showed that cholera was communicable, and initiated quarantine regulations in the Port of New York.

Finally, the interest Sayre took from the outset in the management of fractures and dislocations exemplifies that this field was hardly ever separated from that of classical orthopaedics as that subject developed in the United States, unlike the situation in Europe, where, as in England, it was not possible to divert the management of injuries from the general surgeons into specialist clinics until the Second World War and after.

Henry Gassett Davis (1806–1896) had some clinical training at Bellevue and graduated at Yale in 1837. For some 15 years he practised at Worcester and elsewhere in Massachusetts, developing an interest in skeletal disease and deformities. During this period, around 1856–7, he devised an elastic material for weight and pulley traction which replaced Gross's adhesive strapping. (Samuel David Gross (1805–1884), professor of surgery at Jefferson Medical College, Philadelphia, had revolutionized the treatment of fractures of the long bones by the application of adhesive tape.) It was Davis's method that had been adapted by Gurdon Buck in 1860 and rapidly became standard equipment in the medical corps of the Union Army in the Civil War. It was used for the treatment of fractures, flexion deformities, joint infections, even club-feet, and became known as the 'American method', but this is confusing since the term was also applied to Davis's combination of brace traction and immobilization for the management of hip disease, aiming at 'support without pressure and motion without friction... the treatment itself, concisely defined, consists in abstraction of the joint affected by continued elastic extension... Nature will not yield to violence, but only to gradual force.' He also invented ambulatory hip and spinal braces, which he alleged were pirated by Sayre and Bauer. His scoliosis brace had elastic straps pulling on the convexities.

In 1855 he settled in New York and specialized in orthopaedics and fractures. The practice grew rapidly and he opened a private hospital on Madison Avenue at 37th Street 'for the purpose of carrying out in the most appropriate manner the treatment of diseases and injuries of joints, including old dislocations and deformities.' He was also a pioneer in the sanatorium regime for phthisis.

In 1893 he reported on 59 years' experience in the open evacuation of suppurative arthritis, washing out the joint with tepid water and injecting 'a French preparation of chlorine', using a tent to keep the wound open and allow healing from the depths. This was, essentially, what was to become the Carrel–Dakin hypochlorite irrigation of wounds in World War I. In 1867 he had published his *Conservative Surgery as Exhibited in Remedying some of the Mechanical Causes that Operate Injuriously both in Health and Disease*, the second most important American orthopaedic text after Bauer's. He practised in New York for only 14 years and retired to Massachusetts in 1869 at the age of 62. Shands says that Davis was a giant among the early pioneers, and that his methods revolutionized orthopaedic treatment, 'If one person deserves the title of 'Father of American orthopaedic surgery', it is Henry Gassett Davis, about whom most of us today know little[39].'

Charles Fayette Taylor (1827–1899), from Vermont, attended lectures at New York College in 1855 and qualified in 1856 at the University of Vermont after what seems to have been only a year's study. Then he travelled to London to visit M Roth, a pupil of Peter Henry Ling, the famous Swedish exponent of remedial exercises, and introduced this system on his return to New York. In 1861 he published his *Theory and Practice of the Movement Cure*, designed to 'emulate the Physical Nobleness of the old Norse heroes and to banish disease by the beautiful System Ling originated.' This he thought a near-universal remedy for spinal curvature, muscular paralysis, circulatory and bowel disorders, phthisis, gynaecologic diseases and other troubles. Nevertheless, he came to recognize that rest was the best treatment for many orthopaedic conditions and devoted himself to brace-making. He studied spinal diseases with John M Carnochan, then professor of surgery at New York College. Dismayed by the ineffectiveness of the current treatment of Pott's disease, he devised and discarded one appliance after another, taking ten years to perfect his special brace or 'surgical assistant' with which he successfully treated the young daughter of Theodore Roosevelt, senior, sister of the future President Franklin Roosevelt. This long spinal brace with shoulder-straps is in essence, still widely used. He also advocated the gradual correction of club-foot by leverage and, in 1867, published a monograph on *Infantile Paralysis and its Attendant Deformities.*

A few years later, Roosevelt and others founded the New York Orthopaedic Dispensary at 1299 Broadway, in Taylor's charge from 1866 to 1882. He did not want the dispensary to become a hospital, and when this actually happened after the foundation moved to E 59th Street and became the New York Orthopaedic Dispensary and Hospital in 1873 (now known as the New York Orthopaedic Hospital and affiliated with the Columbia University – Presbyterian Medical Center since 1950), Taylor soon resigned and confined his activities to his own small private institution next door. He was succeeded at the hospital by Shaffer, who had been Knight's assistant at the opening of the Hospital for the Ruptured and Crippled and transferred to the New York Orthopaedic Hospital soon after its extension.

Taylor was very conservative, against operation, used no drugs and took a special interest in the psychological aspects of orthopaedic disease and the treatment of functional disorders; this was doubtless useful at a time when spinal symptoms, especially in women and especially after railway accidents, were often hysterical. Electrotherapy, in his view, was something charlatans seized on to prey on the credulity of the public. He, too, has been designated as the father of American orthopaedics, a child with several putative fathers.

De Forest Willard (1846–1910) repeated Little's history, suffering from poliomyelitis in infancy and being treated for resultant club-foot by Achilles

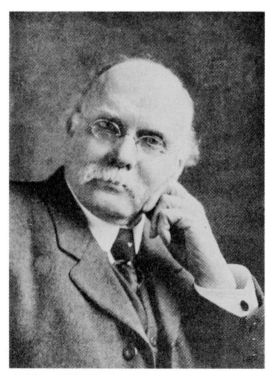

Figure 188   DeForest Willard (1846–1910)

tenotomy as a young man in 1864. He became lecturer in orthopaedic surgery at the University of Pennsylvania in 1877, clinical professor in 1889 and full professor in 1893. He came to specialize in paediatric surgery, both general and orthopaedic, and his best-known publication, *The Surgery of Childhood, including Orthopaedic Surgery* (Lippincott, Philadelphia 1910) dealt with these aspects, so that its orthopaedic value was underestimated. He established orthopaedic wards, a physiotherapy department and a brace shop at the University of Pennsylvania Hospital, and in 1898 promoted a splendid vocational training centre for crippled children. He was a pioneer in peripheral nerve suture and grafting[40]; nerve suture had occasionally been attempted in Europe for centuries, but its general entry into surgery was effected in the American Civil War, an early advocate being Silas Weir Mitchell (1829–1914), whose pioneer *Injuries of Nerves and their Consequences* was published in Philadelphia in 1872. Willard was also an early practitioner, possibly the first, of costotransversectomy for abscesses in Pott's disease[41] and an advocate of Listerism at a time, around 1880, when opposition to the new system was still widespread. He was the fourth President of the American Orthopaedic Association.

Virgil P Gibney (1847–1927), of Kentucky, trained at Louisville and then Bellevue Hospital Medical College and graduated from the latter in 1871, following Shaffer as resident to Knight at the Ruptured and Crippled. As already noted, after 13 years, in 1884, the publication of his best-known book, *Diseases of the Hip*, led to disagreement with Knight, resignation and then, ironically, after a passage in Europe and return to establish a small private hospital, his appointment after Knight's death. His main contribution was to change the Hospital for the Ruptured and Crippled from an institution for crippled children to a hospital fully equipped and staffed for modern orthopaedics, separating the hernia department from the orthopaedic section. It was Gibney, with Shaffer, in that same year of 1887, who organized the first meeting of the American Orthopaedic Association and was to become its President. He led the group of those who championed the surgical, as opposed to the conservative, aspects of orthopaedic treatment, even though he was himself cautious by nature and never deserted conservative methods. In 1882, he was a cofounder of the Polyclinic Medical School and was Professor of Orthopaedic Surgery until 1894, when he became the first professor at Columbia University College of Physicians and Surgeons until succeeded by Russell Hibbs in 1917. The two decades of 1890–1910 marked the real development of modern orthopaedic surgery in the USA and Gibney's contribution was as important as any. He was reappointed President of the AOA in 1912 on its 25th anniversary and remained head of the Hospital for the Ruptured and Crippled until 1925, when he was succeeded by Royal Whitman. (Whitman was followed for a short period by his son, Armitage, later by Philip D Wilson from 1934 to 1955, during which period the institution was renamed the Hospital for Special Surgery and affiliated to the Cornell-New York Hospital Medical Center. The chiefs, after Wilson, were in order, T Campell Thompson, Robert Lee Paterson and Philip D Wilson, Jr). A man of immense energy and application, Gibney wrote 176 papers and was regarded at the time of his death, both by his American

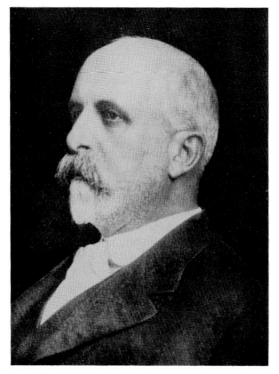

Figure 189   Virgil P Gibney (1847–1927)

colleagues and overseas figures such as Robert Jones, as a great man.

Newton Melman Shaffer (1846–1928), born in New York State, began his medical studies at the age of 17 under Knight at the Hospital for the Ruptured and Crippled on the day it opened on 1st May 1863. He graduated at the University Medical College of New York in 1867 and in 1871 joined the New York Orthopaedic Dispensary under Taylor, succeeding the latter as surgeon-in-chief in 1876. Meanwhile in 1872, St Luke's had become the first major general American hospital to recognize orthopaedics as a speciality with a separate service and Shaffer was appointed to run the department in addition to his superintendence of the New York Orthopaedic Hospital. In 1882 he became Clinical Professor of Orthopaedic Surgery at the NY University Medical College until 1886, and later professor at Cornell. He remained at the NY Orthopaedic Hospital until 1891, when he retired to give way to Russell A Hibbs (1869–1932). Hibbs was followed by Benjamin Farrell. In 1940, under Alan de Forest Smith, the hospital was affiliated to the Columbia-Presbyterian Medical Center, absorbing the renowned fracture service of the Presbyterian Hospital. Smith was succeeded by Frank Stinchfield, who was to become prominent in promoting research and maintaining standards of orthopaedic practice nationwide. At this time he lobbied the state legislature to fund a hospital for the continued treatment and vocational

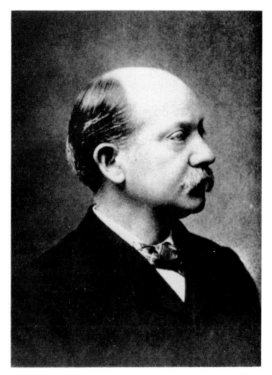

Figure 190   Newton M Schaffer (1846–1928)

care of crippled children, founded first at Tarrytown and then moved to West Haverstraw. This became the New York Rehabilitation Hospital and Shaffer was its superintendent surgeon-in-chief until 1910.

He was a founder member of the AOA and its second President after Gibney; he was also a founder member of the New York Orthopaedic Society. It was largely his chairmanship of a committee at the International Medical Congress in Berlin in 1890 that led to world acceptance of orthopaedics as a recognized speciality. He was always a 'mechanician' and relegated operations to general surgeons on the hospital staff, so much so that ultimately most of the orthopaedic operations at St Luke's were being done by general surgeons and the true aims of the hospital were being obscured; in the end, the Board had to dismiss the general surgeons. Shaffer was a forceful combative man; hence the break with Ridlon described below. Basically, he remained a conservative to the end of his life, 'Orthopaedic surgery is that department of surgery which includes the prevention, the mechanical treatment and the operative treatment of chronic or progressive deformities for the proper treatment of which special forms of apparatus or special mechanical dressings are necessary.' He was critical of the 1890 textbook of Bradford and Lovett because it included resection and amputation and regretted that Listerism had encouraged surgeons to attempt operations for which they were not trained. He defined the 'Shaffer foot', an

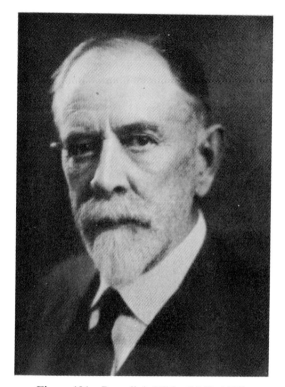

Figure 191   Russell A Hibbs (1869–1932)

early stage of ideopathic pes cavus, wrote on *The Hysterical Element in Orthopaedics* in 1880, and published two books – *Brief Essays on Orthopaedic Surgery* in 1898 and *Selected Essays on Orthopaedic Surgery* in 1923.

John Ridlon (1852–1936) graduated from the New York College in 1878 and became instructor in orthopaedics at New York University Medical School and an assistant at the NY Orthopaedic Hospital and Dispensary. In 1881 he became assistant to Shaffer at St Luke's. In 1888 he visited Hugh Owen Thomas at Liverpool and became a lifelong friend of Thomas and later of Robert Jones. 'Returning to New York, I personally made in the cellar of my home at 337, W 57th Street, the first Thomas splint ever made in this country and put it on a patient in my service at St Luke's Hospital, a child with hip disease who had been six months with the flexion deformity not reduced at all from 90 degrees. It was completely corrected in two weeks. Then my consultant, Dr Newton M Shaffer, chanced to discover it and ordered me to remove it (and to resume the 'American method' of traction with motion). I refused, and the result was that the trustees did not reappoint me at the end of the year. This led to Thomas's publication, at his own expense, of the monograph entitled *An Argument with the Censor of St. Luke's Hospital*, and the mailing of a copy to every distinguished surgeon in the world.'

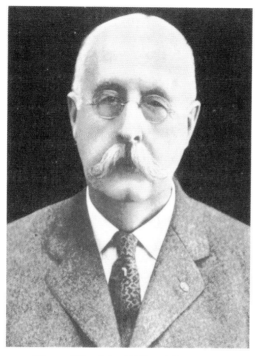

Figure 192   John Ridlon (1852–1936)

In fact, the *Argument* had been published in 1876 as a review of the treatment of hip disease and only acquired its more aggressive title in 1889. It was not only a counterblast to Shaffer's treatment of his friend; it also summarized his feelings about American orthopaedic surgeons. Some, like Shaffer, Thomas vituperated for disagreeing with his principle of absolute rest for diseased joints; others, like Judson, he vilified for pirating his views without acknowledgement; a few, like Bauer, he respected. Of what use were mere statistics when his own reliable rule of detecting the onset of disease and cure in hip disease was ignored? 'As soon as American surgeons master the details of the simple hip flexion test, the American method of treating hip joint affections will be relegated to the history of surgery!' He demolished Shaffer's arguments on the results of treatment published in the New York Medical Journal of 1887, paragraph by paragraph 'Better results would have followed if the patient had received no treatment whatever'. Thomas catalogued the American gamut of surgical sectaries, each with a plan of treatment and all in opposition, as 'extensionists, posterior fixationists, anticoncussionists, distractionists, plaster of Parisists, profrictionists and do-nothingists.' Also, 'the gentleman who undertakes the responsibility of Censor without competent knowledge deserves the neglect which too often falls to the lot of the meritorious' (i.e Thomas himself). We have deviated, but not unprofitably. At one of the earliest meetings of the newly-formed American Orthopaedic Association a sober critic admitted Thomas's excellent results but ascribed them, first, to their having been obtained in private practice, and, second, to English mothers tolerating a degree of uncleanliness in their children, due to their never being removed from their splints, which would be unbearable to their American counterparts!

Ridlon moved to Chicago, where he was instructor at Northwestern University and became professor in 1889 for 16 years. The early years there were difficult, it was hard to build a practice, and in 1891–2 he wrote to Robert Jones in dejection and received by return a lifesaving contribution of a thousand dollars, plus continuing non financial help and advice. When he published his orthopaedic textbook in 1889, he gave Jones's name as co-author though the latter's contribution cannot have been very great, as Ridlon says in the preface that it was written to preserve what was of most value in Thomas's original teachings.

Ridlon served as secretary of the infant American Orthopaedic Association for 16 years, playing one man against another and manipulating its affairs and openly boasting of his president-making powers, interrupted only by his own presidency in 1897. 'In 1890 I proceeded to elect A B Judson as President and myself as Secretary...I served as Secretary for 16 years and one year as President. I was counted as 'Boss' of the Association because I elected every officer except Weigel.'

We have referred to the establishment of the Hospital for the Ruptured and Crippled under James Knight in 1863 and of the New York Orthopaedic Dispensary under Taylor in 1866, and some attention should now be given to St Luke's Hospital. This was opened in 1858 at Fifth Avenue and 54th Street and had an orthopaedic department from the outset. Although a general hospital, the 2nd Annual Report (1859–60) states, 'The ward devoted to the treatment of children is a new and most important feature of the hospital...diseases of the spine and hip have claimed a large share of attention. For the spine, the support invented by Dr H G Davis of this city has been a most valuable ally and more recently the splint invented by the same gentleman for hip disease has been used with thorough success'. The 7th Annual Report (1864–5), referring to the wretched state of children admitted with hip disease and the marked improvement effected in the ward, asserts that 'the modern treatment of hip disease by means of the weight and pulleys was inaugurated in the children's ward of this hospital'. Many of these patients were tuberculous and cases of Pott's disease averaged 14 a year. In the 1860s a country branch was established at St Johnland on Long Island.

Charles Fayette Taylor was on the staff of both the New York Dispensary and St Luke's and, as the Dispensary had no beds of its own until 1873, children requiring hospitalization were admitted to St Luke's nearby, an additional burden. A designated orthopaedic surgeon was not appointed until 1872, when Shaffer was given the post and, as we know, served as Attending Orthopaedic Surgeon between 1873 and 1888; when Taylor resigned from the Dispensary in 1876, Shaffer became surgeon-in-chief at that institution also. Ridlon was appointed 'assistant to the House Surgeon' in June 1878, House Surgeon a year later and assistant to Shaffer in 1881. His departure has been recorded.

At the time of Shaffer's appointment, the 15th Annual Report states, 'The children's ward has had 118 inmates; the great majority are of spinal complaints and hip joint diseases...with a highly competent gentleman in that department skilled in this branch of surgery St Luke's has become to a considerable extent an orthopaedic Institution for children.' The hospital was transferred to 113th Street in 1896. Adult patients were not admitted until 1930, and these included fractures, mainly hip fractures in elderly women. In 1890, Thaddeus Halsted Myers became Attending Orthopaedic Surgeon until his death in 1925, followed by Edwin Pyle (1925–30), Mather Cleveland (1930–50), who had only three beds when first appointed, and then by David M Bosworth for the period 1951–9.

One must not ignore a rather maverick figure, one of those general surgeons whose energy and initiative have contributed so much to orthopaedics. **John B Murphy** (1857–1916) was somewhat of an outsider, the poor son of Irish immigrants. Apprenticed to a general practitioner, he then qualified at Rush Medical College, Chicago, and travelled to Europe to study under Billroth in Vienna and others in Germany, returning to practise general surgery in Chicago in 1884. A man of fanatic vigour and innovation, he made some outstanding contributions to orthopaedic surgery. Long before this became a separate discipline, and while many still restricted themselves to appliance treatment, Murphy devised surgical approaches to every type of orthopaedic condition, not merely in a spirit of adventure but based on a personal and experimental study of the anatomy and physiology of bones, joints and tendons[42]. He developed interpositional (fascial) arthroplasty of the hip, knee and elbow, shoulder and wrist, for the first time in the US. He used wire tension bands for olecranon fractures and devised an operation for recurrent dislocation of the shoulder and used nail fixation for malleolar fractures. He was one of the first really great American orthopaedic *surgeons*, as distinct from mere orthopaedists. His arrival on the surgical scene, almost from nowhere, his development of an enormous practice and his energy in attacking the most diverse fields of surgery all invite comparison with Doyen, in Paris, at much the same period.

We now consider a small but influential group of New England orthopaedic surgeons centred on Boston, taking them in order of birth.

Edward Hickling Bradford (1848–1926) was characterized by Sir Arthur Keith as 'the chief link between the old school and the new[43].' From Harvard Medical School he went to the Massachusetts General Hospital and in 1874 began a two year stay in Europe, spending some time with Thomas, and then had a brief spell with Taylor in New York. Back in Boston he tried general practice, was influenced by Buckminster Brown, and returned to Taylor at the New York Orthopaedic Dispensary. By 1876 he was in Boston again, at the House of the Good Samaritan under Buckminster Brown, whom he succeeded in 1880 as surgeon-in-chief. Shortly after, he was appointed also to the Boston City and Boston Children's Hospitals, but always as a fine general surgeon with a main interest in orthopaedic surgery. As chief of orthopaedics at the Children's hospital, he attracted many brilliant young men, Robert W Lovett, Elliott G Bracket, Robert B Osgood, Arthur T Legg and James W Sever.

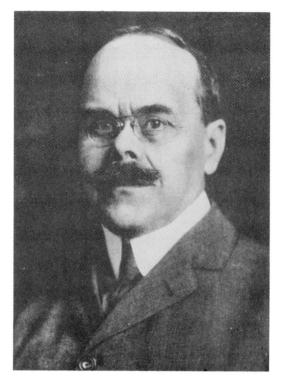

Figure 193   Edward H Bradford (1848–1926)

In 1903 he became first John Ball and Buckminster Brown professor of orthopaedic surgery at Harvard Medical School, a post he held to 1912, and was Dean of the School during 1912–18. Meanwhile, in 1894, after visiting the *Pio Istituto dei Rachitici* in Milan, he had founded the Boston Industrial School for Crippled and Deformed Children; later he initiated the Massachusetts State Hospital School for Crippled Children at Canton, Massachusetts, an infirmary and training centre for cases of skeletal tuberculosis, poliomyelitis and spastic paralysis in that order of frequency. Sadly, he was almost totally blinded in a bicycle accident in his late fifties.

His *Treatise on Orthopaedic Surgery*, written with Robert W Lovett and published by William Wood in New York in 1890, was the standard text of his day and the most advanced of the time, with some 800 illustrations and over 200 pages on hip disease. It described techniques for laminectomy and hip disarticulation and was the first to discuss prevention as well as treatment, but it relegated fractures and dislocations to books on general surgery. It was reissued in 1899, 1905, 1911 and 1915 and was later edited by Robert Jones and Lovett.

Bradford wrote on congenital dislocation of the hip[44], scoliosis[45], club-foot[46], tenoplasty[47] (including 37 transplants by 1897, the extension of muscles by silk sutures e.g. of the trapezius into the deltoid). For club-foot he used wrenching followed by plaster, also Achilles tenotomy and plantar fasciotomy, 'The literature of the treatment of club foot is ... that of unvarying success ... and yet in practice there is no lack of half-cured or relapsed cases ... In club foot, half-cures are practically no cures at all. The great test of the cured club foot is the position of the foot in walking. There should not be the slightest attempt to return to deformity at any period[48].' He invented the Bradford frame for the treatment of spinal disease and a traction table to reduce congenital dislocation of the hip, for which he also practised open reduction with division of the hourglass constriction.

Robert Williamson Lovett (1859–1924) was a Harvard graduate who did general surgery at the Boston City Hospital for a year and was then attracted to New York by the developing orthopaedic services of Sayre, Taylor, Shaffer and Gibney. He was one of the original invitees to the inaugural meeting of the American Orthopaedic Association in 1877 and became President 11 years later. After only a few months in New York, he resumed his Boston post but at the turn of the century resigned to join Bradford at the Children's Hospital, where he initiated clinics for poliomyelitis, scoliosis, spastic paralysis, etc. He became surgeon-in-chief of the Massachusetts Hospital School for Crippled and Deformed Children and of the private Peabody Home for children with skeletal tuberculosis. He wrote on scoliosis[49] and collaborated

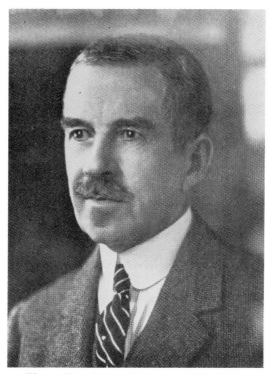

Figure 194   Robert W Lovett (1859–1924)

with Robert Jones in a new text, *Orthopaedic Surgery*, developed from his work with Bradford, which appeared in 1924; and he actually died in that year while visiting Jones in Liverpool.

Elliott G Brackett (1860–1943) was, as has so often been the case, directed to the practice of orthopaedics by a crippling condition in his youth. He was administrative chief of orthopaedic services in the US Army in World War I and described one of the very early good hip reconstruction operations in the 1920s, when this and the Whitman reconstruction were the two commonest procedures for chronic hip disease. In 1921 he assumed editorship of the *American Journal of Orthopaedic Surgery* from Winnett Orr and changed its name to the *Journal of Bone and Joint Surgery*.

Joel Goldthwait (1867–1961) was a great Boston orthopaedist of the early decades of the 20th century, with a major interest in posture but also inventor of a well known procedure for recurrent dislocation of the patella. In 1909, he became head of the first orthopaedic department to be established at the Massachusetts General Hospital; there had been no previous orthopaedic facilities for adults, though John Ball Brown had established a children's service earlier. He is known for his historic paper on the treatment of lumbar disc prolapse by operation in 1911[50]. This related to a man who developed bilateral sciatica followed by paraplegia after a lifting strain, and in whom

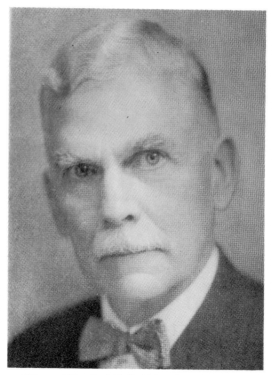

Figure 195   Joel E Goldthwait (1867–1961)

a laminectomy from L1 to S3 was performed by Harvey Cushing with partial recovery. Goldthwait had already postulated disc prolapse as a theoretic possibility, but with associated 'lumbosacral instability' as the causal factor, to be treated by manipulation. (It may be convenient to add here that the neurosurgeon, Walter Dandy, operated in 1929 for 'a loose cartilage from the intervertebral disk, simulating tumor of the spinal cord[51]', and indeed these lesions were long taken to be chondromata[52–55] until the historic paper by Mixter and Barr, also from the Massachusetts General Hospital, in 1934[56], reporting 19 operations for disc prolapse; 4 cervical, 4 dorsal, 10 lumbar and 1 sacral. They showed the value of myelography and that lateral foraminal lesions might have a negative myelogram. Their first operations were transdural, but later Love used a lateral extradural approach.)

Royal Whitman (1857–1946) was for many years chief of service at the Hospital for the Ruptured and Crippled, now the Hospital for Special Surgery, in New York City. He is best known for two particular interests. The first was in flat-foot[57] and the operative management of paralyzed feet (which led to his extensive adoption of astragalectomy, a technique he had originally despised). The second was his reconstruction of the hip, originally devised for ununited fracture but extended to pathologic dislocation and arthrosis (then called arthritis deformans). His initial paper[58] states the

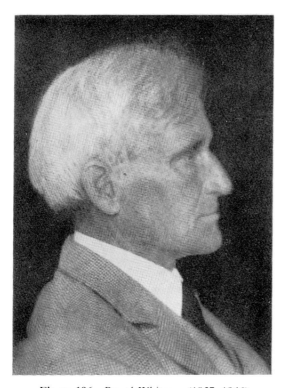

Figure 196   Royal Whitman (1857–1946)

essentials: that it was not only superior to arthrodesis, where fusion could never be guaranteed, but also to simple resection even when the implanted neck stump was covered with a fascial flap, for then the trochanter impinged on the acetabular rim whereas Whitman transplanted it downwards with its muscles, incidentally increasing stability and abduction power.

E G Abbott (1870–1938) of Portland, Maine, specialized in treating scoliosis by suspension in a hammock with lateral pressure pads applied to the convexities of the curve, followed by the application of a plaster jacket. This correction was thus applied mainly via the ribs, which Sir Arthur Keith thought a superficial method 'not affecting the deep essential deformity of the spine' (Keith emphasized the importance of rotation and hence of the discs). Abbott's method recalls that of Andry in 1743:

> 'If the Spine be crooked in the Form of an S, the best method you can take to mend it is to have recourse to a Whalebone Bodice, stuffed in such a manner that the stuffed parts exactly answer to the Protuberances which ought to be repressed, and these Bodices must be renewed every three months at least. One thing very necessary to be observed is, that in proportion as these Protuberances diminish, the stuffing must be increased, without which all your Pains will be lost…'

The last 19th century figure we shall mention here is that of **Thomas G Morton** (1835–1903), a Philadelphian, active in the Civil War, who founded the Philadelphia Orthopaedic Hospital. He described his eponymous metatarsalgia in 1876[59], stating that the anatomic relations of the 4th and 5th metatarsophalangeal joints were such that the digital branches of the lateral plantar nerve were pinched between the metatarsal heads, and that he had cured a case by excision of the 4th joint. Of course, he had identified the wrong space; the neuroma and its bursa lie between the heads and necks of the 3rd and 4th metatarsals, and it is interesting that this had been recognized as long before as 1845 by Lewis Durlacher, chiropodist to the British Court, as 'another form of neuralgic affection occasionally attacking the plantar nerve on the sole of the foot, between the 3rd and 4th metatarsophalangeal joints… the spot where the pain is produced can… be exactly covered by the finger. The pain becomes very severe while walking, or whenever the foot is put to the ground[60].'

One cannot avoid adding here that **Albert H Freiberg** (1868–1940), a Cincinnati surgeon and President of the American Orthopaedic Association in 1910, described 'infraction' of the head of the second metararsal in 1914[61]. But this involved the second metatarsophalangeal joint and led to local thickening and grating thought to be due to injury. (Four of his six cases were young girls who had had provocative trauma. Three had loose bodies, removed in two by dorsal arthrotomy, and the others were treated by a felt pad or steel sole-plate; no other operations and no excisions were done).

Once we enter the 20th century, American orthopaedics offers such a plethora of famous names that some ruthlessness (and individiousness) is inevitable in selection. No attempt at a general and representative portrayal of the period can be given in the space available.

Robert Osgood (1873–1956) of Boston was one of the group of orthopaedic surgeons who worked in England with Robert Jones in World War I. He was chief of orthopaedic surgery at Massachusetts General Hospital afterwards, following Brackett, and director of Children's Hospital from 1922 after Lovett. An early radiologist, he developed skin cancer. Osgood was a close associate of Sir Harry Platt in England when they worked together under Robert Jones and a background eminence in promoting the formation of the British Orthopaedic Association.

William Stevenson Baer (1872–1931), a Johns Hopkins graduate of 1898, was the first head of orthopaedics at that hospital and served the department, eventually as chief, for 31 years. He initially worked as a surgical intern under Harvey Cushing, who had had experience in fracture treatment at the Massachusetts General and in orthopaedics at the Boston Children's Hospital, and Cushing recommended Professor Halsted in 1900 to second Baer in setting up an orthopaedic clinic. (It is interesting that Halsted was one of

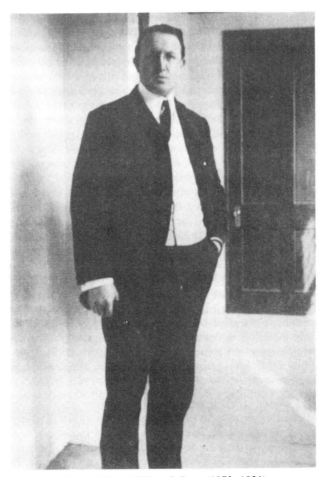

Figure 197   William S Baer (1872–1931)

the very first to plate fractures, under the influence of Hansman in Hamburg, at much the same time as Arbuthnot Lane.) Baer also went to Boston to learn his trade, returned to organize the new department at Johns Hopkins, and was appointed assistant in orthopaedic surgery in 1901–7 and associate professor in 1910, but not a full visiting surgeon until 1920. Baer yearly visited the leading orthopaedic surgeons in Europe; Lorenz in Germany, Putti in Bologna, Calvé in France, Robert Jones in England.

Baer was a stimulating teacher. He is known for his interest in interposition arthroplasty, using membrane from the pig's bladder, with the best results in the temporomandibular and hip joints[62]; but in the late 1920s this was overtaken by the Smith-Petersen cup arthroplasty for the latter. He was an enthusiast of manipulation of the sacroiliac joint for low back pain and sciatica and treated over a thousand cases (at this time Smith-Petersen was fusing this innocuous joint and claimed equal success). He also treated arthritis with vaccines from lymph node cultures. In 1917 he became orthopaedic consultant to the AEF on the Western Front, with Brackett and Osgood, and became impressed with the healthy granulation of untreated wounds infested with maggots. This had been noted previously by Paré in the 16th century and by Larrey in Napoleon's Syrian campaign, while J F Zacharias, surgeon in the Confederate Army in the Civil War, deliberately used maggots to cleanse hospital gangrene. Baer experimented with cultured maggots from 1927 and, once he had learned to sterilize them (after causing two cases of tetanus), got excellent results in chronic osteomyelitis until the sulphonamides arrived in the 1930s.

Baer's residents between, say, 1915 and 1931, included some famous names; Isadore Zadek, of New York, who returned to the Hospital for the Ruptured and Crippled; I William Nachlas, with his shelf operation for congenital dislocation of the hip; Ralph K Ghormley, who was with Lovett in Boston from 1922 to 1929 and then became chief of orthopaedics and eventually professor at the Mayo Clinic from 1938 and 1958; Guy W Leadbetter (1923), who became professor at the George Washington Clinic and described his reduction test for hip fractures and osteotomy of the femoral neck for ununited fractures: Harold R Bohlman (1928), who developed the metal hip prosthesis with Austin Moore in South Carolina in 1943, the forerunner of most present-day prostheses (p. 597).

Baer's successor was **George Eli Bennett** (1885–1962), whose career at Johns Hopkins is sometimes considered Baer's greatest contribution to that institution. A New Yorker who graduated in Maryland and was a resident at the Ruptured and Crippled under Gibney in 1909–1910, Bennett returned to Baltimore in 1910 to work with Baer as director of the orthopaedic outpatient service, took over Baer's practice in World War I and directed the Children's Hospital School from 1931 to 1955 after Baer's death. In 1931 he was asked to return to the Hospital for the Ruptured and Crippled as chief surgeon (this was before the arrival of Philip Wilson). His experience in the severe poliomyelitis epidemics of 1917 and 1946 led him to establish the first respirator unit for bulbar palsy in the world. He worked with the American Academy of Orthopaedic Surgeons to organize undergraduate training, also research, was active in recruiting orthopaedic surgeons in

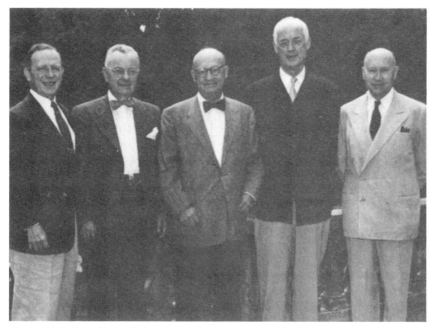

Figure 198   Members of the Class of 1918, Johns Hopkins University School of Medicine, who later became distinguished orthopaedic surgeons (*left to right*) I William Nachlas, Baltimore; Albert H Brewster, Harvard University, Boston; J Albert Key, Washington University, St Louis; Ralph K Ghormley, the Mayo Clinic and Joseph H Kite, Emory University, Atlanta, Georgia

World War II, and President of both the Academy and the American Orthopaedic Association (in 1939–40 and 1941–42 respectively). An important contribution, in WWI, was his transfer of the fibula to the tibia for gross discontinuity of the latter, and he also had a great reputation in the treatment of athletic injuries and was the favourite consultant of many baseball players.

Charles Leroy Lowman (1879–1977) was a California graduate who studied orthopaedics in Boston and, in 1909, founded the Los Angeles Orthopaedic Hospital as a small outpatient clinic and continued there for 63 years. At one time he was the only orthopaedic surgeon between San Francisco and New Orleans and did a 'circuit' by train to treat children throughout the south-west. He devised the insertion of fascial straps to reinforce the power of persistent active segments in the abdominal wall weakened by poliomyelitis, even extending these to the limbs; transplants of fascia passing from the rib-cage to the pelvis hypertrophied and lifted the lower limb from the ground so that wheelchair cases became able to walk with crutches.

There was, in fact, a movement to spread orthopaedic facilities from the established east to the middle and far west of the country; Bauer's early move to St Louis; Ridlon to Chicago. The great **Arthur Steindler** (1878–1959), who had trained under Lorenz in Vienna, came to America in 1907, worked under Ridlon until 1910 and then settled in Iowa, where, as professor, he organized the most advanced state service for crippled children in the USA. He pioneered the application of biomechanics to orthopaedics, and was the first to write in detail on the mechanism of locomotion. His book, *Orthopaedic Operations* of 1943 included various ingenious procedures, such as the plantar stripping for pes cavus and the proximal transplant of the common flexor origin at the elbow for paralysis of the elbow flexors.

We must not forget the pathologists. An early contributor was **Samuel Weissel Gross** (1837–1889), surgical pathologist and lecturer at Jefferson Medical College, who helped to clarify ideas on bone sarcoma – an ancient term, which had been used by Abernethy for tumours 'having a firm and fleshy feel' and by Virchow for lesions with immature connective tissue cells. Gross went in detail into the varied patterns of cytology and matrix in different types of lesion, reproduced in their metastases, noted the method of spread and advised radical amputation, though with a place for occasional local excision[63].

Another figure in the early decades of this century was **Kolodny**[64,65], while in Boston in 1921 **Ernest A Codman** developed the first Registry of Bone Sarcoma in collaboration with the American College of Surgeons. Other names are those of **Charles F Geschickter** and **M M Copeland** of Johns Hopkins, while Joseph Colt Bloodgood of Baltimore (1867–1935) was one of the first to describe giant-cell tumour of bone and **James Ewing** of Bellevue described the reticulum-cell sarcoma that bears his name. S Otani of Mount Sinai Hospital categorized solitary eosinophil granuloma. We should note, too, the definition of the Hand–Schüller–Christian disease in the early century. Arthur Schüller was German; Alfred Hand was a Philadelphian and Henry A Christian worked at Harvard. This led to recognition of the lipoid granulomatoses of bone and of the bony changes in Gaucher's disease. An interesting episode was the observation by **William Bradley Coley** (1863–1936) that bone sarcoma sometimes regressed during erysipelas (something observed earlier by Paget in England), and he treated these tumours by streptococcus injections over many years at the Hospial for the Ruptured and Crippled.

Henry L Jaffe (1896–1979) was the most distinguished bone pathologist of modern times, developing a system for the logical evaluation of lesions of bone which has governed developments in this field ever since. In 1928 he became pathologist to the Hospital for Joint Diseases, a post he held to retirement in 1964. His main contributions relate to the endocrine glands and bone, the development, structure and pathology of the skeleton, and specific skeletal diseases. He wrote *Tumors and Tumorous Conditions of Bones and Joints* in 1958 and *Metabolic, Degenerative and Inflammatory Dieases of Bones and Joints* in 1972. He worked on the role of the parathyroids in osteoclastic bone resorption, and on biochemical factors (especially alkaline phosphatase) in rickets, Paget's disease and osteitis fibrosa. With Lichtenstein, he defined the nature of osteoclastoma in 1932, of osteoid osteoma in 1935, giant-cell tumour in 1940, eosinophil granuloma in the same year, pigmented villonodular synovitis in 1941, chondroblastoma in 1942, nonossifying fibroma in that year, chondromyxoid fibroma in 1948 and aneurysmal bone cyst in 1952. Jaffe brought order to the chaos of bone pathology and was often the final arbiter in difficult lesions sent from the world over.

Louis Lichtenstein (1906–1977) was pathologist for 12 years at the Hospital for Joint Diseases and was later consultant on bone tumours to the California Tumor Registry. He wrote on many aspects and recognized new entities, such as 'histiocytosis X', providing a unified concept for eosinophilic granuloma and the Letterer–Siwe and Hand–Schüller–Christian diseases. His books include *Bone Tumors* and *Diseases of Bones and Joints*.

A note about publications. We shall refer more than once to the meeting at Shaffer's house in New York on 29th January 1887 which founded the American Orthopedic Association, and it bears repetition since this was the first organized group of orthopaedists anywhere in the world. Shaffer spoke of 'the need for such an association, not only to bring together American orthopaedic surgeons, but also to secure a better recognition in Europe for American orthopaedic surgery[66]'. Therefore, there had to be a journal, and its original title was the *Transactions of the American Orthopedic Association*, whose first volume appeared in 1889. In 1903, this was replaced by the *American Journal of Orthopedic Surgery*. In 1918 the editor, Mark Rogers, moved that, as an orthopaedic association had recently been formed in Britain, the American Orthopedic Association should offer the use of its *Journal* as the official organ of the infant British body; and thereafter, from 1919, the cover title was *The Journal of Orthopaedic Surgery*, official publication of the two associations. (The various spellings of 'orthopaedic' and 'orthopedic' at different times are faithfully rendered.) This omission of *American* from the title emphasized the Anglo-American bond and was, of course, born of the comradeship of World War I. The editor of this first volume of the combined journal was H Winnett Orr of Nebraska. Soon the collaboration settled down with Brackett as Editorial Secretary for the AOA, with J L Porter, E W Ryerson and R B Osgood on his editorial committee; the British opposite numbers were Harry Platt as Editorial Secretary for the BOA, plus a committee formed by A S B Bankart, R C Elmslie, E W Hey Groves.

In 1922 the title was changed again, to the *Journal of Bone and Joint Surgery*, still a joint publication, but in 1948 the British produced a separate British volume of the journal, stated on the cover as 'representing the science and practice of orthopaedic surgery in the USA and the Commonwealth of British Nations'. The old *American Journal of Orthopedic Surgery* was not widely read; in 1921, 32 years after the appearance of the first volume of the Transactions, there were only 797 subscribers. Brackett's drive with the new *Journal of Bone and Joint Surgery* increased this five-fold by his death in 1942. In 1935, the *Journal* also became the organ of the American Academy of Orthopedic Surgery (founded in 1932 as a wider grouping than the AOA). Later still, it came to embrace the orthopaedic associations of Australia, Canada, New Zealand, South Africa, the Western Orthopedic Association and, between 1951 and 1975, the American Society for Surgery of the Hand.

The second great editor after Brackett was William Rogers, and it was Rogers who negotiated with the British over their issue of the *J.B.Jt.Surg.* (*B*), not without resistance in the US; but the British wanted their own journal and felt that circulation of an essentially American journal in the UK gave an insufficient audience. The combined journal was an immediate and lasting success.

From 1958, the third great editor was Thornton Brown, who wrote that 'an orthopedic surgeon could with some assurance assume that, if he read the Journal completely, he would keep up to date, at least with respect to major clinical and research advances in his specialty.' But the Journal was not confined to English–speakers; it was read world-wide and exerted a unifying influence. Now the world has some 60 orthopaedic journals! Nevertheless, after the appearance of *Clinical Orthopaedics* in 1953, it is safe to say that the *Journal of Bone and Joint Surgery*, *Clinical Orthopaedics* and *Acta Orthopaedica Scandinavica* became the leading English language orthopaedic journals of the later 20th century.

We must also mention the *Manual of Orthopaedic Surgery*, first issued by the AOA in 1949 to teach residents the elements of orthopaedic history-taking and examination. This has been revised periodically and includes a standardized system of measuring joint movements – 'an amazing compilation of what I would term 'physical diagnosis' in orthopedics,' as Mark Coventry of the Mayo Clinic called it[67].

A fascinating and informative survey of the evolution of orthopaedic surgery in the USA in the first half of the 20th century was given at the midpoint of the century by Leo Mayer[68]. **Leo Mayer** (1884–1972) was born in Alabama but educated at New York and Harvard, graduating from Columbia, and was an intern at the Mount Sinai Hospital in 1909–12. He did postgraduate work with Fritz Lange in Munich and collaborated with Konrad Biesalski on tendon transplantation (see p. 193), Mayer's work on tendons presaging that of Sterling Bunnell. In the early years of World War I he was in charge of a Red Cross hospital in Germany and wrote a monograph on the orthopaedic management of gunshot injuries. With America's entry into the war, he went to work with Fred Albee at the New York Postgraduate Hospital and soon became attending orthopaedic surgeon at the Hospital for Joint Diseases and associate professor of orthopaedic surgery at the New York Postgraduate Medical School. Mayer did pioneer work in reconstructive tendon operations for poliomyelitis and in clarifying the natural history of bone tumours. From 1929 to 1954 he was an associate editor of the *Journal of Bone and Joint Surgery* and was also prominent in organizing rehabilitation and vocational training centres.

The American Orthopaedic Association had been founded at the meeting at Shaffer's house in January 1887: ten of those present were in favour, two against, two abstained. Its first formal meeting was in June of that year at the New York Academy of Medicine, with Gibney as first chairman, Lovett as temporary secretary (soon replaced by Sayre) and 35 invited members. The proceedings of the first 15 years, published in the *Transactions*, reflect the conflict between the old brace mechanics (Shaffer wanted orthopaedic surgeons to confine themselves to mechanical therapy, 'To mingle surgery and mechanics is to endanger both') and such younger men as Russell Hibbs, who replaced Shaffer as head of the New York Orthopaedic Hospital in 1898, who wanted them to be combined. There was also the continuing

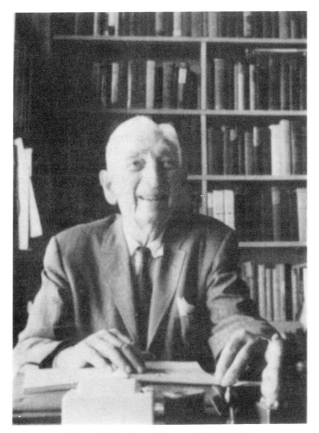

Figure 199   Leo Mayer (1884–1972)

conflict with the general surgeons. As Phelps wrote in 1894, 'The orthopaedist was always at war with the general surgeons[69].'

When, in 1891, Gibney quoted an eminent general surgeon as saying, 'The next work on orthopaedic surgery will likewise tell us all about fractures and dislocations,' it was because this was intended as a sneer. (It took a long time to convince the general surgeons that traumatology was a proper sphere for orthopaedic surgeons, and well on in the next century we find Robert Jones still faintly apologetic about the matter*.) However, the specialists won the battle in a fair fight and perhaps the generalists were not unhappy

---

*In 1913, Jones wrote a paper on 'An orthopaedic view of the treatment of fractures' for the American *Journal*, saying that 'every fracture is potentially a deformity and if it becomes a deformity will lead to impairment of function.' The question was not between manipulation and operation: it was 'what means we must adopt in each individual case to give our patients the surest, safest and most complete restoration of function.'

to be relieved of the burden. That orthopaedics came to include fractures was partly due to Whitman's work on the 'unsolved fracture' of the femoral neck, and this arose from his work on hip fractures in children[70-72], who, by definition, were orthopaedic patients (as so long in France) whereas this was less admitted for adults with fractures. Incidentally, this work was done without the help of X-rays, on clinical grounds alone, and established the principles of abduction, internal rotation and traction.

Ketch, in his presidential address for 1897, summarized the papers of the first ten years: there were 292, of which 114 were on skeletal tuberculosis (49 spine, 35 hip, 19 knee), 43 on club-foot, 20 on scoliosis and 14 on congenital dislocation of the hip. Oddly, for the late 19th century, only nine dealt with rickets, six with poliomyelitis and one or two with osteomyelitis. Fractures, low back pain and bone tumours were barely mentioned, and perhaps this is related to the remarkable paucity of references to the newly discovered X-rays. Mayer points out that Lovett, in his presidential address of 1898[73], never once mentioned X-rays, nor did he in his 1900 paper on scoliosis[74]. This may have been because of the lack of fine detail in the films of that period; in fact, the X-ray was often regarded as fallacious.

The treatment of skeletal tuberculosis at that time was mainly conservative; the 'American method' of traction with movement still conflicted with the rigid fixation of Thomas and Robert Jones. There was also conflict with the management of abscesses. Ridlon said 'Leave them alone; not one in a hundred will cause trouble if you just fix the joint', but there were also the aspirators, drainers and excisionists. Excision of the tuberculous hip was now recognized as legitimate, and had first been done by Sayre as far back as 1854; but even by 1890 mortality was around 50 per cent and function in the survivors was poor. The advent of Listerism led to attempted sterilization at operation with carbolic, alcohol or iodoform, with occasional poisoning, sometimes fatal (and mercuric chloride was used to irrigate the wounds during the Indian and Spanish-American Wars). Knee excision was in much better case because it usually resulted in fusion, whether this was intended or not[75]; nevertheless, there was an ideal concept that operation ought to lead to recovery with movement and sound ankylosis was not regarded as a primarily desirable outcome.

In 1891, Hadra proposed wiring the spinous processes for Pott's disease, having had some success in doing so for unstable neck injuries[76]. The mortality of the tuberculous hip over a five-year period was around 10 per cent[77] and late flexion–adduction deformity was commonly corrected by osteotomy in the last two decades of the 19th century[78,79]. The groundwork of the pathology of tuberculous arthritis was laid by Edward H Nichols of Harvard in the 1890s[80] and, as we know, very nearly the final answer to the problem of skeletal tuberculosis was afforded by Waxman with the discovery of streptomycin soon after World War II.

While the American treatment of club-foot at the end of the century was excellent, that of congenital hip dislocation was less so. The Americans invited eminent Europeans to discuss methods, particularly Adolf Lorenz, who, after some vacillation, eventually came down on the side of the 'bloodless' method and against Hoffa's operations[81]. Early US experience was variable and mostly unsuccessful, but eventually Bradford began to get good results and noted the effects of anteversion and the importance of rotation osteotomy[82-84]. Scoliosis remained what Phelps called a 'spectre', not to be cured by any known treatment once bony changes had occurred. In 1900, Lovett showed that lateral flexion was inevitably associated with torsion in cadaver experiments (but this had been known for a very long time[85]).

By 1900 (see Chapter 33), tendon transfer, tenotomy and fusion were commonplace for poliomyelitis and spastic paralysis, and it was often considered that the best results in the foot were obtained by astragalectomy and calcaneo-tibial fusion[86].

There was a great range of attitudes to surgery. The conservatives, like Shaffer, never operated and called in a general surgeon when intervention was inevitable, especially for amputation. Others operated freely. Thus, Goldthwait did 38 operations for internal derangement of the knee by 1900[87], while Bradford's procedure for recurrent dislocation of the patella was very much as performed today[88]. What was essentially the modern Keller operation was being done by Steele for hallux valgus in 1898[89]. Others at the turn of the century operated for ununited fractures of the femoral neck by freshening the surfaces and inserting nails, screws, bone or ivory pegs[90,91].

Despite the immense amount of hard clinical work and the investment in academic research programmes, the American Orthopaedic Association and its members received little kudos in the medical world generally. In his presidential address of 1900, Sherman pointed out that only 38 out of 76 universities listed orthopaedic teaching in their curricula and that this was really thorough in only five[92]. Things suddenly began to change, just at the time when Augustus Wilson, in his presidential address of 1902, advocated the replacement of the *Transactions* by the *American Journal of Orthopedic Surgery*[93]. There was then a period of exponential growth, linked with advances in X-rays, pathology (especially tumoral), techniques in bone-grafting, tendon and joint operations, in the management of trauma, all aided by the increase in organizations, many of them lay, interested in the orthopaedic management of the crippled child and adult, and by the accelerating influence of the two world wars. In World War I, there had been only two colonels in charge of orthopaedics: Brackett at the US headquarters of the Surgeon–General and Goldthwait in the European theatre. In World War II, Norman Kirk was the Surgeon–General of the Army and very senior orthopaedic officers were everywhere.

In the vital transition period between 1903 and 1918, technical advances were not all that counted. There was the acknowledgment of community responsibility for cripples, rehabilitation, workmen's compensation, the founding of many orthopaedic societies, contact with foreign orthopaedic surgeons, the expansion of university teaching, the emphasis on restoration of function. Mayer says that, had the first world war occurred 15 years earlier, orthopaedic surgery could not possibly have played the part it did. One very important factor was the extension of orthopaedics from children to adults; this was a really novel development in the first decade of the 20th century. Brackett said, in 1905, 'It is within the remembrance of even most of the younger men when the orthopaedic work was almost entirely confined to children[94].' In the same year Gibney urged that the adult cripple 'should receive the same scientific treatment that has so long been meted out to the children,' and this meant that a mass of new material came forward for investigation: low back syndromes, tumours, shoulder and hip problems and many others[95].

Thus, there was the interest taken in the matter of low back pain by Goldthwait, Osgood and others, leading to the study of congenital anomalies, resection of the transverse process of L5, sacroiliac fusion, lumbrosacral fusion, the ideal that gluteal tendinitis might be the cause of sciatica. Fusion gained increasing popularity with developments in bone-graft surgery, which originated with the work of Albee and Hibbs in Pott's disease[96,97] and was transferred to mechanical problems. Bone grafting then began to be further adapted by Albee and others to the treatment of ununited fractures[98] and even fresh fractures[99], and then to the fusion of arthritic joints as in osteoarthritis of the hip[100].

All the bone graft work initiated by Albee had originated with Pott's disease, which continued to baffle orthopaedic surgeons in the early years of this century. Many tried tuberculin, as early as Ridlon in 1907[101]; others used vaccines and sera, all vaguely based on the work of Almroth Wright at St Mary's Hospital in London and his 'opsonic index' (which crops up in Shaw's *The Doctor's Dilemma*) but with little success. Mayer quotes the essentially disgruntled remarks of Ely in 1911, 'This entire subject forms a reproach on surgery...surely one might expect to find in regard to it among intelligent medical men a practical consensus of opinion...to which one may resort for light...No such scientific opinion exists as to any phase of the disease[102].' This impatience was already producing an answer, for in that same year of 1911 Russell Hibbs and Fred Albee, both in New York and working independently, published their papers on spinal fusion for tuberculosis. The *idea* of fusion, or at least stabilization, was not new for Lange, in Germany, in 1910 had implanted steel rods paravertebrally[103]. By 1916, Albee was able to report 539 cases of Pott's disease so treated with arrest in over 80 per cent; and somewhat earlier, Ryerson, describing 26 personal cases[104], called the operation 'the acme of conservative treatment', which is exactly what Girdlestone at Oxford used to say in essence, that it saved *time*. (It is iconoclastic now to have to report, based on experience with chemotherapy, that the best results of fusion are when it fails and allows natural collapse and consolidation, suggesting that fusion gave good results because of the accompanying fixation and general treatment.) Fusion was extended to the tuberculous hip and knee. Albee developed his electric saw and applied grafting to a wide range of conditions[105].

On a converse course, there was a development of interposition arthroplasty of the hip, knee and elbow, marked by the use of autogenous fascia or animal membranes, fostered by Baer[106-108] and aided technically by Murphy's ingenious instrumentation for the hip joint[109]. Perhaps the best exponent of the fascial interposition method, both in the operating theatre and in writing was Willis Campbell, who gave the definitive account in his *Operative Orthopaedics* in 1939.

There were many experimental studies and technical innovations in other fields. The paralyses due to poliomyelitis presented a damaging and recurrent problem. Lange in Berlin had been using tendon transplantation, with prolongation by silk threads if necessary to secure attachment to bone, and the construction of silk ligaments, and was invited to address the American Orthopaedic Association in 1910[110-113]. The work that Leo Mayer had initiated with Biesalski on physiologic tendon transplantation[114] and tenodesis crossed the Atlantic and was also taken up by Gallie and others in Canada[115]. Whitman's astragalectomy for paralytic calcaneus in 1901 rapidly became popular (partly because it is still so useful in the Third World for many foot deformities[116]). But the masterly contributions to the corrective surgery of congenital or acquired foot deformities were made by Michael Hoke of Atlanta in the first two decades of the century; his 'operation for stabilizing paralytic feet' of 1921, a subtalar fusion plus resection and replacement of the head of the talus was well on the way to formal triple fusion and was really conceived and practised years earlier than the date of publication[117,118].

In the first decades, too, it began to be felt that it was time to exorcise the 'spectre' of scoliosis. Lovett had done some research into the mechanisms of curvature, angulation and rotation and now, in 1913, Abbott introduced his method of hammock reclination in flexion with rotational and lateral compression and got an enthusiastic reception in Europe, though his results were questioned by a committee of the American Orthopaedic Association just as a French commission had investigated those of Guérin (p. 250)[120]. Abbott insisted in 1917 that his method could produce complete correction[121], yet it did not catch on because it was stressful to the patient and tended to produce deformities of the ribs and pressure sores. 1917 also marks the appearance of what was to become a famous name, that of Marius Smith-Petersen, describing his new approach to the hip joint[122].

The full value of X-rays was now being recognized. Earlier, as we have noted, attitudes tended to be dismissive. Now, betwen 1900 and World War I, a flood of reports began to clarify previously obscure conditions; rickets[123], hip tuberculosis[124], chondrodystrophy[125], multiple exostoses[126], adolescent coxa vara[127], infraction of the second metatarsal head[128], and many others, including the 'quiet hip disease' (i.e. Perthes' disease) reported by Allison and Brook in 1915 as 'osteochondritis deformans juvenilis'[129].

It should be noted that nearly all the contemporary orthopaedic publications appeared in the *American Journal of Orthopedic Surgery*. They seem not to have been wanted elsewhere, in the staider journals of general surgery, and at the same time the new journal provided an outlet for the burst of new work; it is a matter of observation that men are often reluctant to carry out clinical studies or research if there is little hope of publication.

At this time, too, there was a growing sense of the responsibility of the orthopaedic surgeon to the community. Brackett had urged in 1905 that young orthopaedists should settle in growing communities where they were needed[130]. This may well have been necessary advice then, when many parts of the United States were unprovided, though there is now the opposite risk of overprovision and its attendant hazards. Goldthwait stressed the importance of posture from early life[131,132] and the lessons were applied by the American Posture League founded in 1914. Domestic hygiene was also studied in relation to skeletal tuberculosis and education facilities developed for crippled children. The first state hospital for these (as distinct from earlier charitable institutions) was provided by the legislature of Minnesota in 1897 under the influence of A J Gillette, a founding member of the AOA. Yet, in 1909 he had to complain in an editorial in the *American Journal of Orthopedic Surgery* that state provision over the US was still woefully deficient, and indeed nonexistent in many states. Another forceful advocate of state cripple care was Winnett Orr of Nebraska, where a state orthopaedic hospital was already in existence when he wrote in 1911[133].

The social view was of course advanced by the development of compensation law and practice, and also by the growth of social services attached to hospitals. State care was paralleled and for long overshadowed by the rapid growth of hospitals and care organizations based on private charity, as when Hoke of Atlanta started the negotiations with a masonic order in 1914 that led to the first Shriners' Hospital in Louisiana in 1922 and many others since (in South as well as in North America). Throughout this period (we are speaking of the decade leading up to 1914) there was a growth of orthopaedic clubs and societies; in Boston in 1896, Chicago in 1910, the orthopaedic sections of the New York Academy of Medicine and of the American Medical Association in 1902 and 1912 respectively. There was also a slow but steady expansion of orthopaedic teaching in the medical schools. By 1910 the Association was able to record that 41 out of 110 undergraduate schools taught orthopaedic surgery as a separate subject (35 professors; 64 hours) or combined with general surgery in 51 (13 professors; 47 hours).

THE CIVIL WAR

The medical and surgical aspects of this conflict were recorded in greater detail than those of any previous war in *The Medical and Surgical History of the War of the Rebellion*, prepared under the direction of the Surgeon–General, US Army, Washington 1870–6. This is extraordinarily thorough although, written necessarily from the Union side, cannot be complete. It lists the various surgical procedures and their results, often detailed for individual patients by name and illustrated by photographs and by drawings of the specimens that were collected for the army medical museum. It is an extraordinary achievement.

To proceed by anatomic regions, gunshot wounds of the spine were treated by removal of fragments of balls or shells and of any damaged bony processes. There is a fascinating discussion of the merits and demerits of formal trephining, which includes a historical review. Trephining had been mentioned by Paré and Heister (*q.v.*) in mediaeval times. In 1814, Henry Cline of St Thomas's Hospital in London had performed a laminectomy for an injury at T7-8 pressing on the cord with fatal outcome. Tyrell, also in England, had operated twice, in 1822 and 1827, again uselessly. It is mentioned in Astley Cooper's *Treatise* of 1842. The first to trephine the spine in the USA was John Rhea Barton in 1824 and there were a number of other cases, nearly all failures. The operation was advocated by the Anglo-Parisian Brown-Séquard in a course of lectures given in Philadelphia in 1860, in which he said that from animal experiments it was 'quite evident that the laying bare of the spinal cord is not a dangerous operation.' However, Brown-Séquard was a physician who encouraged surgeons to operate on the neurological lesions in which he was interested (see p. 339). Bernhard Heine at Würzburg had experimented similarly and reported in 1864 that most of his animals died. Malgaigne called it 'a desperate and blind operation'. The Surgeon–General concludes that the removal of loose bony fragments is reasonable, but not formal trephining.

There is a reference to the history of excision of the clavicle, which is dated as far back as 1732 (Renner). In 1823, Charles McCreary of Kentucky had excised the tuberculous clavicle in a boy of 14, who survived many years with excellent function (indeed the clavicle is a dispensable bone). Most of the Civil War cases were partial excisions and complicated by severe neurovascular lesions.

Causalgia is noted, though not by name, treated sometimes by excision of a neuroma, often by amputation. We may ourselves insert here that Silas Weir Mitchell (1829–1914), a Philadelphian who graduated at Jefferson Medical College in 1850 and travelled in Europe and attended Claude Bernard's lectures, joined the Union Army in 1863 and worked in a Philadelphia hospital where the Surgeon–General set aside some beds for nerve injuries and central nervous system injuries. The books Mitchell published, alone and with others[134,135], contain the first use of the term 'causalgia' and describe the terrible suffering, the burning pain and glossy skin, never in the trunk, rarely in the arm or thigh, usually in the hand or foot, the exquisite hyperaesthesia, worse when the skin was dry, a syndrome he believed hitherto undescribed.

852 amputations at the shoulder are recorded with 117 deaths (13.7%). Larrey in the Napoleonic Wars had claimed 90% successes, and Guthrie in the Peninsular War had 19/19 successes in the field, but most of his cases were done later in hospital, and most died. The Civil War results are classified on the basis of primary, delayed and late operations; it is evident that delay tended to give poorer results. Even for amputations at the lower third of the arm the mortality was over 40% and oddly, but uniformly, amputations near the elbow (and knee) had a higher mortality than those higher in the limb, a fact noted often in the medical history of war and as far back as John of Mirfield in England in the 14th century, and probably due to the complexity and relative lack of protection of the structures at this level. Wiring of a compound fracture of the humerus was done on four occasions.

There were many elbow excisions for gunshot wounds, 626 in all with a mortality of up to a third; even when the patients survived, it was often necessary to amputate. Excision might result in either ankylosis or a flail joint, and ankylosis was more likely when the excision had been partial. Even 10% of primary forearm amputations, at any level, proved fatal and the rate rose to a third if the operation were delayed. It is clear that, in all these limb injuries, it was better to take the risk of combining the initial shock with that of an immediate operation than to delay intervention until the condition of the patient and his wound had deteriorated.

Because of reluctance to disarticulate at the shoulder and hip (the mortality for the latter was 83.3%) excision of the head of the humerus or femur was frequent; the former often succeeded, but excision of the hip, at whatever stage, was nearly always fatal. For gunshot fractures of the femur, rather over a third were amputated. We note the malign prognosis of knee wounds, due to suppurative arthritis and popliteal artery damage (the sinister nature of the latter runs like a litany through the histories of latter-day wars).

Until this war, i.e. to around mid-century, there had been a general insistence on immediate amputation for gunshot fractures of the femur; but in the War of the Rebellion this was widely and rapidly modified in favour of splintage and drainage with intent to preserve the limb unless vascular damage made ablation imperative, though a pro-amputation school persisted. This conservatism applied especially to upper third fractures, probably because the results of amputation were so terrible. Various methods were used for splintage, often on a Pott's double inclined plane to flex the hip and knee, or with an *anterior* curved splint held in suspension; there was also traction, sometimes applied with a pulley on the very stretcher, or as Buck's traction in hospital. Only one femoral wiring is recorded, and that fatal. Attempts at preserving the limb with a knee injury, however, either by observation or excision, were usually unsuccessful; amputation, even with a mortality of around 50% was better. In the leg, amputations were by flap or guillotine almost equally; the tendency to bony protrusion in the latter could be lessened by sawing off the crest of the tibia and by applying skin traction to the back of the stump.

At the ankle there was quite frequent success with Syme's amputation, in its later form of tibial section $\frac{1}{2}$–$1\frac{1}{2}$ inches above the joint, together with the malleoli. The Pirogoff amputation was performed to about an equal extent, the tuberosity of the os calcis being applied to the sawn surface of the tibia. While there was a tendency for the Syme's flap to necrose, this was more than matched by the frequency of necrosis or nonunion of the calcanean fragment in the Pirogoff amputation. In both cases, reamputation was frequent.

Hospital gangrene was a problem and a favourite remedy was a strong solution of bromine in potassium bromide, used either for fumigation of the ward or for topical application. Another application was 'chlorinated soda', which is suggestive of Dakin's solution. The bromine seems to have given good results, though some preferred creosote (carbolic) for deep wounds. Because it was recognized that gangrene was acquired in hospital, vaporization of bromine or chlorine in the wards was frequently used.

WORLD WAR I

War with Germany had been seen as inevitable early in 1917. In the *Journal* for March of that year, Goldthwait reported the setting up of committees by the AOA and the orthopaedic section of the AMA to prepare plans for a large number of hospitals to treat soldiers returned from the front, and for reconstructive surgery and subsequent rehabilitation and vocational management, 'the lines followed to be similar to those which have been worked out so admirably in England under the guidance of Colonel Robert Jones.' When America declared war on 7th April 1917, a cable came from Britain to the AOA via the US government asking for six base hospitals and 20 orthopaedic surgeons to help the British, serving under Jones, and in less than three weeks Goldthwait sailed with 20 younger men to Liverpool. The important thing was that both governments now recognized (as the British certainly had not done at the start of the war) the importance of specialized orthopaedic management of wounds and their aftercare and segregation. However, a remark made by Goldthwait to Leo Mayer quoted by the latter in 1959[136] is worth noting, 'Naturally, much of the work was in the field of traumatic surgery, with which few of the orthopaedic men had had much experience,' underlining the painful learning experience of the British in 1914, that the ordinary civilian surgeon had virtually no idea of how to treat the wounds of modern warfare.

Goldthwait studied the work in England and France, planned the requirements of a future American Expeditionary Force, returned to the US and worked out the organization of the Orthopaedic Department of the Army in Washington. He returned to Europe in October 1917 with 45 surgeons, some skilled, some hurriedly trained in the essentials, plus a handful of orthopaedic nurses and occupational therapists, all initially assigned to work with the British under Robert Jones and later transferred to American hospitals to be replaced by new arrivals. At least, the Americans were able to *start* with the Thomas splint on the battlefield, a lesson the British had had to learn the hard way. Again, just as with the British, the general surgeons had to acknowledge that they were unfitted for the treatment of limb injuries and handed these over to orthopaedic colleagues where (and this was far from everywhere) these were available. There were not enough American hospitals in France, so by the late summer of 1919 large numbers of injured, especially with femoral fractures in splints, were ferried out almost directly from the front to the States.

We need not go into much further detail on this, already partly dealt with in Chapter 2, and we can save any sententiousness by merely quoting a 1919 letter from Charles Parker of Chicago to the editor of the *American Journal* cited by Mayer, 'This is truly the era of orthopaedic surgery and the enormous impetus given it by war practice is certain to be reflected in civil practice with results of inestimable value to the multitude of potential cripples constantly repleted from the vast army of citizens engaged in the peaceful pursuits of our normal industrial life.'

Brackett had been made director of military orthopaedics as a major in the autumn of 1917 and stressed that the essential aim, after saving life, was the restoration of function and self-respect. By 1918 he was a Lieutenant-Colonel with over 600 officers; also in 1918, Major Robert W Lovett stressed the value of the curative workshop[137].

SPECIAL FIELDS

To catalogue in detail the achievements of American orthopaedic surgeons in the various fields of the discipline would be unforgivably to overlap the treatment of these matters elsewhere. However, even at the risk of some duplication, a very summary review must be undertaken.

In *arthroplasty*, we have already mentioned the work of John Rhea Barton in 1826 (p. 387), but no vigorous attack was mounted on the problem until Murphy of Chicago developed his pedicled interposition flap of fat and fascia (he thought the fat important for vascularization) and the instrumentation appropriate, especially reamers for the hip. This work was based on rigorous research and experiment[138,139]. Murphy was a general surgeon. Of the orthopaedists interested, we have referred to Baer of Baltimore, who used pig's bladder for interposition in the hip, knee, jaw, elbow, etc., with the best results in the temporomandibular joint[140,141]. Baer reopened some of these joints and found the membrane absorbed by a smooth-lined cavity: 'The membrane is transformed into a fibrous tissue which covers the denuded bone and...a joint-like space is formed.' Overall, Baer's results were not brilliant and were greatly improved by MacAusland of Boston, who used carefully defatted fascia to cover only one of the new joint surfaces, with excellent results in the elbow[142]. The principal advocate of interpositional arthroplasty was **Willis Campbell** of Memphis, Tennessee (1880–1941).

Campbell, a Mississipian, went to Memphis as an anaesthetist and paediatrician, but lack of success led him to study in Boston, New York,

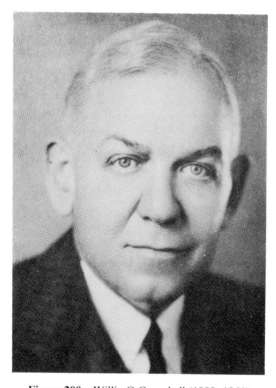

Figure 200   Willis C Campbell (1880–1941)

England and Europe and he restarted as an orthopaedist in Memphis in 1909. In 1911 he organized the department of orthopaedic surgery in the University of Tennessee College of Medicine and was professor for over 30 years. In 1921 he opened the Willis Campbell Clinic at the university medical centre, and this became a complete orthopaedic hospital with residency training that anticipated that laid down a decade later by the American Board of Orthopaedic Surgeons. Later there was a new building elsewhere. Campbell helped found the American Academy of Orthopaedic Surgeons in 1931 and its Examination Board, was its first president, was active in SICOT, made the Campbell Clinic a world-famous centre and wrote a textbook which became and remains a bible. His arthroplasties were based on animal experiment and on examination, X-rays and reoperation on treated patients years later, where there was a joint cavity with fluid and a smooth fibrous or fibrocartilaginous layer which might, he hoped, eventually become true articular cartilage. The best exposition of this work is by Campbell himself in his book *Operative Orthopaedics* of 1939.

Campbell[143] acknowledged the pioneer work of Barton, Textor (1782–1860) of Würzburg, Esmarch, Verneuil and Ollier in attempting to restore movement to ankylosed joints, and credits the first use of accepted interpositional techniques to Helferich's pedicled flap of muscle and fascia in an ankylosed temporomandibular joint. He emphasized that arthroplasty was not to be confused with excision; it was designed not to induce pseudarthrosis, but to restore function. Nor was conformity to the original anatomy essential; it might be artistically desirable but, in practice, could diminish the prospects of success. At the knee, for instance, a single large condyle at the lower end of the femur and a shallow concave tibial surface would give an adequately functional hinge joint. Campbell used a free autogenous transplant of fascia lata from the thigh in a double layer, the smooth surface facing internally, but he did at one time try a vitallium sheath over the lower femur[144]. Smith-Petersen's work with interpositional mould arthroplasty for the hip is treated at p. 599.

Arthrodesis is a term originated by Eduard Albert (1841–1900) of Vienna in 1881[145]. In the USA, its application to paralytic deformities of the foot is associated with the names of Davis for pes cavus in 1913[146], Hoke of Atlanta[147] and Ryerson's triple fusion of 1923[148]. Russell A Hibbs (1869–1932) had laid down the principle of stiffening the tuberculous knee as far back as 1911, resecting only the anterior part of the joint and using the patella as a graft[149], while Albee had progressed in 1915 to an inlaid cortical graft[150]. Others used transfixion nails or wires, and even the three-flanged Smith-Petersen pin when that arrived[151]; while Milgram in 1929 delightfully adapted a method of the German, L Roeren, by coring out a cylindrical block across the joint-line, rotating it through 90° and reinserting it[152]. Perhaps the most important contribution here was Key's description of compression arthrodesis, long before Charnley, in 1932[153].

Arthrodesis of the hip had originally been sought to arrest tuberculosis and therefore the original techniques were mostly extra-articular and involved some form of bone-grafting[154–156]. It is unnecessary to expand here on subsequent developments for fusion of the non-tuberculous knee and hip e.g.

the hip with arthrosis or rheumatoid disease; but we must stray from America long enough to mention the sounder architectural principle of Trumble[157] in Australia, with his ischiofemoral graft in compression, and as modified in England by Brittain of Norwich by the addition of subtrochanteric osteotomy[158]. Fusion of the spine followed a similar course. Originally devised by Hibbs and Albee for tuberculosis, it was largely abandoned as Pott's disease was eliminated by hygiene or chemotherapy and adapted to the treatment of mechanical instability of arthroses, as dealt with below.

Bone-grafting   As Leo Mayer has well written, 'Originated by a great French surgeon, Ollier, is his famous *Traité Experimentale et Clinique* (1867), activated by the brilliant contribution of Macewen of Glasgow in his monograph *The Growth of Bone* (1912), this branch of surgery has reached the peak of its development through the efforts of a group of American orthopaedic surgeons. The story is as exciting as a novel in which ardent rivals, men of blood and brawn, contend for mastery. Even today (Mayer was writing in 1950), after forty years of intense effort, all is not yet decided, but orthopaedic surgery has advanced because of the conflicting views.'

In 1911 two New York orthopaedic surgeons, Fred Albee and Russell Hibbs, independently published papers on spinal fusion for Pott's disease by bone-grafting. Albee's graft was a massive cortico-cancellous strut placed between the split spinous processes and ignoring other structures, while Hibbs carefully rawed the laminae and small articulations and used the fragments without any extraneous graft. Albee sneered at these as 'chicken-feed'; both went their own way and both obtained good results. Albee went on to apply his technique to fractures and reconstructive procedures, favouring the inlay technique with each layer of the graft fitted in at the level of the corresponding layer of the host. Hibbs, unimpressed, extended his method to joint fusion. Albee's method worked; there was no doubt of that; in 1930 he reported nearly 90 per cent of cures in 754 nonunions[159]. Yet, at this very time, Phemister of Chicago showed that merely wrapping osteoperiosteal grafts round the bone or laying a full-thickness graft on one or both sides was effective; the inlay was unnecessary[160].

Willis Campbell[161] put his money on an inlay full-thickness graft for nonunion, fixed with bone-pegs, to provide both osteogenesis and stability, admitting his debt to Henderson, who had begun work on the subject back in 1914 and published a formal paper on the massive onlay graft in the same year as Albee, fixing his graft with screws of beef-bone[162]. Less than 20 years later, in 1943, Boyd of the Campbell Clinic reported a cure-rate of nearly 95 per cent in 500 cases of nonunion[163]. The development of inert alloys soon led to the screw fixation of onlay grafts, as by Albert Key[164].

Though Albee never abandoned his principles of the coapted, unscrewed inlay graft of autogenous bone, others were using homologous grafts and this led to the establishment of the first bone-bank by Inclán of Cuba in 1940–2, using refrigeration in citrated blood or saline[165]. We may add that absolutely the opposite pole in treatment is represented by the use of cancellous bone, in which British plastic surgeons played a part in World War II.

Poliomyelitis   An immense amount of interest has been devoted to poliomyelitis from the beginnings of orthopaedics in America due to the extensive recurrent epidemics of the disease which persisted until the development of the Sabin and Salk vaccines of 1954 and 1960; a wholly American contribution that relegated tendon procedures almost entirely to the fields of hand surgery and nerve injury. At the time of the great epidemic of 1916, measures were available to assess muscle power[166], Soutter had developed his release for hip flexion contracture[167], later modified by Campbell as transference of the crest of the ilium[168], and Mayer had shown how to correct fixed pelvic obliquity by division of tight structures and how to stabilize the corrected pelvis with facial transplants from the lower ribs to the pelvis[169,170]. This last procedure had also been developed by Lowman in 1931[171]. Whitman, Hoke, Ryerson and others were developing or had developed their stabilizing operations on the feet by fusion of tarsal joints; Campbell and others had originated bone-block procedures to check deformity at the knee and ankle; and fusion was applied to the knee and hip (but rather rarely) and more often to the shoulder and wrist.

There was also available by the 1920s a wide range of tendon transplants, associated in Europe with the names of Nicoladoni and Biesalski. Nicoladoni's work dated back to 1850 and his ideas were introduced into the USA on a systematic scale by Parrish of New York City in 1892; at the turn of the century, Goldthwait in Boston was transplanting hamstrings into the quadriceps and Parrish, Goldthwait and Millikan had established tendon transplantation in the United States. Biesalski, in collaboration with Leo Mayer, while the latter was still in Germany, had written his *Die physiologische Sehnenverpflanzung* (Physiologic tendon transplantation) in 1916, a book extensively summarized in America by Mayer[172]. Mayer also worked on transplantation of the trapezius for deltoid paralysis[173] (a problem that was never really solved), and valuable work on transplants for the foot was done by Peabody, especially on transplantation of the tibialis anterior or posterior through the interosseous membrane[174]. Arthur Steindler, in 1919, developed the proximal transplantation of the common flexor origin for paralysis of the elbow flexors with excellent results[175]. Sterling Bunnell developed his techniques for restoration of thumb opposition with a sublimis tendon rerouted around the pisiform in 1938[176] and the sublimis transfer for intrinsic palsy in the hand in 1942[177].

Finally, there was the arrival in America, just after World War II, of Sister Kenny from Australia with her much-debated hot pack treatment for painful muscle spasm in the early stage of poliomyelitis. This excited much controversy, was rejected by most orthopaedists, and defended by a few[178]; but it was not unconnected with the advocacy by Ransohoff of New York of the use of curare or other relaxants to allow early passive (and painful) movement in the acute stage.

This is a convenient point to deal with *tendon surgery* in general and of the hand in particular. This is well treated by Mayer in his 1950 review because of his personal interest. To recapitulate, Fritz Lange (1864–1952) in Germany had revived Nicoladoni's concept of tendon transplantation (see p. 211), using silk strands to prolong the insertions where needed in the early 1900s, and gave an account of his work to the AOA in 1910. It was this that had stimulated Mayer to spend the year of 1912–13 at Lange's clinic at Munich, where he improved Lange's results by learning how to safeguard tendon gliding mechanisms and wrote the joint work with Biesalski, mentioned above. In 1918, Sterling Bunnell published a paper on the repair of tendons in the fingers[179], which, as Mayer rightly says, was the germ of what eventually became one of the most important surgical monographs of the century: *Surgery of the Hand* (Philadelphia 1944, Lippincott). The essence of his teaching was respect for the gliding mechanism at all times: respect in handling the tendon, for its pulleys and its line of pull, for its blood supply and appropriate tension and adequate skin cover. This book remains the bible of tendon surgeons; but it must be remembered that it was preceded by another bible, the classic *Infections of the Hand* by Allan B Kanavel of Chicago (1874–1938) in 1933.

The residual paralyses of poliomyelitis were a great stimulus to transplantation and many ingenious techniques were devised[180–182]. Those interested in the detailed state of play in this field 50 years ago will find a very full account of contemporary procedures in Campbell's *Operative Orthopaedics* of 1939. This experience was extended to palsies following injury or nerve damage. In 1922, Charles L Starr described his military experience to the British Orthopaedic Association, dealing particularly with transfers for radial nerve palsy, using the method we seem to owe originally to Robert Jones[183]. As poliomyelitis came under control by immunization, so the field of tendon work in trauma expanded. Bunnell emphasized preliminary nerve repair, particularly of the digital nerves and plastic soft tissue procedures, and showed how to substitute for inactive intrinsic and opponens muscles in the hand, how to suture tendons with the aid of his pull-out stitch, and how to construct his simple but essential lively postoperative splints.

The topic of *congenital dislocation of the hip* is discussed elsewhere in historical perspective (ch. 23). In Europe, in 1887, Paci had reported what may have been the first manipulative reduction[184]. This was what Lorenz came to call 'bloodless reduction', as opposed to open operation, and as Mayer points out, the history of the treatment of this condition is one of great swings of opinion between the two methods in which fashion tended to replace objective assessment. Albert Hoffa (1859–1907) of Würzburg and Berlin favoured the open method (though a caustic comment at the time was that, before operation, his patients walked like ducks, and afterwards like operated ducks!), and so did Adolf Lorenz (1854–1946) of Vienna. Both toured America as apostles, but very soon Lorenz turned to the closed method and advocated it to the AOA in 1896[185]. Bradford, in Boston, made an exhaustive series of clinical and pathological studies[186–188]. He found the manipulative technique unsuccessful, due perhaps to anteversion, for which he suggested (but does not seem to have actually performed) rotation osteotomy, worked with operation for a time and eventually resumed the closed method. Most surgeons in the early 20th century used manipulation, but it was recognized by some as dangerously traumatic[189] and stigmatized by Galloway in Canada in 1920 as 'blind, irrational and deplorably uncertain in results[190].' Galloway therefore adopted open operation and this was soon also adopted at the New York Orthopaedic Hospital, where the closed method was not securing permanent reduction and often required supplementary rotation osteotomy[191].

At an AOA symposium in 1935, Freiberg[192] stressed the importance of early diagnosis and gentle reduction, the latter essentially bound up with the former. There was a clear leaning to open reduction at this time[193], when a number of papers also appeared on the importance of constructing a shelf to deepen the acetabulum[194-196]. The degree of obliquity of the acetabular roof was defined by Kleinberg's 'acetabular index' in 1936[197]. By mid-century it was clear that the keys to success were early diagnosis, gentle manipulative reduction and operation when this failed to give concentric replacement. Simple abduction in infancy gave the best results and was the only way to obtain perfect hips; once manipulation took the stage, the incidence of avascular necrosis shot up[198].

A field where American contributions helped to realize an old orthopaedic dream was that of *correction of unequal leg-length*. At various times in the 18th and 19th centuries surgeons had mused that one might compensate for

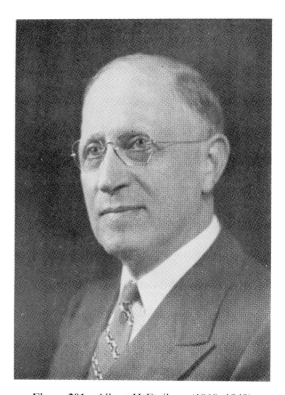

Figure 201   Albert H Freiberg (1868–1940)

shortening due to fracture or congenital hip dislocation by deliberately fracturing the sound femur and letting it override, and one or two bolder spirits seem to have done so. We may recall that Alessandro Codivilla (1861–1912), director of the Rizzoli Institute near Bologna in Italy, devised skeletal traction on the lower limb using a calcanean pin, and employed this method to lengthen the femur after osteotomy, and this was developed by his great successor, Vittorio Putti[199–201] and, in America, by Abbott who osteotomized the tibia and fibula[202]. Warren White preferred shortening of the sound femur[203]. Both lengthening and shortening had their problems. Lengthening was tedious and painful and the bone, if atrophic after poliomyelitis, did not always unite. Shortening involved the hazards of an open operation on the sound side. Compere noted the possible disastrous complications of lengthening: nerve palsy, fracture, malunion or nonunion, osteomyelitis, necrosis of soft tissues or bone and vascular lesions[204]. Willis Campbell regarded it as 'an extremely formidable procedure, involving a long period of disability and much suffering...an operation...rarely justified[205].'

There was therefore a marked tendency towards shortening procedures, but prior to Phemister's introduction of surgical arrest of epiphyseal growth in 1933 little could be done to correct inequality in growing children. Phemister[206] devised a simple and relatively safe method of removing a block of bone on both sides straddling the knee epiphysis of the femur and/or tibia, taken so that the epiphyseal plate traversed it nearer one end of the block, curetting the whole growth-plate as much as possible, turning the block(s) upside-down and replacing them to act as grafts. There was the risk of valgus, varus or recurvatum deformity, and also that of ending up with a sound leg that was still too long or even too short because of difficulty in timing the fusion. Success was therefore predicated on devising tables of growth expectancy, based on the fundamental child studies of Baldwin in Iowa[207]; and this, in turn, led to the work initiated by Wingate Todd on human growth at the Western Reserve University in Cleveland and to the concept of skeletal age as laid down in the monumental *Radiographic Atlas of Skeletal Development of the Hand and Wrist* by Greulich and Pyle in 1950[208]. Armed with this, and with curves of the predicted correction from arrest of the distal femur or proximal tibia (or both) in either sex and at different ages, correction of a given discrepancy could be timed accurately enough to give a reasonable prospect of equalization at the end of growth.

Others whose studies helped establish prediction of the outcome included Green and Anderson[209]. But a method that would retard epiphyseal growth only as long as it was applied was obviously desirable. In 1945, Haas[210] showed that such temporary slowing could be obtained by encircling the growth-plate with a wire loop (the irony was that he was seeking a method for *stimulating* epiphyseal growth, as it was known that the implantation of foreign materials at the metaphysis could do so). In 1949, Blount and Clarke showed that staples inserted to straddle the epiphyseal line would almost entirely stop growth, which resumed on their removal, so that correction could be done on younger children without risk of under- or over-correction[211].

It has to be added that the *idea* of epiphyseodesis to treat angulation, inequality and even spinal curvature originated with Ollier in Lyons in 1879, though he does not seem to have put it into practice (p. 261).

In the second decade of this century, Boston saw a growth of interest in mechanical derangements of the low back and congenital malformations of the lumbosacral region, associated particularly with the name of Joel Goldthwait.

In 1911, Goldthwait wrote a classic paper on *The lumbosacral articulation: an explanation of many cases of 'lumbago', 'sciatica' and paraplegia*[212]. This is fascinating because it postulates disc protrusion on entirely theoretical grounds, but attributes it to strain caused by displacement of the small vertebral articulations or of the sacroiliac joint; and he reported a case with typical positional pain treated (unsuccessfully) by excision of the 5th lumbar spinous process – an operation that still had some vogue even in the 1940s. He speculated that protrusion at higher levels might cause the paraplegia sometimes attributed to transverse myelitis.

In the same year, Middleton and Teacher, in Glasgow, reported the case of a man who developed paraplegia after heavy lifting caused a crack in his back. At autopsy, the lumbar enlargement of the cord was found to have been damaged by 'a mass of firm white tissue which looked rather like the pulp in the centre of the intervertebral discs' at the level of T12-L1, and they found that they could reproduce this lesion by compression of a cadaveric spine. They quoted a much earlier report by Kocher of 1896, of a man who fell 100 feet and died of multiple injuries, the autopsy showing smashing and extrusion of the disc at L1-2.

The situation remained confused for a time, as much attention was being given to dividing the 'spastic piriformis', removing quite innocent sacralized transverse processes and fusing harmless sacroiliac joints, not to mention injecting air or saline in or around the sciatic nerve or stretching it under anaesthesia. (This last *could* help, in ignorance, as it sometimes shifted the relation of a root to a disc prolapse.) Meanwhile, fundamental studies by Schmorl[213,214], Beadle[215] and others focussed attention on the pathogenic role of the discs, while at the same time surgeons were removing space-occupying lesions from the lumbar canal often regarded as 'chondromata'[216–218] or 'fibromata'[219]. It was one of those times when a surgical disovery was 'in the air', and in 1934 **Mixter** and **Barr** from the Massachusetts General Hospital reported a series of 19 cases of *Rupture of the intervertebral disc with involvement of the spinal canal*[220]. 'Investigation...has shown a surprisingly large number of these lesions, classified as chondromata, to be in truth not tumors of cartilage but prolapses of the nucleus pulposus or fracture of the annulus.' This paper laid down principles that still apply. They operated on cervical and lumbar lesions by laminectomy, stressed the diagnostic value of lumbar puncture and lipiodol myelography, dealt with midline lesions transdurally (still the safest approach to large midline prolapses) and treated lateral lesions by extradural dissection carried out well into the foramen if necessary.

We need not rehearse subsequent developments: the discussions on the role, if any, of adjuvant fusion, the tendency to over-operate when, as Jackson-Burrows in England put it, it was discovered that the intervertebral disc contained not a nucleus pulposus but a glittering nugget of gold, the resurgence of conservative management, the advent of discography[221] and of chemonucleolysis with papain[222,223]. What matters is that here centuries of confused speculation and dubious pathology were dispelled by the clear demonstration of an entity that was obviously causal and could be surgically dealt with. The foundations for this advance were laid in many countries; but the coping-stone was added in the USA.

As to *scoliosis*, we have mentioned Abbott's work of 1917 on correction by pressure which had to be abandoned because of sores and rib deformation. Hibbs did the first fusion for this condition in 1914 and reported 59 cases in 1924[224]. Preliminary correction was often by plaster jackets applied in suspension or extension, and subsequently wedged or opened out with turnbuckles. An important paper by Hibbs, Risser and Ferguson in 1931[225] laid down the principles of X-ray measurement of the scoliosis angles, the use of Risser's turnbuckle jacket and operation through a windowed plaster, and ten years later the Research Committee of the AOA stated that this method yielded better results than any other. Nevertheless, two thirds of the results were only fair or poor: the fusions were certainly often sound, but sometimes so effective as to prevent the development of compensatory curves[226]. An important contribution by John Cobb of New York in the 1940s showed that 95 per cent of idiopathic scolioses did not deteriorate after a fixed level determined by successive radiographs as stationary, that braces and exercises were ineffectual, and that the deteriorating minority could be managed by turnbuckle jacket correction and grafting with bank-bone plus prolonged postopertive recumbency. Cobb's very precise method of radiographic measurement of scoliosis angles has become standard.

The introduction of the Milwaukee brace and of halo traction by Blount and others was an important advance, especially in the ultimate version of the latter incorporating pins in the skull and pelvis. This was timely since paralytic scoliosis had become a major problem after the great epidemics of poliomyelitis that swept the USA after World War II, and its treatment by conventional cast correction and spinal fusion often had catastrophic effects on cardiopulmonary function, already compromised. This was now supplemented, in places supplanted, by methods of internal instrumentation developed by Dwyer and others in Australia[227] and by Paul Harrington[228] in Houston. Harrington (1911–1980) first tried screw fixation of the facet joints in the overcorrected position, but the improvement was transient. He therefore developed internal fixation by hook purchase on the posterior elements coupled to distraction or compression rods, or both. The results were good and the method subsequently applied to idiopathic scoliosis and even fractures of the spine. (We have mentioned that, in 1910, Fritz Lange of Munich read a paper to the AOA on *Support for the spondylitic [tuberculous] spine by means of buried steel bars attached to the vertebrae*[229]. Lange thought there was a place for inorganic 'heteroplastic' materials as internal splints, especially in Pott's disease; he began by wiring the spinous processes, noted the electrolytic complications of dissimilar metals, and ended with zinc-plated steel rods sutured to the spinous processes over the laminae plus a plaster jacket.) Others tried the effect of unilateral spinal epiphyseodeses.

If we may step back in time, it was an immigrant from Germany to Texas, **Berthold Ernest Hadra** (1842–1903), who did the first, or first-reported, spinal fusion in 1891, using silver wire to fix the spinous processes of the 6th and 7th cervical vertebrae in a man of 30 who had injured his neck a year before, and later applied this to Pott's disease and fixed the transverse processes if the spines were fractured[230]. This has been described by Bick as 'probably the most original American contribution to orthopaedic surgery.' 'What do we do in other fractures,' wrote Hadra, 'if the usual means do not suffice? We do the most natural thing in the world; we fix them to each other by direct means – clamps, nails, wires, sutures and so on. Now, there is no good reason why vertebral fractures should not enjoy similar advantages.' This was not absolutely the first case of vertebral fixation, for Hadra mentions an earlier operation by a Dr W T Wilkins of which he had been ignorant at the time, who fixed a defect between T12 and L1 in a neonate with carbolized silk ligatures. Hadra was a modest man and did not claim his method as a panacea. 'It is simply a method of holding the broken or diseased parts together better than any other method, and with less annoyance to the patient...in many cases it may do so by itself, in others it will be a desirable addition to other operations, in others again it will be as fruitless as all other methods at our disposal...if only a small portion of the advantages set forth could be attained, it would constitute a very desirable addition to the present means to combat such formidable and intractable ailments.' The idea spread rapidly to American and European centres. Lange used it, trying various suture materials in place of wire. Hadra's technique remained unchanged until the advent of Hibbs' fusion and is still employed in essence for traumatic lesions, especially atlanto-axial instability. When Hibbs came to write his preliminary report in 1911[231], he had based his work on experience in fusing the tuberculous knee with a patellar graft. His method of careful subperiosteal denudation and use of the spinous processes as bridging grafts has been referred to; and he adds, prophetically, in his last sentence, 'In the lateral curvatures, it would seem to offer a means of preventing a progress of that distressing deformity.' Albee's massive tibial cortical graft between the split spinous processes was a contemporary competitor, but time gave the palm to Hibbs.

As regards *fracture treatment*, this became a field for orthopaedists earlier in the USA than in Europe, partly because orthopaedics as a separate discipline was established earlier in America. Although general surgeons have not usually exhibited reluctance in unloading fractures on anyone willing to undertake the work (in some great London teaching hospitals the fracture clinics were conducted by medically unqualified practitioners up to and beyond the mid 19th century), there was some resistance in the USA. The first specific hospital fracture service was set up by Scudder at the Massachusetts General Hospital in 1917, and he and others there published *An Outline of the Treatment of Fractures* in 1922 which became the official manual of the American College of Surgeons.

A helpful factor was Whitman's work on hip fractures in children, establishing the importance of full abduction and extension so that the acetabular rim levered the trochanter into position[232-234]. Whitman extended this principle to adults and was famous for his long hip abduction plaster casts which were highly polished and retained for many months, leading to bony union in a fair percentage of cases. In 1932, Leadbetter modified this by effecting reduction by traction in right angled flexion and internal rotation, completed by abduction and full extension (for intracapsular fractures), his test of success being that when the heel was allowed to rest on the surgeon's hand the limb did not relapse into external rotation; this too was followed by a hip spica, giving bony union in 70 per cent of cases[235,236].

Little need be said here of Smith-Petersen's introduction of his triflanged nail in 1931[237], epoch-making as it was, the apotheosis of the many 19th century attempts by so many in the Old and the New Worlds to peg, pin or nail this fracture. It was originally inserted after open exposure until the Swede, Johansson, showed that the nail could be cannulated and inserted blindly over a guide-wire under X-ray control[238].

It is interesting that, even several years after these events, in 1935, Kellogg Speed of Chicago was able to write a famous paper on *The Unsolved Fracture*[239] which makes only cursory mention of the new method, but gives a rather pessimistic review looking back to Sir Astley Cooper of Guy's Hospital in London (p. 94) who believed that bony union of intracapsular fractures rarely if ever occurred and that this was due to damage to the nutrient retinacula of the neck[240]. Speed said that the mechanical treatment of this fracture had been put on a rational basis by Whitman 45 years before, but that this work had received scant recognition, and that surgeons were still largely ignorant of methods of reduction or how to apply a proper cast. He regarded operative methods as mere reflections of this failure and lists disparagingly a series of procedures ranging from Murphy's nailings of 1902 through Delbet's screw and guide to the flanged nail. He was very critical of Hey Groves' method of removing an ununited femoral head and bolting it on to the neck because 'it violated one of the sacred sources of blood supply to the head via the ligamentum teres', not now considered important. Even Whitman's method came in for criticism, since the pressure exerted on the head might cause its necrosis. He ends, 'The fracture is still unsolved,' one more example of a recurrent feature in the history of orthopaedics as of other disciplines, that an *ex cathedra* statement that the solution of some problem is impossible, or undesirable, or even sacrilegious, almost inevitably presages its imminent arrival. And yet Speed's appellation, 'the unsolved fracture', is still largely true in the sense that we do not achieve sound union in much more than half the cases. Instead, we have either a prosthesis or an internal fixation with a high incidence of necrosis – so much so that even total hip replacement is urged as primary treatment by some.

Objective assessment by the American Academy in 1939–41[241-242] indicated a rate of bony union exceeding 70 per cent, but with a considerable risk of avascular necrosis and arthrosis. Great as this advance was, especially in allowing early ambulation and avoiding months of immobilization, it was not a panacea and further improvement of results had to await the arrival of the prosthetic femoral head. In 1937, Lawson Thornton of Atlanta fixed a plate to the Smith-Petersen pin for trochanteric fractures, and this 'blade-plate' was developed by Blount, Jewett, McLaughlin and others.

We should note the exhaustive histologic and biochemical studies of fracture healing in man and animals made by Urist and various colleagues in the 1940s[243-246]. The importance of the introduction of biologically inert metals such as vitallium for internal fixation by Venables and Stuck and others is referred to elsewhere (p. 593). We should note, too, that the compression method of osteosynthesis was anticipated by Eggers in 1948 with his slotted plate[247], and that methods of intramedullary fixation were being used by Rush as early as 1939[248] and that Roger Andersen and others in 1943 had introduced (or rather, historically, reintroduced) the use of the external fixator with transfixion pins held by a rigid bar[249].

Whitman's early work on hip fractures marked the turning-point of the battle with the general surgeons over fractures in general, and after the world wars American orthopaedists increasingly arrogated this field to themselves, so that the discipline in their country differed notably in character from that in Europe. As Valentin points out, one need only compare a volume of the American edition of the *Journal of Bone and Joint Surgery*, with its many articles on fractures, with a volume of the *Zeitschrift für Orthopädische Chirurgie* or the *Revue d'Orthopédie* to prove this point.

It had not been an easy progress where operations were concerned, for in many areas conditions in the 1870s and 80s were entirely primitive. Of the Middle West at this time it has been said: 'Operations in rural districts, even for the simplest of lesions, were practically unknown. In those days all wounds suppurated. It was the common practice for the surgeons in that day to operate garbed in the Prince Albert coat...the only fitting garment for the professional man. The cuff was turned up by the more fastidious...the surgeon threaded the needles with silk and then stuck them in the lapel of his coat so as to have them readily accessible when needed. He held his knife in his teeth when not in actual use...Injuries which today seem comparatively trivial were treated by amputation. The experience was that if amputation was not done, death from infection would most likely follow, an end not obviated, however, in many cases by amputation because the wound made by the amputation often became infected and killed the patient. The vessels were tied by silk threads cut long so that they could be pulled out after the end of the vessel sloughed off: that is, if the patient did not die of secondary haemorrhage'. Even in a large New York public hospital like the Bellevue, the situation was no better. 'From 40–60 per cent of amputations of limbs proved fatal, the nurses were ignorant and often worthless,' so Wyllie stated in 1876[250].

To select a handful of names from the long list of famous American orthopaedic surgeons is a hopelessly invidious task. The few now mentioned are those whose work has had a particular appeal for the present writer.

Nicholas Senn (1844–1908) was a child immigrant with Swiss parents to Wisconsin. A Chicago graduate in 1868, he was an intern at Cook County Hospital, went on to the Milwaukee Hospital; and spent the year of 1877 at Munich with Professor Nussbaum, an advocate of Listerism. He was then professor of surgery at the College of Physicians and Surgeons in Chicago and became professor at Rush Medical College in 1888. Enormously busy, he served in the Spanish-American War, was President of the American Medical Association and chairman of the editorial board at the inception of *Surgery, Gynecology and Obstetrics* in 1905. On the basis of experimental work in cats he maintained that a reduced intracapsular fracture of the femoral neck produced intermediate but not external or provisional callus, and because impacted fractures did so well it was obvious that fixation with a steel pin inserted in the trochanter only and incorporated in a windowed spica to apply indirect compression on the fracture, or by an ivory or bone nail transfixing the head also, must be helpful. When he advocated such nailing of hip fractures to the American Surgical Association in 1883, the reception was so hostile that he resorted to reduction and a plaster spica like Whitman. Thomas was aware of Senn's proposition, but thought that even if mechanical fixation were obtained bony union would not necessarily follow.

Ernest Amory Codman (1869–1940) was a typical Bostonian, a Harvard graduate of 1895, the year of the discovery of X-rays. He enthused over their use in the diagnosis of bone disease, describing the 'reactive triangle' in malignant tumours (though this is not a really specific sign), and continued the work of the Bone Tumor Registry of the American College of Surgeons with Joseph Bloodgood and James Ewing. His interest in shoulder lesions led to a book[251] recommending the suture of rotator cuff ruptures and deploring the lack of interest in this field (though time has proved him largely wrong on the need for repair in most cases). He was rather a dilettante and this book is charmingly and amusingly written. He described 'epiphyseal chondromatous giant cell tumor' of the proximal humerus (now known as chondroblastoma) recognizing it as benign, 'yet I am not satisfied with such a long cumbersome name...we must find a name which will not tie the tongue, but it should associate adolescence with this puzzling lesion[252].' Jaffe did so. This suggests a digression into the history of bone sarcoma in general and giant-cell tumours in particular. 'Sarcoma' was a very old term, one defined by Hunter's pupil, John Abernethy, in his classification as 'a kind of tumour with a firm and fleshy feel[253].' Another ancient term was 'spina ventosa', literally a bag of wind i.e. a bony shell around a haemorrhagic cyst, although it was also applied to tuberculous dactylitis. Hey[254] had thought that this indicated that tumours originated in haematomas, and Dupuytren[255] took this up with *fungus hématode*, though he had been anticipated by Astley Cooper in 1818 with 'fungus medullary exostosis', providing drawings of what were obvious giant-cell tumours of long bones[256]. Thus, until the mid-19th century the main groups of bone tumours were osteosarcoma (bone becoming fleshy) and spina ventosa (hollowish cystic haemorrhagic central lesions). Histologic study was initiated by Johannes Müller in 1838[257] and more so by Lebert in Paris in 1845[258], who laid down that microscopy was essential to classification, and that the solid bone tumours previously generally classed as osteosarcoma were distinguishable among themselves on histologic grounds. Thus, there was a *tumeur fibroblastique* with fusiform cells and multinucleate giant-cells (the first record of the latter in tumours), apt to recur, curable by amputation and different from secondary carcinoma in bone (cancer encephaloides).

Paget in his 1845 *Lectures on Surgical Pathology* called these 'myeloid' because they were soft and red like marrow; hence 'myeloma' or 'myeloid sarcoma', which could also occur in nonosseous tissues. In 1860, Nélaton wrote an entire book on these *tumeurs à myéloplaxes*[259], which he thought always benign and peculiar to bone, neither belief true. Virchow thought them malignant, a form of *Riesenzellsarkome*. The classic paper on sarcoma of the long bones was that of **Samuel Gross** of 1879[260], based on a study of 165 cases, of which 70 were grouped as giant-cell sarcomata, certainly the least aggressive of the bone sarcomata but not altogether innocent; indeed, a quarter were malignant, but it was difficult to distinguish between true giant-cell lesions and other types of tumour containing some giant-cells but bone also. With the arrival of Listerism, he thought that local resection or curettage could replace amputation in some cases, and resections (especially of tumours of the lower radius) and curettage were reported by many surgeons towards the end of the century[261-264]. **Joseph Bloodgood** (1867–1935) was a surgeon at Johns Hopkins and director of surgical pathology. From the mid-1890s he analyzed his own cases and those in the literature, 52 in all, concluding that this was a benign lesion to be treated conservatively rather than by amputation and labelled it 'giant-cell tumour' and not sarcoma; but his diagnosis was based on the clinical, radiological and gross appearances rather than the histology. He used curettage, carbolic irrigation and a gauze pack and did a bone-graft of the cavity a few weeks later. It seems strange now, but the idea then spread that this was not a tumour at all, but a reparative or reactive granulomatous process to dead bone in low-grade infection 'chronic nonsuppurative haemorrhagic osteomyelitis', and even Codman accepted this and thought the giant-cells phagocytic migrants from the blood until the work of the registry and of Coley and others showed them to be true neoplasms.

Credit here is also due to **Ewing** in the 1920s, who used a multiple clinical-radiological-histological approach, saw a definite X-ray pattern and recognized a spectrum of aggressiveness, though he asserted that the tumour never metastasized[267-269]. He used a histologic grading system to predict its behaviour. He advocated treatment by irradiation alone; and many radiologists before World War II and even later, like Brailsford in England, felt confident enough of their diagnosis to dispense with the imagined dangers of open biopsy. When Henry Jaffe became director of the laboratories at the Hospital for Joint Diseases in 1925, he took a hand in clinical decision-making and separated off the giant-cell tumour variants or 'brown tumours' or xanthomas[270]. We now know that even low-grade lesions may metastasize or recur locally after curettage in more malignant guise, i.e. Jaffe's grading was not reliable.

Philip Duncan Wilson (1886–1969) was an outstanding orthopaedic surgeon and surgical statesman. An Ohioan, he graduated from Harvard, interned at the Massachusetts General Hospital, and had just returned to Columbus when he was invited to join the Harvard group of surgeons assembling at Boston under Harvey Cushing to embark for Europe and serve in the American Ambulance at Neuilly in 1915. His companions included Smith-Petersen and Elliot Cutler. Later, he served in the American Expeditionary Force, eventually in charge of amputations. In 1919 he joined Goldthwait

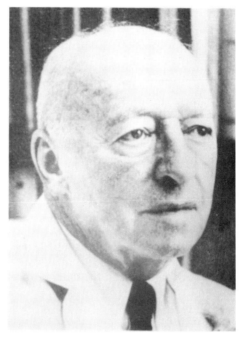

Figure 202   Philip D Wilson (1886–1969)

on the staff of the MGH, whose orthopaedic department was then directed by Brackett, and the John Bent Brigham Hospital where he developed posterior capsuloplasty for flexion contracture of the knee and arthroplasty of the elbow. It took some time for orthopaedics at the MGH to embrace trauma, and for a period fractures were treated by both general and orthopaedic surgeons. In 1925, he wrote *Fractures and Dislocations* with W A Cochrane, later the first orthopaedic surgeon to the Edinburgh Royal Infirmary.

Wilson never became chief of orthopaedics at the MGH – this went to Smith-Petersen – but in 1934 became surgeon-in-chief to the rather stagnant Hospital for the Ruptured and Crippled in New York, which he reorganized and relocated and renamed as the Hospital for Special Surgery, affiliated to Cornell Medical School, where he was Clinical Professor for a short time. The hospital acquired fame as a postgraduate training centre. In 1940, Wilson brought the vanguard of the American Hospital in Britain to that country and returned for tours of duty.

Wilson promoted the care of cripples in New York and elsewhere, helped found the American Academy of Orthopaedic Surgery, and was President of the Vienna meeting of SICOT in 1963. From the British point of view, he was, as Harry Platt has well written, 'the outward symbol of the "special relationship" between the orthopaedic surgeons of the two countries created in the days of war by Sir Robert Jones and nurtured by Robert Osgood.'

Paul Budd Magnuson (1884–1968), born in Minnesota, and of Swedish descent, graduated in Pennsylvania and even as a student undertook such research as experimental bone-lengthening in dogs, for which he devised an electric circular bone-saw. After graduating in 1909, he assisted John B Murphy in Chicago and then built his own practice in the slaughterhouse area, where he acquired enormous experience in trauma. After assisting Brackett in the organization of orthopaedic services in World War I, he became Professor of Surgery and Director of Bone and Joint Surgery at North-Western University, wrote a textbook, *Fractures*, and enriched many fields, especially in 'debridement' of the osteoarthritic knee-joint[271] (removal of osteophytes and damaged menisci, shaving of cartilage to the bare bone if necessary, narrowing of the patella but no formal synovectomy) as well as in recurrent dislocation of the shoulder and bone-grafting. After World War II he reorganized the Veterans Administration hospitals by linking them with the medical schools, a policy contested by the administration which led to his resignation. He became something of a medical politician and founded the Rehabilitation Institute of Chicago, assimilated with North-Western University. Magnuson was one of the 'wise men' of American surgery.

Mather Cleveland (1889–1979) served in the first world war, first as an ambulance man, and then as a surgeon, and in 1930 was assigned just three beds on appointment as orthopaedic surgeon and eventually director of orthopaedics at St Luke's Hospital in New York City. On this basis he built the first orthopaedic department in a general hospital in New York, and this became one of the oustanding orthopaedic departments of the whole country. He pioneered the treatment of skeletal tuberculosis at Sea View Hospital, Staten Island, and in World War II was a military orthopaedist in the USA and the European theatre.

If Willis Campbell was one of the great names in orthopaedic surgery in the South during the early 20th century, the other was that of **Michael Hoke** (1874-1944), a quietly-spoken intellectual of Atlanta. He wrote on arthrodesis of the paralysed foot, operation for flat-foot, well-leg traction and helped found the Scottish Rite Hospital for Crippled Children in Atlanta in 1915. For four years he was medical director at Warm Springs, where he treated Franklin Roosevelt after his paralysis and provided his calipers.

Fred H Albee (1876–1945) of New York has been described by Shands as probably the most aggressive and egocentric orthopaedic surgeon of his time, features not unknown in this speciality. Trained at Harvard and the MGH, he first practised in Connecticut but left in 1906 to work as a radiologist and assistant to Gibney at the Hospital for the Ruptured and Crippled and became assistant professor and head of orthopaedic surgery at Cornell University. He was also attached to the University of Vermont and the New York Postgraduate Medical School. When he discovered what an electric saw could do in bone surgery, his star ascended quickly. He did a great deal for state rehabilitation services during and after World War I and was one of the American orthopaedic surgeons best known abroad; but his aggression made him not too well-liked. He was a founder-member of SICOT and Shands says that Baer travelled to Paris from New York in 1929 for just two days for the organizational meeting of SICOT with the express purpose of keeping Albee out of the Presidency! His autobiography,

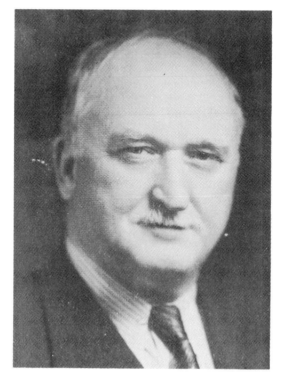

Figure 203   Fred H Albee (1876–1945)

A Surgeon's Fight to Rebuild Men (New York, E P Dutton 1943) is not marked by diffidence, but contains a fascinating photograph of Robert Jones, Royal Whitman, Albee and Hey Groves in a little group at the joint meeting of the American and British Orthopaedic Associations in July 1929, when Albee was president of the former and Hey Groves of the latter.

Winthrop Phelps (b.1894) professor of orthopaedic surgery at Yale University Medical School and director of the Children's Rehabilitation Center at Baltimore, made immense contributions to the management of cerebral palsy. The clinical aspects of his work are detailed elsewhere. What Phelps did was to bring order into the classification and hope into the management of what had, until 1900, been considered a hopeless condition, and to establish definite lines of treatment, rehabilitation and vocational training that excited interest and emulation the world over.

Howard C Naffziger (1884–1961) of the University of California produced in 1938 a study of the 'scalenus anterior syndrome'[272] that seemed important at the time but has not retained all, or much, of its validity. This he considered to be a cervical rib syndrome without a cervical rib, based on an abnormal relation of the shoulder-girdle to the chest-wall and/or a postfixed brachial plexus. The concept was not entirely new. In Britain a historic paper by Stopford and Telford in 1919–20[273] referred to the treatment of such symptoms by removing part of the normal first rib and dividing the scalenus, and others confirmed this[274–276].

Relevant work was done by **Alfred Washington Adson** (1887–1951), the son of immigrant Norwegian parents in Iowa. He graduated at the University of Pennsylvania in 1914 and was head of neurosurgery at the Mayo Clinic during 1921–46. He made many contributions to understanding of the cervical rib and scalenus anterior syndromes. He was not the first in this field, but he was the first to approach the region from the front through the posterior triangle and to stress the role of the scalenus. His pathognomic sign of the scalenus syndrome was that turning the head to the affected side and deep inspiration while sitting upright obliterated the radial pulse; and if this was positive he did a scalenotomy at once because the development of atheroma in the subclavian artery behind the muscle carried a risk of rupture or aneurysm or thrombosis[277].

Adson noted in these cases the anatomic variation from the normal, the descent of the shoulder-girdle in adult life ('widows who take to washing' as a British surgeon put it), that scalenus section alone could suffice without removing the cervical rib, and that the sympathetic irritation might cause gangrene of the fingers. But we now know that many of these cases were really carpal tunnel syndromes.

While **Marius Smith-Petersen**'s work on hip arthroplasty is discussed elsewhere, we should note that in 1945, with others, he described what seems to have been an absolutely novel procedure for correction of flexion deformity of the spine by osteotomy in what he called 'rheumatoid arthritis' but was actually ankylosing spondylitis[278]. This involved excision of spinous processes and of any ossified ligamentum flavum, osteotomy of the articular processes, leverage correction by angulation of the operating table, use of the spinous professes as grafts and plaster fixation.

The great contributions of **Austin Moore** (1899–1963) to metal hip arthroplasty are dealt with elsewhere (p. 598).

David Marsh Bosworth (1897–1979), a Vermont graduate, originally an anatomist, resident to Russell Hibbs at the New York Orthopaedic Hospital and an intern and lasting friend of Mather Cleveland, succeeded the latter as orthopaedic director at St Luke's. He was an inventive and ingenious surgeon, wrote many papers, and was Visiting Professor at the University of Vermont from 1940 until his death. He was also professor of orthopaedic surgery at the New York Polyclinic Medical School and lecturer at Bellevue Medical College, as well as consultant at 22 hospitals in New York and environs, a domain he covered in his own plane. His main contributions were in skeletal tuberculosis and hip disorders.

We should, perhaps, note that the surgeon most responsible for the development of arthroscopic surgery of the knee was the short-lived **Richard L O'Connor** (1933–1980). A graduate of DePaul University, Indiana, in 1955, he was first a general practitioner in Colorado but did an orthopaedic residency in Louisville and began orthopaedic practice in California in 1968. In 1970–71 he trained in arthroscopy with Watanabe in Tokyo and introduced arthroscopic surgery to California, developing new instruments for meniscectomy. He was rather a lone pioneer, a founding member of the

International Arthroscopy Association and author of a textbook in 1977.

At various places we have referred to **D B Phemister** (1882–1951), a graduate of Rush Medical College in Chicago in 1900 who joined the department of surgery at Cook County Hospital in 1908. After two years' postgraduate study in Europe, he became in 1926 the first chairman of the new medical school of Chicago University and held the post for 22 years. He worked on bone tumours, aseptic necrosis and fracture healing. His work on bone-grafting of fractures is mentioned elswhere; here we add his work on conservative surgery in the treatment of bone tumours, his 1940 paper dealing with seven sarcomata treated by segmental resection and bone-grafting with several long-term cures[279].

Earl D McBride (1891–1975) was a man from the mid-west who graduated in New York, trained at the Hospital for the Ruptured and Crippled (we see over and over again how central a position this institute held in training) and returned to practise in Oklahoma City in 1920, where orthopaedic surgery at that time was virtually unknown. His private clinic became the internationally renowned Bone and Joint Hospital. McBride is now remembered mainly for his operation for hallux valgus and for his system of rating disability and his deep understanding of the disabled.

Alfred Rives Shands (1899–1981) was the son of the first orthopaedic surgeon in Washington DC. A Virginia graduate of 1922, he trained at Johns Hopkins (1922–7), founded the orthopaedic department at Duke University in 1930, where he wrote his *Handbook of Orthopaedic Surgery* and became director of the Du Pont Institute in Wilmington, Delaware in 1937. He is famed for his work with crippled children, orthopaedic training and research and in orthopaedic history (*The Early Orthopaedic Surgeons of America*).

Marshall Urist is probably best known for two things: his research into the pathophysiology of bone and his editorship of *Clinical Orthopaedics and Related Research*. A graduate of Johns Hopkins and a natural polymath, he collaborated with Franklin C McLean at Chicago for many years on aspects of fracture healing, was an orthopaedic resident at Johns Hopkins and an outstanding chief of orthopaedics at 22 General Hospital in World War II. After a period with Smith-Petersen at Massachusetts, he returned to research into osteogenesis at Chicago and continued this at the University of California, Los Angeles to produce a flow of research on bone induction and calcium metabolism; his group produced nearly 200 papers in all. His work overlaps into many and surprising fields and he proved just the right editor for a notably reflective and selective (and eclectic) journal which has been immensely helpful to orthopaedists the world over. What appears in its pages represents the 'state of the art' as defined by those best authorized to present it. The value of the historical perspective it provides has been mentioned in the preface.

We must also pay tribute to two medical orthopaedic historians. **Edgar M Bick** (1902–1978), professor of clinical orthopaedic surgery at the School of Medicine of the City University of New York, a battlefield military surgeon in the European and African theatres in 1942–5, not only was awarded the distinguished service medal of the Association of Bone and Joint Surgeons but selected the *Classics* – the reprints of epochal papers by famous figures of the past – for *Clinical Orthopaedics* for over ten years. Many of these have been assembled and published in book form. He was, of course, also author of *A Source-Book of Orthopaedics*, also acknowledged in the preface as a staggeringly rich mine of information about the history of our discipline. It is difficult to understand how Winnett Orr and John Ridlon could have agreed so concertedly that it was a poor work when it first appeared; both tended to carp, felt that Robert Jones was not the man to propagate Thomas's teachings, and Ridlon had never completed his project of editing Thomas's works. Perhaps they felt outdone, as every reader must who surveys this source-book.

Then there is **Leonard F Peltier** (b.1920), a Minnesota graduate, certified in both general and orthopaedic surgery, assistant professor of surgery at the University of Minnesota in 1952, now professor at the University of Arizona in Tucson, who won awards in 1960 from both the American Association of Bone and Joint Surgeons and the American Academy of Orthopaedic Surgeons. An amateur (in the proper sense) of the history of surgery, since 1979 he has been the *Classics* editor of *Clinical Orthopaedics* and his scholarship in this area has shown him to be a worthy successor to Bick.

REFERENCES

1. Duncan, L.C. (1970). *Medical Men in the American Revolution* (New York, Kelley)
2. Lorenz, A. (1937). *Ich dürfte helfen.* (Leipzig)
3. Packard, F.R. (1931). *A History of Medicine in the United States.* (New York)
4. Brown, J.B. (1938). *Boston Med. Surg. J.,* **18**, 139
5. Brown, J.B. (1844) *Reports of cases in the Boston Orthopaedic Infirmary.* (Boston)
6. Brown, J.B. (1850). *Reports of cases treated at the Boston Orthopaedic Institution* (Boston)
7. Sayre, L.A. (1876). *Lectures on orthopaedic surgery and diseases of the joints,* p. 4. (New York and London)
8. Detmold, W. (1938). *Am. J. Med. Sci.,* May
9. Mütter, T.D. (1839). *A Lecture on Loxarthrus, or club foot.* (Philadelphia)
10. Brown, B. (1846). Orthopaedic Surgery in Europe. *Boston Med. Surg. J.,* 429
11. Brown, B. (1868). *Cases in Orthopedic Surgery, read before the Massachusetts Medical Society. With photographic illustrations of the cases represented.* (Boston)
12. Barton, J.R. (1835) Views and treatment of an important fracture of the wrist. *Medical Examiner,* **1**, 365
13. Barton, J.R. (1827). *Am. J. Med. Sci.,* **3**, 279 and 400
14. Chelius, M.J. (1847). *A System of Surgery.* (London)
15. Barton, J.R. (1837). *Am. J. Med. Sci.,* **21**, 332
16. Bick, E.M. (1976). *New York State J. Med.,* July 1192
17. Detmold, L.G. (1830) *De emeticis.* (Göttingen)
18. Cleveland, M. and Winant, E.M. (1948). Lectures on Regional Orthopedic Surgery. No. II. p. 228. Presented at the *American Academy of Orthopedic Surgery,* Ann Arbor 1948
19. Dupuytren, G. (1834). *Lancet,* **ii**, 222
20. Detmold, W.L. (1850). Abscess in the substance of the brain: the lateral ventricles

opened by an operation. *Am. J. Med. Sci.* **19**, 86

21. Keith, A. (1919). *Menders of the Maimed* p. 175. (London)
22. Thomas, H.O. (1887). *Contributions to Medicine and Surgery.* (London)
23. Sayre, L.A. (1883). *Lectures on orthopaedic surgery and diseases of the joints,* 2nd edn. (New York)
24. Bauer, L. (1889). *Medical Chips,* **2**, 181
25. Bigelow, H.J. (1846). Insensibility during surgical operations produced by inhalation. *Boston Med. Surg. J.,* **35**, 309, 379
26. Velpeau, A.A.L.M. (1839). *Nouveaux éléments de médecine opératoire,* 2nd edn., Vol. I, p. 32 (Paris)
27. Carnochan, J.M. (1850). *On the etiology, pathology and treatment of congenital dislocations of the head of the femur.* (New York)
28. Buck, G. (1857). An improved method of treating fractures of the femur. *Trans. New York Acad. Med.,* **2**, 233
29. Crosby, J. (1851). *New York Med. J.,* January
30. Jones, A.R. (1953). *J. Bone Jt. Surg.,* **35B**, 661
31. Beekman, F. (1939). *The Hospital for the Ruptured and Crippled.* (New York)
32. Shands, A.R. (1970). *The Early Orthopedic Surgeons of America.* (St Louis, C V Mosby)
33. Sayre, L.A. (1854). *Exsection of the head of the femur and removal of the upper extremity of the acetabulum for morbus coxarius.* (New York, Holman Gray)
34. Sayre, L.A. (1876) Report on Pott's disease or caries of the spine, treated by extension and the plaster of Paris bandage. *Trans. Am. Med. Assoc.,* **27**, 573
35. Sayre, L.A. (1876). The treatment of rotary lateral curvature of the spine with practical demonstrations *Trans. Med. Soc. New York,* 126
36. Bigg, H.R.H. (1905) *General principles of the treatment of spinal curvatures.* p. 165. (London)
37. Sayre, L.A (1863). A new operation for artificial hip joint in bony ankylosis, two cases. *Trans. Med. Soc. New York,* 111–27
38. Bradford, E.H. (1889). Presidential address, 3rd Annual Meeting of the American Orthopaedic Association. *Trans. Am. Orthop. Assoc.,* **2**, 1–10
39. Shands, A.R. (1969). *Bull. Hosp. Jt. Dis.,* **30**, 119–22
40. Nicholson, J.T. (1966). Founders of American Orthopedics. *J. Bone Jt. Surg.,* **48A**, 582
41. Bick, E.M. (1948). *A Source Book of Orthopedics.* p. 273. (Baltimore, Williams and Wilkins)
42. Siegel, I.M. (1979). *Int. Surg.,* **64(1)**, 83
43. Keith, A. (1919). *Menders of the Maimed.* (London)
44. Bradford, E.H. (1909). Congenital dislocation of the hip, results of treatment at Boston Children's Hospital. *Am. J. Orthop. Surg.,* **7**, 57
45. Bradford, E.H. and Brackett, E.G. (1893). Treatment of lateral curvature by means of pressure correction. *Boston Med. Surg. J.,* **5**, 183
46. Bradford, E.H. (1893). Operative treatment of resistant club foot. *Trans. Am. Orth. Assoc.,*
47. Bradford, E.H. (1897) Tenoplastic surgery. *Ann. Surg.,* **26**, 153
48. Bradford, E.H. and Tubby, A.R. (1912). *Deformities, including diseases of the bones and joints, a textbook of orthopaedic surgery.* 3rd edn. (London, MacMillan)
49. Lovett, R.W. (1900). The mechanics of lateral curvature of the spine. *Trans. Am. Orthop. Assoc.,* **13**, 251
50. Goldthwait, J.E. (1911). *Boston Med. Surg. J.,* **164**, 365
51. Dandy, W.E. (1929). *Arch. Surg.,* **19**, 660
52. Clymer, G., Mixter, W.J. and Mella, H. (1921). *Arch. Neurol. Psychiat.,* **5**, 213
53. Stookey, B. (1929). *Arch. Neurol. Psychiat.,* **20**, 275

54. Elseberg, C.A. (1928). *Surg. Gynecol. Obstet.*, **1**, 46
55. Bucy, P. (1930). *J. Am. Med. Assoc.*, **94**, 1552
56. Mixter, W.J. and Barr, J.S. (1934). *New Engl. J. Med.*, **211**, 210
57. Whitman, R. (1888). Observations on 45 cases of flat-foot with particular reference to etiology and treatment. *Boston Med. Surg. J.*, **188**, 598
58. Whitman, R. (1924). The reconstruction operation for arthritis deformans of the hip joint. *Ann. Surg.*, **80**, 779
59. Morton, T.G. (1876). *Am. J. Med. Sci.*, **71**, 37
60. Durlacher, L. (1845). *A Treatise on Corns, Bunions, the Diseases of Nails and the General Management of the Feet.* (London)
61. Freiberg, A.H. (1914). *Surg. Gynecol. Obstet.*, **19**, 191
62. Baer, W.S. (1909). The use of animal membranes in producing mobility in ankylosed joints. *Bull. Johns Hopkins Hosp.*, **20**, 271
63. Gross, S.W. (1879). Sarcoma of the long bones. *Am. J. Med. Sci. NS*, **78**, 17 and 338
64. Kolodny, A. (1925). Diagnosis and prognosis of bone sarcoma. *J. Bone Jt. Surg.*, **7**, 911
65. Kolodny, A. (1927). *Bone Sarcoma.* (Chicago, Surgical Publishing)
66. Preliminary meeting (1889). *Trans. Am. Orthop. Assn.*, **1**, 1
67. Coventry, M.B. (1977). *J. Bone Jt. Surg.*, **59A**, 1121
68. Mayer, L. (1950). *J. Bone Jt. Surg.*, **32B**, 461
69. Phelps, A. (1894). Presidential address: The influence of surgical bacteriology and modern pathology upon orthopedic surgery. *Trans. Am. Orthop. Assoc.*, **7**, 31
70. Whitman, R. (1894). Observations on bending of the neck of the femur in adolescence. *Trans. Am. Orthop. Assoc.*, **7**, 270
71. Whitman, R. (1897). Further observations on fractures of the neck of the femur in childhood. *Trans. Am. Orthop. Assoc.*, **10**, 216
72. Whitman, R. (1902). A new method of treatment for fracture of the neck of the femur. *Trans. Am. Orthop. Assoc.*, **15**, 338
73. Lovett, W.R. (1898). Pathology in its relation to orthopaedic surgery. *Trans. Am. Orthop. Assoc.*, **11**, 1
74. Lovett, W.R. (1900). The mechanics of lateral curvature of the spine. *Trans. Amer. Orthorp. Assoc.*, **13**, 251
75. Bryant, (1891). Ten cases of excision of the knee joint for disease and their lessons. *Trans. Am. Orthop. Assoc.*, **4**, 314
76. Hadra, B.E. (1891). Wiring the spinous processes in Pott's disease. *Transactions*, **4**, 206
77. Lovett, W.R. and Goldthwait, J.E. (1889). The abscesses of hip disease. *Transactions*, **2**, 82
78. Vance, A.M. (1889). Femoral osteotomy for the correction of deformity resulting from hip joint disease. *Transactions*, **1**, 149
79. Gibney, V.P. (1894). The correction of the deformity of hip disease. *Transactions*, **7**, 190
80. Nichols, E.H. (1898). Tuberculosis of bones and joints. *Transactions*, **11**, 353
81. Lorenz, A. (1896). The cure of congenital luxation of the hip by bloodless reduction. *Transactions*, **9**, 254
82. Bradford, E.H. (1894). Congenital dislocation of the hip. *Transactions*, **7**,
83. Bradford, E.H. (1900). Congenital dislocation of the hip. *Transactions*, **13**, 124
84. Bradford, E.H. (1902). Congenital dislocation of the hip. *Transactions*, **14**, 284
85. Lovett, W.R. (1900). The mechanics of lateral curvature of the spine. *Transactions*, **13**, 251
86. Dane, J. (1902). Remarks on arthrodesis of the ankle for infantile paralysis. *Transactions*, **15**, 29

87. Goldthwait, J.E. (1900). Knee joint surgery for non-tubercular conditions. *Boston Med. Surg. J.*, **143**, 286

88. Bradford, E.H. (1895). Slipping patella. *Trans. Am. Orthop. Assoc.*, **8**, 228

89. Steele, A.J. (1898). *Transactions*, **11**, 17

90. Davis, G.G. (1900). An operation for ununited intracapsular fracture of the neck of the femur. *Transactions*, **13**, 134

91. Thomson, C.E. (1901). Operative case of intracapsular fracture of the hip. *Transactions*, **14**, 361

92. Sherman, H. (1900). Presidential address. *Transactions*, **13**, 1

93. Wilson, A. (1902). Presidential address. The advance of orthopaedic surgery. *Transactions*, **15**, 1

94. Brackett, E.G. (1905) Presidential address. *Am. J. Orth. Surg.*, **3**, 1

95. Gibney, V. (1905). A report of the adult ward of the Hospital for the Ruptured and Crippled for the first two years ending March 1, 1905. *Am. J. Orth. Surg.*, **3**, 178

96. Albee, F. (1911). Transplantation of a portion of the tibia into the spine for Pott's disease. *J. Am. Med. Assoc.*, **57**, 885

97. Hibbs, R.A. (1911). An operation for progressive spinal deformities. *New York Med. J.*, **93**, 1013

98. Henderson, M.S. (1914). The treatment of ununited fractures of the tibia by the transplantation of bone. *Ann. Surg.*, **59**, 486

99. Albee, F. (1914). The inlay bone graft in fresh fractures *New York Med. J.*, **99**, 1020

100. Brackett, E.G. (1915). Operative treatment of osteoarthritis. *Am. J. Orth. Surg.*, **13**, 46

101. Ridlon, J. (1907). A preliminary report upon ten cases of chronic joint disease treated by tuberculin injections by Wright's method. *Am. J. Orth. Surg.*, **5**, 14

102. Ely, L.W. (1911). Joint tuberculosis in children. *Am. J. Orth. Surg.*, **9**, 31

103. Lange, F. (1910). Support for the spondylitic spine by means of buried steel bars attached to the vertebrae. *Am. J. Orth. Surg.*, **8**, 344

104. Ryerson, E.W. (1914). Pott's disease: Albee's bone-grafting operation. *Am. J. Orth. Surg.*, **12**, 259

105. Albee, F. (1916). *Bone graft surgery*. (Philadelphia, Saunders)

106. Baer, W.S. (1918). A preliminary report of the use of animal membrane in producing mobility in ankylosed joints. *Am. J. Orth. Surg.*, **16**, 94

107. Allison, N. and Brooks, B. (1918). Arthroplasty: experimental and clinical methods. *Amer. J. Orth. Surg.*, **16**, 83

108. Henderson, M.S. (1918). What are the real results of arthroplasty? *Am. J. Orth. Surg.*, **16**, 30

109. Murphy, J.B. (1912). Contribution to the surgery of bones, joints and tendons. *J. Am. Med. Assoc.*, **58**, 985

110. Lange, F. (1910). The orthopedic treatment of spinal paralysis. *Am. J. Orth. Surg.*, **8**, 8

111. Bartow, B. and Plummer, W.W. (1911). The use of intra-articular silk ligaments for fixation of loose joints in the residual paralysis of anterior poliomyelitis. *Am. J. Orth. Surg.*, **9**, 65

112. Bartow, B. and Plummer, W.W. (1913). The use of intra-articular silk ligaments for fixation of loose joints in the residual paralysis of anterior poliomyelitis. *Am. J. Orth. Surg.*, **10**, 499

113. Bartow, B. and Plummer, W.W. (1916). The use of intra-articular silk ligaments for fixation of loose joints in the residual paralysis of anterior poliomyelitis. *Am. J. Orth. Surg.*, **14**, 594

114. Mayer, L. (1916). The physiological method of tendon transplantation. *Surg.*

Gynecol. Obstet., **22**, 182

115. Gallie, W.E. and Le Mesurier, A.B. (1922). A clinical and experimental study of the free transplantation of fascia and tendon. *J. Bone Jt. Surg.*, **4**, 600

116. Whitman, R. (1901). The operative treatment of paralytic talipes of the calcaneus type. *Am. J. Med. Sci.*, **122**, 593

118. Hoke, M. (1911). An operative plan for the correction of relapsed and untreated talipes equinovarus. *Am. J. Orth. Surg.*, **9**, 379

118. Hoke, M. (1921). An operation for stabilizing paralytic feet. *J. Orth. Surg.*, **NS3**, 494

119. Freiberg, A.H., Silver, D. and Osgood, R.B. (1914). Report of the Committee on the treatment of Structural Scoliosis to the American Orthopedic Association. *Am. J. Orth. Surg.*, **12**, 5

120. Freiberg, A.H., Silver, D. and Osgood, R.B. (1915). Second Report of the Committee on the treatment of Structural Scoliosis to the American Orthopedic Association. *Am. J. Orth Surg.*, **13**, 6

121. Abbott, R.G. (1917). *Am. J. Orth. Surg.*, **15**, 26, 108, 172, 243, 262

122. Smith-Petersen, M.N. (1917). A new supra-articular approach to the hip joint. *Am. J. Orth. Surg.*, **15**, 592

123. Blanchard, W. (1906). The exceptional rachitic distortions of the legs. *Am. J. Orth. Surg.*, **4**, 207

124. Taylor, R.T. (1903). Hip disease. *Am. J. Orth. Surg.*, **1**, 14

125. Geist, E.S. (1907). Chondrodystrophia foetalis. *Am. J. Orth. Surg.*, **5**, 240

126. Davis, G.G. (1905). Multiple cancellous exostoses. *Am. J. Orth. Surg.*, **3**, 234

127. Freiberg, A.H. (1905). Coxa vara adolescentium. *Am. J. Orth. Surg.*, **3**, 6

128. Freiberg, A.H. (1914). Infraction of the second metatarsal bone. *Surg. Gynecol. Obstet.*, **19**, 191

129. Allison, N. and Brooks, B. (1915). Osteochondritis deformans juvenilis. **13**, 197

130. Brackett, E.G. (1905). Presidential address. *Am. J. Orth. Surg.*, **3**, 1

131. Goldthwait, J.E. (1909). The relation of posture to human efficiency and the influence of poise on the support and function of the viscera. *Am. J. Orth. Soc.*, **7**, 371

132. Goldthwait, J.E. (1916). The opportunity for the orthopedist in preventive medicine through educational work on posture. *Am. J. Orth. Soc.*, **14**, 443

133. Winnett, Orr, H. (1911). Reasons for the state care of the crippled and deformed. *Am. J. Orth. Surg.*, **9**, 218

134. Mitchell, S.W., Morehouse, G.R. and Keen, W.W. (1864) *Gunshot wounds and other injuries of nerves.* (Philadelphia, Lippincott)

135. Mitchell, S.W. (1872). *Injuries of nerves and their consequences.* (Philadelphia, Lippincott)

136. Mayer, L. (1959). Orthopaedic surgery in the United States of America. *J. Bone Jt. Surg.*, **32B**, 483

137. Lovett, R.W. (1918). The problem of the reconstruction and re-education of the disabled soldier. *Surg. Gynecol. Obstet.*, **27**, 169

138. Murphy, J.B. (1905). Ankylosis, arthroplasty, clinical and experimental. *J. Am. Med. Assoc.*, **44**, 1573, 1671, 1749

139. Murphy, J.B. (1913). Arthroplasty. *Ann. Surg.*, **57**, 593

140. Baer, W.S. (1909). A preliminary report of the use of animal membrane in producing mobility in ankylosed joints. *Am. J. Orth. Surg.*, **7**, 1

141. Baer, W.S. (1916). Arthroplasty with the aid of animal membrane. *Am. J. Orth. Surg.*, **16**, 1, 94, 171

142. MacAusland, W.R. (1923). Mobilisation of ankylosed joints *Surg. Gynecol. Obstet.*, **37**, 255

143. Campbell, W.C. (1931). The physiology of arthroplasty, Robert Jones Lecture

at the Hospital for Joint Diseases, New York. *J. Bone Jt. Surg.*, **13**, 223

144. Campbell, W.C. (1940). Interposition of vitallium plates in arthroplasty of the knee. *Am. J. Surg.*, **47**, 639

145. Albert, E. (1881). *Zentralblatt f. Chirurgie.*, **48**

146. Davis, G. (1913). The treatment of hollow foot (pes cavus). *Am. J. Orth. Surg.*, **11**, 231

147. Hoke, M. (1921). An operation for stabilising paralytic feet. *J. Orth. Surg.*, **3**, 494

148. Ryerson, E.S. (1923). Arthrodesing operations on the feet. *J. Bone Jt. Surg.*, **5**, 453

149. Hibbs, R.A. (1911). An operation for stiffening the knee joint. *Ann. Surg.*, **53**, 404

150. Albee, F.H. (1915). *Bone-Graft Surgery.* (Saunders, Philadelphia)

151. Bosworth, D.M. (1946). Knee fusion by the use of a three-flanged nail. *J. Bone Jt. Surg.*, **28**, 550

152. Milgram, J.E. (1931). A modification of the rotation arthrodesis of the knee (Roeren). *Surg. Gynecol. Obstet.*, **53**, 355

153. Key, J.A. (1932). Positive pressure in arthrodesis for tuberculosis of the knee joint. *South Med. J.*, **25**, 909

154. Albee, F.H. (1929). Extra-articular arthrodesis of the hip for tuberculosis. *Ann. Surg.*, **89**, 404

155. Hibbs, R.A. (1926). A preliminary report of 20 cases of hip joint tuberculosis treated by an operation devised to eliminate motion by fusing the joint. *J. Bone Jt. Surg.*, **8**, 522

156. Schumm, H.C. (1920). Extra-articular immobilisation of the hip joint. *Surg. Gynecol. Obstet.*, **48**, 112

157. Trumble, H.C. (1932). Fixation of hip by extra-articular bone graft. *Aust. N.Z.J. Surg.*, **1**, 413

158. Brittain, H.A. (1942). *Architectural Principles in Arthrodesis.* (Baltimore, Williams and Wilkins)

159. Albee, F.H. (1930). Principles of treatment of nonunion of fractures. *Surg. Gynecol. Obstet.*, **51**, 289

160. Phemister, D.B. (1931). Split grafts in the treatment of delayed and nonunion of fractures. *Surg. Gynecol. Obstet.*, **52**, 376

161. Campbell, W.C. (1923). The treatment of ununited fractures. *Am. J. Surg.*, **37**, 1

162. Henderson, M.S. (1923). Nonunion in fractures: the massive bone graft. *J. Am. Med. Assoc.*, **81**, 463

163. Boyd, H.B. (1943). The treatment of difficult and unusual nonunions, with special reference to bridging of defects. *J. Bone Jt. Surg.*, **25**, 535

164. Key, J.A. (1937). Treatment of nonunion of fractures. *Surgery*, **1**, 730

165. Inclán, A. (1942) The use of preserved bone grafts in orthopaedic surgery. *J. Bone Jt. Surg.*, **24**, 81

166. Lovett, R.W. (1916) The spring balance muscle test. *Am. J. Orth. Surg.*, **14**, 415

167. Soutter, R. (1914). A new operation for hip contractures in poliomyelitis. *Boston Med. Surg. J.*, **170**, 380

168. Campbell, W.C. (1923). Transference of the crest of the ilium for flexion contracture of the hip. *South. Med. J.*, **16**, 289

169. Mayer, L. (1931). Fixed paralytic obliquity of the pelvis. *J. Bone Jt. Surg.*, **13**, 1

170. Mayer, L. (1936). Further studies on fixed paralytic pelvic obliquity. *J. Bone Jt. Surg.*, **18**, 87

171. Lowman, C.L. (1931). Plastic repair for paralysis of abdominal musculature.

New Engl. J. Med., **205**, 1187

172. Mayer, L. (1916). The physiological method of tendon transplantation. *Surg. Gynecol. Obstet.*, **22**, 182, 298, 472

173. Mayer, L. (1927). Transplantation of the trapezius for paralysis of the abductors of the arm. *J. Bone Jt. Surg.*, **9**, 412

174. Peabody, C.W. (1938). Tendon transposition: an end-result study. *J. Bone Jt. Surg.*, **20**, 193

175. Steindler, A. (1919). Operative treatment of paralytic conditions of the upper extremity. *J. Orth. Surg.*, **1**, 608

176. Bunnell, S. (1938). Opposition of the thumb. *J. Bone Jt. Surg.*, **20**, 269

177. Bunnell, S. (1942). Surgery of the intrinsic muscles of the hand other than those producing opposition of the thumb. *J. Bone Jt. Surg.*, **24**, 1

178. Pohl, J.F. (1943). *The Kenny concept of infantile paralysis and its treatment.* (Bryce Publishing Co., St Paul, Minnesota)

179. Bunnell, S. (1918). Repair of tendons in the fingers. *Surg. Gynecol. Obstet.*, **26**, 103

180. Ober, F.R. (1932). An operation to relieve paralysis of the deltoid muscle. *J. Am. Med. Assoc.*, **99**, 2182

181. Schwartzmann, J.R. and Crego, C.H. (1948). Hamstring tendon transplantation for the relief of quadriceps femoris paralysis in residual poliomyelitis. *J. Bone Jt. Surg.*, **30A**, 541

182. Irwin, C.E. (1942). Transplants to thumb to restore function of opposition. End-results. *South. Med. J.*, **35**, 257

183. Starr, C.L. (1922). Army experience with tendon transference. *J. Bone Jt. Surg.*, **4**, 3

184. Paci, A. (1888). *Studio ed osservazione sulla lussazione iliaca commune congenita e sua cura razionale.* (Genoa)

185. Lorenz, A. (1896). Cure of congenital luxation of the hip by bloodless reduction and weighting. *Trans. Am. Orth. Assoc.*, **9**, 254

186. Bradford, E.H. (1894). Congenital dislocation of the hip. *Trans. Am. Orth. Assoc.*, **7**, 88

187. Bradford, E.H. (1900). Congenital dislocation of the hip. *Trans. Am. Orth. Assoc.*, **13**, 124

188. Bradford, E.H. (1902). Congenital dislocation of the hip. *Trans. Am. Orth. Assoc.*, **15**, 284

189. Davis, G.G. (1907). A method of reduction of congenital luxation of the hip by manipulation. *Am. J Orth. Surg.*, **4**, 276

190. Galloway, H.P.H. (1920). The open operation for congenital dislocation of the hip. *J. Orth. Surg.*, **2**, 390

191. Farrell, B.P., von Lackum, H.L. and Smith, A. de F. (1926). Congenital dislocation of the hip: report of 310 cases treated at New York Orthopaedic Dispensary and Hospital. *J. Bone Jt. Surg.*, **8**, 551

192. Freiberg, A.H. (1935). Congenital luxation of hip: selection of cases for open reduction. *J. Bone Jt. Surg.*, **17**, 1

193. Farrell, B.P. and Howarth, M.B. (1935). Open reduction in congenital dislocation of the hip. *J. Bone Jt. Surg.* **17**, 35

194. Dickson, F.D. (1935). The shelf operation in treatment of congenital dislocation of the hip. *J. Bone Jt. Surg.*, **17**, 43

195. Gill, A.B. (1935). Plastic construction of an acetabulum in congenital dislocation of the hip: the shelf operation *J. Bone Jt. Surg.*, **17**, 48

196. Compere, E.L. and Phemister, D.B. (1935). The tibial peg shelf in congenital dislocation of the hip. *J. Bone Jt. Surg.*, **17**, 60

197. Kleinberg, S. and Lieberman, H.S. (1936). The acetabular index in infants in

relation to congenital dislocation of the hip. *Arch. Surg.*, **32**, 1049

198. Bost, F.C. *et al.* (1948). The results of treatment of congenital dislocation of the hip in infancy. *J. Bone Jt. Surg.*, **30A**, 454

199. Anzoletti, A. (1954). *Alessandro Codivilla e Vittorio Putti nel ricordo di un loro contemporaneo.* (Bologna)

200. Codivilla, A. (1905). On the means of lengthening, in the lower limbs, the muscles and tissues which are shortened through deformity. *Am. J. Orth. Surg.*, **2**, 353

201. Putti, V. (1927). The operative lengthening of the femur. *J. Am. Med. Assoc.*, **77**, 934

202. Abbott, L.C. (1927). The operative lengthening of the tibia and fibula. *J. Bone Jt. Surg.*, **9**, 128

203. White, J.W. (1935). Femoral shortening for equalizing of leg length *J. Bone Jt. Surg.*, **17**, 597

204. Compere, E.L. (1936). Indications for and against the leg lengthening operation. *J. Bone Jt. Surg.*, **18**, 692

205. Campbell, W.C. (1939). *Operative Orthopaedics* (St Louis, CV Mosby)

206. Phemister, D.B. (1933). Operative arrestment of longitudinal growth of bones in the treatment of deformities. *J. Bone Jt. Surg.*, **15**, 1

207. Baldwin, B.T (1921). The physical growth of children from birth to maturity. (University of Iowa Publications)

208. Greulich, W.W. and Pyle, S.I. (1950). *Radiographic Atlas of Skeletal Development of the Hand and Wrist.* (Stanford University Press).

209. Green, W.T. and Anderson, M. (1947). Experiences with epiphysial arrest in correcting discrepancies in length of the lower extremities in infantile paralysis. *J. Bone Jt. Surg.*, **29**, 659

210. Haas, S.L. (1945). Retardation of bone growth by a wire loop. *J. Bone Jt. Surg.*, **27**, 25

211. Blount, W.P. and Clarke, G.R. (1949). Control of bone growth by epiphysial stapling *J. Bone Jt. Surg.*, **31A**, 464

212. Goldthwait, J.E. (1911). The lumbosacral articulation: an explanation of many cases of 'lumbago', 'sciatica' and paraplegia. *Boston Med. Surg. J.*, **164**, 365

213. Schmorl, G. (1927). *Verh. d. Deutsches Path. Ges.*, **21**, 3

214. Schmorl, G. (1928). *Verh. d. Deutsches Path. Ges.*, **22**, 250

215. Beadle, O.A. (1931) The Intervertebral Discs: observations on their normal and morbid anatomy in relation to certain spinal deformities. London, No 161, Medical Research Council Special Report Series

216. Stookey, B. (1928). Compression of the spinal cord due to ventral extradural cervical chondromas. *Arch. Neurol. Psych.*, **20**, 275

217. Dandy, W.E. (1929). Loose cartilage from intervertebral disc simulating tumor of the spinal cord. *Arch. Surg.*, **19**, 660

218. Bucy, P.C. (1930). Chondroma of intervertebral disc. *J. Am. Med. Assoc.*, **94**, 1552

219. Petit-Dutaillis, D. and Alajouanine, T. (1928). Syndrome unilatéral de la queue de cheval, laminectomie exploratrice et ablation d'un fibrome du disque intervertébrale. *Bull. Mem. Soc. Nat. Chir.*, **54**, 1452

220. Mixter, W.J. and Barr, J.S. (1934). Rupture of the intervertebral disc with involvement of the spinal canal. (1934). *New Engl. J. Med.*, **211**, 210

221. Lindblom, K. (1948). Diagnostic puncture of the intervertebral discs in sciatica. *Acta Orthop. Scand.*, **17**, 231

222. Smith, L. (1963). Enzyme dissolution of the nucleus pulposus. *Nature*, **198**

223. Smith, L. (1964). Enzyme dissolution of nucleus pulposus in humans *J. Am. Med. Assoc.*, **187**, 137

224. Hibbs, R.A. (1924). A report of 59 cases of scoliosis treated by the fusion operation. *J. Bone Jt. Surg.*, **6**, 3
225. Hibbs, R.A., Risser, J.C. and Ferguson, A.B. (1931). *J. Bone Jt. Surg.*, **13**, 91
226. Steindler, A. (1929). *Diseases and deformities of the spine and thorax.* p. 244 (St Louis, CV Mosby)
227. Dwyer, A.F., Newton, N.C. and Sherwood, A.A. (1969). An anterior approach to scoliosis. *Clin. Orthop.*, **62**, 192
228. Harrington, P.R. (1973). The history and development of Harrington instrumentation. *Clin. Orthop.*, **93**, 110
229. Lange, F. (1910). Support for the spondylitic spine by means of buried steel bars attached to the vertebrae. *Am. J. Orth. Surg.*, **8**, 344
230. Hadra, B.E. (1891). Wiring of the vertebrae as a means of immobilization in fractures and Pott's disease. *Med. Times and Register*, **22**, 423
231. Hibbs, R.A. (1911). An operation for progressive spinal deformities. A preliminary report of three cases from the service of the New York Orthopaedic Hospital. *N.Y. Med. J.*, **93**, 1031
232. Whitman, R. (1893) *Med. Record,*
233. Whitman, R. (1897). *Trans. Am. Orth. Assoc.*, **10**, 216
234. Whitman, R. (1902). A new method for fractures of the neck of the femur. *Ann. Surg.*, **36**, 746
235. Leadbetter, G.W. (1933). A treatment for fracture of the neck of the femur. *J. Bone Surg.*, **15**, 931
236. Leadbetter, G.W. (1938). Closed reduction of fractures of the neck of the femur. *J. Bone Jt. Surg.*, **20**, 108
237. Smith-Petersen, M.N., Cave, E.F. and Vangorder, G.W. (1931). Intracapsular fractures of the neck of the femur. *Arch. Surg.*, **23**, 715
238. Johansson, S. (1932). *Acta Orth. Scand.*, **3**, 362
239. Speed, K. (1935). The Unsolved Fracture. *Surg. Gynecol. Obstet.*, **60**, 341
240. Cooper, A. (1823) A Treatise on Dislocations of the Joints. 2nd edn. p. 570 (London)
241. Fracture Committee of the American Academy of Orthopaedic Surgeons (1939). Treatment of fractures of the neck of the femur by internal fixation. *J. Bone Jt. Surg.*, **21**, 483
242. Fracture Committee of the American Academy of Orthopaedic Surgeons. (1941). Treatment of fractures of the neck of the femur by internal fixation. *J. Bone Jt. Surg.*, **23**, 386
243. Urist, M.R. and McLean, F.C.L. (1941). *J. Bone Jt. Surg.*, **23**, 1
244. Urist, M.R. and McLean, F.C.L. (1941). *J. Bone Jt. Surg.*, **23**, 483
245. Urist, M.R (1942). *J. Bone Jt. Surg.*, **24**, 47
246. Urist, M.R and Johnson, R.W. (1943). *J. Bone Jt. Surg.*, **25**, 375
247. Eggers, G.W.N. (1948). Internal contact splint. *J. Bone Jt. Surg.*, **30A**, 41
248. Rush, L.V. and Rush, H.L. (1939). A technique for longitudinal pin fixation of certain fractures of the ulna and of the femur. *J. Bone Jt. Surg.*, **21**, 619
249. Anderson, R., McKibbin, W.B. and Burgess, E. (1943). Intertrochanteric fracture. *J. Bone Jt. Surg.*, **25**, 153
250. Bordley, J. and Harvey, A. McG. (1976) *Two Centuries of American Medicine.* (Philadelphia, Saunders)
251. Codman, E.A (1934). *The Shoulder.* (Boston, Todd)
252. Codman, E.A. (1931) Epiphyseal chondromatous giant cell tumors of the upper end of the humerus. *Surg. Gynecol. Obstet.*, **52**, 543
253. Abernethy, J. (1804) *Surgical observations on tumours.* (London, Longman and Rees)
254. Hey, W. (1803). *Practical observations in surgery, illustrated with cases.* (London)

255. Dupuytren, G. (1839). *Leçons orales de cliniques chirurgicales faites á l'Hôtel-Dieu de Paris.* (Paris, Baillière)
256. Cooper, A. and Travers, B. (1818). *Surgical Essays, Part* 1. (London)
257. Müller, J. (1838). *Über den finern Bau und die Formen der krankhaften Geschwülste.* (Berlin)
258. Lebert, H. (1845). *Physiologie Pathologique aux Recherches Cliniques, Expérimentales et Microscopiques.* (Paris, Baillière)
259. Nélaton, A. (1860) *D'une nouvelle espèce de tumeurs bénignes des os, ou tumeurs à myéloplaxes.* (Paris, Delahaye)
260. Gross, S. (1879). Sarcoma of the long bones: based on a study of 165 cases. *Am. J. Med. Sci.,* **78**, 17
261. Morris, H. (1876) Annotations, *Lancet,* March 18, 440
262. Clutton, H.H. (1894). Three cases of giant-celled sarcoma of the radius. *Trans. Clin. Soc. Lond.,* **27**, 86
263. Krause, F. (1889). Ueber die Behandlung der schaligen myelogenen Sarcoma (Myeloide, Riesenzellensarkoma) durch Ausräumung anstatt Amputation *Verh. Dtsch. Ges. Chir.,* **18**, 198
264. Mickulicz, J. (1895). Ueber ausgedehnte Resectionen der langen Rohrenknochen wegen maligner Geschwülste. *Arach. Klin. Chir.,* **50**, 660
265. Bloodgood, J. (1899). Benign and malignant tumors of bone. *Prog. Med.,* 234.
266. Bloodgood, J. (1812). The conservative treatment of giant-cell sarcoma with the study of bone transplantation. *Ann. Surg.,* **56**, 210
267. Ewing, J. (1919). *Neoplastic Diseases. A Treatise on Tumors.* (Philadelphia, WB Saunders)
268. Ewing, J. (1922). A review and classification of bone sarcomas. *Arch. Surg.,* **4**, 485
269. Ewing, J. (1939). A review of the classification of bone tumors. *Surg. Gynecol. Obstet.,* **68**, 971
270. Jaffe, H.L., Lichtenstein, L. and Portis, R.B. (1940). Giant cell tumor of bone. Its pathologic appearance, grading, supposed variants and treatment. *Arch. Path.,* **30**, 993
271. Magnuson, P.B. (1941) Joint debridement: surgical treatment of degenerative arthritis. *Surg. Gynecol. Obstet.,* **73**, 1
272. Naffziger, H.C. and Grant, W.T. (1938) Neuritis of the brachial plexus mechanical in origin: the scalenus syndrome. *Surg. Gynecol. Obstet.,* **67**, 722
273. Stopford, J.S.B. and Telford, E.D. (1919). *Brit. J. Surg.,* 7, 168
274. Adson, A.W. and Coffey, J.R. (1927). Cervical rib. *Ann. Surg.,* **85**, 839
275. Ochsner, A., Gage, M. and DeBakey, M. (1935). *Am. J. Surg.,* **28**, 669
276. Wartenberg, R. (1936). *Ztschr. ges. Neurol. u. Psychiat.,* **154**, 695
277. Adson, A.W. (1947). Surgical treatment for symptoms produced by cervical ribs and the scalenus anticus muscle. *Surg. Gynecol. Obstet.,* **85**, 687
278. Smith-Petersen, M.N., Larsen, C.B. and Aufranc, O.E. (1945). Osteotomy of the spine for correction of flexion deformity in rheumatoid arthritis. *J. Bone Jt. Surg.,* **27**, 1
279. Phemister, D.B. (1940). Conservative surgery in the treatment of bone tumors. *Surg. Gynecol. Obstet.,* **70**, 355

CHAPTER 16

National Histories – Latin America

To some extent, the problems and development of orthopaedic surgery in Latin America resemble those of Australasia and South Africa. All were vast areas, remote in European terms, colonized from Europe with large immigrant European populations, and their orthopaedic history has been mostly confined to the 20th century. It was natural for them originally to turn to the 'mother country', as generations of Australians did to Britain; but in South America this was not to Spain or Portugal, but to other European countries: to France, for Mexico, to Italy for Argentina because of its huge Italian immigrant population, and to Germany. Later, more especially after World War I, the trend was towards the United States, partly because it was nearer and advance faster there, partly because of the investment of American concern and funds in the treatment of crippled children in the southern half of the continent. But it should also be borne in mind that the Spaniards had established universities in the south as far back as the 16th century, and that some of these had medical faculties before any existed in the north.

This is not to say that there is no history of native South American orthopaedics before the Conquest. As Juan Farill points out[1], in what was to become Mexico, the Aztec kingdom had a well-developed system of medicine with various types of specialists, including bonesetters – *teomiquet-zani* or *tepatiltzili* – who used traction, countertraction, manipulation and immobilization for fractures and dislocations. For ununited fractures, according to a Spanish friar of the 16th century, they scraped the bone and 'inserted into the medullary canal a stick of very resinous wood...in order to set the bone firmly[2].' Fractures were immobilized in wooden splints or by rigid agave leaves bound with leather straps, or by an adhesive resinous paste. Excavations at Teotihuacan revealed Indian frescoes depicting bilateral club-feet and what appears to be a left hemiplegia.

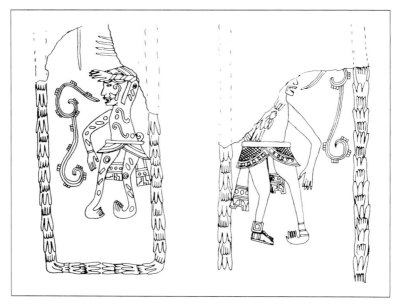

Figure 204 Drawings from the frescoes of excavations at Teotihuacán, Mexico which show (at the left) a boy with bilateral club-foot and (at the right) a case of unilateral club-foot deformity in an older person

MEXICO

Here the first hospitals were established by Cortés himself, in 1524, and in 1536 the clergy founded the *Colegio de Santa Cruz de Tlaltelolco* in which medicine was taught for the first time in the Americas, North or South. The *Universidad de México* was inaugurated in 1533 and soon acquired a bonesetter. Farill says that, also in the 16th century, operations on bones and limbs were performed under analgesia produced by the consumption of mandrake. Nor was more modern Mexico slow to exploit medical advances: the first blood transfusion in the Americas may have been performed there in 1845, ether anaesthesia was used in 1847, a year after Morton in Boston, the first X-rays were taken in 1896, a few months after their discovery.

French influence predominated in Mexico (and other Latin countries) from the late 19th century until after World War I, when it was replaced by the United States, notably by Steindler. Thus, the French school had been very conservative in treating skeletal tuberculosis in children, but the advent of the Hibbs and Albee techniques of spinal fusion changed this. Synovectomy for tuberculosis had been performed in the early years of the 20th century, perhaps under the influence of Volkmann and Mignon, but possibly because, just before 1900 and after, Aureliano Urrutia, later professor of surgery, was a general surgeon with notable interests in orthopaedic surgery, including synovectomy and astragalectomy. In 1920, Manuel Madrazo, who had trained in New York, imported the first Albee electric saw and an orthopaedic table and was the first Mexican to practise exclusively in orthopaedics, so ushering in the modern era of this field in that country.

In 1922 a department for bone and joint disease was opened in the *Hospital General* by Ortiz Tirado by converting a general surgical department, and in 1933 Juan Farill was formally appointed its head. The outsider tends to equate the story of Mexican orthopaedics with this great man and is not far wrong, for he introduced skeletal traction and fixation, pinning of the femoral neck under X-ray control, myelography for disc lesions, arteriography for bone tumours, epiphyseodesis and many other contemporary techniques. This sudden adoption and exploitation of the newest techniques, without any previous gradual evolution of experience and principles, is a characteristic of virgin territories in any field. It has been said of politics in the Third World that the French and Russian Revolutions arrived hand in hand.

When a society for aid to crippled children known as the *Amigos del Niño Lisiado* was founded in 1935, it was natural for Farill to be its first president and he was executive secretary of the International Society for the Welfare of the Crippled during 1942–8. His only failure seems to have been the *Revista de Ortopedia y Traumatología Esqueletica*, which he founded in 1937 but did not survive the first issue.

When the *Hospital Infantil* opened in 1943, it housed two orthopaedic services, directed by Farill and Velasco Zimbron, who started the first cadaveric bone-bank. In 1945 the Internal Association of Shriners founded its first Latin American unit in Mexico, inaugurating an era of orthopaedic collaboration between north and south.

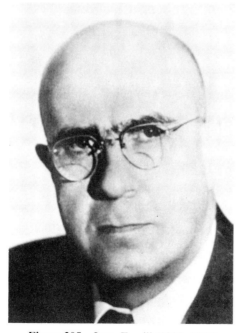

Figure 205   Juan Farrill (1902–1973)

The *Sociedad Mexicana de Ortopedia* was inaugurated in 1944 and published the *Anales de Ortopedia y Traumatología* from 1950 on. In 1944 also, Mexico followed the Austrian example with Böhler in that the *Instituto Mexicano del Seguro Social* founded the *Hospital de Ortopedia y Traumatología*, directed by José Dominguez. In 1948 the inaugural meeting of the *Sociedad Latino-Americana de Ortopedia y Traumatología* was held at Acapulco with Farill as President.

Academic recognition began with instructional courses in the hospitals by Farill and others. In 1944 he became the first professor in the orthopaedic department of the university faculty.

ARGENTINA

Here, orthopaedics naturally developed in first Buenos Aires, later in Rosario de Santa Fé and Córdoba. The strongest early influences were Italian, French and German and were of a conservative nature; later, more interventionist British and US approaches prevailed. But with its enormous Italian immigrant population, it was natural to turn to Italy for guidance, and in 1905 Luis Tamini, recently graduated, went to study at the Rizzoli Institute in Bologna under Codivilla, later at Zürich under Schulthess. Back at home, he was given charge of orthopaedic cases (though there was as yet no department) at the *Hospital de Clínicas*. At the same time, Alejandro Castro was combining paediatrics with orthopaedics on the French style at the *Hospital de Niños*, where there were many cases of bone tuberculosis, and created a true school of clinical orthopaedics.

Tamini was to become the first professor of orthopaedics, in 1923 and was the first exclusively orthopaedic surgeon in Argentina. A great surgeon practising orthopaedics at the *Hospital de Clínicas* was Alejandro Posadas, one of whose pupils, Enrique Finocchietto (1881–1948) was to acquire fame as an orthopaedic surgeon. Finocchietto graduated in 1904 with a thesis on club-foot, studied in Europe and, with other Argentinians, worked in France during World War I as senior surgeon at the Argentine Hospital in Paris.

Even after the first quarter of the century, however, Argentine orthopaedics was relatively underdeveloped and still largely in the hands of the general surgeons, especially as regards fractures.

Then, in 1925, interest was aroused by a lecture tour by Vittorio Putti and a scholarship was created to allow Argentinians to study in Bologna The first to do so was **José Valls** (1896–1977), who, perhaps more than anyone, is identified with the rise of modern Argentinian orthopaedics. When he returned he was made head of the department of orthopaedics and traumatology in the Italian Hospital of Buenos Aires in 1926, with the same pitifully small allocation of beds – in this case, six – that we have noted in infant orthopaedic departments elsewhere, but with a disciple, Carlos Ottolenghi, who was also to become famous. Between them, they created one of the foremost departments in the world, one which trained not only young Argentine orthopaedists but others from Chile, Peru, Venezuela, Colombia, Ecuador and Mexico. In the 1930s they pioneered regional lymph-

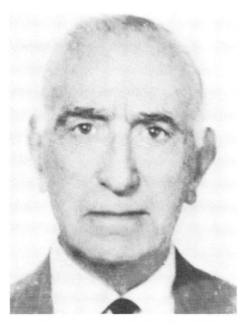

Figure 206 José Valls (1896–1977)

node biopsy for the diagnosis of osteoarticular tuberculosis[3]. Valls did so much in so many fields that only the most important can be named; his work on bone tumours, especially diagnosis by aspiration biopsy, including the vertebral bodies, done with Ottolenghi and Fritz Schajowicz, the last a pathologist imported by Valls from Vienna in 1938. For 46 years Valls was editor of the *Revista de Ortopedia y Traumatología*.

Carlos E Ottolenghi (1904–84) was a Buenos Aires graduate of 1926 who followed Valls to Bologna in 1929 and, like him, joined the staff of the Italian Hospital and was chief of service in 1944–75. In 1963–70 he was professor of orthopaedics and traumatology at the university in Buenos Aires, developing a national orthopaedic school. He was a founder-member of the Argentine Society for Orthopaedics and Traumatology and of the Latin American Society and in 1970 created the Ottolenghi Foundation for the Progress of Orthopaedics and Traumatology which established a research centre.

The second holder of the Bologna fellowship was Julio Dellepiane Rawson (1895–1930), whose organization of the service at the *Hospital Rivadivia* was interrupted by his untimely death. In 1930 Valls inaugurated the *Revista de Ortopedia y Traumatología*, the first Latin American orthopaedic journal. In 1936, with others who had trained under Putti, he founded the *Sociedad Argentina de Ortopedia*; the words *y Traumatología* were not added to the title until 1949, confirming the hesitation in, or obstruction to, including fractures in orthopaedic treatment that were seen elsewhere as orthopaedics emerged from general surgery.

Valls succeeded Tamini as professor at the latter's death in 1938, teaching mainly at the Durand Hospital for 25 years, and giving up the chair at La Plata which had been created in 1936. The La Plata chair was filled by **Enrique Lagomarsino** (1900–1946), a dynamic organizer and researcher, co-author with Valls in 1943 of a book on the treatment of femoral neck fractures but removed by early death. Premature death was impending for another brilliant young man, **Julio Soronto** (1903–1947), who had realized that, as in Australia, medical services in remote parts of a vast country could only be ensured by air and developed the equivalent of the Flying Doctor Service, the *Socorro Médico Aéreo*.

Marcelo Fitte (1894–1949) studied in Europe, especially with Ombredanne and devoted an outstanding talent to scoliosis and poliomyelitis, directing the department for infantile paralysis at the *Hospital de Niños* for ten years and urging that these patients should be treated by orthopaedists from the outset. In other fields at the Children's Hospital, the French tradition of combining paediatric with orthopaedic surgery was maintained for many years.

Hydatid disease of bone is not rare in Argentina and was documented by Ivanissevich in 1934[5].

Rosario de Santa Fé is the second city of Argentina and a chair of orthopaedics was founded there in 1930, first held by Marcos Steinleger. Two brothers, **Artemio** and **Lelio Zeno**, greatly contributed to developments in the city. Artemio fostered the separation of orthopaedics from general surgery and the training of younger men. Lelio was more inclined to regard traumatology as part of general surgery and, in 1931, was invited to plan the first Russian institute of traumatology in Moscow in collaboration with Professor Sergius Judin, chief of surgery at the Sklyfasowsky Institute. He pioneered overhead skeletal traction for elbow fractions in children[6] and translated Böhler's book into Spanish.

Córdoba, the 'Oxford' of Argentina, the site of the first university, had as professor of surgery in the 1920s **Juan Martin Allende**. He visited the Rizzoli Institute in 1925 and was sufficiently impressed to recommend this new field to his brother, Guillermo, who in turn studied under Putti and practised orthopaedics exclusively, taking the first chair when it was founded in 1940. Allende was a leading figure, especially in training, and in 1947 Cordoba founded its own *Sociedad de Ortopedia y Tramatología*.

CUBA

Orthopaedics here is largely identified with **Alberto Inclán** (1888–1965), and Inclán with the early massive use of banked bone grafts[7]. In fact, the first orthopaedic departments were started around 1904, by Enrique Porto at the *Hospital Nuestra Señora de las Mercedes* after study under Sayre and Whitman had led him to devote himself to this field, and by Armando Guerrero. Inclán began under Porto at the *Mercedes* in 1916 and created his own emergency service at the municipal hospital in 1920. In 1925 the University of Havana created a chair and appointed Inclán, who returned to the *Mercedes* to build up the first Cuban orthopaedic organization, and in 1933 he founded the *Revista de Cirugía Ortopédica y Traumatología*, later to become the organ of the *Sociedad Cubana de Ortopedia y Traumatología*, founded in 1944 with Inclán as president. In 1956, the *Revista* merged with the journal of the Latin American Orthopaedic Association. Inclán was a dynamic and meticulous worker, a Havana graduate of 1910, who studied under Whitman at the Hospital for Special Surgery in New York in 1911–13. He wrote over 60 papers, is best known for his work on refrigerated bone and was internationally honoured, but became isolated in the Castro years.

URUGUAY

The link with one particular man is seen again in Uruguay, where the protagonist was Jose Luis Bado. Until 1935, orthopaedics was performed by general surgeons, whether for children or adults (the two tended to be separate, the former related mainly to congenital deformities, skeletal tuberculosis and osteomyelitis, the latter to injuries). In the early part of the century French influence predominated and affected the first professor of clinical surgery, Alfredo Navarro, appointed in 1897. Because he had been taught by Kirmisson in Paris, among others, he had a particular interest in locomotor disorders and treated them along the lines of the French school. As early as 1908, at the Children's Hospital in Montevideo (*Hospital de Niños Pereyra Rosell*), two wards with 60 beds were allotted to paediatric orthopaedic surgery as an entity with Prudencio de Pena as director (where he remained for 30 years). A similar combined department was set up at the *Hospital Pedro Visca*.

Jose Luis Bado (1903–1977) is one of the great figures in Latin American orthopaedics. He trained for two years under Putti and on his return was designated director of a new department for orthopaedics and trauma at the *Clínica Quirúrgica* As Bado says, this was an entry point for Putti's spirit into Uruguay[8]. Bado was thus the first specialized orthopaedic surgeon, and in June 1941 inaugurated the new *Instituto Traumatológico*, built by the social security authorities, later to become the *Instituto de Ortopedia y de Traumatología*. In such a small country, this became the national centre, though other services existed for children and a special government institute for occupational injuries.

1948 saw the foundation of the *Anales de Ortopedia y Traumatología de Montevideo*. Bado became the first professor of orthopaedics in 1951 and was a founder-member of the Latin American Society. Bado was not just an excellent orthopaedic surgeon and organizer. He devoted imense effort to training and he was also an exponent of the philosophy of orthopaedic surgery and author of a dozen books. Few orthopaedic surgeons *think* deeply about their art; they are too busy getting on with it; but Bado was of the right temperament and had been taught by Putti and that was something that permanently influenced a man's way of life.

CHILE

In Chile the speciality dates only from about 1925. Before then most surgeons had been trained in France, so there was the familiar pattern of a department of paediatric/orthopaedic surgery, based on children's hospitals (*Hospital de Niños Roberto del Rio*) and the first chair in this combined field was allotted in 1929 to **Eugenio Diaz Liva** (1880–1945), who had been trained under Broca, Kirmisson, Calot and Ménard. Other combined departments grew up at other children's hospitals. Liva, the father of Chilean orthopaedics, was succeeded by Arnulfo Johow, and the passage of social security legislation led to the establishment of the *Instituto Traumatológico de Santiago* in 1937, headed by Professor Teodoro Gebauer, who graduated in 1927, trained in Europe and then trained large numbers of Chilean traumatologists. Centres in other parts of this long straggling country were founded by the social insurance authorities. In 1936, Putti visited the country as part of a tour of South America and bestowed two scholarships for study at Bologna which led to a spread of Italian influence.

BRAZIL

We are told that the medical faculty at Rio de Janeiro petitioned the government for an orthopaedic institute in 1841, and that this was not granted until 1911[9]. True, a chair in paediatric surgery was founded in 1888, held by **Candido Barata Ribeiro** (1843–1910), who was interested in skeletal problems, including the forcible correction of Pott's kyphosis. Another distinguished orthopaedist, or would-be orthopaedist, was **Joaquin Pinto Portella** (1860–1934), whose travels in Europe in 1888 led him to write an account of his impressions with a plea for Brazilian doctors to pay attention to this new speciality, 'so that some might dedicate themselves to it as earnestly and thoroughly as European and American orthopaedists.' In that same year he wrote an article on *The Necessity for the Foundation of Orthopaedic Institutes and Maritime Hospitals in Rio de Janeiro* which was very productive. An orthopaedic department was based at the *Santa Casa* in 1911 and a special *Hospital São Zacharias* created in 1914, with 15 children's beds and operating and plaster facilities.

The university at Rio established a chair in paediatric/orthopaedic surgery in 1911, held until 1925 by **Nascimento Gurgel** (1876–1928). This was obviously under French influence, one result of which was that the teaching institutions had no accommodation for adults with orthopaedic disorders: it was not until 1944 that the combined clinic became the *Clínica Ortopédica e Traumatológica* for children and adults of both sexes. Even in 1911, when medical and surgical paediatric chairs were separated, the latter included orthopaedics.

In 1925, progress suddenly accelerated when new chairs of paediatric/orthopaedic surgery were created at three peripheral centres: São Paulo, **Rezende Puech** (1884–1939); Recife, **Barros Lima**; and Bahia, **Durral de Gama**. At the same time, **Barbosa Vianna** (1890–1946) succeeded Gurgel. The foundations of the modern era were laid in the ensuing 15–20 years. Orthopaedic teaching found its place in the medical schools, departments were created in many hospitals, the *Sociedade Brasileira de Ortopedia e Traumatología* was founded in 1935, and two journals, the *Arquivos Brasilieros de Cirugia e Ortopedia* and the *Revista Brasileira de Ortopedia e Traumatología.*

Puech was an outstanding man, though largely self-taught, and built a special orthopaedic hospital of 150 beds, the *Pavilhão Fernardinho Simonsen* in the grounds of the *Santa Casa* for children under fifteen. He did much for the planning and lustre of orthopaedic hospitals and services in Brazil before his early death.

Lima, in Recife, founded the first Brazilian hospital for skeletal tuberculosis, the *Sanitorio Infantil para Tuberculose Cirurgica* and was largely responsible for the *Arquivos.* He helped organize state aid to hospitals but never abandoned general surgery and reverted to a chair in surgery in 1947.

The *Sociedade* had 22 founder-members and was the first such orthopaedic association in Latin America. Its early years were difficult, partly for geographic reasons in a vast country, where, as in Australia, developments in the several states were largely autonomous and professional meetings on a national scale were difficult before the development of easy air travel. Putti addressed its first meeting in São Paulo in 1936 – the first such in Latin America – and encouraged the treatment of fractures by orthopaedic surgeons in general hospitals. By mid century, the subject was being taught in most medical schools.

The best internationally-known Brazilian orthopaedic surgeon was **Francisco de Godoy-Moreira**. After general surgical training at São Paulo he studied under Biesalski in Berlin and Putti in Bologna, and when he returned in 1934 he founded the *Instituto Ortopedico e Clinica de Fraturas.* In 1940, he succeeded Puech in the chair and two years later became director of the 120 bed department in the new *Hospital das Clínicas*; this was soon overwhelmed by work and a magnificent new institute replaced it in 1945. Godoy-Moreira was the first Brazilian orthopaedic surgeon to gain true international status, and his contributions were very numerous, notably on fractures of the neck of the femur treated by osteosynthesis with a lag screw[10].

The *Pavilhão Fernandinho* became the nucleus of another São Paulo centre, eventually directed after Puech by **Domingo Define**, who had trained under Glaessner in Berlin and Putti in Bologna, and as an assistant to Puech himself. Define had a strong academic bent and became professor in orthopaedics in the new medical school and a profuse author. In Rio, **Achilles de Araujo** succeeded Vianna as professor of orthopaedics and traumatology in 1948; but long before that, in 1919, at the *Hospital Sao Zacharias*, he had performed the first Albee spinal fusion. In 1930 he founded the orthopaedic clinic of the *Hospital Evangelico*; his energies helped create the *Sociedade* and he personally founded the *Revista.*

REFERENCES

1. Farill, J. (1952). Orthopaedics in Mexico. *J. Bone Jt. Surg.*, **34A**, 506
2. de Sahagun, B. (1946). *Historia General de las Casas de Nueva España.* (Mexico, Edit. España)

3 Ottolenghi, C.E. (1933). Diagnóstico de la tuberculosis ósteoarticular por la biopsia ganglionar. *Rev. Ortop. Traumatol.*, **3**, 1

4. Valls, J., Ottolneghi, C.E. and Schajiwicz, F. (1942) *La biopsia por aspiración en el diagnóstico de las lesiones óseas*. (Buenos Aires)

5. Ivanissevich, O. (1934). *Hidatidosis ósea*. (Buenos Aires)

6. Zeno, L.O. (1934). Fracturas supracondileas del humero: tratamiento tipificado. *Rev. Ortop. Traumatol.*, **3**, 452

7. Inclán, A. (1942). The use of preserved bone grafts in orthopaedic surgery. *J. Bone Jt. Surg.*, **24**, 81

8. Bado, J.L. (1952). Orthopaedics in Uruguay. *J. Bone Jt. Surg.*, **34A**, 539

9. de Camargo, F.P. and Wertheimer, L.G. (1952). 50 years of progress in orthopaedics and traumatology in Brazil. *J. Bone Jt. Surg.*, **34A**, 513

10. Godoy Moreira, F.E. (1938). O tratamiento operatorio das fracturas do collo femural. Seus principios fundamentales e sua solucão technica. *Brasil*, **52**, 1027

CHAPTER 17

National Histories – Russia

In the 18th century, when Peter the Great was intent on modernizing Russia, he imported many western European surgeons, as well as artists and engineers. There was always a strong German influence but it is noteworthy that English (or Scottish) surgeons were actively engaged in Russia before and after Peter's reign. Thus, the Medical College founded by Catherine the Great in 1763 actually derived from the old Apteka, or Pharmaceutical Institute, established by James Frensham in 1581, and included a Medico–Chirurgical Academy. 1799 saw the founding of the St Petersburg Military Medical Academy, later to become the field of activity of Nikolai Pirogov; it was established by a Scot, James Wylie, who was its President for 30 years. Wylie gained a reputation by amputating both of General Moreau's legs on the battlefield and refraining from amputating the Emperor's leg; he was right both times and saved their lives.

At this time, Russian medicine was largely equivalent to military medicine and not very much of a learned profession; 'This is not surprising. A society composed of 40 million unlettered slaves, a frivolous aristocracy of about 250 000 playing at soldiers, and two million impoverished civil servants and priests, would not lend itself to reflection and experiment. Foreign scholars were essential ... although the incoming medical men ... had to submit to the Academy examination and had to promise not to poison the Czar[1].' Wylie transformed the Russian Army medical services and stopped the practice of wounded officers taking medical men off the field to look after them, to the neglect of the common soldier.

Early in the 19th century, five universities had developed medical faculties; Moscow (1755), Kiev (1833), Kharkov (1805), Kazan (1804) and Dorpat (1802). In Russia, as elsewhere, traumatology and orthopaedics had to develop within the framework of general surgery. If there is a founder of modern Russian surgery, especially in the military – and therefore largely orthopaedic – field, it must be **Nikolai Ivanovich Pirogov** (1810–1881), an infant prodigy, trained in Moscow, whose doctoral thesis was on ligation of the abdominal aorta. He worked at Dorpat in his early years, became professor of surgery there at the age of 26, engaged in animal experiments and wrote on Achilles tenotomy in 1838[2]. In 1841 he moved to the chair of clinical surgery at the St Petersburg Military Medical Academy, which he occupied for 14 years. There, he was head of a surgical department of 1000 beds and personally conducted some 12000 autopsies.

In 1851 he published a famous work on topographic anatomy, based on sawn sections of frozen cadavers. In the same year, in his book *Chirurgische Hospital-Klinik*, he described a plaster-of-Paris dressing in more or less its modern form and used this or other occlusive dressings extensively in the Crimean War in 1854, in which he also aimed at replacing amputation by excision wherever possible. He also wrote on *Plastic Surgery of the Foot* and his well known amputation just above the ankle, in which the tuberosity of the os calcis was brought round and applied to the sawn underside of the tibia, rivalled Syme's amputation at the same site in popularity throughout the world, notably in the American Civil War (p. 424). In 1847, interestingly, he and Syme had been the first Europeans to use ether anaesthesia, and Pirogov used both ether and chloroform extensively in the Caucasian War and other conflicts as the Russian state expanded. He developed triage on the battlefield, classifying the injured into the mortally wounded, the severely wounded who needed immediate operation, the less severe whose operation could be postponed to the next day, and the lightly wounded. In 1870, he was invited by the Red Cross to inspect conditions during the Franco-Prussian War.

According to Matthies, K Gibentahl was the first in Russia, and possibly anywhere, to use plaster for immobilizing fractures of the limbs, in 1815, and also elaborated numerous operations on the locomotor system. Matthies also tells us that E O Mukhin, in 1806, published a book entitled *The ABC Book of Osteocorrection*. In 1839, I V Rklitsky was performing subperiosteal resection of the bone. In the 1830s, R Chernosvitov devised hinge-splint prostheses for the lower limbs. Other Russian developments during the 19th century included work on the microscopy of bone regeneration (I A Bredikhin), subperiosteal amputation (S F Feiktisov 1863), osteoplastic procedures in animals (N P Nikolsky 1870) and osteosynthesis (I I Nasilov 1875). In 1893, roughly the contemporary of Hansmann in Germany, Lambotte in Belgium and Lane in England, V I Kuzmin was performing osteosynthesis with nickel pins. The whole of the development of Russian traumatology and orthopaedics was greatly influenced by the work of such western European surgeons as Kocher, König, Langenbeck, Hoffa in Germany and Austria as well as Farabeuf and Dupuytren in France. Thus, in 1865, Berend in Berlin was invited to provide an 'orthopaedic teaching system' for the University of Kiev and produced for this an atlas with a hundred photographs of various aspects of orthopaedic disease and treatment, together with examples of splints and appliances[3].

We may also recall that the terrible experiences of Napoleon's Russian campaign resulted in hitherto unparalleled expertise in traumatology. Larrey, as senior surgeon to the *Grande Armée*, during the retreat across the Beresina, did 234 amputations for frostbite in a single night; and it was before sleeping that he wrote in his diary the pregnant words, 'The muscles left in the stump should be used for the movements of an artificial hand', words that germinated in the minds of Vanghetti and Sauerbruch and others and promoted them to conceive and, in the first world war, actually to perform, the first kineplastic procedures on amputation stumps.

Traumatology and orthopaedics have never really been regarded as separate disciplines in Russia but as part of a whole. The emergence of this unified discipline from within the confines of general surgery was marked by the establishment, by G I Turner, of the first orthopaedic department at the Petersburg Medico-Surgical Academy in 1900. Henry Turner (in the anglicized form) became professor of orthopaedics at the Military Academy of Medicine, was a well-known figure on the international orthopaedic scene, and retained his post after the 1917 Revolution and his completion of 50 years' service was officially celebrated. Two other centres were set up before 1917; the Orthopaedic Institute of R R Vreden in Petersburg in 1906 and the Medico-Mechanical Institute in Kharkov by K F Bergner, M I Sitenko and N P Novachanko. These were the foundations of the Russian school, which did not really develop fully until after the Revolution.

The first world war and the Revolution resulted in so many wounded (Pirogov had defined war as a 'traumatic epidemic') that the new Soviet government had to set up institutes in a number of cities. These included one in Kazan in 1918, now the Kazan Research Institute of Traumatology and Orthopaedics; the All-Ukraine State Orthopaedic Institute in 1919, now the Kiev Research Institute of Orthopaedics; and the Sverdlovsk Institute in 1931. In 1921, at Lenin's initiative, a Therapeutic and Orthopaedic Institute was set up in Moscow which became what is now the Central Institute of Traumatology and Orthopaedics named after **N N Priorov** (1885–1961), and this has since led the field in Russian traumatology and orthopaedics. Many famous surgeons have trained or worked there: Priorov himself, V D Chaklin, V A Chernevsky, T P Vinogradova, A E Rauer, F M Khitrov and V N Blokhin among them. This Institute engages in training and treatment, coordinates research, and supervises the national provision of equipment and appliances.

Vasily Dmietrievich Chaklin (1892–1976) is a fairly representative figure of this period. A Kharkov graduate, he became head of the Sverdlovsk Institute of Orthopaedics and Traumatology in 1931 and was director of the Moscow Prosthetic Research Institute between 1944 and 1948. In 1949 he was appointed director of the Moscow Orthopaedic Hospital and of the Children's Orthopaedic Clinic within the Central Institute of Traumatology and Orthopaedics. Here, he worked on problems of tissue compatibility, combined autogenous with heterogeneous bone-grafting and wrote extensively on scoliosis. Chaklin was a warm and great man, with many international contacts.

After World War II, institutes of traumatology and orthopaedics were established in Riga, Minsk, Donetsk, Tbilisi, Yerevan, Baku, Tashkent, Novosibirsk, Kurgan, Irkutsk, Prokopiev, Saratov and Gorky. As of now, there are some 20 such institutes in Russia, and there are some 97 departments at medical and training institutes and universities. The separation of orthopaedics from general surgery seems to have been less traumatic in Russia than in other countries, An orthopaedic section was established at the XVII Russian Surgical Congress in 1925, time was allotted to orthopaedic presentations, and the first Soviet Society of Traumatologists and Orthopaedists was set up in Leningrad in 1926. In 1963, all the local societies were amalgamated into the All-Union Scientific Society of Traumatologists and Orthopaedists, whose first national congress was held in Moscow in the same year.

The largest relevant periodical is the monthly *Orthopaedics, Traumatology and Prosthetics*, founded by Sitenko in Kharkov in 1927. There are also orthopaedic reports within such surgical journals as *Vestnik khirurgii im. I I Grekova, Khirurgiya, Klinichskaya*, the *Kazansky Meditsinsky Zhurnal* and others, while the Moscow Institute publishes *Current Problems of Traumatology and Orthopaedics* twice a year.

Russian work in this field has been marked by a spirit of innovation and by the free adaptation of engineering techniques. Sivash's integral endoprosthesis for the hip-joint was introduced in 1956 and endoprosthetics for fractures (mainly of the hip) and tumours has flourished. At the same time, indeed much earlier, there has been a particularly Russian interest in massive homografts of bone, joints and half-joints (see p. 552), extending back even to before World War I. The Moscow Central Institute established laboratories for low temperature tissue preservation shortly after World War II and reports on joint transplantation by Volkov and Immamaliev appeared in the West in the 1960s[4-6], though the first Russian papers in this field date as far back as 1913 and 1914. The Russians were largely pioneers in the storage of massive cadaver bone or osteoarticular grafts at very low temperatures.

We must also recall the various forms of compression–distraction appliances, notably that of Ilizarov, which have helped so much in problems of bone lengthening and shortening, sometimes with the aid of fully implanted devices.

REFERENCES

1. Schuster, N.H. (1968). English doctors in Russia in the early 19th century. *Proc. Roy. Soc. Med.*, **61**, 185
2. Pirogov, N. (1840). Über die Durchschneidung der Achillessehne als operativ orthopädische Heilmittel. (Dorpat)
3. Berend, H.W. (1865). Ein orthopädische Lehr-Apparat für die Kaiserliche Russische Universität Kiew. *Allg. Med. Centr. Ztg.*, **34**, 261
4. Volkov, M.V. and Immamaliev, A.S. (1966). Problème de l'homoplastie des articulations et des parties osseuses articulaires. Presented at the *10th Congress of SICOT*, Paris 1966
5. Immamliev, A.S. (1969). The preparation, preservation and transplantation of articular bone ends. In Apley, A.G. (ed.), *Recent Advances in Orthopaedics*. p. 209 (London, Churchill)
6. Volkov, M.V. (1970). Allotransplantation of joints. *J. Bone Jt. Surg.*, **52B**, 49

CHAPTER 18

National Histories – China

In modern China the development of orthopaedic surgery was much influenced by the Japanese occupation before and during World War II. There were also American associations; because of the activities of medical missions, the American funding of Chinese institutes and the training of postgraduates in the USA. Chinese orthopaedics, interrupted by invasion and war, underwent a vast expansion after 1949, especially in the cities and in industry and is marked by an integration of traditional Chinese medicine with Western practice. Before 1960, the bulk of the work related to bone and joint tuberculosis. An Orthopaedic Society was founded in 1980 and the Chinese Journal of Orthopaedics in the same year. There is also now a Journal of Microsurgery, a bone tumour registry, a Chinese Hand Club and a Chinese Bioengineering Society.

Two men are regarded as the main founders of modern orthopaedic surgery. **Chi-Mao Meng** (1897–1980) was a Beijing graduate of 1920 and an MD of Rush Medical College in Chicago in 1925. At various times before the second world war he worked under Smith-Petersen in Boston, with Steindler in Iowa and in Italy and Austria. He became associate professor of orthopaedics at Beijing University Medical College, was a founder-member of the Orthopaedic Group in 1931, was an energetic and capable clinician and heavily engaged with trauma, especially during the Korean War. He used the McMurray osteotomy for fresh femoral neck injuries (because there were no Smith-Petersen pins). He devised an ingenious abduction osteotomy of the upper femur for old unreduced congenital hip dislocation in adults; the division was intertrochanteric, the upper fragment was curetted to create a cavity, and the superolateral apex of the main fragment was abducted and impacted into this cavity and fixed by screws. He used the patella as a central bone-peg in arthrodesis of the knee and treated chronically infected gunshot wounds of the elbow by excision through a split triceps incision. He founded the division of hand surgery at the Beijing Chi-Shin-Tan Hospital.

Hsien-Chi Fang (1906–1968) obtained his MD at the Beijing Medical

469

College in 1933, was an orthopaedic resident in Boston in 1938, and became assistant professor of orthopaedics at the Beijing University Medical College. This was closed by the Japanese in 1942, so he moved to Tianjin and founded the Tianjin Orthopaedic Hospital, where he trained orthopaedists even during the occupation. He cared for Korean War casualties and organized orthopaedic training in the new China, expecting his trainees to develop services in their own regions. He used to say, 'A good surgeon is a physician who wields a scalpel with dexterity', which is equivalent to Trotter's 'A surgeon is a physician who uses his hands'. He concentrated on the extirpation of the local skeletal tuberculous focus, aiming at recovery with movement after a year rather than several years of immobilization ending in probable ankylosis[1]. In over 3000 cases, his cure-rate exceeded 90 per cent. He internally fixed fractures, often dispensing with plaster. He also integrated traditional methods, replacing open fixation often by manipulative reduction with traction and with wooden splints and paper pressure pads over the shafts of the bones only, leaving the joints above and below free for early movement and muscle contraction. Thus, the femur was treated by tibial pin traction plus splints and pads applied to the thigh only, while for forearm fractures splints and pads were applied between the bones to tauten the interosseous membrane and so maintain reduction, a method known to the ancient Egyptians.

A day that deserves to be marked with a white stone is 2nd January 1963, when a machinist, Wang Toun-Po, aged 27, severed his right forearm an inch above the wrist. He was operated on an hour later; the radius was plated and screwed and the vessels repaired, taking seven and a half hours[2]. This, the first ever reimplantation of a hand severed above the wrist, was a complete success. Although severe swelling required decompression incision on the dorsum, the ultimate functional result was excellent and he was able to return to work, write and play table tennis. Between 1963 and 1983 there were 1131 reimplantations of limbs and 2604 of digits in China, with success rates of 83.9 per cent and 76.5 per cent respectively. The work had to be organized locally because of problems of transport over a distance, and later microsurgery became available. The problem of the preoperative duration of ischaemia was reduced by cold storage of the part, and reimplantation of a limb was successful in one case after 36 hours. Such late cases tended to have problems of swelling and toxic absorption which might be fatal; here, hyperbaric oxygen proved helpful. (The Chinese example was soon followed in the West; but it should be noted that it has been claimed that the first successful arm reimplantation was in fact performed by Malt and McKhann in Boston in 1962[3].)

Yan-Qing Ye (b.1906) pioneered modern Chinese orthopaedic surgery after the 1930s. A graduate of Qi-Lu University Medical School in 1930, he did research in Shanghai, obtained the MCh Orth diploma at Liverpool in 1935 under McMurray, and became a member of the Chinese Orthopaedic Group in 1937. He was involved in treatment in the 1937 Japanese invasion and became chief of general surgery and orthopaedics at the Lester Chinese Hospital. To this, in 1939, was added work at the Marshall-Jackson Polyclinic. In 1940 he became professor of orthopaedic surgery at the

Shanghai Women's Medical College, and in 1943 associate professor at the St John's University School of Medicine. In the new China of 1958 he became Vice-Director of the newly-formed Shanghai Institute of Traumatology and Orthopaedics and, in later years, chairman of the Chinese Orthopaedic Association and Vice-Editor of the orthopaedic section of the Chinese Medical Encyclopaedia.

Yan-Qing Ye began nailing fractured hips in 1940 and Küntscher nailing in the 1950s. He devoted much attention to fracture-dislocations of the spine with cord injury, using immediate open reduction and fusion without, as a rule, laminectomy. He treated skeletal tuberculosis conservatively before the arrival of chemotherapy, and afterwards by radical local excision, lateral rachotomy and synovectomy. He was interested in traditional Chinese medicine, especially manipulation, transmitted – he thought – to Europe by the Mongols, and applied it to modern use. He also did basic research on bone metabolism and microstructure and, at 80, was still Director of the Shanghai Institute.

REFERENCES

1. Fang, H.C. *et al.* (1957). The treatment of bone and joint tuberculosis by radical excision of the local tuberculous focus. A clinical report of 941 cases. *Chin. Surg.*, **5(2)**, 90

2. Chen, Z.W., Chien, Y.C. and Pao, Y.S. (1963). Salvage of the forearm following traumatic amputation. *Chin. Med. J.*, **82**, 632

3. Malt, R.A. and McKhann, C.F. (1964). Replantation of severed arms. *J. Am. Med. Assoc.*, **189**, 716

CHAPTER 19

National Histories – Japan

The first department of orthopaedic surgery in Japan was founded in 1906, at the University of Tokyo, the second, in Kyoto, soon after. The Japanese Orthopaedic Association was founded in 1926. Before World War II, the predominant foreign influence had been German; afterwards it was American. At the 56th annual meeting of the Association in 1983 there were over 10 000 members, but only half of these were certified specialists.

In 1927, Hayashi anticipated von Rosen in stressing the importance of the earliest diagnosis in congenital dislocation of the hip[1]. The reimplantation of severed limbs and digits using microsurgery has been an important field[2], as has hand surgery, pioneered at Jyushu University by Jinnaka[3,4] and by Mizuno[5], professor of orthopaedics at Osaka. A bone tumour registry was founded for western Japan by Amako in 1954 and later extended to the rest of the country.

Truly country-specific disorders are very rare, but Japan does seem to have a near-monopoly of ossification of the posterior longitudinal ligament of the spine as an inherited condition that may cause cord damage[6].

We have noted elsewhere (p. 572) the great Japanese contributions to arthroscopy of the knee. In 1918, Kenji Takanagi used a cystoscope in cadaver knees and devised an arthroscope. In 1957, **Masaki Watanabe** produced his 'No 21 arthroscope' and published an Atlas of Arthoscopy[7]. In fact, Watanabe's work had been stimulated by **Kenji Takanagi** (1888–1963), professor at Tokyo University, who must be accorded priority in this field. Takanagi had been spurred on by the poor results of arthrography and reported his first results at the 64th meeting of the Japanese Orthopaedic Association in 1932 and later used intra-articular cinematography[8,9]. He was the original designer of the instrument, but Watanabe improved it and took colour pictures and produced the Atlas. Takanagi went on to use the instrument for other joints and also for myeloscopy (in spina bifida). Watanabe was doing arthroscopic meniscectomies as early as 1962. We should also refer to Takanagi's pupil **Isahusu Miki** (1904–1966) who became professor of orthopaedics in Tokyo in 1944 and made innumerable contributions, including early clinical electromyography and the management of osteoclastoma.

REFERENCES

1. Hayashi, K. (1927). Congenital dislocation of the hip. *J. Jap. Orthop. Assoc.*, **2**, 13
2. Tamai, S. (1984). *Clin. Orthop.*, **184**, 24
3. Jinnaka, S. (1940). *Orthopedic Surgery.* (Tokyo)
4. Jinnaka, S. (1941). *Orthopedic Operations*
5. Mizuno, S. (1970). *Short Lectures on Orthopedic Surgery.* (Tokyo)
6. Tsuyama, N. (1984). Ossification of the posterior longitudinal ligament of the spine. *Clin. Orthop.*, **184**, 71
7. Watanabe, M., Tekeda,S. and Ikeuchi, H. (1979). *Atlas of Arthroscopy.* 3rd edn. (Tokyo, Igatu-Shoin)
8. Takanagi, K (1932). *J. Jap. Orthop. Assoc.*, **7**, 241
9. Takanagi, K. (1939). Arthroscope. *J. Jap. Orthop. Assoc.*, **14**, 359

CHAPTER 20

SICOT

On 25th November 1913, Robert W Lovett wrote from Boston to Hans Spitzy in Vienna and Vittorio Putti in Bologna saying that the existence of international societies in other fields of medicine justified the need for an international orthopaedic association, and one with its own journal. This was not the first word on the subject for the three had evidently already constituted themselves as an *ad hoc* executive committee.

Further letters were exchanged but the correspondence was brought to a halt by the events of July 1914. The idea was resurrected in 1923 and then laid aside again when Lovett died the following year. In 1929, Putti was in London at a joint congress of the American and British organizations and mentioned the matter to Fred Albee. Albee was never a man for wasting time; the society was founded at a meeting in Paris on 10th October of the same year and its first Congress was held, also in Paris, in October of 1930.

Albee had written to the most eminent orthopaedists throughout the world, meeting with general enthusiasm except from the British – Robert Jones, Rowley Bristow and Harry Platt – who dragged their feet. Despite these delaying tactics, a founding meeting was held at the Hotel Crillon, attended by the following: Philip Erlacher and Hans Spitzy (Austria); Jean Delchef (in spirit, he was laid up with gout!), Paul Lorthioir and Adolphe Maffei (Belgium); Ramon San Ricart (Spain); Fred Albee, William Baer and Henry Meyerding (USA); Louis Ombredanne, Louis Rocher and Etienne Sorel (France); Thomas Fairbank (UK); Riccardo Galeazzi and Vittorio Putti (Italy); Murk Jansen (Netherlands); Patrik Haglund and Henning Waldenström (Sweden); Alfred Machard (Switzerland); Jean Jiano (Rumania); and Jan Zahradnicek (Czechoslovakia).*

---

*This list is from the official history: *SICOT, 50 years of achievement*, E Van der Elst, Ed., Springer-International 1978. However, Fairbank, who was there, states that Lange and Biesalski of Germany, and Nové-Josserand of Lyons, were also present.

Albee and Putti pushed the matter through, despite the reasoned objections of the British; that there were too many similar associations already, that younger men would be excluded (for membership was to be limited to 100), that multiple nationalities would make useful discussion impossible. Putti joked about England's 'splendid isolation' and Albee noted, 'Everyone in favour but the English.' Yet, despite Albee's major part, he never held a major position in the new society,* which was initially called the *Société Internationale de Chirurgie Orthopédique* (SICO). There must have been a good deal of magnanimity around, for the unanimous choice for president was Sir Robert Jones, who had led the opposition; but, after all, he was the most eminent orthopaedic surgeon in the world at that time.

It was not until the Third Congress, at Bologna in 1935, that Putti, against the opposition of the German members, succeeded in adding *et de Traumatologie* to the title of the society, henceforward SICOT. (In some countries general surgeons obstinately refused to let go their control of traumatology; this was why the Germans were against its inclusion, which they feared as a bar to true orthopaedic independence.**)

After 1929 the Society has held a congress in different capitals every three years in times of peace. Though Albee had urged the production of a journal from the outset, the society initially published only the reports of its congresses, though this itself was a very considerable undertaking managed by Delchef, Secretary-General and mainstay of SICOT for a quarter of a century. 'But for him,' said Bryan McFarland of Liverpool, 'the Society might well have died.' Then, in January 1977, *International Orthopaedics* made its appearance, and was to be issued several times a year. The main credit for this was due to Robert Merle d'Aubigné of Paris.

Of course, recent decades have seen the origin of 'superspecialized' societies, concerned with regional problems – the lumbar spine, the hip, the hand and so on. There is also the relatively new *Société International de Recherche Orthopédique et de Traumatologie* (SIROT), *World Orthopaedic Concern* (WOC) concerned with problems of the Third World, and the joint organization of the English-speaking orthopaedists of the world.

---

*Partly, or mainly, because Baer had attended this meeting specifically to prevent Albee from holding major office; he knew his man!

**The German delegation had originally been in favour but changed its opinion overnight as the result of a direct instruction from Hitler, probably at the instigation of the general surgeons.

Section 3

Special Subjects

CHAPTER 21

Amputations and Prostheses

Amputation, however and why ever achieved, is a very ancient phenomenon that goes back to prehistory, for neolithic man is known to have survived amputation, almost certainly traumatic, ritualistic or punitive, rather than therapeutic.* Fingers are sometimes missing from the imprints of hands made on cave-walls. Amputation is not mentioned in the Old Testament or in the Egyptian medical papyri; but the Babylonian code of Hammurabi, of about 1700 BC, inscribed on the famous Black Stone, now in the Louvre, specifies that if the physician, operating with a bronze lancet, causes the death or loss of sight of a lord, the physician's hand is to be cut off; and the same penalty applied to a brander who cut off a slave-mark without the owner's consent.

Punitive amputation of the hand has been part of the Islamic code to the present time, but is far from having been specific to Islam. In 1579, on a stage set up in the market-place at Westminster, John Stubbs, a religious writer, and William Page, his publisher, 'had their right hands cut off by the blow of the butcher's knife with a mallet struck through their wrists', for having produced a pamphlet criticizing Queen Elizabeth's marital ambitions. 'Stubbs, so soon as his right hand was cut off, put off his hat with the left and cried aloud, 'God save the Queen!''

It is probable that the artificial limbs that have been found with mummies having congenital or traumatic absence of limbs were purely cosmetic and never used in life. There is an account by Herodotus of one Hegesistratus, a prophet condemned to death in Sparta in 484 BC, who amputated his own tethered foot to escape and, when recaptured, had managed to acquire a

---

*There is one other type of amputation, for which it is difficult to coin an adjective, and of which there is only one example: the Red Hand of Ulster. In a famous (and legendary) boat race between an O'Neill and a McDonnell, the O'Neill, to save the race, cut off his own hand and threw it ahead of both boats to the winning post.

wooden one. There is mention of artificial limbs for kings and queens in Irish and Hindu legend, but these replaced limbs lost in battle.

Certainly, therapeutic amputation for disease of the hand or foot is mentioned in Plato's *Symposium* of 385 BC as a matter of course, but the earliest clinical description of deliberate amputation is that by Hippocrates in *De Articulis*, for vascular gangrene, performed through the ischaemic tissue, the wound left open to heal by granulation. Hippocrates also describes disarticulation at the knee, and he refers to the use of cautery for haemostasis, and this was continued for centuries until quite recent historical times, and is often mentioned by famous surgeons discussed elsewhere in this book; Galen, Avicenna, Albucasis, Salicet, Guy de Chauliac.

In early times, the main risks were shock, haemorrhage and sepsis, and amputations of the thigh or upper arm were usually fatal; but, to offer some perspective, let us recall that an elective operation on a toe at the Bellevue Hospital in New York in the 1870s could have the same outcome (p. 437). In pre-anaesthetic days, amputation was always a brutal torment; but that was a fact of life, a man like Josiah Wedgwood in the 18th century in England could *ask* for a swollen troublesome limb to be cut off.

Cautery was often useless for large vessels, and though Celsus in the first century AD used ligatures, as did others after him, it is not clear that this was actually for amputations. (Celsus, incidentally, removed gangrenous limbs through the nearest viable tissue, dividing the bone higher than the soft tissues, which were allowed to fall together.) Ambroise Paré's introduction of the ligature in amputations in 1529 was therefore really a reintroduction, at a time when gunpowder was causing violent injuries for which amputation had to be routine treatment. As to the level of section, Paré wrote, 'Art bids to take hold of the quicke, and to cut off the member in the sound flesh; but the same art wisheth us to preserve whole that which is sound, as much as in us lies...for unless you take hold of the quicke flesh in the amputation, or if you leave any putrefaction, you profit nothing by amputation, for it will creepe and spread over the rest of the body...wherefore you shall cut off as little as that which is sound as you possibly can: yet so that you rather cut away that which is quicke, than leave behind anything that is perished[1].'

The invention of the tourniquet is sometimes ascribed to figures such as Botallus or Fabricius Hildanus ab Aquapendente in the 16th century, but Paré deliberately used a thick ligature or fillet round the root of the limb, 'to prohibit the fluxe of blood by pressure and shutting up the nerves and arteries'. It also dulled the sense of the part. His recommended level of below-knee amputation was 'some five fingers' breadths under the knee', to permit a better artificial limb, equivalent to the modern hand's breadth below the tibial tuberosity which gives a five-inch stump. Paré says he had learned from Galen how to bind up the vessels. At first, he always had the conventional hot irons and cauteries in readiness, 'until at length, confirmed by happy experience...I bid eternally adieu to all of these.' He saw no reason to bow to tradition or authority in this, 'Let no man say to us, that the Ancients have always done thus.' He treated phantom pains with strongly irritant ointment applied to the back.

The tourniquet has also been ascribed to Morel, in 1674, at the siege of

Besançon, and to Petit in 1718, but it was Esmarch's rubber bandage of 1873 that made amputation, and bloodless operations in general, really practicable and safe, so much so that in 1908 Schulthess, of Zurich, referred to it as a precious gift from the German Empire to humanity[2]. Esmarch is dealt with elsewhere (p. 199), and here we need only repeat his dates (1823–1908), that he was an assistant to Langenbeck, a military surgeon in the various Prussian wars of his century, and in 1873 described his technique of preoperative exsanguination with an elastic rubber bandage followed by a rubber tourniquet. This meant that one could 'operate precisely as in the dead subject', reducing blood loss and facilitating inspection of diseased areas. He noted the possibility that the firm strapping of a limb for any considerable period might be followed by dangerous circulatory disturbance in the part, and that infected limbs should not be exsanguinated[3].

The first reputed successful above-knee amputation is said to have been done by William Clowes in 1588, but Paré, in his *Oeuvres* in 1575, figures an above-knee prosthesis and had done the first elbow disarticulation in 1536. Haemorrhage was always a problem, though John Hunter pointed out in 1786 that, in most cases, shock, vasospasm and clotting would put an end to bleeding before it proved fatal. The various styptics used – oil of turpentine, alum, vitriol, though intended to control bleeding, had their main virtue, if any, in antisepsis. Boiling oil, and Paré's discovery that it was unnecessary, we refer to elsewhere.

All the early amputations were circular. Paré used adhesive strips to approximate the wound edges, as did von Gersdorff (1455–1517), who also used animal bladders to cover the stump, but in 1679, Yonge and Lowdham introduced the use of flaps for easier closure, often postponed to prevent a haematoma. Liston in the 19th century used cold water compresses, followed by closure with adhesive tape, but primary closure was always hazardous, and even in the mid 19th century some still considered it good practice to leave the wound open to granulate. Speed was of the essence in preanaesthetic days. Assistants restrained the patient, who was given analgesic drugs, rum or brandy, or, in the USA, may have had a very black cigar stuck in his rectum. A surgeon should be able to remove a thigh in 30 seconds and complete the operation in three minutes. 'Time me, gentlemen!' the operator used to say to the watching students.

Of course, the mortality until the midcentury was formidable, estimated by Malgaigne in 1842 as 62 per cent for thigh amputations in the Paris hospitals, while Pirogoff lamented the lack of survivors in the Crimean War. Then there was the habitual *dirtiness* of surgeons, with their old, filthy, blood-encrusted garments. Even in the 1870s, Bigelow and his assistants at the Massachusetts General Hospital had their sutures stuck on their lapels, even held them in their mouths (see also p. 437). Some surgeons did have good results; Monro, in 1752, in Edinburgh, reported 99 amputations with only eight deaths, and Alanson in Liverpool had 35 cases in 1782 without a single death.

We note elsewhere that amputation on the battlefield was almost routine for severe sabre or gunshot wounds up to the American Civil War, when voices were raised in favour of conservatism (p. 424). The first successful amputation at the shoulder is believed to be that by a Bostonian, John Warren, in 1781, and Dominique-Jean Larrey, Napoleon's surgeon-in-chief, often amputated at both hip and shoulder and sometimes, as after the Battle of the Beresina, removed over 200 limbs at one session. According to Bick, Norman Kirk states that Larrey performed eleven shoulder disarticulations in 24 hours at one stage of the 1812 campaign, with nine complete recoveries. In 1806, successful amputation at the hip-joint was performed by one Walter Brashear, of Kentucky, but Herman Melville, in his novel *Whitejacket*, portrays the much more sinister outcome of a similar procedure performed by an American naval surgeon. All the famous military surgeons – Guthrie on the British side against Napoleon, Pirogoff in the Crimea – were formidable amputationists. They had to be. Many types of amputation of the foot were developed by, among others, Lisfranc, Hey, Chopart, Pirogoff and Syme. The two last were both popular in the American Civil War (p. 424) and the Syme had an interesting history of regained popularity in World War I (p. 368), but on the western rather than the eastern side of the Atlantic.

We have said that early amputations were of guillotine or circular nature, as they had been with Paré, though some surgeons saw that the deeper layers should be divided at successively higher levels. Flaps were introduced by, among others, Verduin in Amsterdam in 1696 and by various French surgeons in the early 18th century. Liston, in 1837 in England, put the flap operation in fairly modern form as we now know it, on the map, at much the same time that Malgaigne, in Paris, designed the racquet incision. Possibly the earliest description of a through-knee amputation is that of Nathan Smith in the USA in 1825[4], and Velpeau reported a series of such procedures which he considered provided end-bearing stumps[5]. In 1857, Gritti[6] described a section through the femoral condyles in which the patella (freshened) was applied to the raw surface to give an end-bearing stump, modified in England by Stokes in 1870[7] to give the Gritti–Stokes amputation, but one that has never been very popular with limb-manufacturers.

The last century has seen discussion, cooperation and a certain amount of controversy, between surgeons and artificial limb-makers as to the optimum sites for amputation. It has not always been easy to integrate the views of both parties; the surgeons have had a natural preference for the longest length of stump; the limb-makers pointed out that shorter stumps made it possible to more easily incorporate useful artificial joints within the new limb.

The earliest surviving prosthesis, possibly Etruscan, was discovered at Capri in 1858; it was made of bronze and wood for a thigh amputation and was unfortunately lost in the bombing of the Hunterian Collection at the Royal College of Surgeons of England during World War II. Wooden peg-legs have been known from very early times, were described by Paré for knee disarticulation, and are well designated by Vitali *et al.* as 'the prostheses of the peasants and the poor.'

The medieval rich, the *Ritter* or knights, got their armourers to produce prostheses suited to their armour, often functional, always decorative; these differed from those more habitually afoot; a horseman might have a limb with a rigid semiflexed knee for riding astride, but this was of iron and heavy, while the cheaper wooden limb of the foot-soldier tended to be more functional, articulated and lighter. Verduin, in 1696, constructed what may have been the first above-knee limb, with a leather socket and thigh corset and hinged side-steels.

A famous historical prosthesis was the 'iron hand' of Götz von Berlichingen (1480–1562), a renowed German freebooter, romanticized by Goethe, and useful in peace and war. It replaced a right hand lost at the siege of Landshut in 1509; the first crude model Götz called his 'claw', but it was followed by an elegant articulated model with fingers that could be flexed passively and with ratchet locking. In myth, there had been the iron leg of Queen Vishpla, mentioned in the Rig Veda, fitted after she had lost her limb in battle to enable her to fight on; likewise the Silver Hand of the Irish King Nuadhat assigned to around 500 BC.

To return to fact, Pliny tells us that Marius Sergius also lost his right hand, in the Second Punic War of 218–202 BC, and wore an iron hand. The German Alt-Ruppin hand, dating to around 1400 AD, was also iron, with a fixed opposed thumb, flexible fingers with ratchet locking and a mobile wrist. All these hands were heavy and had to be operated by the other hand, and the ordinary working tool for many centuries was the more useful, if repulsive, hook.

As for legs, the Prince of Homburg (1633–1708) had his right leg blown off fighting for the Swedes at the siege of Copenhagen; it was left dangling by a single tendon, which he severed himself. He was supplied with an artificial limb a metre long, weighing 5 kg and composed of two wooden sheaths, held together by bone-glue and two wooden dowels. There were anatomically placed metarsophalangeal and ankle joints, and a spring to

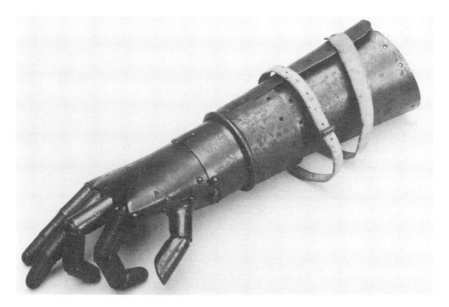

Figure 207   The 'iron hand' of Götz von Berlichingen

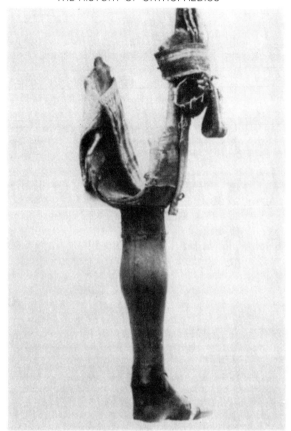

Figure 208   The 'silver leg' of the Prince of Homburg

hold the foot at 15° flexion. This – rather, three like it – he wore for the 50 years after his injury during many campaigns; it is often, wrongly, called the Silver Leg. It is the oldest known prosthesis to usefully combine different materials and, with a mechanism to replace the calf muscles and to give a normal roll to the foot, it is without parallel in the 18th and 19th centuries.

Around 1800, James Pott, a London mechanic, constructed an ingenious leg prosthesis with artificial tendons for the knee and ankle, later to be known as the Anglesey limb because Pott was patronized by the Marquis of Anglesey after Waterloo.

From early in the 19th century, the idea developed of using the remaining healthy muscles to activate a prosthesis; it haunted, among others, Larrey, probably because of the mountains of arms and legs he had had to amputate for Napoleon's *Grande Armée*. Originally, this concept was simple and unambitious. In 1818, a Berlin dentist, Peter Bailly, used the shoulder-girdle muscles to activate a below-elbow prosthesis, and this principle was extended by others to produce elbow flexion, while the precursor of the present-day shoulder harness was devised by de Beaufort in 1867. However, in the

Abyssinian campaigns of the late 19th century a number of Italian soldiers had their hands cut off by tribesmen, and Vanghetti[9] formed the concept of utilizing the muscles remaining about the stump to act as motors for the prosthesis (see p. 651). He seems himself to have remained a theorist, but he did persuade a colleague, Ceci, to attempt some of these 'cinematic' or 'kineplastic' procedures just before the turn of the century and they were much discussed around 1900[10]. Galeazzi[11] took an interest before the first world war, which inevitably reawakened interest. It was worked on by Putti[12] in Italy, but more notably by Sauerbruch[13] in Germany, who reported on 1500 cases in 1920. The actual techniques were varied. The simplest method was to construct skin-lined tunnels through the muscles, which activated rods traversing the tunnels and connected to cords, levers and pulleys activating the hinged joints of prostheses or other mechanical devices useful at work or at home. Further steps were taken by Bosch-Arana in the Argentine in 1918–20[14,15] and by Kessler in the USA a little later[16]. The Krukenberg, or 'chopstick' forearm, constructed by splitting the limb longitudinally and skin-grafting the cleft, took a different path since nothing but living tissue was required to effect grasp. However, despite the energetic efforts of a few, enthusiasm for any of these procedures always remained essentially local; patients did not much like the look of their redevised stumps, or like others to look at them.

Erth, Dederich and others in Germany, in the 1950s, used 'myodesis' to attach muscles to bone. Much research was done after World War II on various types of powered, mainly upper limb, prostheses; and the Russians, around 1960, were the first to produce a useful myoelectrically controlled hand. All such work, of course, gained enormous impetus from the thalidomide tragedy[17–19].

In the USA, an enormous effort was invested in the development of better artificial limbs after World War II, an effort originating, at least in part, from the appointment of Major-General Norman T Kirk as Surgeon General of the Army in 1943, for Kirk had been closely concerned with amputations in the first world war, had written on the subject in standard works, and issued directives on amputation in forward areas in World War II. It was Kirk, in 1943, who laid down that a modified guillotine amputation was to be performed as distally as possible, but with the soft tissues cut at successively higher levels, the bone last and highest of all, with strapping extension to the skin of the stump, a generally satisfactory procedure which allowed for elective reamputation under calmer conditions.

At home, the National Academy of Sciences had an advisory committee, which was replaced by the Prosthetics Research Board in 1955, and this lasted in one form or another up to 1976, while the Army and Navy had their own prosthetic departments and the Veterans Administration had a Rehabilitation Engineering Center. Perhaps the most immediately useful results of all this research were the emergence of the suction socket in 1946, the patellar-tendon bearing prosthesis[20], and the immediate postoperative fitting of temporary lower limb prostheses. There was also an endeavour, from around 1960, to preserve the knee-joint in elderly patients with vascular gangrene, and this actually reversed the ratio of above-knee to below-knee amputations in the United States from 70:30 in 1965 to 30:70 in the 1980s, with an enormous improvement in results.

In Britain, the experience of World War I was marked by some initial conflict of interests between the surgeons and the limb-makers, but this was eventually ironed out after considerable discussion and optimum sites for amputation agreed that were (reasonably) acceptable to both parties. A centre for the care of amputees had been set up at Queen Mary's Hospital, Roehampton, to the west of London, in 1915 and privately-owned artificial limb manufacturers provided with workshop facilities there. Later, much of this work was transferred to a government department, the Ministry of Pensions; and later still, after the second world war, arrangements were further changed by the development of the National Health Service in 1948.

We should add that the first successful hindquarter amputations, were done by Jaboulay[21] and by Girard in France[22] in the 1890s. Its main proponents in Britain in more recent years were Gordon Taylor and Philip Wiles of the Middlesex Hospital in London; in 1935 they reported five cases with two deaths and found the overall mortality in the literature to be over 55 per cent[23].

THE CRUTCH

An erudite paper on this topic, by Sigmund Epstein of New York, appeared in 1937: *Art, History and the Crutch*, and is well worth reading[24]. Epstein provides some very useful references[25-28].

The earliest known staff with an axillary crossbar was carved on an Egyptian tomb portal of 2830 BC, while a burial stele of the temple of Astarte in Memphis, of around 800 BC, shows an individual with a flexed, short, wasted equinus leg obviously due to poliomyelitis, carrying a similar staff. Crutches, staffs (or spears) to support the wounded are depicted in Etruscan, Greek and Pompeian art, and the Echternach Codex of 991 AD shows a cripple with a crutch. Amputation or loss of limbs became ever more frequent in the Middle Ages, due to the effects of artillery, surgery, self-mutilation, torture, leprosy, ergotism and other causes of gangrene. Cripples with crutches are depicted on the bronze door of the Baptistry in Florence in a panel showing the healing of the sick. There is a Duccio painting and a work by John of Arderne: *De arte physicale de cirurgia* of 1412, with a sketch. Crutches were integral to the design of paintings by Fra Angelico, as in his Vatican fresco of St Laurence giving alms, and there is a painting by Hieronymus Bosch of St Martin, the patron saint of cripples, showing throngs of cripples with crutches, peg-legs, knee-pads and so on.

A very useful review of the historical aspects of amputations is to be found in *Amputations and Prostheses* by Vitali, Robinson, Andrews and Harris. Baillière Tindall, London (1978). Also helpful is the *Atlas of Limb Prosthetics* of the American Academy of Orthopaedic Surgery, CV Mosby, St Louis (1981).

REFERENCES

1. *The Apologie and Treatise of Ambroise Paré*, translated by Thomas Johnson, 1634 (Keynes, G. ed.) University of Chicago Press, 1952
2. Schulthess, W. (1908) *Rev. d'Orthop.*, 2nd series, Vol. 9 (Paris)
3. Esmarch, J.P.A. (1876). *German Clinical Lectures.* (London, New Sydenham Society)
4. Smith, N. (1825). Amputation at the knee joint. *Am. Med. Rev.*, **2**, 370
5. Velpeau, A. (1830). Mémoire sur l'amputation de la jambe dans l'articulation du genou et description d'un nouveau procédé pour pratiquer cette opération. *Arch. Gén. Med.*, **84**, 44
6. Gritti, R. (1857). Un nuovo metodo denominato amputatione del femore ai condili con lembo patellare. *Omodei Annali Univ. Med.*
7. Stokes, W. (1870). On supra-condyloid amputation of the thight. *Med. Chir. Trans.*, **53**, 175
8. Paré, A. (1654). *Instrumenta Chirurgiae et Incones Anatomica.* (Paris)
9. Vanghetti, G. (1898). *Amputazione, disarticulazione e protesi.* (Florence)
10. Ceci, A. (1905). Amputazione plastico-orthopediche secondo Vanghetti. Presented at *Congr. Ital. di Chir.* October 1905
11. Galeazzi, R. (1911). Sulla protesi cinematice. Presented at *9th Congr. Soc. Ortop. Ital.*
12. Putti, V. (1917) Plastiche e protesi cinematiche. *Chir. Org. di Muovimento*, **1**, 5
13. Sauerbruch, E.F. (1916). *Die willkürlich bewegliche Künstliche Hand.* (Berlin)
14. Bosch-Arana, G. (1918). Las amputaciones cineplasticas. *Prensa Med. Argentina*, March 30
15. Bosch-Arana, G. (1920). *Las amputaciones cineplasticas.* (Buenos Aires)
16. Kessler, H.H. (1935). *The crippled and disabled.* (Columbia University Press)
17. Hirsch, C. and Klasson, B. (1974). Clinical aims and desires for today's arm prosthesis. In Herberts, P., Kadefors, R., Magnusson, R. and Petersen, I. (eds.) *The control of upper extremity prostheses and orthoses.* pp. 58–62. (Springfield, Illinois, Charles C. Thomas)
18. Herberts, P., Almström, and Caine, K. (1976). Clinical applications study of multifunctional prosthetic hands. *J. Bone Jt. Surg.*, **60B**, 552
19. Northmore-Ball, M.D., Heger, H. and Hunter, G.A. (1980). The below-elbow myoelectric prosthesis. *J. Bone Jt. Surg.*, **62B**, 363
20. Callander, C.L. (1935). A new amputation of the lower third of the thigh. *J. Am. Med. Assoc.*, **105**, 1746
21. Jaboulay, M. (1894). La désarticulation interilio–abdominale. *Lyon méd.*, **75**, 507
22. Girard, Ch. (1895). Désarticulation de l'os iliaque pour sarcome. *Congr. Franc. Chir.*, **9**, 823
23. Gordon-Taylor, G. and Wiles, P. (1935). *Brit. J. Surg.*, **22**, 671
24. Epstein, S. (1937). Art, History and the Crutch. *Ann. Med. Hist.*, **9**, 304
25. Darenberg, C.L. (1865). *La médecine dans Homère.* (Paris)
26. Dumesnil, R. (1935). *Histoire illustrée de la Médecine.* (Paris)
27. Meyer-Steinegg, T. and Sudhoff, K. (1928). *Die Geschichte der Medizin im Überblick mit abbildungen.* 3rd edn. (Jena)
28. Richer, P. (1902). *L'Art et la Médecine.* (Paris)

CHAPTER 22

Club-foot

As mentioned elsewhere (p. 31), club-foot and its management had been excellently described by Hippocrates (for those fortunate infants who had not been dealt with by exposure). Valentin tells us that Montfalcon, writing in 1820, was able to say that 'the principles of treatment recommended by Hippocrates are very similar to those so often successfully employed in the machines of Venel and Scarpa: one should not proceed forcefully, but restore the feet gently to their natural conformation, and it was in this manner that the father of medicine proceeded in his bandaging...the oracle of Cos will always retain the merit of having recognized the nature of deformities of the feet and the requirements presented by their management[1].'

Trendelenburg, too, wrote in 1924, 'Were we able...to attend the polyclinic of an Asclepian temple, we should be amazed by the similarity of practice there to that of our own hospitals, particularly as it existed before the introduction of anaestheseia and asepsis. Were a woman to emerge from the temple with her crying baby on her arm, whose club-foot the priest physician, working like a modeller in wax, had bent aright and held in the corrected position with adhesive plaster strips, flannel bandages, a stiff leather sole and a strap on the side of the little toe, we could scarcely regard this bandage as not having been applied by the hand of one of our contemporary surgeons or orthopaedists, who very probably consider themselves the inventors of this technique[2].'

As to aetiology, there was a sustained belief in embryonic influences from the time of Fabricius Hildanus ab Aquapendente (1560–1634). He was well aware that equinovarus might be no more than persistence of an embryonic stage of development, 'All embryos in the mother's womb customarily have the feet bent more or less inwards; and if the nurses be negligent, it is easy for them to growth thus and the varus persists, but if they diligently strive to pull the feet in the opposite direction by wrapping bandages around them they are easily corrected. Whereas, if the joints of the feet are distorted from an external cause, and the varus results immediately, we cannot restore the position gradually manually[3].'

This makes a clear distinction between congenital and acquired varus; and it may be relevant that the first reported case of astragalectomy was performed by Hildanus himself in 1607 for a compound dislocation of the bone in the Reverend Meister Wolfbrand, of Duisburg. The developmental theory was supported by later authors, so Aquapendente's early thesis was quite consistent with the 19th century concept of 'arrested development', a concept invoked to explain the origin of many congenital disorders, believed to be due to persistence of an embryonic stage. There was at the same time, in the Middle Ages and even later, a continued belief in the influence of maternal shocks or impressions sustained during pregnancy at the sight of such deformities; as we have seen (p. 180), this was one of the reasons advanced in the 19th century in Germany for clearing cripples from the streets and segregating them in institutions, so that the good burgers' wives should not be so frightened. This belief was not altogether unshared by the doctors, one of whom declared, in Germany in 1795, 'We are not justified on logical grounds in bluntly declaring such an effect to be impossible[4].'

It was simultaneously accepted that there was a hereditary factor, as multiple cases tended to occur in families, so much so that if, in such a family, a child was born who was *not* club-footed, the husband might look thoughtfully at his wife. Recent genetic research has amply confirmed this. As Ruth Wynne-Davies points out[5], congenital talipes equinovarus can be inherited as a multifactorial disorder, in that its incidence in first degree relatives is 20–30 times that in the normal population, and that there is a greater concordance in monozygous twins and also great racial variation The present writer's own observation is that club-foot is very much commoner in black inhabitants of Southern Africa than elsewhere (though this may be partly factitious since most cases tend to be channelled to the very few orthopaedists available).

Another suspected cause favoured in the early 19th century was a neuromuscular influence, due to disordered innervation arising in intrauterine life[6]. There might be actual structural defects of the central nervous system, as in anencephalics or spina bifida (especially spina bifida occulta) or an irritability leading to intrauterine spasm. This latter theory of 'convulsive muscular contraction' as the cause of club-foot and many other deformities, congenital or acquired, was adopted in a rather obsessional way by many French workers from Andry onward[6-8]. Well on in the century, Little[9] and Adams[10], in London, certainly believed in abnormal fetal spasm; but they may not have distinguished between congenital and paralytic deformity, since poliomyelitis was not then recognized as an entity. Adams' dissections had shown the absence of muscle groups, but in spina bifida cases. A primary muscle *imbalance* was often postulated[11,12], but it was also recognized that once the deformity was corrected, the muscles worked normally, that in fact this was an index of cure. It was all very difficult. Were the muscular changes, genuine enough, only secondary to a primary structural deformity, or was it the other way round?

There was also a school that attributed the deformity to purely external mechanical causes, operating via the posture of the fetus or of the mother or by pressure due to oligohydramnios, and this goes as far back as Ambroise

Paré, 'This vice sometimes comes from the mother's belly, who, during her pregnancy, has remained too long seated with her legs crossed; or if the mother has the same defect; or because of the nurse not having held the child straight[13].' Many blamed an unnatural position of the feet in the womb, favouring contracture of the muscles on the side of the deformity; or there might be amniotic adhesions, so often inculpated as the causes of obscure lesions. Deficiency of liquor amnii long remained a favourite postulate. Even the great Sir Arthur Keith, in England in the 1920s, pointed out that the feet were inverted up to the 7th month of pregnancy pressed against the belly-wall, and often remained so at birth[14,15]. He thought that the human club-foot was equivalent to the normal ape foot, and was a retarded development or atavism.

In his excellent monograph of 1928[16], based on a prize essay for the British Orthopaedic Association, Brockman stated that all mechanical theories must be regarded as invalid. But Brockman's own view, that there was a congenital subluxation of the head of the talus, analogous to congenital dislocation of the hip, and due to a congenital atresia of the inferior and medial calcaneonavicular ligaments, a primary failure of development of the socket and of *all* the tissues of the foot, with secondary contracture of the plantar and both tibialis muscles, is also impossible to sustain since proper correction and maintenance will give a normal foot.

There was no lack of pathology. In the late 18th century, Camper[17] had noted deformity of the talus and os calcis and regarded these as the primary deviations and muscle contracture as secondary. In the 19th century, one dissection followed another[18-20] – Scarpa clearly saw that there was a talonavicular dislocation but that the position and shape of the talus itself remained normal. Little's historic treatise, originally published in Berlin in 1837: *On the Nature of Club Foot and Analogous Distortions* in the English version of the original Latin of his doctoral dissertation[21], reported many personal dissections in the Anatomical Institute of that city.

Brockman made an important and essential classification into three types: the common variety in otherwise normal children, more frequent in boys, only rarely associated with abnormalities of the central nervous system, of varying severity and resistance to treatment; talipes in arthrogryposis multiplex congenita, a condition that had been recognized by Adams in 1852, but not named as such until 1923[22]; and the deformity associated with congenital absence of the tibia. He also made a clear distinction between true talipes and metatarsus varus.

TREATMENT

'In the newborn child it is desirable to convert the feet to their natural state, that not being difficult; but it is difficult to maintain them so converted.' Thus the Milanese surgeon, Giovanni Battista Palletta (1748–1832) in 1826[23]; and that has always been the crux of the matter. Bick writes, 'Although almost every orthopaedic surgeon of note since ancient times had designed shoes and braces to correct this deformity, very little change in the fundamental principle of therapy has occurred[24]. This may be true enough; but, unfortunately, we know little or nothing of the history of the subject between the times of Hippocrates and the Middle Ages. And then Vidus Vidius (c. 1500–1569), commonly known as Guido Guidi, professor at the *Collège de France*, stated in his posthumously published *Opera omnia*, 'The feet are guided, both manually and by bandaging, so as to be restored to their natural state: suitable shoes provide the most force... however, at first, both iron rods and sheets are used to train the leg towards the opposite side[25].'

Certainly, the methods of management were bound to be conditioned by the anatomy, as always in orthopaedics. Here, innovations were in techniques and materials, in this case the iron splints that were not available to the Greeks. Two roughly contemporary figures interested in the problem were Francisco Arceo (or Arcaeus) (c. 1493–1573) and Gabriele Falloppio (1523–1562). The earliest illustration of the use of an iron splint is given in a book by Arcaeus published posthumously in Antwerp in 1574 *De recta curandorum vulnerum ratione et aliis eius artis praeceptia, libri duo.* He gives a detailed account of the actual management in his collected works, originally in Latin and reissued in German a hundred years later, with the subtitle: *Of the cure of a valgus* (sic) *foot in a male boy from the womb*[26].

Preliminary hot baths and poultices were often used to soften the parts, and after a week or two the child was taken on the knee of an assistant with

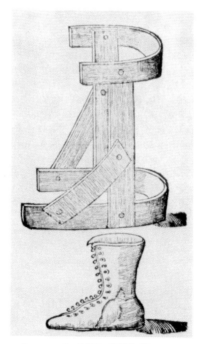

Figure 209   Franciscus Arcaeus (c. 1493–1573): De recta curandorum vulnerum et aliis eius artis praeceptis libri duo, Antwerp, 1574

his arms and legs fastened. The surgeon then restored the lame foot to its proper shape 'with great force' and applied a soft towel or bandages soaked in ointment, and adhesives, and a wooden sole was fastened to the sole with a bandage wound from within outwards, and malleable wooden splints were bandaged overall. Subsequent metal splintage and special shoes were also used. Falloppio favoured gradual correction, day by day, 'If restoration cannot be done completely the first time, it is repeated a second, third, fourth, fifth or even sixth time, but nothing is to be done with violence... the second precept is that it is not enough for the joint to be restored to its place and natural and proper condition, but that it should be drawn rather to the opposite side... the ancients used shoes of the kind called *pelopatides* i.e. rigid shoes for walking on clay[27].'

Paré, Glisson, Hunter, Venel and Scarpa were among the many who devised appliances. However, it is difficult to understand why, until the end of the 19th century, treatment was deliberately delayed until early childhood; Hippocrates himself had urged that treatment be begun at the earliest moment, and correction in early infancy has probably been the greatest single advance in management; yet, even now, there are those who would delay for the first 4–6 weeks of life. The other oddity is that there have never lacked those ready to state that the problem had been entirely solved and that complete cure could more or less be guaranteed, an assertion that still rings untrue today.

In the Middle Ages, the management of talipes and other deformities was the province of barber-surgeons, quacks and charlatans, bonesetters, truss-makers and mountebanks at fairs; not until the 18th century did treatment pass into medical hands. This is well exemplified by a passage that bears repetition, from the English surgeon and anatomist, William Cheselden (1688–1752) in 1740 (see p. 84):

> Children are sometimes born with their feet turned inwards, so that the bottom of the foot is upwards: in this case the bones of the tarsus, like the vertebrae of the back in a crooked person, are fashioned by the deformity. The first knowledge I had of a cure of this disease was from Mr Presgrove, a professed bonesetter, then living in Westminster. I recommended a patient to him, not knowing how to cure him myself. His way was by holding the foot as near the natural posture as he could, and then rolling it up with straps of sticking plaster, which he repeated from time to time, as he saw occasion, until the limb was restored to a natural position, but not without some imperfection, the bandage wasting the leg and making the top of it swell and grow larger. After this, having another case of this kind under my care, I thought of a much better bandage, which I had learnt from Mr Cowper, a bonesetter at Leicester, who set and cured a fracture of my own cubit when I was a boy at school. His way was, after putting the limb in the proper posture, to wrap it in rags dipped in the whites of eggs and a little wheat flour mixed; this drying grew stiff, and kept the limb in a good posture. And I think there is no way better than this in fractures, for it preserves the position of the limb without strict bandage, which

is the common cause of mischief in fractures. When I used this method in the crooked feet, I wrapt up the limb almost from the knees to the toes, and caused the limb to be held in the best posture till the bandage grew stiff, and repeated the bandage once a fortnight[28,29].

These remarks well illustrate contemporary relations between the medically qualified and unqualified, Cheselden had been treated by one of the latter in childhood and later referred one of his own patients to another without question i.e. bonesetting was legitimate and these practitioners usually better fitted than doctors to treat fractures and deformities, although doctors were beginning to take over. Even so, throughout the 18th century, especially with increasing experience of dissection of club-feet, authorities expressed scepticism as to the possibility of really being able to correct this deformity completely and permanently.

Aquapendente, in the 17th century, improved on the splints of Arcaeus and Paré of a century earlier. Splints now began to reach above the knee, and Levacher de la Feutrie of Paris, in 1772, illustrates one such with a hinge[30]. But the outstanding contribution was that of the Swiss orthopaedic pioneer, Jean-André Venel (1740–1791) at his institute at Orbe (see p. 295) This was the famous *sabot de Venel*, which utilized the leverage of a rod fastened to a sole-plate and attached to the outer side of the leg, a mechanical principle that has formed the basis of most club-foot appliances over the last 200 years, as, for instance, the 20th century splint of Denis Browne at Great Ormond Street Hospital for Sick Children in London. Venel himself never

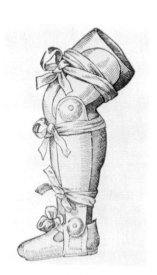
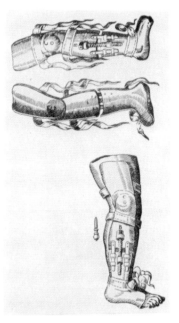

Figure 210   Fabricius Hildanus: *Wundartzney*, Frankfurt, 1652. Appliances for club-foot

wrote any account of this, for while he was projecting a work to be entitled
*Nouveaux moyens de prévenir et de corriger dans l'enfance les déjettements,
courbures et difformités des pieds, des jambes et des genoux, même ceux de
naussance* (New methods of preventing and correcting in childhood the
distortions, curvatures and deformities of the feet, legs and knees, even those
from birth), he succumbed to pulmonary tuberculosis at the age of 51. We
know that he obtained excellent results because he took plaster casts of his
patients before and after treatment, and reproduced these in a 1789 prospectus
of his institute. The splint was only part of the programme, which included
warm baths and manipulation, gradual and repeated, with the infant best
admitted for the duration of the treatment.

A German surgeon, Johann Matthias Wantzel (1777–1800) was himself
treated for bilateral congenital talipes by Venel with excellent results, but he
too died (by suicide) before publishing his planned account of the appliance.
There almost seems, Valentin says, to have been a malignant fate attached
to this history, for the plates for the work had already been engraved and
were eventually published by Brückner in 1795[31]; but Brückner (1769–1797),
who treated many small children by this method, died of tuberculosis before
his 28th birthday. The French adopted and 'improved' Venel's splint[32,33]
and, of course, the Swiss remained faithful to it in Lausanne, not only at the
beginning of the 20th century, but in essence right up to the 1950s[34].

Cheselden's method of bandaging was improved on by Jacob van der
Haar in Amsterdam towards the end of the 18th century, who began with
corrective adhesive bandaging but added a wooden half-shoe 'and bent the
upper and outer part, *which acts entirely as a lever*, outward towards the
fibula and knee while I fastened it with a sticking-plaster stuck on linen.
Thereby, both feet were immediately brought into their proper position and
retained there. This bandage was first applied by me and later by the mother,
but it was not renewed until it had become soiled by the urine, which was
prevented as far as possible[35].'

All techniques based on adhesive bandages suffered from the long
drying and hardening time; matters improved markedly when the German,
Dieffenbach (1792–1847), applied to club-foot the type of plaster cast
previously used for fractures and demonstrated this in France in 1834.
Brockman says that a type of plaster bandage was also used by Guérin, in
Paris, for club-foot around 1836[36], but these bandages were awkward to use
and remained so until the Dutchman, Antonius Mathysen (1805–1878),
invented the first modern plaster-of-Paris bandage in 1852 (p. 570). Mathysen
was more interested in its use for fractures, but the bandage was adapted to
club-foot by a compatriot, Blumenkamp[37], in the following year, while a
little later, in 1856, a Belgian, Maximilien Michaux (1806–1890)[38], reported
on a series of cases so treated but with the feet taken out of the splint daily
for manipulation.

There had been other earlier approaches. In the late 18th century, the
medically unqualified Timothy Sheldrake, 'Truss-maker to the Westminster
Hospital and Mary-le-bone Institution' in London, wrote a series of books
on his practice, including one on club-foot in 1798[39]. Sheldrake travelled
throughout Britain to treat patients, many children of the eminent, and

opined that club-foot was curable in 2–3 months in most cases if taken in time, though he did not leave the children free until they were old enough to walk. (It was Timothy's younger brother, William, who had bungled the treatment of Byron's club foot when the poet was at school in Dulwich in south-east London.) Sheldrake seems to have relied mainly on bandaging, and it was for deformities elsewhere in the limb that he introduced the use of spring correction. The idea of the spring was grasped at by the Italian, Antonio Scarpa (1752–1832) who incorporated it with Venel's method in an elegant and effective appliance. 'None of the appliances is more suitable than the steel spring because it acts continuously by means of its own elasticity... without ever ceasing to act, in such a manner that it prevails[18].'

The use of the spring seems to have reached Scarpa, not directly from Sheldrake, but via a chance discovery on a visit to Typhesne, in Paris, in 1781; chance because both Sheldrake and Typhesne took care not to give too clear a public description of their inventions for fear of plagiarism and loss of custom. In fact, all Typhesne ever said on the matter was, 'Nature does not yield to violence, but only to the graduated application of forces,' and Scarpa, so Valentin says, only discovered the secret by bribing Typhesne's housekeeper to admit him to the Frenchman's rooms, where a glimpse of a steel spring lying on a pillow revealed the secret. The Scot, Wishart, refers to Scarpa's method in a publication in 1818[40]. The London surgeon, Richard Barwell (1826–1916) considered that Scarpa had behaved 'in a manner which in England is considered discreditable.' Barwell himself wrote on the treatment of club-foot in 1863[41], and again in 1865[42], stressing the dangers of

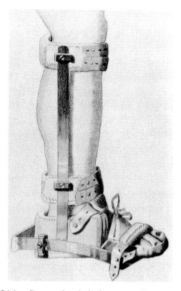

Figure 211   Scarpa's club-foot appliance, *c.* 1800

indiscriminate tenotomy and the importance of the plantar muscles.

Nothing in the way of splints or appliances published after Scarpa's book in 1803 contains anything essentially new, though the Denis Browne splint, introduced in Britain in the 1930s, has always been very attractive, clean and efficient, if efficiently applied[43]. Yet, despite all this ingenuity, the results cannot have been outstanding, for surgeons even at the start of the 19th century still felt helpless (this was the opposite pole to the euphoria mentioned earlier) and, in a leading German clinic in 1835, the Director was driven to assert that true club-foot could never be cured but must be amputated[44]. The stage was therefore set for the arrival of tenotomy as an entirely new factor in practical management, but we should first just mention that Hugh Owen Thomas used immediate forcible correction with his own wrench, a type of osteoclast, and that osteoclasis was also practised by Grattan, of Cork, Bradford in Boston, and Lorenz in Vienna; or else the foot was broken over the apex of a padded triangular wedge. We should also mention, before leaving nonoperative measures, that some, like Julius Wolff (1836–1902)[45], of Berlin, staged the treatment by repeated manipulations and casting and removal of wedges from the outer side of the casts, an anticipation of the method introduced by Hiram Kite, of Decatur, Georgia, USA, in the 1930s[46–48], who used essentially the same method to correct even the most severe deformities without operation, only a simple fusion if the deformity tended to recur.

Tenotomy, then, came when it was needed. The idea was not entirely new, for Moritz Gerhard Thilenius (1745–1809), a physician of Upper Hessen in Germany, on 26th March 1784, had an open transection of the Achilles tendon performed in a 17-year-old girl with a (? paralytic) club-foot, performed by the conventionally subordinate surgeon, here one Lorenz, and with outstanding success[49–50]. Brockman states that the second such operation was performed by Antony Petit in 1799, but gives no details. It is certain that it was repeated by Johann Friedrich Sartorius on 16th May 1806 on a 13-year-old lad with equinus due to calf suppuration, with primary healing and an excellent outcome[51]. And on 18th November 1809, Christian Friedrich Michaelis (1754–1814) operated on a 16-year-old youth and later on eight other patients with various deformities[52].

All these procedures were open tenotomies, and this was regarded as dangerous and had been so regarded from antiquity. Until quite late there had been no clear distinction between tendons and nerves (both were designated *nervus*), and one of Hippocrates' aphorisms states that 'if a portion of bone, cartilage or tendon is cut off from the body, it is never replaced, nor does it ever reunite.' Hippocrates also said of the Achilles tendon, 'This tendon, if bruised or cut, causes the most acute fevers, induces choking, deranges the mind and at length brings death.' It is true that Vesalius did distinguish between nerves and tendons, and that the Nuremberg surgeon, Lorenz Heister (1683–1758) described tenotomy of the sternomastoid for torticollis and methods of tendon suture in 1719[53], but even he believed that damage to the 'nerves or sinews' could cause severe pain and convulsions. Nevertheless, later in the 18th century, there were those, like von Haller of Göttingen in 1752, who maintained that tendons were insensitive and might be sectioned with impunity[54]. In 1745, Pietro Paolo Molinelli (1698–1764) looked at cases of Achilles tendon injury and concluded that 'a surgeon may boldly expose this tendon, cut it and separate it from the adjacent parts[55].' What seemed to matter was exclusion of the outside air when dividing a tendon. We recall that John Hunter (1728–1793) himself sustained a ruptured Achilles tendon while dancing, in 1767. Soon after his death, his brother-in-law, Everard Home (1763–1832), wrote:

> It was in this year (1767) that by an exertion in dancing…he broke his tendo achillis. This accident…led him to pay attention to the subject of broken tendons. He divided the tendo achillis of several dogs by introducing a couching needle through the skin at some distance from it…the dogs were killed at different periods to show progress of union, which was exactly similar to that of a fractured bone when there is no wound in the skin.'

The idea was to draw the skin to one side, before approaching the deeper structures, as did William Bromfield (1712–1792) when extracting a loose body from the knee in 1773[56].

Jean-Mathieu Delpech (1777–1832), the great orthopaedic surgeon of Montpellier, was the first to advocate and practise subcutaneous tenotomy clinically[57–59], though he seems to have operated only on a single case, in 1816, that of a 9-year-old child with congenital equinovarus, in whom he made a tiny incision medial to the tendon, which he transected with an angled knife without damaging the overlying skin.* He was criticized, notably by the Parisians, but maintained that 'we are entirely convinced that this operation is very practicable at every site where tendons are opposed to the natural attitude of the limbs, whatever the origin of the deformity, and that it is a further resource for the cure of club feet.' Although Delpech had ushered in a new era in orthopaedics, it was not until 15 years later that Louis Stromeyer (1804–1876) followed suit and operated on his first case in February 1831[60], and that the report of this in a French journal[61] led to Delpech's Parisian colleagues conceding that there might be some merit in his work.

Stromeyer did not hesitate to divide the tibialis posterior and flexor hallucis longus tendons also, and made some observations on the operation which are still pertinent enough to aggressive orthopaedic methods as to bear repetition, 'The appliances used for extension after the operation are of great importance and I cannot sufficiently warn against engaging in cures of this kind without being equipped therewith, and without understanding how to go about it.' He warned against 'a too reckless use of tendon and muscle section, for once the first impulse to a general application of orthopaedic operations is spent, I believe that there will be a tendency subsequently to misuse or neglect them.' This emphasis that operation is merely an incident in the management of orthopaedic cases is one that has

---

*There is some uncertainty about this. Some say that he made *two* incisions, each of about 1 cm, one on either side of the tendon.

always been respected by good orthopaedists everywhere, especially in England, by Hugh Owen Thomas, Robert Jones and G R Girdlestone; but not always, sadly, by the young, enthusiastic or just operatively-minded surgeons described by Thomas as 'enterprising surgeons who, inspired by the spirit of the times, prefer to cut mechanically what can be unloosed physiologically[62].' We may add that Thomas, in the 1870s and 80s, treated talipes by repeated manipulation, 'by attention to which it is possible to make a better correction than by knife or saw', and insisted on the importance of maintaining overcorrection while the weakened muscles took up the slack. His wrench was a modification of an engineer's monkey-wrench, which became popular in the USA and is often still used in its original form. It is to be noted that he always began his correction, even at the age of a few weeks, with an Achilles tenotomy – 'an easy and effective operation' – which was not in keeping with his usual conservatism. His aftertreatment consisted of repeated manipulation with interim bandaging in an iron shoe. Thomas had a considerable influence on east coast Americans, if not on his own compatriots. Virgil Gibney[63] stated that the wrench had made it possible to bring any club-foot into good shape, though Bradford, while using the method, contended that the story of unvarying success was denied by the profusion of half-cured or relapsed cases.

We now come to a 19th century episode of great historical and personal interest, worthy of description in some detail, if only because it led to the foundation of orthopaedics as a speciality in Britain. This relates to the encounter between William John Little (1810–1894), of London, and Louis Stromeyer (1804–1876) of Hanover. Little had had poliomyelitis at the age of two and was left with a paralytic equinus deformity of one foot; the case history has been described by both protagonists. No treatment or appliances had been successful; no one, in England or Europe, including Delpech, wanted to operate for fear of sepsis; and, as Keith tells us, 'He found that club-foot was regarded as lying outside the legitimate scope of surgery and, in the opinion of his teachers, was properly confined, as his own case had been, to the care of bonesetters and sprain-rubbers, who treated the condition with manipulations or instruments, often with a fair degree of success[64].' Remember that amputation for club-foot was still being performed in London in the 1840s, even after Little had shown the way to tenotomy.

In 1833, Little, who had qualified in 1832 and was teaching comparative anatomy, went to Berlin to work in the anatomical institute of Johannes Müller (1801–1858) because he had been passed over for a staff post at the London Hospital, before devoting himself to orthopaedics. Müller advised him to consult Stromeyer, the great Dieffenbach gave him a letter of introduction, and he travelled to Hanover, where on 6th June 1836, he was operated on with complete success. Dieffenbach's letter, before the operation, ran, in part;

'Dr Little, from London, a very capable man, desires as I do to learn whether the operative method on which your reputation is partly based can be of any help to him. My own experience is too limited and concerns other deformities, so that I have not enough confidence in

SYMBOLAE AD TALIPEDEM VARUM COGNOSCENDUM.

PARS 1.   GENESIS.

DISSERTATIO INAUGURALIS MEDICA

QUAM IN

UNIVERSITATE LITERARIA FRIDERICA GUILELMA

PRO SUMMIS IN MEDICINA ET CHIRURGIA HONORIBUS

DIE XVII. M. JANUARII A. D. MDCCCXXXVII.

PUBLICE DEFENDET AUCTOR

W. J. LITTLE, ANGLUS,

SOCIUS COLLEGII REGALIS CHIRURG. LONDINENSIS MED. ET CHIR. PRACT. ET IN „THE LONDON HOSPITAL"
ANATOMEN COMP. PUBLICE DOCENS.

OPPONENTIBUS:

G. HOLTHOFF, M. D. PRACT.
J. JACOBSON, M. D. PRACT.
H. W. BEREND, M. D. PRACT.

BEROLINI,
FORMIS NIETACKIANIS.

Figure 212   Title page of Little's Berlin Doctoral Dissertation of 1837

myself in this case...'

His second letter, in October of that year, runs;

> 'Little's return from you marks a new era in my medical life; never
> before has a surgical operation had such an effect on me. Ever since, I
> have spoken freely to other doctors to tell them about your important
> discovery... all that we can drum up in the way of club feet and equinus
> is already marked down for the next opportunity... Little visits me
> daily, he undertakes excursions of several miles and now walks like a
> normal person. Had you no other reward than this, dear Stromeyer, it
> would be great enough to hand your name down gloriously to
> posterity[65].'

Stromeyer's introduction of tenotomy had, in fact, transferred the treatment of deformities from mechanics to surgeons. The former had kept few records, while the doctors rarely condescended to this work and when they did so had not described it in detail. (Whipple, of Plymouth, had done transection at an earlier date in 1836, but it is not clear whether this was an open or a subcutaneous procedure.)

Little was always grateful to Stromeyer for transforming his life. His Berlin doctoral thesis on the treatment of club-foot was subtitled *Tuus et propter Te felix*, and he called one of his sons Louis Stromeyer Little, which rather reminds one of John Sebastian Bach Stopford. When he returned to England in 1837, it was a proselytiser for Stromeyer's method, and he did the first subcutaneous tenotomy in England in February of that same year. When, in 1838, he founded at his own expense the Infirmary for the Cure of Club Foot and other Contractures in Bloomsbury Square, it was at Stromeyer's prompting and because he felt impelled to spread the knowledge of a method, not known to those who had treated him earlier, which had been so beneficial.

There was also the conviction, expressed by John Ball Brown, of Boston (who did what may have been the first subcutaneous tenotomy in the USA in 1839), when he founded the first orthopaedic hospital in America at almost exactly the same time, that 'deformities of the human frame cannot be conveniently or judiciously treated, except in a Hospital or Institution expressly devoted to this object[66].' Little assigned as his principal reasons 'the dispensation of that relief to poor persons afflicted with deformities which they were unable to obtain in existing hospitals, the formation of a school for studying deformities, and instruction in the art of remedying them[67].' The subsequent progress of what was to become the Royal National Orthopaedic Hospital in London is narrated elsewhere (p. 125), and we may note that Syme, in Edinburgh, followed suit.

It must not be imagined that Little, even in the early days, was an uncritical enthusiast of tenotomy, or of operation solely on the Achilles tendon. He was, in fact, a physician on the staff of the London Hospital, something of a neurologist, and best known for his original masterly account of spastic birth palsy given to the Obstetrical Society of London in 1862[68]. He was opposed to regarding a club-foot as 'a mere shapeless mass…requiring to be merely moulded and compressed by mechanical instruments' and regarded operation only as a last resort when rigid muscular contracture demanded tenotomy, a tenotomy which sometimes included the tibialis anterior and posterior and even the long flexor and extensor of the hallux. The tenotome was passed from the point of entry behind the Achilles tendon to emerge through the skin at the other side, and the tendon rather pressed against the blade than using a deliberate cutting action. Correction thereafter had to be gradual and progressive; immediate redressment was inadvisable and dangerous and continued splintage was essential.

In later life, Little confessed to having operated too readily when younger, and pleaded for the nonoperative treatment of club-foot. But this seems to have been an expression of depression, for he retired early after quarrelling with the hospital administrators and retired to the country, where, says Gibney in his 1912 memoirs, a visit showed that he had retired from practice and gone back to the farm. 'I tried to engage him in talk about his deeds in orthopaedic surgery, but he seemed far more interested in ... the construction of earth closets, of which he was, in his declining years, making a profound study[69].'

Little's most important pupil was William Adams (1810–1900), also on the staff of the hospital, and also retiring (in 1872) because of friction. Adams did pioneer work on the pathology of club-foot, and his monograph on its causes, pathology and treatment received the Jacksonian prize of the Royal College of Surgeons of England[70]. He remained an exponent of 'subcutaneous surgery' and gave a Smithsonian lecture on the topic in 1877 in relation to osteotomy for bony ankylosis of the hip[71,72]. Adams advocated early tenotomy to restore muscle balance and thought any changes in the shape of the talus were secondary. There could be no central nervous causes since power was rapidly restored after correction and cure was independent of the aetiology, whatever that might be.

Dieffenbach, in Berlin, was so stimulated by Little's cure that he operated on 350 patients between the October of that year of 1836 and 1841[73]. The method spread rapidly throughout Europe, so much so that Vincent Duval (1796–1876) for instance, who had performed the first Achilles tenotomy in Paris in 1835, now devoted himself entirely to treating club-foot, and this in a city where, only a few years earlier, German visitors had complained of not seeing a single case of club-foot treated in the many hospitals he visited[74,75]. Valentin tells us that in London, Gustav Krauss (1813–1887), who had emigrated from Germany in 1837, often performed Achilles tenotomy[76,77]. Italian enthusiasts included Casimiro Sperino (1812–1894), of Turin, followed by others in rapid succession[78,79].

In the USA, David L Rogers, assisted by the young Lewis Sayre[80], did the first Achilles tenotomy in 1834, but the main influence there for a time was a man of German origin, a pupil of Stromeyer's, William Ludwig Detmold (1808–1894), marking the start of his practice in New York with a series of successful transections that had not hitherto even been attempted by the most enterprising native surgeons. The first American book on the subject was that of Thomas Dent Muetter, in 1839[81]; Detmold published his results a year later[82].

It has to be stated that there was considerable resistance to operation throughout the middle of the 19th century, largely from those who preferred, often because their livelihoods depended on them, various methods of elastic traction, such as the orthopaedic mechanic, Henry Heather Bigg[83] and the orthopaedic surgeon, Richard Barwell[84], both of London. In fact, rubber tubing and steel strips had been used to correct deformity as far back as around 1800.

Some surgeons applied corrective plaster-of-Paris bandaging at the time of tenotomy; others advised delay. Theodor Billroth (1829–1894) found the method dangerous, having had two cases of gangrene[85]. The more impatient began to operate on the bones of the foot. Abel Mix Phelps (1851–1902) in New York performed extensive open release of tendons and ligaments at the inner side of the foot when aspesis made this possible[86] and reported this to the International Medical Congress at Copenhagen in 1888. 'Each contracted part was carefully divided as it showed itself when the parts were put upon the stretch by extending the feet.' Similar procedures have remained part of the orthopaedic repertory for severe or neglected cases, especially in the Third World. The even more impatient began to attack the skeleton. Solly, of St Thomas's Hospital in London, seems to have been the first, at Little's suggestion in 1857, to remove the cuboid, though without notable benefit[87]. Other Londoners performed wedge tarsectomy[88]. Pughe, of Liverpool, resected the head of the talus in 1883[89]. The multiplicity of bone operations at the beginning of the 20th century is indicated in the review of national endeavours in Chapter 33. Many preferred to limit their bone operations to arthrodesis, with excision as required, Agustoni[90], in Italy and Morestin[91], in Paris, found astragalectomy useful in 1888 and 1902 respectively.

As astragalectomy has an interesting history, a little may be said of this here. We have mentioned that Fabricius Hildanus had done this for compound fracture in 1608; and Laming Evans tells us that it was repeated for the same indication by Broglie in 1741, Marrigue in 1782, Dessault in 1788 and, for the first time in England, by Trye of Gloucester in 1789, followed by Hey in Leeds in 1804, Percy in 1811, Evans in 1815 and Astley Cooper in 1820[92]. In Leeds, Smith reported 10 cases in 1821. It was then performed for caries by various surgeons in the mid century, but its first use for club-foot was by Lund in 1872, a bilateral operation done under chloroform and antisepsis[93]. In 1873, Hancock was able to collect 109 operations from the literature[94]. In the 1890s, Lucas-Championnière began with astragalectomy[95] and went on to 'ablation of the totality of the bones of the tarsus[96]'.

What is fascinating is that the great American orthopaedic surgeon, Royal Whitman, stated in 1893 that he had never done an astragalectomy, which he considered an operation of the last resort[97], but he had begun to do so (for paralytic calcaneocavus) by 1901[98], by 1910[99] he had treated 50 cases, in 1915 he did 60 operations for various types of deformity at the Hospital for the Ruptured and Crippled in New York[100], and in 1927 he told Laming Evans that he had operated on many thousands of cases.

In Paris, in 1911, Lamy reported or collected 200 cases, operated mainly for tuberculosis, but also for injury. In 1939, Thompson reviewed 2066 cases from the records of the Hospital for the Ruptured and Crippled, with the best results when done for calcaneocavus[101].

Laming Evans himself stressed the importance of backward displacement of the foot, as initially stressed by Whitman in 1901, to give a good line of weight transmission to the mid-tarsus, and used the method widely for paralysis, spasticity and other neurogenic deformities. As for its application in club-foot, 'Astragalectomy has played so important a part for so many years in the treatment of this deformity that there is little new to say about it' – though it was usually necessary to add a wedge osteotomy. This was in 1926, when Evans wrote a paper on the subject for the Robert Jones Birthday Volume. Yet Brockman, writing at much the same time, regarded the procedure almost with horror; the deformity was unchanged, or relapsed, and the foot was 'dreadful-looking'.

The question has become academic in the west, since most children with resistant talipes are now operated, if necessary, very early in life, as early as a few weeks of age, by open posterior or posteromedial release, astragalectomy being performed, if ever, only for the rigid talipes of arthrogryposis. It is certainly the case, however, as the writer knows from personal experience, that in the Third World, where late cases are common, astragalectomy 'takes all the fight out of the foot' and offers the quickest and most undemanding route to an aesthetic and functionally satisfactory foot.

If, in the west, severe cases were treated for a period by triple fusion of various types, such as Naughton Dunn's, or modifications thereof, with or without wedge tarsectomies, the general rule followed was that laid down by Robert Jones: that no bone operations should be done before maximal correction had been obtained by manipulation or wrenching, and not before the age of 10, and that failed bone operations were more difficult to treat than fresh cases. The more important innovations that have tended to replace this final and definitive procedure include early tendon transplantation of the tibialis anterior or posterior, or both, Dillwyn Evan's fusion of the calcaneocuboid joint after appropriate excision, and the calcanean osteotomy introduced in Australia by Dwyer for the varus component.

Club foot recurs as a theme in life and literature (in *Madame Bovary* by Flaubert and *Of Human Bondage* by Somerset Maugham, among others). When the novelist, Gustave Flaubert, was planning his work, he wished to describe how Dr Bovary, a rural physician, was persuaded by the local pharmacist to perform the new operation of tenotomy on Hippolyte, ostler at the *Golden Lion*; it would gain the doctor renown and cost the patient nothing. So Bovary had to look up the technique, as did his creator – in Duval's *Traité Pratique du Pied Bot*, which had first appeared in 1839. 'Yesterday,' he wrote, 'I spent my entire evening engaged in...studying the theory of club-feet. In three hours I devoured an entire volume of this interesting literature and took notes.' The protagonist of his novel, having to follow suit, sent to Rouen for the book and 'with his head between his hands, buried himself in it every evening and informed himself about equinus malformations, varus and valgus...' and decided to divide the Achilles tendon first, and the tibialis anterior later if necessary.

As we know, gangrene developed after the operation, clearly described as a moist ascending necrosis, due not so much to wound infection as to compression by the metal appliances applied postoperatively, and not removed even when Hippolyte complained of pain. One gains a distinct impression that Flaubert's father, Achille-Cléophas Flaubert (1786–1846), who was a surgeon at the Hôtel-Dieu in Rouen (the house is preserved as a museum), and had treated such a case, also unsuccessfully, had had personal experience of this complication. In the novel, a more experienced surgeon had to amputate through the thigh, Bovary paying for the artificial limb. The crux, for the conservatively minded, is that before the procedure the luckless ostler depended on his hard horny deformed foot more than its normal counterpart and galloped on it like a stag from morning to night. This is an instance of what the present writer has christened 'surgical Bovarism'[102], in which surgeons seek out and operate on untreated and highly functional abnormalities, merely because they *are* technically abnormal, against the patient's better judgment, and often with similar destructive results.

One wonders a little about the novelist's motivation in creating this floundering village doctor, and must remind ourselves that Flaubert père had also, in 1838, performed the first successful bone suture for pseudarthrosis in France, after resecting the bone-ends[103].

REFERENCES

1. Montfalcon (1820). Pied bot. *Dict. Sci. Méd. Paris*, **42**, 387
2. Trendelenburg, F. (1924). *Aus Heiteren Jugendtagen*. (Berlin)
3. Fabricius ab Aquapendente, H. (1592). *Opera cirurgica*. (Frankfort)
4. Brückner, K.A.F. (1795). Über einwärts gedrehte Füsse und deren Behandlung. *J. Erfindungen, Theorien und Widersprüche in d.Natur- und Arznei Wissenschaft*, **3**, (Sect. 12), 35
5. Wynne-Davies, R. (1973). *Heritable Disorders in Orthopaedic Practice*. (Oxford, Blackwell Scientific Publications)
6. Guérin, C. (1876). *Mémoire sur l'étiologie générale des pieds-bots congénitales*. (Paris)
7. Delpech, J.-M. (1828). *De l'Orthomorphie*. vol. I, p. 177 (Paris)
8. Bouvier, J. (1858). *Leçons cliniques sur les maladies chroniques de l'appareil locomoteur*. (Paris)
9. Little, W.J. (1839). *A Treatise on Club Foot*. (London)
10. Adams, W. (1852). *Trans. Path. Soc.*, **3**, 455
11. Boyer, A. (1803). *Leçons sur les maladies des os*. (Paris)
12. Jörg, J.C.G. (1806). *Über Klumpfuss und eine leichte und zweckmassige Heilart derselben*. (Leipzig and Marburg)
13. Malgaigne, J.-F. (1840). *Oeuvres complètes d'Ambroise Paré*. (Paris)
14. Keith, A. (1921). *Human Embryology and Morphology*. (London)
15. Keith, A. (1929). History of the human foot. *J. Bone Jt. Surg.*, **11**, 10
16. Brockman, E.P. (1930). *Congenital Club-Foot*. (Bristol and London)
17. Camper, P. (1782). *Abhandlung über den besten Schuh*. (Vienna)
18. Scarpa, A. (1803). *Memorie chirurgica sui piedi congeniti dei fanciulli e sua maniere di corregere questa difformita*. (Pavia)
19. Coles, A. (1817). On the distortion termed Varus or Club Foot. *Dublin Hosp. Rep.*, **1**, 175
20. Mackeever, T.L. (1820). Dissection of two cases of Club-Foot. *Edinb. Med. J.*, **15**, 220
21. Little, W.J. (1837). *Symbolae ad talipidem varum cognoscendum*. *Diss. Med.*, English translation, London 1839
22. Stern, W.G. (1923). Arthrogryposis multiplex congenita. *Trans. Orth. Sec. Am. Med. Assoc.*, **66**
23. Palletta, G.B. (1826). *Exercitationes Pathologicae*. Part 2. (Milan)
24. Bick, E.M. (1968). *A Source Book of Orthopaedics*. (Reprint of 1948 edition with additional references.) (New York, Hafner)
25. Vidius, V. (1611). *Opera omnia, sive Ars medicinalis*. (Venice)
26. Arcaeus, F. (1674). *Chirurgische Bücher*. (Nuremberg)
27. Falloppio, G. (1606). *Opere genuine omnia*. (Venice)
28. Cheselden, W. (1740). *The Anatomy of the Human Body*. 5th edn. (London)
29. Le Dran, H.-F. (1768). *The operations in surgery. Translated by Mr. Gataker, with remarks by William Cheselden*. 4th edn. (London)

30. Levacher de la Feutrie, T. (1772). *Traité du Rakitis.* (Paris)
31. Brückner, A. (1796. *Über die Natur, Ursachen und Behandlung der einwärts gekrümmten Füsse oder der sogenannten Klumpfüsse.* (Gotha)
32. d'Ivernois, L. (1817). *Essai sur la torsion des pieds (pieds-bots) et sur le meilleur moyen de les guérir.* (Paris)
33. Mellet, F.L.E. (1823). Considérations générales sur les déviations des pieds (pieds-bots). *Thesis,* Paris No 82
34. Nicod, P. (1908). *Le pronostic du pied bot congénital.* (Lausanne)
35. van der Haar, J. (1797). *Uitgezochte genees- en keelkundige Mengelscriften.* (Amsterdam)
36. Guérin, J. (1938). *Mémoire sur l'étiologie générale des pieds bots congénitaux.* (Paris)
37. Blumenkamp, C. (1853). Eenige waarnemingen van behandelnde beenbreuken met her gipsverband. *Geneesk. Courant,* **18**
38. Michaux, M. (1856). Considerations sur les pieds-bots poplitées internes. *Bull. Acad. Med. Belg.,* **15**, 447
39. Sheldrake, T. (1798). *A practical essay on the club-foot and other distortions in the Legs and Feet of Children.* (London)
40. Wishart, J.H. (1818). *Memoir on congenital clubfoot of children.* (Edinburgh)
41. Barwell, R. (1863). *The Cure of Club Foot.* (London)
42. Barwell, R. (1865). *On the cure of club-foot without cutting tendons.* 2nd edn. (London)
43. Browne, D. (1937). Modern methods of treatment of club-foot. *Br. Med. J.,* **1**, 570
44. Stromeyer, L. (1874). *Erinnerungen eines deutsches Arztes.* (Hanover)
45. Wolff, J. (1903). *Über die Ursachen, das Wesen und die Behandlung des Klumpfusses.* (Berlin)
46. Kite, J.H. (1939). Nonoperative treatment of congenital clubfeet. *Southern Med. J.,* **23**, 337
47. Kite, J.H. (1932). The treatment of congenital clubfeet. *J. Am. Med. Assoc.,* **99**, 1156
48. Kite, J.H. (1939). Principles involved in the treatment of congenital club-feet. *J. Bone Jt. Surg.,* **21**, 595
49. Thilenius, M.G. (1789). *Tachenbuch für deutsche Wundärzte.* (Altenburg)
50. Thilenius, M.G. (1789). *Medizinische und chirurgische Bemerkungen.* (Frankfort)
51. Sartorius, J.F. (1811). *Sammlung seltener und auserlesener chirurgischer Beobachtungen und Erfahrungen.* Vol. 3, p. 258 (Arnstadt)
52. Michaelis, C.F. (1811). Über die Schwächung der Sehnen durch Einschneidung als einem Mittel bei manchen Gliederverunstaltungen. *J. prakt. Heilk. Berlin,* **33** (No.26, Part II) 4
53. Heister, L. (1719). *Chirurgie.* (Nuremberg)
54. Sudhoff, K. (1922). *Klassiker der Medizin.* (Leipzig)
55. Molinelli, P.P. (1745). De vulnerato Achillis tendinis. *Comment. Acad. Sci. Bonon.,* **2**, 189
56. Bromfield, W. (1773). *Chirurgical observations and cases.* (London)
57. Delpech, J.-M. (1816). *Précis élémentaire des maladies réputées chirurgicales.* (Paris)
58. Delpech, J.-M. (1828). *Chirurgie clinique de Montpellier.* Vol. II, pp. 177 and 231 (Paris and Montpellier)
59. Delpech, J.-M. (1828). *De l'Orthomorphie,* Vol. II, p. 328. (Paris)
60. Stromeyer, L. (1833). Die Durchschneidung des Achillessehne, als Heilmethode des Klumpfusses, durch zwei Fälle erläutert. *Mag. ges. Hielk.* (*Rust*), **39** (NF15), 195

61. Stromeyer, L. (1834). *Arch. Gén. Méd.*
62. Le Vay, D. (1956). *Life of Hugh Owen Thomas.* p. 82. (Edinburgh and London, Livingstone)
63. Gibney, V.P. (1889). *Trans. Am. Orthop. Assoc.*, **1**, 74
64. Keith, A. (1919). *Menders of the Maimed.* (London)
65. Valentin, B. (1934). *Dieffenbach an Stromeyer, Briefe aus den Jahren 1836–1846.* (Leipzig)
66. Brown, J.B. (1845). *Reports of cases in the Boston Orthopaedic Institution or Hospital for Cure of Deformities of the Human Frame.* (Boston)
67. Little, W.J. (1853). *On the nature and treatment of deformities of the human frame.* (London)
68. Little, W.J. (1862). *Trans. Obstet. Soc. Lond.*, **3**, 293
69. Gibney, V.P. (1912). Reminiscences of the orthopaedic surgeons of the latter half of the 19th century. *N.Y. Med. J.*, **95**, 913
70. Adams, W. (1871). *Club-Foot: Its causes, pathology and treatment.* (London)
71. Adams, W. (1871). *A new operation for bony anchylosis of the hip-joint.* (London)
72. Adams, W. (1878). Subcutaneous surgery. In *Smithsonian Miscellaneous Collections,* Vol. 15, Lecture VI. (Washington)
73. Dieffenbach, J.F. (1841). *Über die Durchschneidung der Sehnen und Muskeln.* (Berlin)
74. von Ammon, F.A. (1823). *Parallele der französischen und deutschen Chirurgie.* (Leipzig)
75. Berend, H.W. (1842). Die orthopädische Institute zu Paris nach eigner Anschauung und mit Rücksicht auf den jetzigen Standpunkt der Orthopädie Überhaupt. *Ma. Ges. Heil. (Rust),* **59**, 496
76. Krauss, G. (1839). Remarks upon Club-Foot and its cure. *Lond. Med. Gaz.,* **24** (NS2), 342
77. Krauss, G. (1839). *Cure of Club-foot, bent knee and wry-neck,* (London)
78. Antoldi, G. (1842). *Della cura dei piedi torti mediante la tenotomia.* (Mantua)
79. Sani, F. (1844). *Alcune operazione di tenotomia e miotomia.* (Rome)
80. Sayre, L.A. (1876). *Lectures on Orthopedic Surgery and Diseases of the Joints.* (New York)
81. Muetter, T.D. (1839). *A Lecture on Loxarthrus, or club foot.* (Philadephia)
82. Detmold, W.L. (1840). *An essay on club-foot and some analogous diseases.* (New York)
83. Bigg, H.H. (1869). *Orthopraxy: the mechanical treatment of deformities, debilities and deficiencies of the human frame.* 2nd edn. (London)
84. Barwell, R. (1863). *The Cure of Club-Foot.* (London)
85. Billroth, T. (1837). Über die Geraderichtung der Klumpfüsse unmittelbar mittels der Sehnendurchschneidung und die Anwendung des Gipsgusses. *Med. Annalen (Heidelberg),* **3**, 611
86. Phelps, A.M. (1881). A case of double talipes equinovarus treated by open incision and fixed extension. *New Engl. Monthly,* **11**, 195
87. Solly, S. (1857). *Med. Chir. Trans.,* **40**, 119
88. Bryant, T. (1878). *Trans. Clin. Soc. Lond.,* **12**, 36
89. Pughe, R.N. (1883). *Liverpool Med. Chir. J.,* **3**, 353
90. Agustoni (1888). 23 casi d'estirpazione dell'astragalo per la correzione dei piede torto. *Arch. di Ortop.,* **3**, 4
91. Morestin (1901). Pied plat invéteré et irreducible traité par l'astragalectomie. *Bull. et Mém. Soc. Anat. Paris,* **76**
92. Laming Evans, E. (1928). *Robert Jones Birthday Volume.* (London, Oxford University Press)
93. Lund, E. (1872). Removal of both astragali in a case of severe double talipes.

Br. Med. J., **2**, 438

94. Hancock (1873). *On the operative surgery of the foot and ankle joint.* (London, Churchill)
95. Lucas-Championnière, J.M. (1890). Traitement des pieds bots par l'ablation de l'astragale. *J. Méd. Chir. Prat.*,
96. Lucas-Championnière, J.M. (1900). Traitement des formes graves du pied bot par l'ablation de la totalité des os du tarse. In 13*th International Medical Congress*, Paris
97. Whitman, R. (1893). *Trans. Am. Orthop. Assoc.*, **6**, 169
98. Whitman, R. (1901). The operative treatment of paralytic talipes of the calcaneus type. *Am. J. Med. Sci.*, **122**, 593
99. Whitman, R. (1908). *Ann. Surg.*, **47**, 264
100. Whitman, R. (1915). *Med. Record*, July 24
101. Thompson, T.C. (1939). Astragalectomy and the treatment of calcaneovalgus. *J. Bone Jt. Surg.*, **21**, 627
102. Le Vay, D. (1976). *Scenes from Surgical Life.* (London, Peter Owen)
103. Vaultier, R. (1954). La Médecine dans *Madame Bovary*. *Presse Méd.*, **62**, 823

CHAPTER 23

Congenital Dislocation
of the Hip

That Hippocrates was well acquainted with this condition is very clear from his *De Articulis*, 'Those suffer the greatest injury in whom, while still in the womb, this joint has been disclocated.' And, 'However, it sometimes happens that an outward dislocation of both hips is found in one case from birth and in another as the result of disease.' Nevertheless, although very energetic and often successful attempts were made by the Greeks to reduce traumatic dislocations, there is no evidence that these were employed – at any rate successfully – for the congenital lesion.

Little was to be added to this until the 16th century, when Ambroise Paré explains that reduction is often impossible because the socket is too shallow, an argument repeatedly advanced later to prove the absurdity of contemplating anatomic restitution:

'It happens also that some have the cavities of their joints not deep, and that the rims of their sockets or cavities are much flattened, whereby the heads of the bones do not enter deeply into them, and that the ligaments which hold the bones in their joints are not firm but greatly relaxed and soft in their conformation[1].'

This is a remarkably penetrating analysis of two main elements of the pathology, and it justified the remark of a contemporary, Jean-Baptiste Verduc (d.1700):

'Before applying extension, enquire well what is the nature of the luxation; for if it is a person lame from birth, your extension will serve only to expose your ignorance[2].'

This was to spare patients from the vain efforts of doctors; the bonesetters were notoriously unsuccessful in this condition. Another contemporary, Theodor Zwinger (1658–1724) relates the prognosis to the promptitude of treatment and stresses the genetic factor:

'But if the bone remains thus dislocated a long time, then callus formed
in the joint prevents all hope of reposition. It is worthy of note that to
the mother of this lame child there were born three sons lame from
femoral luxation, though the same number of daughters were brought
into the world not lame[3].'

Andry was familiar with the condition, strikingly describing the gait of those
affected as *dandinant* (waddling), and advised strengthening baths and a belt
or girdle encircling the abdomen and well-padded over the hips[4].

In Holland, in the late 18th century, Petrus Camper, who was interested
in geographic pathology, noted the regional distribution of the disorder:

'This affliction is very common, particularly in our young girls, so that
among every 28 persons at Franecker one is lame...and not only among
the common townsfolk but in various of the first houses of this university
city, as evidence that this affliction cannot be ascribed to lack of either
care or remedies[5].'

In 1783, the Milanese, Giovanni Pattista Palletta, gave a very accurate
account of the autopsy findings in a 15-day-old boy with a double displacement[6] and many years later, in his *Exercitationes Pathologicae*[7], minutely
described the state of the head, socket, capsule and round ligament.

Then, in the early 19th century, we come to Dupuytren's historic treatise
of 1826, *Original or congenital displacement of the heads of the thigh-bones*[8],
historic despite the inaccuracy of its initial premise: 'It is a sort of displacement
of the upper extremity of the femora of which I have found no indication in
the authors, despite my searching for one.'

The important thing was his grasp of the pathology:

'This displacement consists in a transposition of the head of the femur
from the cotyloid cavity on to the external iliac fossa of the ilium, a
transposition which exists from birth and which appears due to a defect
in the depth or completeness of the acetabulum, rather than to accident
or disease. The class of dislocations to which it belongs is that in which
the bone is thrown upward and outward...a variety which I shall name
original or congenital dislocation to distinguish it from the two forms
mentioned above (i.e. traumatic and pathologic)...I have been able to
study (the post-mortem appearances) in only a few instances...all the
muscles which have their attachments either above or below the
acetabulum were drawn up towards the crest of the ilium...the upper
and inner part of the head of the bone has sometimes lost a little of its
roundness, a circumstance apparently due to contact with a surface
unsuited for articulation. The cotyloid cavity is either altogether absent
or presents only a small osseous irregular prominence, where neither
traces of diarthrodial cartilage nor vestige of synovial or other capsule
nor fibrous margin is to be found, but which is surrounded by some
tough cellular tissue and covered by the muscles which are inserted into
the lesser trochanter. Once, in two or three subjects submitted for my
examination, I met with the round ligament of the joint very much
elongated, flattened above and, as it were, worn at certain points by the

pressure and friction of the head of the femur. The head of the bone itself is lodged in a hollow, somewhat analogous to that which is developed round it in traumatic dislocations upwards and outwards. This new cavity, which is very superficial and almost without a rim, is situated...above and behind the acetabulum, at an elevation proportional to the site of the head of the femur. In fact, the only perceptible difference that I have been able to detect between these congenital cases and longstanding traumatic dislocations...is that in the former the arrangement of the parts appears to have subsisted for a longer term, and gives the impression of having been the primitive condition, or that which was assumed at the very earliest period of existence.'

Dupuytren described the typical stature, the lordosis, the gait – in which the patient tried to throw his weight over the affected hip but was defeated by the instability that produced the effect Trendelenburg was later to label – the ability of the surgeon to telescope the limb. He restated Verduc's point: if the condition were mistaken for a displacement consequent on disease, vain and tedious treatment might be inflicted on the patient, or the parents might be accused of battering their child. But the history 'does not include any of those marked symptoms which characterize that painful and cruel disease of the hip-joint (i.e. suppurative arthritis) which usually leads to spontaneous dislocation of the femur.' At that period, diagnosis was delayed until walking; and as walking itself tended to be delayed, discovery often took three or four years.

Therapeutically, Dupuytren was nihilistic and his main motive in writing this paper was 'the desire to save practitioners from grave errors of judgment and patients from treatments as useless as they are rigorous...What is the use of traction exerted on the lower limbs? Supposing that it were possible so to restore these limbs to their length, is it not obvious that, the femoral head finding no cavity disposed to receive it and capable of retaining it, the limb would lose the length afforded it by the traction as soon as it was left to itself!'

Some further remarks on Dupuytren's views will be found at p. 256. Although other causal factors operate – seasonal, birth posture and birth order – the idea of a primary aplasia of the acetabulum implicit in Dupuytren's account was to be confirmed by later writers and geneticists. Lorenz, in his last summing-up, in 1920[9], of a subject which had occupied him throughout a long career, spoke of a 'dysarthrosis ilio-femoralis congenita', postulating arrest at an early stage of development; as the head had never been in the acetabulum, the term dislocation could not apply. (This was a total misconception, since workers like Pierre Le Damany, in France, had demonstrated the earliest and reversible stage in infancy as far back as 1910 [see p. 268].)

In recent times, Ruth Wynne-Davies[10] has stressed the hereditary aspect, as evidenced by the racial factor, the connective tissue abnormality, the acetabular dysplasia and the fact that the concordance in monozygotic twins is 20 times that in dizygotic twins.

Other ideas on aetiology included Guérin's theory of 'convulsive muscular contraction', popular in France for decades in the 18th and 19th centuries as the cause of numerous orthopaedic disorders. This theory was to have unfortunate results, for, writing in 1841[11], he said, 'It is necessary to perform subcutaneous section of all the contracted muscles' and proceeded to do just that, sparing hardly any of the muscles spanning the pelvis and femur, so further impairing the ability to retain the head in the socket even if reduced. At much the same time, in 1842, Parise postulated a hydrops of the joint in intrauterine life, stretching and weakening the capsule.

Roser, in 1864[12] and subsequently[13], explained the commoner incidence in girls by attributing the dislocation to persistent severe thigh adduction *in utero*, a position less tolerated by male foetuses because of the pressure on the genitals, a view unlikely to find favour in the present-day climate of feminist opinion. Misguided as this may have been, Roser rendered two valuable services: he described Nélaton's line in 1846[14], a year before Nélaton himself, pointing out that the diagnosis of dislocation was made easy if the trochanter was found above the line from the anterior superior iliac spine to the ischial tuberosity, and he stressed that the early diagnosis of such dislocations was the first condition of their curability, 'I believe that many, even most, of these cases would still be curable if the disorder were detected in the newborn and if the necessary abduction appliance were applied at once. I believe that with plaster boots held apart by a crossbar or crossboard the object would be most simply obtainable.' All earlier efforts had been doomed to failure because recognition had been achieved too late. And this in 1879! It is in the highest degree unfortunate that Roser's views coincided with the rise of operative treatment, which so fascinated many that simpler measures were ignored; it should be borne in mind that the hazards of forcible manipulative reduction were probably even greater than those of a simple open operation.

If Dupuytren was a nihilist, he nevertheless employed a girdle very much like Andry's, and one may assume that, like everyone else, he advised a raised shoe for the shortening. His declaration that reduction was impossible had the effect of similar pronouncements throughout history – that anaesthesia, the prevention of poliomyelitis, trips to the moon, were impossibilities: it stimulated the endeavour to prove him wrong. Even in his own department, in 1828, shortly after Dupuytren's thesis, a Dr Bilonière wrote a dissertation which certainly mentions his master's girdle but goes on to refer to the case of an 8-year-old girl whom Dupuytren had transferred to the Institute of Jalade-Lafond and Vincent Duval at Chaillot, in Paris, to be managed by continuous traction in their *machine oscillatoire*, or extension bed. To his surprise, the good effects produced by a few months' continuous traction lasted over several weeks. Bilonière cautioned against results in a single case; but 'this case is important in itself and may become even more so because of the consequences it may have[15].' Lafond himself gave no details of his late results and Dupuytren's pessimism remained unaltered.

However, the situation was changing, thanks to the demonstration of the morbid anatomy by Dupuytren in Paris in 1826 and by Vrolik (1775–1859) in Amsterdam in 1839[16], who illustrated the flattened deformed femoral head and the coxa vara. It was now clear where the femoral head lay and

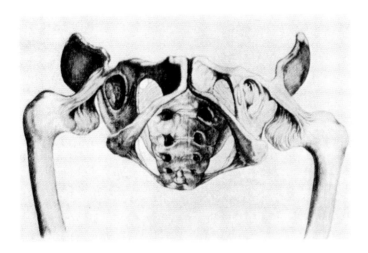

Figure 213   Gerard Vrolik: the pathology of congenital dislocation of the hip,
Amsterdam 1839

whither it had to be reduced, and another Frenchman, Francois Humbert
(1776–1850), asserted with Jacquier in 1835[17] that he had succeeded in
reducing a congenital dislocation in an 11-year-old girl at a single session of
forced traction on a machine in under an hour. It seems probable that
Humbert was producing, not a true reduction, but a transposition of the
femoral head into the obturator foramen or sciatic notch; but even this was
a great step forward, for it lengthened and stabilized the limb and it showed
that the situation could be changed for the better. There was now some
hope.

For 2000 years a true reduction of the congenitally dislocated hip had
haunted the imagination of surgeons; what Humbert had done was really to
conceive its practicability – the essential first step in any human project –
and only a few years later, in 1841[18] and 1847, Pravaz in Lyons brought
about the long-desired result. Pravaz reported on 19 cases in a book of
1847[19]. After some nine months of traction, when the head had reached the
level of the acetabulum, reduction was effected by daily abduction with
pressure on the trochanter, while maintaining the extension; and even then
traction was continued while the child spent the next two years in a small
carriage, self-propelled, the *char à engrenage et à bielles* (car with gear and
cranks) so that the active movements 'ground out' the acetabulum, followed
by a walking-aid with an axillary crutch mounted on the side-arm.

In his own country, Pravaz was opposed by Boyer and Bouvier, the latter maintaining that the great obstacle to reduction – the constriction of the capsule – was impassable, but as the years passed the experience of others provided support. Malgaigne, in 1862[20], said he did not doubt that reduction was sometimes possible, and might even be easy. Pravaz's results were confirmed by a commission of the *Académie de Médecine*, by Nélaton, and later by Lorenz. In Würzburg, Jakob Heine bestirred himself in the matter, having attended Pravaz' dissertation, and in 1842 reported on 11 cases, though without claiming unequivocal success. In the United States, John Murray Carnochan (1817–1887) comprehensively reviewed the method and his own dissections, the first proper account in America[21]; but, according to Valentin, the first there to apply the method was Buckminster Brown in Boston, and then not until 1885, but with complete success, after 15 months' traction, in a 4-year-old girl with bilateral deformity. (It is strange that Bick does not refer to this and indeed mentions Brown, so important in American orthopaedic history, only once and very briefly in his *Source Book*.)

In England, in 1866, Bernard Edward Brodhurst (p. 130) used Pravaz's method in a 12-year-old boy, combined with section of the trochanteric muscles, though he thought that 'in children under two years of age, it will probably not be necessary to have recourse to this operation. Through extension alone the head of the femur may be restored to and retained in the acetabulum; but after this age there is great difficulty in preventing the escape of the bone from the cavity[22].' Also in London, William Adams reported a series of cases similarly treated[23].

Pravaz's son, Jean Charles Theodor (1831–1892) followed his father as director of the orthopaedic institute at Lyons and himself wrote on the subject in 1864[24]. The method fell into desuetude, no doubt becaue it was tedious and prolonged.

After this there seems to have been a fallow period, though marked by

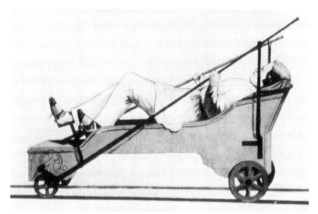

Figure 214   Pravaz: self-propelled carriage for the after-treatment of congenital dislocation of the hip. (Pravaz, Ch.-G. (1847) *Traité théorique et pratique des luxations congénitales du fémur*)

some novel treatments; though mentioned elsewhere, we shall repeat them here. Around the mid century, it occurred independently to Joseph Anton Mayer in Würzburg in 1852[25,26] and to Francesco Rizzoli in Bologna in 1849[27] that a patient with old shortening of one leg due to a femoral fracture could be restored to equality of leg-length if a fresh fracture of the opposite femur were allowed to heal with shortening. It now occurred to Mayer to treat a 9-year-old girl with congenital hip dislocation by removing an appropriate segment from the healthy femur, while Rizzoli had a special osteoclast, his *macchinetta ossifraga*, made by the Lollini brothers in 1847 to break the healthy femur to correct limp due to shortening of one leg, though it is not clear whether this included congenital dislocation. There were those who condemned such procedures as unethical, but after the turn of the century it was adopted with enthusiasm by German workers for limb inequality and has of course since become a commonplace, mainly for the effects of poliomyelitis.

Then again, before 1850, Guérin[28] in Paris attempted to deepen the postero-superior rim of the acetabulum by subcutaneous scarification of the ilium down to the bone, and this early shelf operation was followed by procedures developed by Hueter[29] in 1877, König[30] in 1891 and Schönbron in 1892; these were of a rather different nature, since they consisted of turning down an osteoperiosteal flap from the ilium and fastening it to the capsule, sometimes even while the head was still displaced or had even been excised. Such resection became not uncommon in the 1870s and 80s. One gains the impression that, as Lorenz commented, this was a last-ditch procedure; the intention had been to replace the femoral head, and when this proved impossible, it was resected for the sake of doing something. One knows the feeling. Nevertheless, this was not a total failure, for it led to the concept of deliberately deepening the acetabulum, as performed by Margary in Italy in 1884[31], and was perhaps the forerunner of the Colonna arthroplasty.

The great step towards modern management was due to Agostino Paci (1845–1902) of Pisa (p. 291), an outstanding 19th century Italian orthopaedist, who in 1886 demonstrated manipulative reduction by leverage of the head over the posterior acetabular rim as for traumatic dislocations[32] and demonstrated this to an international congress in Rome in 1894. This was a return to the old Humbert–Jacquier method of single-stage forcible reduction, secured by flexion, then moderate abduction, external rotation and final extension of the limb; of course, it had the advantage of anaesthesia. Whether this procedure actually routinely produced true reduction rather than transposition is debatable. What it did lead to was a long-running dispute with Hoffa[33] and Lorenz[34] in the 1890s as to the priority and efficacy of the method, a dispute pursued during lecture tours of the United States. Both originally asserted that Paci's reduction was impossible, both then changed their minds, and later Hoffa tended towards operative reduction while Lorenz used his 'bloodless method' wherever possible. It was all rather esoteric. Lorenz's programme began with forced extension and continued with flexion, forced abduction to a right angle, and wound up with external rotation and gradual reextension. Manipulative reduction was in vogue, for Calot[35] reported much the same method as Lorenz at much the same time, though without all the publicity, for Lorenz secured and held pride of place and continued to publish on the subject up to his master-work of 1920, though suggesting earlier subcutaneous adductor tenotomy in resistant cases.

In his book of 1900, dealing with results in 450 cases, he acknowledged three deaths, 13 fractures, a dozen major nerve palsies and one total gangrene of the limb; there were also stiffness and some anterior transpositions. In 1905 he claimed good anatomic results in 52.6 per cent of cases, and of course by this time such claims had to be backed up by radiographic confirmation.

Hoffa claimed only 30 per cent of successes with manipulation; but this was because he tended not to persevere but to operate on his failures, giving the success rate for the combined methods as 80 per cent. Lorenz strongly advocated the bloodless method, and many in Europe and England, and most in the USA, followed him. Hoffa took the middle position. Sherman of San Francisco, in 1903[36] pointed out the physical impossibility of manipulative reduction without serious damage in many cases, and that it was often far from bloodless internally in older children. Also in the USA, and in the same year, Davis[37] proposed reduction with the patient prone, which seemed sensible as the displacement was backwards and gravity would aid reduction, and this was revived by Denis Browne in London in the 1930s.

All these workers were aware that success depended on early diagnosis. After three years of age it became increasingly difficult and different upper limits were set for manipulation, a common one being eight years for unilateral and five for bilateral cases, after which open operation would be called for. If manipulation was successful, it was standard to hold the reduction in the 'frog' position of 90° abduction, 90° flexion and 90° external rotation in a plaster spica, though many varied this.

The discovery of X-rays by Roentgen in 1895 was important for two reasons: it confirmed the diagnosis and also reduction; and it could be used to demonstrate early cases of dysplasia and subluxation before dislocation developed, using various indices of the slope of the upper acetabulum and the position of the femoral head. These indices included the various guidelines drawn through salient points and also any break in the symmetry of Shenton's line, first described in 1911.

The arrival of the X-ray also settled an age-old controversy, somewhat akin to the problem of the philosopher's stone. Before then, as Valentin points out, 'commissions were appointed, investigations instituted...all without yielding a tangible result, simply because within the diagnostic limitations of the time, an assured decision was not possible, the opponents being unable to visibly demonstrate successful reduction as can be done so simply by radiography today[38].' Lorenz was lucky in that his technique came just at the right time to coincide with Roentgen's discovery. 'Then, and only then, the doubters – and they were powerful not only in numbers but also in importance – fell silent.'

It was recognized before 1900, by Schede[39], that redislocation was common, and usually due to anteversion of the femoral neck, and he tried to correct this by a subcutaneous subtrochanteric external rotation osteotomy of the shaft; but, in the infancy of metal fixation, there was no way of holding the correction. In 1913, Reiner[40] practised supracondylar femoral osteotomy as a preliminary to reduction, which was performed when the osteotomy had united. So did Russell Hibbs in New York, in 1915[41]. Others performed a manual supracondylar osteoclasis *after* reduction had been held for some time[42,43].

Bone operations for congenital dislocations have a longer history than is often recognized, for as early as 1835 Bouvier[44,45], in Paris, was performing subcutaneous femoral osteotomy (for unreduced cases, of course) to improve gait and stability, partly by correcting the adduction as Barton had done in 1826 for vicious ankylosis (p. 381), and this example was followed by others: Pravaz in 1847, Brodhurst in London in 1866 and Gant, also in London, in 1872 (though the last-named used an open procedure). We have referred earlier to the practice of resecting the femoral head, which remained particularly popular in Germany until the end of the 19th century and even later (p. 192), for almost any type of hip disease; but this only added to the shortening and instability, though it did correct fixed adduction. The idea of reconstruction of the shallow acetabulum, which Dupuytren had regarded as the irremovable obstacle to reduction, we owe to Poggi[46] in Italy (p. 290) in 1880, who deepened the socket and reshaped the femoral head. This was taken up in the 1890s with enthusiasm (and rivalry) by Hoffa and Lorenz in Germany, who must be regarded as developers rather than innovators on this field at least.

Moreover, König's early shelf operation of 1891 was also a way of deepening the socket and led to standard methods of acetabuloplasty, using an iliac flap turned down and held in place by iliac or even tibial grafts, as practised in France and Britain, and in the US by Smith-Petersen and others from the early years of the 20th century, and sometimes applied to other conditions[47–51]. Writing in 1939, Willis Campbell[52] asserted that a shelf operation was required in virtually every case operated after the age of four, either after open reduction or, in neglected cases, in the displaced position, but with the head transferred above the acetabulum to correct the lordosis. He recognized that the shelf might be absorbed if skin or pin traction were not maintained. Sometimes the acetabular rim was turned down like a bucket-handle, the gap being filled with grafts.

Before going any further, it may be useful to refer to the findings of an American commission in 1923 (Goldthwait, Adams and De Forest Willard), which reported on cases treated in the USA and Canada. The commission was impressed by the frequency of late destructive changes or misshaping of the head, even though many of these cases had good clinical function, and they related this to the violence of manipulative reduction.

In 1926, a report from the New York Orthopaedic Hospital by Benjamin P Farrell, Herman von Lackum and Alan de Forest Smith found that there was only a 50 per cent immediate success rate with closed reduction, and an overall rate of only 30 per cent. Early diagnosis would help, but operation was essential in some cases. 'Practically every congenital dislocation of the hip within a reasonable age limit can be reduced by operation, and in that way improved...a much larger percentage should be reduced by open operation than were so treated.' Nevertheless, many operated cases were left

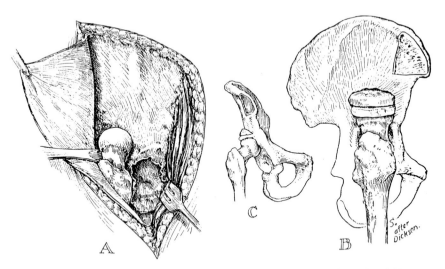

Figure 215   Dickson shelf operation. *A*. Exposure of dislocated hip and mobilisation of head of femur, permitting forward transference of head onto ridge between anterior and posteriorplanes of pelvis. *B* and *C*. Flap of bone turned down from crest of ilium over head of femur and held in place by wedge graft. (Figures 215–221 are reproduced from Willis Campbell's *Operative Orthopedics* St Louis, Mosby, 1939)

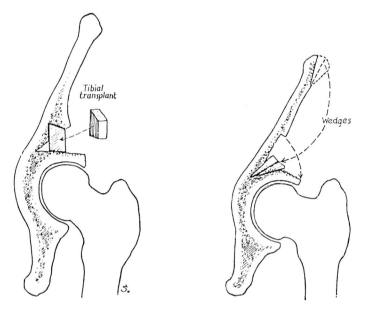

Figure 216   *Left* Albee shelf operation (1915). *Right* Gill shelf operation

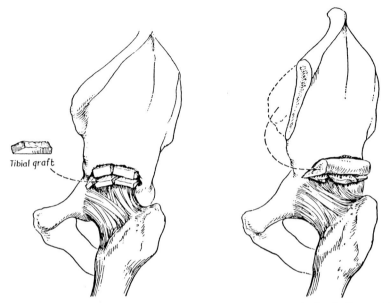

Figure 217   *Left* shelf operation of Compere and Phemister. *Right* shelf operation of Ghormley

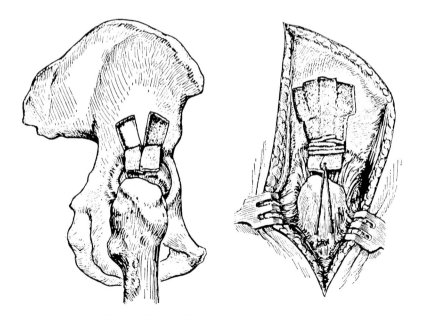

Figure 218   Shelf operation of Lowman

with considerable stiffness. In the same year, Herbert Galloway[53] wrote in the *Journal of Orthopedic Surgery*, 'The results in young children are...uniformly satisfactory...but let it be clearly understood that my claim that the open operation is simple, safe and reliable applies particularly to children under three years of age who have never been subjected to treatment by manipulation or otherwise.' Nevertheless, 'I believe that by some form of operation substantial improvement can be secured in practically every case and at any age.'

In 1926, Putti relied mainly on manipulation and operated only in 5 per cent of cases, in older children with severe displacement or anteversion. Even at this late date, he wrote, 'Anterior transposition may...produce results which are functionally just as satisfactory as those which are anatomically perfect,' an unexpected remark from one who was himself such a perfectionist. But this was not an unshared view, for in 1922 H A T Fairbank, in London, had found open operation possibly necessary between the ages of three and six, but rarely later, whereas anterior transposition might give 'remarkably good functional results' in the short term.

To return to Tennessee and the Campbell Clinic, Campbell was so influential on so many surgeons that it is worth reporting his views in some detail. Looking back to these, as they were set out in 1939, one is forcibly reminded of the gross pathological changes that used to be associated with delay in recognition and treatment:

> 'Congenital dislocation of the hip arises from a lack of embryonic development of the joint. Since the osseous changes as demonstrated by the roentgenograms are not conspicuous at birth, diagnosis is exceedingly difficult...A brief summary of the changes present after the lapse of three or four years is as follows:
>
> > (1) The acetabulum is shallow, triangular in shape, and may be filled with cartilaginous or fibrous tissue.
> >
> > (2) The head of the femur is poorly developed, irregular, and small and, in comparison, the neck is thick and short.
> >
> > (3) Anterior torsion of the neck of the femur may be 45° or more at

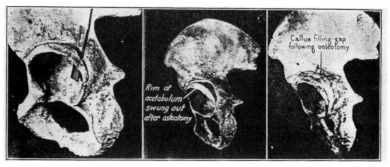

Figure 219   Bucket-handle acetabuloplasty for repair of defects in acetubular roof
(Nachlas)

birth and...may approach 90° after three or four years and causing the flat surface of the neck to come into contact with the pelvis.

(4) The capsule, in particular, is abnormal, being extremely thick, and...its posterior superior surface is usually adherent to the ilium. An hour-glass contracture or a fold of the thickened inferior capsule may form an insurmountable barrier to closed reduction. On reduction, the inferior fold may precede the head into the acetabulum and cause recurrence of the dislocation.

(5) The ligamentum teres may be elongated and thickened, or, rarely, may be entirely absent.

(6) The abductor muscles are shortened and unable to function, as the trochanter is high on the ilium. This loss of gluteal power and of bony support to the head of the femur are responsible for a positive Trendelenburg sign.

(7) The soft tissues which pass from the pelvis to the thigh, particularly the hamstring and adductor muscles, are contracted.'

This is a pathology now utterly strange to most orthopaedic surgeons working in the West, used to screening of the newborn and to early or even only suspected diagnosis (and often, also, to overtreatment or unnecessary treatment in consequence). Nor, as one might expect, is it readily found in the Third World, for there congenital dislocation is uncommon. Yet, at the time when Campbell was writing, and discussing Putti's success at the end of the 1920s in large-scale population screening and early treatment, he argued that such measures might be practicable and justifiable in some countries, but not where the condition was rare, as in the USA, where the time and expense would not be warranted, and where 'the condition is seldom discovered or the child presented for treatment until walking is begun.' Also, Campbell was then still describing one-stage reduction under general anaesthesia as practised by Lorenz and others, and makes little reference to preliminary traction.

Nor did he worry unduly about anteversion, 'The majority of surgeons regard correction of anteversion of the neck as necessary only in extreme cases; growth and exercise will gradually accommodate for and overcome a moderate deformity.' Still, for some children under three years of age, when anteversion was such as to produce redisplacement when abduction was reduced, Krida's manual supracondylar osteoclasis might be needed[54]. Nothing is said about rotation osteotomy.

When open reduction was required for older children 50 years ago then preliminary traction was advisable. The procedure had remained essentially that of Hoffa until 1926, when Hey Groves[55] in England sutured the longitudinally incised capsule transversely to correct its laxity and the constriction and drove a pin through the trochanter into the ilium above the socket and incorporated it in the cast for a time to stabilize the reduction. Groves' principles led to the famous operation devised by Colonna in 1936[56]. Its first stage involved subcutaneous tenotomies or gluteal stripping, with skin or skeletal traction to bring the head down. A few weeks later the hip was exposed through an anterolateral incision, the great trochanter reflected, and the capsule dissected free and used to cover the head, which was reduced into the reamed acetabulum and the trochanter reattached, Hey Groves had anticipated this, for in 1927 he released the capsule and also used it to envelop the head in the reamed acetabulum, but with a pull-through suture through an opening in the acetabular floor to tighten the capsule in its new position as a socket lining.

Before and just after World War II, a number of salvage procedures were designed for old irreducible dislocations, some of which are discussed under their authors. The essential principle was established by von Baeyer[57] in 1918; the unstable head was left *in situ* and an osteotomy was performed below the trochanters and the proximal shaft inserted in the acetabulum – the bifurcation operation. This was modified, while respecting its objective, by Lorenz[58] in his intertrochanteric osteotomy of 1919; and then Schanz[59], in 1922, performed the section at the level of the ischium, leaving the upper fragment of the femur adducted against the side of the pelvis. Such procedures may very properly now be regarded as antediluvian, yet may still be occasionally indicated for the odd neglected congenital or pathological dislocation, though it might be that arthrodesis or even total replacement would find more favour.

We must certainly refer to the introduction in recent decades of the Salter innominate osteotomy for congenital subluxation or dislocation[60], the ultimate extension of the shelf operations listed earlier, and to the adaptation of Chiari's pelvic osteotomy to acetabular dysplasia in young subjects[61]. Very recent elaborations of the Salter technique include double, triple and 'dial' innominate osteotomy[62-64].

Perhaps the greatest contributor to the general management of congenital

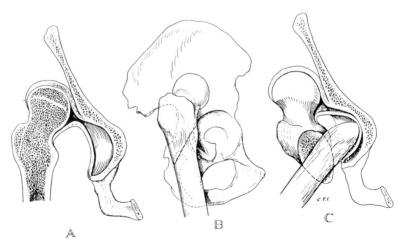

A   B   C

Figure 220 Lorenz bifurcation operation, derived from von Baeyer's procedure
of 1918

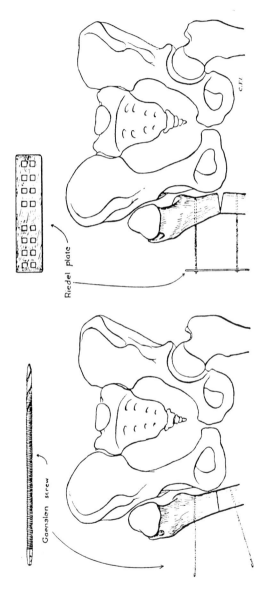

Figure 221 Schanz osteotomy (at level of tuberosity of ischium) for irreducible dislocation of hip. Fragments controlled by Gaenslen screws. After osteotomy, screws fixed by Riedel plate

dislocation of the hip in this century was Vittorio Putti at the Rizzoli Institute in Bologna, after World War I; if we note the great contributions of Italian surgeons, it is because of the endemic nature of this condition in northern Italy. Putti was one of the first – Le Damany in Britanny, much earlier, was truly the first (p. 268) – to institute large-scale screening of the newborn, alerting both doctors and parents, and devised the simple triangular abduction pillow which was the forerunner of the Pavlik and other harnesses[65-67].

It is true that, just before and after World War II, Ortolani[68] in Italy (1937), von Rosen[69] in Malmö, Sweden (1957) and Barlow[70] in England (1962) greatly developed screening programmes for early diagnosis and heightened the index of suspicion; yet it may not be too unkind to note that this has led to as much unnecessary, though harmless, treatment as there was previous neglect. If such programmes eliminate the need for more or less violent procedures of reduction, which have been shown later to produce avascular changes and deformation in the femoral head giving rise to arthrosis in what had seemed to be anatomically satisfactory reduction, then that is their justification. As shown by Severin and others in the 1940s and 50s, the functional results may remain excellent for a long time, but the radiological changes will eventually have their effect.

There is little need to rehearse here the advances of recent years: the use of arthrography to delineate the configuration of the joint, the inclusion of excision of the limbus as part of open reduction at an increasingly early age in cases of any difficulty, the early resort to rotation osteotomy. We are now as surprised to see a late case of dislocation as our forerunners were to see an early one and have infinitely better means of dealing with the disorder at any stage.

ACKNOWLEDGEMENT

It is a pleasure for me to acknowledge how much I owe to Bruno Valentin's *Die Geschichte der Orthopädie* (Georg Thieme, Stuttgart 1961) for information on the history of this subject.

REFERENCES

1. Malgaigne, J-F. (1840). *Oeuvres complètes d'Ambroise Paré*. (Paris)
2. Verduc, J.B. (1710). *Pathologie de Chirurgie*. 4th edn. (Paris)
3. Zwinger, T. (1710). *Theatrum praxeos medicae*. (Basel)
4. Andry, N. (1941). *L'Orthopédie*. (Paris)
5. Camper, P. (1784). *Über das Hinken der Kinder*. (Leipzig)
6. Palletta, J.B. (1783). *Adversaria Chirurgica*. (Milan)
7. Palletta, J.B. (1820). *Exercitationes pathologicae*. (Milan)
8. Dupuytren, G. (1826). Mémoire sur un déplacement originel ou congénital de la tête des fémurs. *Répert. Gén. Anat. Physiol. Path. Clin. Chir. Paris*, **2**, 82
9. Lorenz, A. (1920). *Die sogenannte angeborene Hüftverrenkung*. (Stuttgart)
10. Wynne-Davies, R. (1973). *Heritable Disorders in Orthopaedic Practice*. (Oxford, Blackwell)

11. Guérin, J.R. (1841). *Recherches sur les luxations congénitales.* (Paris)
12. Roser, W. (1864). Zur Lehre von den Spontanluxationen. *Arch. Phys. Heilk.*, 542
13. Roser, W. (1879). Über angeborene Hüftverrenkung Verh. dtsch. Ges. Chir., 8th Congress. *Arch. Klin. Chir.*, **24**, 309
14. Roser, W. (1846). Bonnets Ansichten Über die Gelenkkrankheiten mitgetheilt und mit Anmerkungen versehen. *Arch. Phys. Heilk.*, **5**, 132
15. Caillard-Bilonière, A.J. (1828). Sur les luxations originelles ou congénitales des fémurs. *Thesis* Paris No. 223
16. Vrolik, G. (1839). *Essai due les effets produits dans le corps humain par la luxation congénitale et accidentelle nonréduite du fémur.* (Amsterdam)
17. Humbert, F. and Jacquier, N. (1835). *Essai et observations sur la manière de réduire les luxations spontanées ou symptomatiques de l'articulation iliofémorale.* (Bar-le-Duc and Paris)
18. Pravaz, C.G. (1841). Mémoire sur le traitement des luxations congénitales du fémur. *Bull. de l'Acad.*, **7**
19. Pravaz, C.G. (1847). *Traite théorique et pratique des luxations congénitales du fémur.* (Lyon)
20. Malgaigne, J-F. (1862). *Leçons d'Orthopédie.* (Paris)
21. Carnochan, J.M. (1850). *On the etiology, pathology and treatment of congenital dislocations of the head of the femur.* (New York)
22. Brodhurst, B.E. (1866). On congenital dislocations of the femur. *St. George's Hosp. Rep.*, **1**, 217
23. Adams, W. (1885). On the treatment of hip-joint disease by extension with motion. *Br. Med. J.*, **2**, 859
24. Pravaz, J.C.T. (1864). *De la curabilité des luxations congénitales du fémur.* (Lyon)
25. Mayer, J.A. (1852). Die Osteotomie, ein neuer Beitrag zur operativen Orthopädik. *Illustr. med. Ztg.* (*Munich*), **2**, 1 and 65
26. Mayer, J.A. (1855). *Das neue Heilverfahren der Fötalluxation durch Osteotomie.* (Würzburg)
27. Rizzoli, F. (1849). Nuovo metodo per togliere le claudicazione, derivante dall' accavallamento, e reciproca unione dei frammenti del Femore. *Novi Comm. Acad. Sci. Inst. Bononiensis, Bologna,* **10**, 245
28. Malgaigne, J-F. (1848). *Rapport sur les traitements orthopédiques de M. Jules Guérin.* (Paris)
29. Hueter, C. (1877). *Klinik der Gelenkkrankheiten mit Einschluss der Orthopädie.* 2nd edn. (Leipzig)
30. König, F. (1891). Osteoplastische Behandlung der kongenitalen Hüftgelenksluxation. *Verh. Dtsch. Ges. Chir.*, 20th Congress p. 75
31. Margary, F. (1884). *Arch. Ortop.* (*Milano*), 381
32. Paci, A. (1888). *Studio ed osservazione sulla lussazione iliace commune congenita e sua cura razionale.* (Genoa)
33. Hoffa, A. (1896). Zur unblutigen Behandlung der angeborenen Hüftgelenksverrenkung. *Arch. Klin. Chir.*, **53**, 3
34. Lorenz, A. (1896). Über die Stellung der funktionellen Methode der Belastung des eingerenkten Schenkelkopfes mit den Körpergewicht zu den anderen unblutigen Behandlungsmethoden der angeborenen Hüftverrenkung. *Wien. Klin. Wschr.*, **36**
35. Calot, F. (1903). La technique du traitement non-sanglant de la luxation congénitale de la hanche. *Ann. Chir. et Orth.*, **12**
36. Sherman, W.O. *Trans. Am. Orthop. Assoc.*,
37. Davis, C.G. (1903). The forcible reposition of congenital dislocation of the hip. *Am. Med.*, **5**, 30
38. Valentin, B. (1961). *Die Geschichte der Orthopädie.* (Stuttgart, Thieme)
39. Schede, F. (1892). Über die blutige Reposition veralteter Luxationen. *Arch. f.*

Klin. Chir., **43**

40. Reiner, M. (1910). Über die preliminäre Detorquierung. *Ztschr. f. Orth. Chir.*, **25**, 775
41. Hibbs, R. (1915). *Trans. Sect. Orth. Surg. Am. Med. Assoc.*, 48
42. Froelich, M. (1921). L'antetersion de l'extremité supérieure du fémur dans la luxation congénitale de la hanche: sa correction. *Rev. d'Orthop.*, **8**, 214
43. Krida, A. (1928). Congenital dislocation of the hip. The effect of anterior distortion: a procedure for its correction. *J. Bone Jt. Surg.*, **10**, 594
44. Bouvier, S.-H.-V. (1858). *Leçons cliniques sur les maladies de l'appareil moteur.* (Paris)
45. Bouvier, S.-H.-V. (1864). Rapport sur la curabilité des luxations congénitales de la hanche. *Gaz. des Hôp.*, **10**
46. Poggi, (1880). Contributi alla cura cruenta della lussazione congenita coxofemorale unilaterale. *Arch. di Ortop.*, **7**, 105
47. Albee, F. (1915). The bone graft wedge. Its use in the treatment of relapsing, acquired and congenital dislocations of the hip. *N.Y. Med. J.*, **102**, 433
48. Smith-Petersen, M.N. (1936). The treatment of malum coxae senilis, old slipped upper femoral epiphysis, intrapelvic protrusion of the acetabulum and coxa plana by means of acetabuloplasty. *J. Bone Jt. Surg.*, **18**, 869
49. Lance, (1925). Constitution d'une butée ostéoplastique dans les luxations et subluxations congénitales de la hanche. *Presse Med.*, **33**, 945
50. Ghormley, R. (1931). Use of anterior superior spine and crest of the ilium in surgery of the hip joint. *J. Bone Jt. Surg.*, **13**, 784
51. Compere, E.L. and Phemisyer, D.B. (1935). The tibial peg shelf in congenital dislocation of the hip. *J. Bone Jt. Surg.*, **17**, 60
52. Campbell, W. (1939). *Operative Orthopaedics.* (St Louis, Mosby)
53. Galloway, H.P.H. (1920). Open operation for congenital dislocation of the hip. *J. Orth. Surg.*, **2**, 390
54. Krida, A. (1928). Congenital dislocation of the hip. The effect of anterior distortion: a procedure for its correction. *J. Bone Jt. Surg.*, **10**, 594
55. Hey Groves, E.W. (1926). Some contributions on the reconstructive surgery of the hip. *Br. J. Surg.*, **14**, 486
56. Colonna, P.C. (1936). An arthroplastic operation for congenital dislocation of the hip – a two stage procedure. *Surg. Gyn. Obstet.*, **63**, 777
57. von Baeyer, H. (1918). Operative Behandlung von nicht reponierbaren angeborenen Hüftverrenkungen. *Münch. Med. Wschr.*, **65**, 1216
58. Lorenz, A. (1919). Über die Behandlung der irreponibilen angeborenen Hüftluxation (Bifurkation des oberen Femurendes). *Wien. Klin. Wschr.*, 41
59. Schanz, A. (1922). Zur Behandlung der veralteten angeborenen Hüftverrenkung. *Münsch. Med. Wschr.*, **69**, 930
60. Salter, R.B. (1961). Innominate osteotomy in the treatment of congenital dislocation and subluxation of the hip. *J. Bone Jt. Surg.*, **43B**, 518
61. Colton, C.L. (1972). Chiari osteotomy for acetabular dysplasia in young subjects. *J. Bone Jt. Surg.*, **54B**, 578
62. Steel, H.H. (1973). Triple osteotomy of the innominate bone. *J. Bone Jt. Surg.*, **55A**, 343
63. Sutherland, D.H. and Greenfield, D.L. (1977). Double innominate osteotomy. *J. Bone Jt. Surg.*, **59A**, 1082
64. Eppright, R. (1981). Dial osteotomy. In American Academy of Orthopaedic Surgeons Instructors Course
65. Le Damany, P. (1908). *Z. Orthop. Chir.*, **21**, 129
66. Le Damany, P. and Sauget, J. (1970). *Rev. Chir. (Paris)*, **45**, 502
67. Le Damany, P. (1912). *La luxation congénitale de la hanche.* (Paris)

68. Ortolani, M. (1937). *Pediatria (Naples)*, **45**, 129
69. von Rosen, S. (1957). *Acta Orthop. Scand.*, **26**, 136
70. Barlow, T.G. (1962). *J. Bone Jt. Surg.*, **44B**, 292

CHAPTER 24

Scoliosis

In my opinion, the problem of the treatment of scoliosis is the main problem of the orthopaedics of the future. (Hoffa, A. (1897). *Berl. Klin. Wchschr.* 4).

Scoliosis is remarkable for the stubbornness with which throughout the ages this deformity has defied explanation. (Osmond-Clarke, H. (1955). *J. Bone Jt. Surg.*, **37B**, 3).

Our knowledge of the aetiology of idiopathic scoliosis is negligible; probably less is known of it than of any other disease so common, or so visually evident. In consequence of this lack of factual knowledge there are, as always, numerous hypotheses. (James, J.I.P. (1967). *Scoliosis.* Edinburgh and London, Livingstone).

To those orthopaedic surgeons who have only occasional contact with scoliosis the whole picture is one which approaches bewilderment. (Nicholson, O.R. (1975). *J. Bone Jt. Surg.*, **57B**, 129).

It is regrettable that the last two decades have not seen a single major advance in the treatment of scoliosis based on a scientific understanding of the aetiology and mechanisms of curve progression. The efficacy of early detection and surgical techniques cannot be denied but orthopaedic surgery is not relieved of the responsibility of pursuing the causation and pathogenesis of scoliotic curva-ture...A sacrifice of spinal mobility is not a final acceptable solution to the malady. (Taylor, T.K.F., Gosh, P. and Bushell, G.R. (1981). *Clin. Orthop.*, **156**, 79).

The Greeks had no pathology, if plenty of natural history. Therefore, Hippocrates and his successors treated scoliosis by the same vigorous or violent means that they employed for simpler deformities due to injury or disease, though probably with fewer disastrous results. These methods included traction and countertraction on the Hippocratic bench, the *scamnum*, with or without the operator exerting leverage or sitting or standing on the hump, suspension on a ladder and dropping from a height: all pictured for us by the Byzantines and transmitted by Vidus Vidius in Paris in 1544 (p. 29)! Like other types of spinal deformity, lateral curvature was thought to

be an instance of *spina luxata*; the Latin legend to one of Vidius's figures
runs:

> Harmless it is indeed if anyone sit on that part where is the hump of
> the back: and also, if a man maintain himself erect standing on the back
> where the hump is and gently agitate it with his feet, nothing forbids
> this: as to how much is sufficient to the purpose, any wrestler will be
> familiar with this[2].

The basic methods of treatment throughout the ages have consisted of
traction, support and more or less vigorous redressment, plus exercises and
massage; internal *distraction* is an entirely recent development. And yet we
have seen (p. 29) that, more than once, Hippocrates expressed a yearning to
be able to do just that, to insert his hand in the body cavities and directly
straighten the spine. It is poignant to see from here someone having the
right idea before the right techniques were available, like Leonardo with his
flying machines and Langenbeck with his hip nails before X-rays and stainless
steel and Themistocles Gluck in the 1890s with his ivory joint replacements
but no adequate cement.

Everyone tried suspension, from Hippocrates to Glisson in the 17th
century and Erasmus Darwin at the end of the 18th. Century after century
the attempts continued. In Münich in the late 19th century, Nussbaum used
head suspension from a hook on the door of his lecture-room; but once a
patient fell down dead and then the hook remained unused. The German,
Johannes Scultetus (1595–1645) (p. 56) recommended procedures transmitted
from antiquity quite unaltered: 'How the backbone which is yielded outwardly
is to be made straight[3].' Denis Fournier (d.1683) of Paris pictures the
Byzantine machines of Oribasius – which differed little from the medieval
rack – and coined the term *apocataostéologie* for correction of the bones of
the body[4,5]. Deventer (1651–1724) in Holland (p. 307), though primarily an
obstetrician, took a special interest in spinal deformities and also used
suspension, from axillary straps[6]. Francis Glisson (1597–1677), Professor of
Physic at Cambridge (p. 66), author of the first book on rickets by name[7],
thought that all scoliosis was rickety (some then undoubtedly was) and
devised an appliance for combined head and axillary suspension, what the
French called the *escarpolette anglaise*; an *escarpolette* is a child's swing, and
indeed the patients, mostly children, did swing gently to and fro and found
it pleasurable.

The great Paré (1510–1590) (p. 222), who attributed scoliosis to habitual
malposture, used a corset of thin iron sheets, perforated for lightness, which
Valentin considers the oldest attempt to treat spinal curvature with a corset[8]
(but claims to priority always tend to be fallacious). Many came to use these
and often they were worn day and night; elsewhere (p. 68) we relate how the
young Edmund Verney was sent from England to Utrecht in 1653 to be
treated for scoliosis by one Skatt, to whom thousands flocked, and there
wore his quilted iron corsets continuously despite the sores. The archetypal
corset was the 'iron cross' devised by Lorenz Heister in Germany (1583–
1758)[9], yet it had been previously described by Pierre Dionis (d.1718) in
Paris, whose works Heister had translated in Augsburg in 1722[10]; but it was

not original to either of them. The cross was a modification of a simple backboard such as was later used for clavicular fractures and is pictured by Benjamin Bell, the Edinburgh surgeon, in his *System of Surgery* of 1788.

Nicholas Andry (1658–1717) (p. 233) thought scoliosis was due to asymmet-

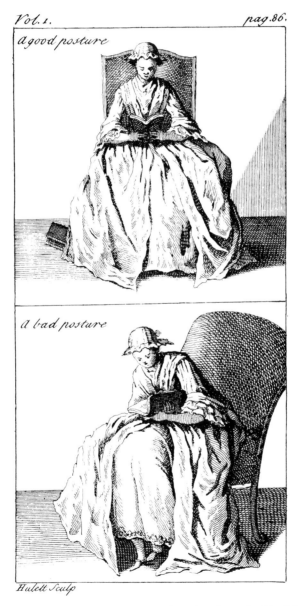

Figure 222 Andry: the effects of posture on the spine (from the English translation of Orthopaedia, 1743)

ric muscle tightness, so ushering in an era of French belief in 'convulsive muscular contraction' as the cause of many deformities, epitomized by Guérin in Paris in the 19th century with his extraordinary multiple myotomies and fasciotomies for scoliosis. What Andry actually did, in the way of rest, suspension, posture, padded corsets, etc., was sensible enough and his attention to the minutest details of seating, desks and tables is praiseworthy[11].

The 18th and 19th centuries saw an explosion in the development of every possible kind and elaboration to exploit the principles of spinal support and traction (often in combination) as well as the pocketbooks of the parents of the rising bourgeoisie, concerned, as always, for the wellbeing, posture – and marriageability – of their adolescent daughters.* There were special extension chairs, starting with Dionis in 1707. Initially, these were simply for patients in some form of corset, held upright by straps fastened to the chair, but then they became more ambitious, as when Ulhoorn (1692–1749) in Holland in 1641, attached an iron post and hook for head traction. There were the chairs, pictured elsewhere, of Levacher de la Feutrie (p. 242)[12] and of Erasmus Darwin (p. 534) (1731–1802), grandfather of Charles Darwin. Erasmus noted – it was not original – that 'if one measures young persons very accurately, it will be found that they are half-an-inch taller in the morning than in the evening. This arises from the fact that the cartilages between the

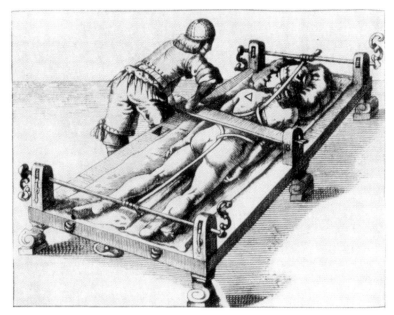

Figure 223 Johannes Scultetus: 'How to correct and straighten the outwardly deviated spine: (From the Wund Artzneyisches Zeug-Hauss, Frankfurt 1666)

---

*In 1776, at Yverdon, Venel wrote a monograph entitled *Essai sur la santé et sur l'éducation médicinale des filles, destinées au mariage*

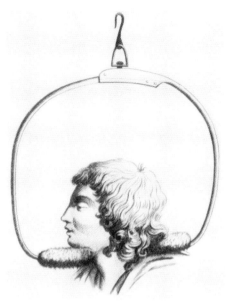

Figure 224 Erasmus Darwin's 'neck swing' for scoliosis (*Zoonomia*, London 1796)

vertebral bodies are compressed during the day by the weight of the body and the shoulders'. Hence his 'neck-swing' and suspension chair and hence his use of day and night traction. At night, the neck-swing was attached to the bed-head, which was raised a foot or more; by day, it was fixed to a mast over the chair[13].

The combination of a corset with traction led to the elaboration of some quite extraordinary appliances, designed to allow the execution of social and educational and even travel activities. They involved the concept of pelvic bearing and of the use of the 'jury-mast' or *arbre suspensoir*, associated particularly with the names of John Shaw[14] and Timothy Sheldrake in England (p. 81) and the Levacher brothers, Delpech, Augustin Roux and Magny[16] in France (pp. 237). Sometimes these were combined with axillary crutches, as by Antoine Portal in Paris in 1772[17], when he exhibited the first such appliance to the *Académie Royale des Sciences*. Robert Chessher (1750–1831) at Hinckley in England, used traction via his 'Hinckley collar' and cords and pulleys so as to be able to apply a brace in the upright corrected position, about a century before Sayre did the same in New York using plaster of Paris. However, body-weight was always an aggravating factor. There was a strong argument for treatment in recumbency. In Switzerland, towards the end of the 18th century, Jean-André Venel (1740–1791) who has a far better claim than Andry to be the father of orthopaedics, introduced the extension bed which provided traction and countertraction by night and during rest periods by day. 'This method is exclusively my own and the basis of my particular treatment.' It had the advantage of applying traction with gravity eliminated in the horizontal position and the relaxing warmth of the bed. The extension was effected via a tight cap provided with a hook, also

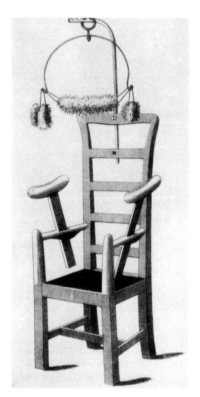

Figure 225 The 'neck-swing' attached to the extension chair (*Zoonomia*, London 1796)

via loops under the armpits, all fixed to the head of the bed, while counterextension was obtained by a pelvic girdle with straps passing down and fixed to leather pads at knees and ankles to the lower end of the bed[18]. The trouble was that every proprietor of a provincial orthopaedic institution in France or Germany had to be in the fashion, just as everyone nowadays has to be seen to own an arthroscope. He had to have an extension bed and to patent his own modifications to it. Many such were introduced in Germany; by Schreger in 1810[19], Heine at Würzburg in 1826[20] (using an X-spring and an adjustable inclined plane), by Langenbeck in 1829[21] with added lateral traction devices, and by Stromeyer in 1838[22] (who also used it for the aftertreatment of tenotomy for torticollis. In France, Jalade-Lafond in 1827[23] introduced his *lit oscillatoire* and other enthusiasts included Delpech[24], Maisonabe[25] and Bouvier[26] (see p. 252). In 1829, Dieffenbach in Berlin compiled a catalogue of extension beds and chairs and suchlike which ran to 70 pages[27]. Valentin quotes Claude Lachaise in Paris in 1827;

> Such is currently this sort of orthopaedic frenzy that not only is there no mechanic–bandagist who does not claim to possess a mechanical bed superior to those of all his colleagues, but in defiance of the most

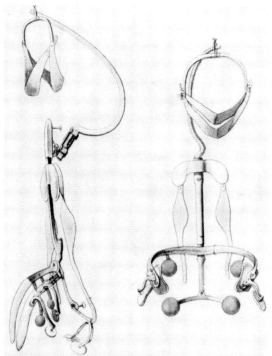

Figure 226   John Shaw: *Engravings illustrative of a work on the nature and treatment of the distortions to which the spine and the bones of the chest are subject.* London, 1824. Plate VI, Figure 2 'Hinckley Collar'

positive laws there exist sanatoria of this type directed by men who are entire strangers to medicine: some headmistresses, seeing that this furore for getting oneself put straight conspired against their interests by depriving them of their pupils, procured mechanical beds and thus transformed their boarding-schools into veritable infirmaries[28].

There is a similarly caustic remark by Julius Konrad Werner, of Königsberg in East Prussia, in 1837;

An extension bed is nothing more for the orthopaedic physician than the operating table for the operator, a surface on which he treats the misshapen in the supine position. Just as it can hardly be called music when a monkey beats on the keys of a piano, so orthopaedics can hardly be mentioned when a person who is not an orthopaedic physician lays a cripple on an extension bed and manipulates him on the same; and a cripple is as little likely to become straight if one gives him an extension bed as a child is to become musical if one plays him some notes[29].'

By 1870, or therabouts, the tide had turned and the extension bed had been abandoned, after criticism as a relic of the Inquisition. Just how far therapeutic furore could go is shown by an appliance devised by Max

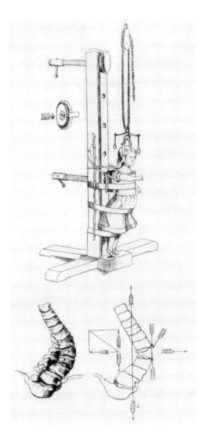

Figure 227   Max Langenbeck (1818–1877): perhaps the ultimate in correction of scoliosis, Göttingen, 1850

Langenbeck (1818–1877) of Göttingen in 1850 (cousin of the more famous Bernhard of Berlin), who abandoned the supine position for a device, 'adapted, as it were, from the torture-chamber', in which the victim was fastened upright to a post while a padded board across the convexity was thrust forward by a screw, constraining the spine to yield at its convexity[30].

It was recognized early on that lateral pressure was also a requirement and this was effected by elastic metal plates, as in the appliances of David van Gesscher (1736–1810) in Amsterdam in 1792[31] and Eduard Grafe (1794–1859) in Berlin in 1818[32], while Borella[33] (1784–1954) showed a most elegant combination of axillary crutch distraction with screw-plate pressure on the hump in an appliance demonstrated to the Royal Academy in Turin in 1821. This last was reproduced by John Shaw in London in 1824, in the *Atlas* accompanying his textbook, but with the comment, 'A good proof of the mania for complicated machinery'.

In 1835, J Hossard, a surgical mechanic in Paris, seized a principle first laid down by Delpech to patent his *ceinture à inclinaison*, or *ceinture à*

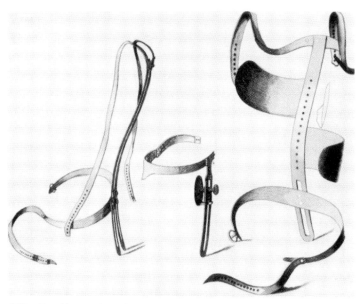

Figure 228 David van Gesscher: scoliosis correction with metal plate pressure on convexities, Amsterdam, 1792

léviers[34]. Here, a well-fitting girdle had attached an adjustable back-bar running diagonally upwards away from the convexity. Its upper end was a fixed point for straps to pull the curvature to the opposite side. Since exertion was required to stay balanced, the long spinal muscles became active corrective factors. This had an interesting outcome. Hossard was asked to demonstrate his method to the *Institut de France*, which appointed Guérin and Bouvier as assessors. Hossard showed them a very deformed young woman, of whose back casts were taken, and produced her again not long after without a trace of curvature. All were astounded; but Guérin thought there had been skulduggery and showed by mixing true cripples with those he had taught to feign scoliosis that the distinction was virtually impossible. Hossard sued Guérin, and that the latter was in the right did not save him from heavy damages. Moreover, Guérin rather slavishly imitated Hossard's girdle, while careful not to infringe the patent rights. Nor was the principle a bad one, for it conformed to the spiral nature of the curve and promoted active muscle contraction in cure.

Poor Guérin! Himself a litigious individual, his suits did not succeed. He himself was investigated by the Faculty for transgressing the boundary between surgery and orthopaedics. Malgaigne, in 1844, argued that Guérin's operative treatment for scoliosis by myotomy, over which Valentine Mott so enthused when visiting Europe from the United States (p. 377), made the patients worse. The Academy concurred, Guérin sued him and Velpeau and won, but gained no credit. 'His myotomies for spinal curvature,' wrote

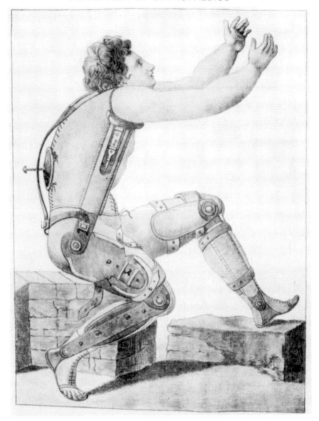

Figure 229   Bartolommeo Borella: correction of scoliosis by axillary crutch distraction and screw-plate pressure on hump, Turin, 1821

Stromeyer, 'and other extravagances injured him as much as his patients'. Yet, if Guérin's soft tissue operation was finished in France, this was not so elsewhere in Europe. Dieffenbach was by no means negative, while Berend from Berlin, a most judicious observer, who watched Guérin work in 1842 and followed up the patients, found the results 'often amazing and, in certain cases, unattainable by any of the other conventional methods hitherto... I was sufficiently satisfied not to hesitate to perform the operation myself in my own institute[35]'. There was also vigorous support from Roger and Carbonai in Italy, where there was furious debate in 1845–6, and it is not often realized that a figure as recent and as eminent as Joseph Trueta used an essentially similar method.

At this point it is indispensable to say a word about pathogenesis, not that we shall be able to come to any conclusions. As Bick has pointed out, between Galen in the 2nd century and Glisson in the 17th little was added to the description given by Hippocrates and the only change lay in abandonment of the violent methods of the Greeks. Valentin goes so far as to say that not until 1779, when Percival Pott's work first appeared, was

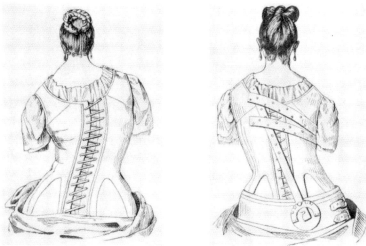

Figure 230   Hossard: *ceinture à léviers*, Paris, 1835

there any proper distinction between scoliosis, kyphosis and tuberculous caries, all these lesions being regarded as vertebral luxations. Scoliosis was attributed to swaddling, tight stays, an asymmetric flow of tumours. Andry thought it postural, with muscle contracture, and many, like Guérin, saw the primary lesion as onesided muscular overactivity, or, conversely, weakness. In 1866, Meyer saw the problem as one of local imbalance[36]. Glisson had thought it rachitic. In 1828, in his *De l'Orthomorphie*, Delpech pointed to the role of the intervertebral discs. Others in the 19th century blamed asymmetric growth, bad physical habit or weak ligaments. Some argued that there is normally a mild physiological right thoracic curve due to the arch of the aorta, and that scoliosis merely exaggerates this. The morbid anatomy, particularly the torsion (which had been remarked on by Mery in Paris in 1707)[37], was worked on in the late 19th century by Nicoladoni[38,39] and Albert[40] in Vienna and notably by the Swiss, Schulthess[41]. At the turn of the century, Goldthwait[42] and Bradford[43] and Brackett[44] in Boston settled for a postural aetiology. There was also for long much advocacy of the patchy and occult effects of poliomyelitis as causal; but the incidence of scoliosis has not noticeably declined since the vaccine was introduced. The advent of X-ray revealed the role of congenital anomalies, mainly hemivertebra; others noted the influence of neurofibromatosis.

It would be hard to argue that we are any further forward in this matter. However, Ruth Wynne-Davies[45] in Edinburgh has shown that *infantile* idiopathic scoliosis, at least, is multifactorial, but that there is a definite, though variable, genetic predisposition. Thus, the incidence in first degree relatives is 30 times that in the general population and there is an association with plagiocephaly, mental retardation and congenital heart disease, but there is also, as in congenital dislocation of the hip, a link with breech deliveries and winter births, while the condition is virtually absent in North America, possibly because infants there are usually laid prone. Familial cases of ordinary scoliosis have also been reported[46]. A basic problem has always been the inability reliably to produce an experimental model, though a close approach has been made by Langenskiöld in Sweden in 1962 by excising the heads of the ribs on one side[47].

We have described treatment by corsets and traction, whether erect or in recumbency. There has also, of course, been a wide range of treatments by remedial exercises, gymnastics, mechanotherapy and massage; but Greek gymnastics (*gymnos* = naked) was a matter of general physical development and the specific use of orthopaedic gymnastics for spinal curvature had to await the early 19th century. Then there began the European craze for 'institutes', often orthopaedic in name only but sometimes permitting genuine scientific observation and treatment. These were the forerunners of the true orthopaedic hospitals, as detailed particularly in the chapter on Germany (p. 179). Very often, these seem to have been finishing-schools for young ladies and the remedial exercises mere exercises in deportment carried out under pleasant conditions in the open air; many of the lateral curvatures treated must have been purely postural; the girls were taught not to slouch. Of course, some of the curvatures were genuine scolioses and some were tuberculous; John Shaw (p. 95) was an enthusiast for exercise therapy, but Shaw was well aware that only minor curves were amenable and that serious misdiagnoses were possible.

There was Pravaz's *balançoire orthopédique*[48]; his girls exercised in rational garments and tights on apparatus in the garden. At Montpellier, Delpech had his famous institute in the 1820s, coupling these simple measures with a high degree of observation and surgical endeavour; Delpech realized that the prolonged use of corsets or extension beds led to muscle wasting and relied on the gymnasium and swimming pool to counteract this. We have referred elsewhere (p. 252) to Bouvier's girls, who were made to leap about on crutches, like kangaroos, to the point where they could not progress unaided. The German contribution, and the German enlistment of Swedish gymnastics at the midcentury, is detailed in Chapter. The Ling system was introduced to England by Mathias Roth (1819–1891)[49] and into America by George H Taylor, medical director of the 'Remedial Hygienic Institution of New York City[50]'. The apotheosis of the Swedish system was the Zander institute with its battery of patient-operated machines, the contemporary equivalent of latterday 'pumping iron'.

There were also creeping exercises. The best known, named after Rudolf Klapp (1873–1948) were, until only a few decades ago, world-famous; but crawling had been recommended much earlier – by Pietro Moscati in Milan in 1770[51] and by Pravaz[52] later, the underlying idea being that human beings deserved their spinal ills for having abandoned the quadripedal position, a moralizing attitude that has not entirely disappeared.

We should add that, though there is no evidence at all that any kind of exercises have any effect whatever on the primary curve of scoliosis, it may be that exercises can help to develop compensatory curves and hence maintain overall balance. This was argued by Arthur Steindler of Iowa in his *Diseases and Deformities of the Spine* (St Louis 1929), in which Steindler pays a tribute to Schulthess of Zürich as 'the greatest clinical observer of scoliosis of all times'.

There was also the plaster jacket applied in suspension, as popularized by Lewis Sayre (1820–1900)[53] in New York towards the end of the 19th century. It is rather sad that Sayre's book omits to acknowledge that suspension dates back to Hippocrates, or at the very least to Glisson, nor was his overhead 'jury-mast' at all new, as we have seen. Bick says that not until Sayre was suspension used as a corrective while a support was applied, rather than as a treatment in itself; but even this is not the case, since the essential notion of applying a corset while the spine was straightened by overhead traction goes back to Chessher in 1800 (p. 88). The only novel element was the maintenance of correction in a plaster jacket, yet according to Valentin even this was not really new. Walter Heineke (1834–1901), a professor of surgery at Erlangen, had treated many cases by 'forcible correction and redressment in plaster bandages', but abandoned the method because of inevitable disappointment and even deterioration, publishing only the briefest reference[54].

For Sayre, suspension was from a head halter and also from axillary straps, and lateral traction bands over the convexities were also used as required. Others, particularly Bradford and Brackett in Boston[55], used traction in recumbency on a frame, sometimes with the patient on his side, the frame angled or a pad or sling applied to the convexity, all followed by a plaster jacket. We have seen elsewhere that, in the 1890s, Calot[56] in France was routinely employing forcible correction under anaesthesia for the kyphosis of Pott's disease; and, incredible as it may now seem, he and the likeminded[57] applied this to scoliosis – but not for long. Attempts to correct the deviation by less violent mechanical pressure date back to Deventer, Glisson, Levacher and Langenbeck, using pads, plates, slings and springs to pull or push the convexities into place. In the 19th century attempts were made to sophisticate this technique by the addition of spirally acting 'derotating' forces acting from the shoulder and pelvic girdles. These reached their apotheosis with E G Abbott of Portand, Maine, just before the first world war[58]. The patient was pulled and untwisted on a special table and a cast applied that often extended from both upper arms to both thighs. In the 1920s, Galeazzi in Milan used a somewhat similar method in which direct leverage was applied to the spine and at about the same time McCrae Aitken in England was using plaster jackets applied with the patient supine, with hips and knees flexed, with side slings pulling on the convexities, and with due attention to the emphasis laid by Hoke, of Atlanta, on the rotary component. By the end of the first decades of the 20th century a general pessimism was beginning to set in as regards the possibility of influencing the primary curve, for X-rays now showed how often a hailed 'improvement' was only apparent. In addition, the era of operative treatment was well established.

We refer elsewhere to the historic 1911 paper of Russell Hibbs, of the New York Orthopaedic Hospital, in which he described the first spinal fusion operation. This referred to three cases of tuberculosis; but the paper was entitled *An operation for progressive spinal deformities* and Hibbs postulated that it could also be applied to scoliosis and did so apply it in 1914. By then, according to Bick, the idea had already taken root, for a similar procedure had been suggested by Calot, and de Quervain and Ombrédanne had used the spine or medial border of the scapula as a graft, others parts of the ribs from the convexity (with simultaneous aesthetic improvement). It will be recalled that Albee had introduced his operation for fusion by insertion of a tibial graft into the split spinous processes in 1911 also, and also for Pott's disease, and this could be and was adapted to scoliosis, though technically difficult as a thick straight graft would not fit.

These were formidable operations for children or adolescents, the blood-loss often severe; hence an enthusiasm for bankbone or beefbone as grafts. Also, the long follow-ups sometimes cast doubts as to the solidity of the fusion, sometimes to the extent that reexploration was necessary to check on this.

A useful mutation in progress in the late 1920s was the advent of the Risser plaster jacket, which was split transversely at the apex of the curve, hinged there with flat metal hinges, and opened up by turnbuckles on the side of the concavity in stages, fusion being performed through a window in the jacket when X-rays showed maximal correction[59]. A review of 265 cases so treated at the New York Orthopaedic Hospital was published in 1938[60]. The results were generally good. Writing in 1939, Willis Campbell noted, 'In the majority of cases it promises a far brighter outcome than can be anticipated by the use of conservative means alone[61]'. (It is interesting that Campbell pictures a turnbuckle correction cast developed by Lovett and Brewster in 1924[62]; though it does not appear that they used this other than as a means of correction, it is the direct precursor of the Risser jacket.) Campbell used thin flexible tibial strip grafts to allow for the curve and his pre- and postoperative photographs show just how excellent a correction could be obtained. This general method remained standard for many years until it was ousted by the direct internal instrumentation of Harrington and Dwyer.

One longstanding problem was the measurement of the degree of scoliosis. Without an accurate method, it was impossible to keep proper records or to demonstrate improvement, or deterioration. When Dieffenbach's nephew, Johann Julius Bühring (1815–1855) opened his Berlin clinic in 1850, he had a female superintendent, a Fräulein Weichenthal, who invented a contrivance 'to obtain a direct impression of the contours of the human back with mathematical precision and true to nature'. This consisted of a glass sheet divided into squares in front of which the patient was placed; specified points were marked with a plumbline and the curvature transferred to paper by tracing[63]. Schulthess and others later used the same principle towards an objective analysis, which was finally achieved by John Cobb at the Hospital for Special Surgery in New York in the 1940s with the now standard angular measurements from the X-rays[64].

Cobb's findings, and those of others[65], indicated that the curve did not deteriorate once the iliac apophyses were set, that most cases coming to a clinic did not deteriorate, that most cases of structural scoliosis will stabilize at a not grossly deforming angle by the age of 15, and that fusion is not often indicated. This replaced the emphasis on nonoperative methods, and eventually led to the Milwaukee brace and then to the halo-pelvic traction developed by Dewald and Ray in 1970[66] and elaborated by O'Brien and others[67]. These began to be coupled with the anterior operative approach of Dwyer in 1969[68] and the direct internal instrumentation of Harrington in the USA (initially for paralytic scoliosis)[69]. It was a paradox that these new methods of correction were so effective, and the new internal instrumentation so directly powerful, that operation now began to be extended to severe cases that might otherwise have been left alone, and even to an older age-group altogether.

It seems right to end this section with a tailpiece from Bick, written many years ago but as applicable as ever,

> Admission of a present dissatisfaction with treatment is only permissible if it does not lead to complacency. This is not quite the time to halt some 300 years of an accumulative attempt to solve the intricate mechanical problem of early correction of scoliosis... but it is generally agreed that the nature of the factors involved in idiopathic scoliosis is such as to preclude the possibility to complete restitution of the spine to normal by any method yet devised.

This remains true today as it was 2500 years ago. However, it is fair to add that when Moe, in 1971[70], chided the defeatist attitude to the maintenance of correction which had made scoliosis 'the Cinderella of orthopaedic surgery', he added that the future was brightened by the promise of internal and external metal fixation; and it is a fact that permanent major correction can now be obtained, and the patient can be discharged at as little as a week after operation and with little or no external support, thanks to anterior or combined anterior and posterior surgery with metal implants.

REFERENCES

1. Vidius, V. (1544). *Chirurgia è Graeco in Latinum conversa.* (Paris)
2. Brockbank, W. (1958). Three manuscript precursors to Vidius's *Chirurgia. Med. Hist.,* **2**, 191
3. Scultetus, J. (1666). *Wund-Artzneyisches Zeug-Hauss.* (Frankfort)
4. Fournier, D. (1671). *L'oeconomie chirurgicale, pour le r'Habillement des Os du Corps Humain. Contenant l'Ostéologie, la Nosostéologie, l'Apocataostéologie et le Traité des Bandages.* (Paris)
5. Fournier, D. (1668). *Explication des Bandages.* (Paris)
6. von Deventer, H. (1739). *Beschryving van de Ziektens der Beenderen. En inzonderheyd, van de Rachitis of engelsche Ziekte.* (Leiden)
7. Glisson, F. (1650). *De rachitide, sive morbo puerili, qui vulgo The Rickets dicitur Tractatus.* (London)
8. Paré, A. (1582). *Les Oeuvres de M. Paré.* (Paris)
9. Heister, L. (1719). *Chirurgie.* (Nuremberg)
10. Heister, L. (1722). *Des berühmten französichen Chirurgen Pierre Dionis, Chirurgie oder chirurgische Operationen.* (Augsburg)
11. Andry, N. (1741). *L'Orthopédie, ou l'art de prévenir et de corriger dans les enfants, les difformités du corps. Le tout par des moyens à la portée des Pères et des Mères, et de toutes les Personnes qui ont des Enfants à elever.* (Paris)
12. Levacher de la Feutrie, T. (1772). *Traité du Rakitis.* (Paris)

13. Darwin, E. (1796). *Zoonomia*. (London)
14. Shaw, J. (1874). *Engravings illustrative of a work on the nature and treatment of the distortions to which the spine and the bones of the chest are subject.* (London)
15. Sheldrake, T. (1783). *An essay on the various causes and effects of the distorted spine.* (London)
16. Roux, A. (1782). Utrum deformitatis a Rachitide oriundae, dum ipsa Rachitis curatur. Thoracibus, Ochreis et aliis machinamentis debeant. *Thesis*, Paris 18th March
17. Portal, A. (1776). Mémoire où l'on prouve la nécessité de recourir à l'art pour corriger et prévenir les difformites de la taille. *Mem. Acad. Roy. Sci., Paris*, 482
18. Venel, J-A. (1789). Description de plusieurs nouveaux moyens méchaniques propres a prévenir, borner et même corriger, dans certains cas, les courbures latérales et la torsion de l'épine du dos. *Hist. et Mém. Soc. Phys., Lausanne*
19. Schreger, B.G. (1810). *Versuch eines nächtlichen Streckapparatus für Rückgratgekrümmte.* (Erlangen)
20. Heine, J.G. (1826). *Hausordnung des orthopädischen Carolinen-Instituts zu Wurzburg*
21. Langenbeck, C.J.M. (1810). *Extensionsmaschine gegen Krummungen des Ruckgrats. Bibliothek für die Chirurgie.* (Göttingen)
22. Stromeyer, L. (1835). *Heilanstalt für Verkrümmte.* (Hanover)
23. Jalade-Lafond, G. (1827). *Recherches pratiques sur les principales difformités du corps humain et sur les moyens d'y remédier.* (Paris)
24. Delpech, J-M. (1828). *De l'Orthomorphie.* (Paris)
25. Maisonabe, C.A. (1834). *Orthopédie.* (Paris)
26. Bouvier, S.-H.-V. (1834). *Orthopédie.* In *Dictionnaire médicale et chirurgie practicale.* (Paris)
27. Dieffenbach, J.F. (1829). *J.F. Henkels Anleitung zum chirurgischen Verbande, von neuem bearbeitet und mit Zusätzen vermehrt von JFD.* (Berlin)
28. Lachaise, C. (1827). *Précis physiologique sur les courbures de la colonne vertebrale.* (Paris)
29. Werner, J.K. (1837). *Erster Bericht über die orthopädische Heilanstalt zu Königsberg*
30. Langenbeck, M. (1850). *Klinische Beiträge aus dem Gebiete der Chirurgie.* (Göttingen)
31. Van Gesscher, D. (1792). *Aanmerkingen over de wangestalten der Ruggrat en de Behandeling der ontwrichteingen en Breuken van het Dyebeen.* (Amsterdam)
32. Malsch, G. (1818). *De nova machina Graefian distorsiones spinae dorsi ad sanandas nec non disquisito deformitatum istarum.* (Berlin)
33. Borella, B. (1821). Cenni d'Ortopedia. *Mem. Accad. Sci. Torino*, **26**, 163
34. Hossard, J. (1835). *Traitement des déviations de la taille sans lits mécaniques, systéme d'inclinaison employé a l'établissement ortopédique d'Angers.* (Angers)
35. Berend, H.W. (1842). Die orthopädischen Institute zu Paris. *Mag. ges. Heilk. (Rust)*, **59**, 496
36. Meyer, H. (1866). Die Mechanik der Skoliose. *Virchows Arch. Path. Anat.*, **35**, 225
37. Méry, J. (1707). Observations faites sur un squelet d'une jeune femme agée de 16 ans, morte à l'Hôtel-Dieu de Paris, le 22 février 1706. *Acad. Roy. Sci. Paris*, 472
38. Nicoladoni, C. (1882). *Die Torsion der skoliotischen Wirbelsäule.* (Stuttgart)
39. Nicoladoni, C. (1909). *Anatomie und Mechanismus der Skoliose.* (Berlin and Vienna)
40. Albert, E. (1890). *Zur Theorie der Skoliose.* (Vienna)
41. Schulthess, W. (1905). Die Pathologie und Therapie der Rückgratsverkrummungen. In *Handbuch orthopädisches Chirurgie.* (Jena)

42. Goldthwait, J. (1916). Opportunity for the orthopaedist in preventative medicine through educational work on posture. *Am. J. Orth. Surg.*, **14**, 443

43. Bradford, E.H. (1899). The seating of schoolchildren. *Trans. Am. Orth. Assoc.*, **12**

44. Brackett, E.G. (1902). The school in its effect upon the health of girls. *Boston Med. Surg. J.*, **145**

45. Wynne-Davies, R. (1975). Infantile idiopathic scoliosis. *J. Bone Jt. Surg.*, **57B**, 138

46. Robin, G.C. and Cohen, T. (1975). Familial scoliosis. *J. Bone Jt. Surg.*, **57B**, 146

47. Langenskiöld, A. and Michelsson, J.E. (1962). The pathogenesis of experimental progressive scoliosis. *Acta Orth. Scand.*, (suppl.), 59

48. Pravaz, C-G. (1827). *Méthode nouvelle pour le traitement des déviations de la colonne vertébrale.* (Paris)

49. Roth, M. (1851). *The prevention and cure of many chronic diseases by movement.* (London)

50. Taylor, G.H. (1860). *An exposition of the Swedish movement cure.* (New York)

51. Moscati, P. (1770). *Delle corpore differenze essenziale che passano fra la struttura de' bruti e la umana.* (Milan)

52. Pravaz, C.G. Mémoire sur la somascétique dans ses rapports avec l'orthopédie. *Mém. Acad. Roy. Méd. Paris*, **III**, 69

53. Sayre, L.A. (1877). *Spinal disease and spinal curvature. Their treatment by suspension and the use of the plaster of Paris bandage.* (London)

54. Heineke, W. (1876). *Compendium der Operations- und Verhandlehre.* 2nd edn. (Erlangen)

55. Bradford, E.H. and Brackett, E.G. (1893). Treatment of lateral curvature by means of pressure correction. *Boston Med. Surg. J.*, **128**, 463

56. Calot, F. (1897). *Note sur la correction opératoire des scolioses graves.* (Paris)

57. Delore, G. (1895). Du redressement de la scoliose par le massage force. *Lyon Méd.*, **26**

58. Abbott, E.G. (1912). Correction of lateral curvature of the spine. *New York Med. J.*, **95**, 833

59. Hibbs, R.A., Risser, J.C. and Ferguson, A.G. (1931). Scoliosis treated by the fusion operation. *J. Bone Jt. Surg.*, **13**, 91

60. Smith, A. de F., Butte, F. L. and Ferguson, A.B. (1938). Treatment of scoliosis by the wedging jacket and spine fusion. *J. Bone Jt. Surg.*, **20**, 825

61. Campbell, W. (1939). *Operative Orthopaedics.* (St Louis, Mosby)

62. Lovett, R.W. and Brewster, A.H. (1924). The treatment of scoliosis by a different method from that usually employed. *J. Bone Jt. Surg.*, **6**, 847

63. Bühring, J.J. (1851). Die seitliche Rückgratsverkrümmung. In *Erstem Jahresbericht aus dem orthopädischen Institut am Ausgange der Schönebergerstrasse zu Berlin.* (Berlin)

64. Cobb, J.R. (1943). Treatment of scoliosis. *Conn. Med. J.*, **7**, 467

65. McElvenny, R.T. (1941). Principles underlying the treatment of scoliosis. *Surg. Gyn. Obst.*, **72**, 228

66. Dewald, R.L. and Ray, R.D. (1970). Skeletal traction for the treatment of severe scoliosis. *J. Bone Jt. Surg.*, **52A**, 233

67. O'Brien, J.P. *et al.* (1971). Halo-pelvic traction. *J. Bone Jt. Surg.*, **53B**, 217

68. Dwyer, A.F., Newton, N.C. and Sherwood, A.A. (1969). An anterior approach to scoliosis. *Clin. Orthop.*, **62**, 192

69. Harrington, P.R. (1973). The history and development of Harrington instrumentation. *Clin. Orthop.*, **93**, 110

70. Moe, J.H. (1961). Changing concepts of the scoliosis problem. *J. Bone Jt. Surg.*, **43A**, 471

CHAPTER 25

Bone Grafting

There are vague suggestions, but no actual records, that transplants of animal tissues to man were attempted in the time of Hippocrates and the experiment repeated in the late Middle Ages; that it had been tried by the ancient Hindus and Egyptians. Paré is said to have replaced a princess's decayed tooth with one of her beloved. In 1682, Job van Meekren in Holland – whom we meet in connection with congenital torticollis (p. 306) – filled in a defect in a soldier's cranium with a piece of dog's skull[1]; but the Church authorities thought this improper and made him remove it. We also know that, in 1697, Salmon tried replacing large bone splinters or segments in gunshot fractures, sometimes with successful reincorporation, sometimes with suppuration and extrusion[2]. In 1821, there were successful experiments in Germany to replace artificial defects in animal skulls with heterogeneous grafts[3].

The work of Flourens and Ollier in France (p. 260) and Macewen's crucial grafting of a lost humeral shaft in Glasgow (p. 131) yielded practical successes despite heated debate as to whether the graft had survived or merely been replaced. In the late 19th century and early 20th centuries many workers were attempting to use autogenous grafts for defects that were congenital, due to trauma or, more frequently, to osteomyelitis. We refer elsewhere to the fundamental work of Axhausen (p. 199) and Lexer (p. 200) on the substitution of massive bone or osteroarticular segments. The results were disappointing overall, frequently because of sepsis. Various workers tried to transplant epiphyses in animals, from Enderlen[4] and Helferich[5] in 1899, but again with poor results. Henri Judet in France, father of the well known Judet brothers, experimented also with the transfer of joint components in 1908[6], and it may have been filial piety that led his sons to try animal grafts in human surgery nearly 50 years later[7].

The question whether a transplant, including that of an epiphysis (usually the upper end of the fibula) would grow tended to recur, mainly in the context of loss of the femoral head and neck from hip infection in children or for congenital absence of the radius. Some, like Bankart, affirmed that it could; others that it might[8]; yet others that it did not[9,10]. The first clinical report of an unequivocally successful epiphyseal transplant was by Straub in 1929[11]. Experimental work in animals has shown that such transplants certainly survive if transferred by microvascular anastomosis[12].

As far back as 1889, Senn had tried filling bone cavities with chemically decalcified bone, with varying clinical results[13]. There was always the underlying and unsolved question whether bone growth in successful grafting originated in the revascularized graft or in the host bed, and what, if any, was the contribution of the periosteum. But, whatever the theoretical and experimental aspects, bone-grafting was put on the map as a practicality by Fred Albee in New York in 1911 (p. 428). Albee adopted a carpenter's technique, fitting a cortical graft from the tibia as a snug inlay in a cancellous bed, exactly adapted to its new site – periosteum to periosteum, cortex to cortex, medulla to medulla. He used an electric saw, at first with one blade and then with two, and rapidly employed this for spinal fusion in Pott's disease[14]. He wrote a monograph on grafting in 1915[15] and eight years later was able to report his results in 3000 operations[16]. This was at exactly the same time that Hibbs was also fusing the spine with cancellous flaps turned up and down from local structures, the spinous and transverse processes and spinal articulations[17].

It is ironic that it is now thought, certainly since the arrival of antituberculous chemotherapy, that these grafting operations on the tuberculous spine are most successful when they fail and so allow rapid complete natural collapse of the diseased vertebral bodies[18]. It is also ironic that the initial successes should have been with the cortical graft when we now find cancellous chips or iliac strips more useful.

Albee's method suddenly made bone-grafting popular and successful after decades of rather sterile debate, conducted mostly in laboratories. It led, for instance, to a notable running research by Gallie and his associates in Toronto[19]. Why was this? It must have been because of the ease of removing a tibial graft with a power-driven saw; because of the attraction of tight carpentering techniques for the 'handy' orthopaedic surgeon, the practical man averse to theorizing – orthopaedics is not one of the more intellectual disciplines – and because it manifestly *worked*. Grafting in the limbs was initially for nonunion, fibrous or pseudoarthrotic; later it was extended to delayed union and even to fresh fractures known to be likely to present problems. Albee cut a slot for an exactly fitting inlay graft, without screws or pegs; this might come from a normal tibia or be a sliding graft from the fractured bone itself. Many modifications followed. Intramedullary grafts were used, taken either from the adjacent shaft (Haglund 1917)[20] or from the fibula (Ryerson 1931)[21]. Willis Campbell used an onlay graft, fixed with bone-pegs[22]. Henderson screwed his onlay grafts[23]. It was usual to raw the cortex of the recipient bone if there was an ununited fracture, to plough up the fibrous union and ream the medullary canal; but Phemister in 1931[24] simply laid a massive graft as a splint alongside the quite undisturbed recipient shaft and relied on tight soft tissue suture – a method the present writer always found satisfactory.

There were problems. No one really liked taking a graft from a healthy tibia, which might become infected or fracture. Moreover, the graft itself, before it became revascularized by 'creeping substitution' and incorporated, could break at its weak midpoint, so that some surgeons supplemented it with an overlying metal plate. At one time there was a certain vogue for a delayed, two-stage procedure. The graft was removed and then replaced in its bed for a few weeks, when it was found surrounded by highly osteogenic callus. However, the autogenous bone graft was altogether a biological method; it was not like the plate which might hold the bone-ends apart indefinitely unless, by good luck, it broke; and if it is now used far less in its original form, this is because of the arrival of sounder mechanical systems – medullary nailing and the AO method – and because of the wider use of iliac spongy bone. It is interesting now, studying Campbell's *Operative Orthopaedics* of 50 years ago, to note how very little mention is made of metal plates, even for fresh fractures, and virtually none of cancellous grafting.

The fact is that the cortical graft was being used for two very different purposes: fixation and osteogenesis; yet it provided less effective fixation than the new plates developed after 1930 and was less osteogenic than iliac grafts. Cancellous grafting began to become popular during World War II as a method of dealing with a host of nonunions and malunions and found particular favour with plastic surgeons for filling defects in the facial skeleton (Mowlem 1944). The use of spongy bone for grafting had been advocated before this, by Gallie in 1931[19] and Matti in 1932[25], and Ghormley had used it for his lumbosacral fusions in 1933 because it was readily available from the back of the ilium without leaving the operative field. It had also been used for filling cavities after the curettage of benign bone lesions, or in arthrodeses, but it was the urgent requirements of war that brought its general acceptance. Bick has represented this as a return to Macewen, but this is hardly the case, for he simply filled the gap of the missing humeral shaft in his famous case with the fragmented but mainly cortical wedges he had removed in operations on other children for angular knee deformities.

The use of bone as graft material raised a host of questions, some almost theological in their intensity. Obviously, autogenous bone was the ideal, yet exogenous grafts were often necesssary; a child could not supply enough bone for grafting a scoliosis, where bankbone was better because it reduced operating time and blood loss[26]. Exogenous bone might excite an immune response and was certainly dead and probably less inductive of osteogenesis and more slowly incorporated, and where were the grafts to come from, humans or animals? If the former (homografts, allografts), there were various possible sources: the ribs of thoracotomized patients in the era of thoracoplasty for phthisis (but this carried a real risk of infecting the recipient with tuberculosis); amputated limbs and excised femoral heads; parents; cadavers. If such grafts were not used immediately, they would have to be stored; hence the concept of the bone-bank, which is usually associated with the name of Inclán, in Cuba, whose seminal paper on *The use of preserved bone graft in orthopaedic surgery* appeared in 1942[27].

Inclán obtained his bone in the course of various operations and stored it in blood or saline at just above 0°C. The concept was not original. Albee had stored bone, chilled, as far back as 1912[28], and so had Hey Groves in

England[29]. Most orthopaedic surgeons have to remove healthy bone from their patients from time to time and have wished to preserve it, and the early bone-banks of the 1940s and 50s, notably that of Philip Wilson in New York (1947, 1951)[30,31] and others[32] consisted essentially of the bone removed in clinical practice preserved by refrigeration, in Wilson's early work simply in an empty sealed glass container at -10°C to -24°C.

Methods of preservation have been legion. Some have used merthiolated bone, with a failure rate of around 30 per cent[33,34], others boiled or autoclaved cadaveric bone in the 1950s and 60s[35,36], though Gallie had used boiled bone as far back as 1918[37]. It had the advantage of not being antigenic, but it was inert and only slowly replaced, and therefore best for cavities or shaft defects in young patients with an intact periosteal cylinder, for boiling markedly retards incorporation.

Homografts gave rise to various problems. Had they really been incorporated? In the limbs, one could usually tell from the X-rays; after spinal fusion, reexploration might be the only way to distinguish between success and pseudoarthrosis and, at one time, was advocated by James[38] as a routine. Were there immunological problems of antigenicity and rejection? If so, the best compromise solution, while retaining osteogenic potency, seemed to be by deep-freezing or freeze-drying[39,40]. The literature contains few references to the use of irradiated bank-bone, though irradiated freshly removed cadaver bone would seem to offer many advantages. The present writer's small experience was entirely satisfactory. Nevertheless, irradiation may decrease the inductive capacity of the graft and destroy the fibrillary network of its matrix.

Another approach was that of the use of 'prepared' bone and of animal bone (heterografts). As to the former, we have mentioned Senn's decalcified bone of 1889; its value seemed to depend on the chemical agent employed. An alternative was the deproteinized bone of Svante Orell in Sweden in the 1930s[41], in which an 'os purum' was produced by treatment with caustic potash and acetone to remove all soft tissue in an attempt to obviate antigenicity in exogenous grafts; it provided a scaffolding. If it was buried under the tibial periosteum for some weeks, it developed callus and became 'os novum'[42,43]. These techniques did not outlast World War II.

As for animal grafts, if these are fresh they are so antigenic and rejection-stimulating as to be unemployable in orthopaedic surgery unless new developments in the control of immune mechanisms prove otherwise. Preserved beef-bone had its vogue. Both frozen and freeze-dried calf-bone gave unsatisfactory results overall[44,45], but it could also be deproteinized as a 'Kiel graft' of any desired shape and thickness[46]. Results varied; they were better for smallish cavities, much less so for major shaft defects, but improved by mixing with red marrow aspirated from the patient's own ilium[47,48]. What has been called 'anorganic' or 'Oswestry' bone[49,50] was made by extraction with ethylene dioxide or hydrogen peroxide and ethylenediamine, leaving an unimpaired crystalline lattice with a large surface area. This was inert, very slowly absorbed and quite nonantigenic but with little inductive capacity. Therefore it was effective only in a well vascularized bed with many osteoblasts and, again, was best used for packing cavities or a line of nonunion, though it might be used to expand an inadequate supply of the patient's own cancellous bone. We owe a great deal of our knowledge about the fate of bone grafts, fresh or preserved, to the masterly studies and surveys of Burwell[51-53] in England and of Marshall Urist in the USA. Burwell's interim conclusions in 1969 were that, next to autogenous bone, the best source was stored exogenous human grafts and that, when frozen or freeze-dried, this was not only better than merthiolated or boiled material but often as good as an autogenous graft. Exogenous grafts were best used for cavities or when intimately connected with the cancellous bone at the shaft ends and was unsuitable for bridging shaft defects. The graft died but induced osteogenesis indirectly; so the indwelling soft tissues of the graft should be removed to promote its revascularization.

A fairly recent study of the whole field was made by Brown and Cruess in 1982[54]. The question whether bone-growth in grafting originates in the revascularized graft or in the host bed has long been studied and, as far back as 1940, Levander had noted the role of bone marrow in regeneration[55]. Even with iliac grafts few peripheral bone cells survive; it is the cells of the contained red marrow that are the main source of osteogenesis by stimulating the nonspecific mesenchymal cells of the host. Certainly, the old 19th century argument about the role of the periosteum appears to have been settled, in the sense that it has been clearly shown to be a potent *stimulator* of new bone formation[56].

In more recent years, many of these problems have been short circuited by the use of an autogenous graft transferred with its vascular pedicle and anastomosed to a local donor pedicle by a microvascular technique. This has proved extremely useful in the hands of plastic surgeons and for certain stubborn lesions such as congenital pseudoarthrosis of the tibia. Useful early work on this was done by Taylor in 1977[57,58]. As noted elsewhere, large avascular grafts take a long time to revascularize and are therefore structurally weak for a period. It has therefore been suggested that vascular pedicled grafts from the fibula, rib or iliac crest should be used for shaft defects of over 6 cm and also for congenital pseudoarthrosis of the tibia if electrical treatment has failed, and such a graft can combine the bone with the overlying soft tissue if desired[59]. Alternatively, if the graft is mounted on a local muscle pedicle, an anastomosis may not be necessary. Pedicled grafts may be useful for the total transfer of small joints in the hand.

The great advantage of the allograft is its ability to replace articular surfaces, impossible with autogenous grafts except perhaps the upper fibula. Therefore, we should not conclude this section without referring to the transplantation of really massive osseous or osteoarticular segments to replace defects due to trauma or, more often, to malignancies treated by local excision rather than ablation of the limb. Some discussion will be found elsewhere. All this work is largely based on the studies of Lexer (p. 200) in the early years of this century on joint transplantation, work which has proved of continuing interest to Russian surgeons.

In the West, particularly after World War II, it was eclipsed by the use of artificial metallo-plastic prostheses, but recently, thanks to the efforts of Mankin in Boston and others, it is now gaining ground. The Russian references go back to before the first world war[60,61]. The Central Institute of Traumatology and Orthopaedics of the USSR's Ministry of Health established laboratories for the low temperature preservation of organs and tissues in Leningrad in 1952 and in Moscow in 1956. Volkov and Immamaliev reported on joint or half-joint transplantation to the 10th congress of SICOT in Paris in 1966[62] and Immamaliev discussed the subject in a British publication in 1969[63] and Volkov in the *Journal of Bone and Joint Surgery* in 1970[64].

On the whole, the Russians seem to have favoured massive grafts taken from the cadaver in cases of sudden death from injury or heart attack within six hours, to be stored at very low temperatures ($-70°C$ for 24 hours, then at $-30°C$ for up to six months, though this may now have changed). This was considered to diminish antigenicity, especially if storage was for not less than 25 days. Sometimes antibiotic solutions were used for storage; in some cases sterilization was with X-rays.

The surgical techniques employed need not be discussed in detail. They include step interlocking of the shafts, careful capsular reattachment, the use of screws, external fixators or Küntscher nails. There was a wide range of complications: poor fit and fixation, early or late fracture or displacement, infection, absorption (incompatibility), late arthritis or tumour recurrence. Rejection occurred in about 12 per cent of cases and then called for arthrodesis, if this were still technically possible. The best results were with replacement of the whole or part of only one joint surface.

Some American interest was shown in the 1950s in relation to transplants for damaged joints, mainly metacarpophalangeal, in the hand[65,66], and, of course, the transfer of autogenous whole joints has been greatly aided by the advent of microvascular anastomosis[67]. It has to be acknowledged that prosthetic joint replacement, whether in the hip or hand, shoulder or knee, gives immediately good results and is more suited to the ordinary practising orthopaedic surgeon than elaborate autogenous or cadaveric transplantation, difficult to execute and with a high failure rate. Nevertheless, artificial joints can also fail and are never really accepted biologically. For the time being, it would seem sensible to continue with prosthetic methods in older patients with a shortish life expectation and to consider osseous or osteoarticular techniques of replacement after massive local resections, if at all, only in younger patients.

REFERENCES

1. Janeway, H.H. (1910). Autoplastic transplantation of bone. *Ann. Surg.*, 217
2. Salmon, W. (1697). *Ars chirurgica*
3. Merrem and von Walther, Ph. F. (1821). *J. der Chir. u. Augenheilk.*, **2**, 571
4. Enderlen, E. (1899). Zur Reimplantation des resecierten Intermediärknörpels beim Kaninchen. *Dtsch. Ztschr. f. Chir.*, **48**, 1246
5. Helferich, H. (1899). Versuche über die Transplantation des Intermediärknörpels wachsender Röhrenknochen. *Dtsch. Ztschr. F. Chir.*, **1**, 564
6. Judet, H., (1908). Essai sur la greffe des tissus articulaires. *C.R. Acad. Clermont-Ferrand*, **146**, 193 and 600

7. Judet, J. and Judet, R. (1954). Animal grafts in human surgery. *Acta Orthop. Belg.*, **19**, 135

8. Blockey, N.J. (1967). Observations on the fate of fibular transplants for congenital absence of the radius. *J. Bone Jt. Surg.*, **49B**, 762

9. Riordan, D.C. (1955). Congenital absence of the radius. *J. Bone Jt. Surg.*, **37A**, 1129

10. Wilson, J.N. (1966). Epiphyseal transplantation: a clinical study. *J. Bone Jt. Surg.*, **48A**, 245

11. Straub, G.F. (1929). Anatomical survival, growth and physiological function of an epiphyseal bone transplant. *Surg. Gynecol. Obstet.*, **48**, 687

12. Brown, K. *et al.* (1982). 7th Combined Meeting of Orthopaedic Asociations of the English-speaking world. *J. Bone Jt. Surg.*, **64B**, 621

13. Senn, N. (1889). On the healing on aseptic bone cavities by implantation of antiseptic decalcified bone. *Int. J. Med. Sci.*, **98**

14. Albee, F. (1911). Transplantation of a portion of tibia into the spine for Pott's disease. *J. Am. Med. Assoc.*, August

15. Albee, F. (1915). *Bone-graft Surgery.* (Philadelphia: Saunders)

16. Albee, F. (1923). Fundamentals in bone transplantation. Experience in 3000 bone-graft operations. *J. Am. Med. Assoc.*, **81**, 1429

17. Hibbs, R.A. (1911). An operation for progressive spinal deformities. *N.Y. Med. J.*, **93**, 1013

18. Griffiths, D.L. (1987). *Current Orthop.*, **1**, 179

19. Gallie, W.E. (1931). The Transplantation of Bone. *Br. Med. J.*, **2**, 840

20. Haglund, E.J. (1917). New method of applying autogenous intramedullary bone transplants and of making autogenous bone screws. *Surg. Gynecol. Obstet.*, **24**, 243

21. Ryerson, E.W. (1931). The treatment of ununited fractures. *Milwaukee Proc. Inter-State Postgrad. Med. Assem.*, 413

22. Campbell, W.C. (1923). The treatment of ununited fractures. *Am. J. Surg.*, **37**, 1

23. Henderson, M.S. (1923). Nonunion in fractures: the massive bone graft. *J. Am. Med. Assoc.*, **81**, 463

24. Phemister, D.B. (1931). Splint grafts in the treatment of delayed union and nonunion of fractures. *Surg. Gynecol. Obstet.*, **52**, 376

25. Matti, H. (1932). Über freie Transplantation von Knochenspongiosa. *Arch. f. klin. Chir.*, **168**, 236

26. Dodd, C.A.F. *et al.* (1988). Allograft versus autograft bone in scoliosis surgery. *J. Bone Jt. Surg.*, **70B**, 431

27. Inclán, A. (1942). The use of preserved bone graft in orthopaedic surgery. *J. Bone Jt. Surg.*, **24**, 81

28. Pear, L.A. (1955). *Transplantation of Tissues.* (Baltimore, Williams and Wilkins)

29. Hey Groves, E. (1917). Methods and results of transplantation of bone in the repair of defects caused by injury or disease. *Brit. J. Surg.*, **5**, 185

30. Wilson, P.D. (1947). Experience with a bone bank. *Ann. Surg.*, **126**, 932

31. Wilson, P.D. (1951). Follow-up study of the use of refrigerated homogeneous bone transplants in orthopaedic surgery. *J. Bone Jt. Surg.*, **33A**, 307

32. Ehalt, W. (1954). Ergebnisse bei der Verwendung konservierten Knochen. *Arch. klin. Chir.*, **279**, 44

33. Reynolds, F.C., Oliver, D.R. and Ramsey, R. (1951). Clinical evaluation of the merthiolate bone bank and homogeneous bone grafts. *J. Bone Jt. Surg.*, **33A**, 373

34. Arden, G.P. (1956). Experiences with a merthiolated bone bank. *Brit. J. Clin. Pract.*, **10**, 522

35. Lloyd-Roberts, G.C. (1952). Experience with boiled cadaveric bone. *J. Bone Jt.*

Surg., **34B**, 428

36. Williams, G. (1964). Experiences with boiled cadaveric cancellous bone in fractures of the long bones. *J. Bone Jt. Surg.*, **46B**, 398
37. Gallie, W.E. (1918). The use of boiled bone in operative surgery. *Am. J. Orthop. Surg.*, **16**, 373
38. James, J.I.P. (1967). *Scoliosis.* (Edinburgh, Livingstone)
39. Berkin, C.R. (1957). Freeze-dried bone grafts. *Lancet*, **i**, 730
40. Chalmers, J., Lea, L. and Sissons, H.A. (1960). Freeze-dried bone as grafting material. In Parkes, A.S. and Smith, A.H. (eds.) *Recent research in freeze-drying.* (Oxford, Blackwell)
41. Orell, S. (1931). Experimental chirurgische Studie über Knochentransplantate und ihre Anwendung in der praktische Chirurgie. *Dtsch. Z. Chir.*, **232**, 701
42. Orell, S. (1934). Studies of bone implantation, new bone formation, implantation of 'os purum' and transplantation of 'os novum'. *Acta Chir. Scand.*, **74** (Suppl. 31), 1
43. Orell, S. (1937). Surgical bone grafting with 'os purum', 'os novum' and 'boiled bone'. *J. Bone Jt. Surg.*, **19**, 873
44. Kingma, M.J. (1967). Deep-frozen calf bone. Presented at the *10th Congress of SICOT*, Paris
45. Bassett, C.A.L. and Creighton, D.K.J. (1962). A comparison of host response to cortical autografts and processed calf heterografts. *J. Bone Jt. Surg.*, **44A**, 842
46. Maatz, R. and Bauermeister, A. (1957). A method of bone maceration. *J. Bone Jt. Surg.*, **39A**, 153
47. Burwell, R.G. (1951). A study of homologous cancellous bone combined with autologous red marrow after transplantation to a muscular site. *J. Anat.*, **65**, 613
48. Salama, K. and Weissman, S.L. (1978). The clinical use of combined xenografts of bone and autologous red marrow. *J. Bone Jt. Surg.*, **60B**, 111
49. Williams, J.B. and Irvine, J.W. (1954). Preparation of the inorganic matrix of bone. *Science*, **119**, 771
50. Roaf, R. (1966). Experience of using deproteinized bone, especially the assessment of its value heterologically and radiologically. In *Symposium on bone grafting materials.* (Eastbourne, Arrow Pharmaceutical Co.)
51. Burwell, R.G. and Gowland, G. (1962). Studies in the transplantation of bone III. *J. Bone Jt. Surg.*, **44B**, 131
52. Burwell, R.G. (1963). Studies in the transplantation of bone V. *J. Bone Jt. Surg.*, **45B**, 386
53. Burwell, R.G. (1969). The fate of bone grafts. In Apley, A.G. (ed.), *Recent Advances in Orthopaedics.* (London, Churchill)
54. Brown, K.L.B. and Cruess, R.L. (1982). Bone and cartilage transplantation in orthopedic surgery. *J. Bone Jt. Surg.*, **64A**, 270
55. Levander, G. (1940). An experimental study of the role of the bone marrow in bone regeneration. *Acta Chir. Scand.*, **83**, 545
56. King, K.F. (1976). Periostial pedicle grafting in dogs. *J. Bone Jt. Surg.*, **58B**, 117
57. Taylor, G.I. (1977). Free bone transfer. In Daniel and Terzis (eds.) *Reconstructive Microsurgery.* (Boston)
58. Taylor, G.I. (1977). Microvascular free bone transfer, a clinical technique. *Orthop. Clin. N. Am.*, **8**, 425
59. Weiland, A. (1981). *J. Bone Jt. Surg.*, **63B**, 635
60. Petraschew, K. (1913). A case of free transplantation of half a joint. *Abstr. Internat. Surg.*, **17**, 525
61. Pavlov-Silvanski, V.N. (1914). The problem of free plastic surgery of joints. *Khirurg.*, **36**, 62
62. Volkov, M.V. and Immamaliev, A.S. (1966). Problème de l'homoplastie des

articulations et des parties osseuses articulaires. Presented at *10th Congress SICOT*, Paris

63. Immamaliev, A.S. (1969). The preparation, preservation and transplantation of articular bone ends. In Apley, A.G. (ed.) *Recent Advances in Orthopaedics*. p. 209 (London, Churchill)
64. Volkov, M. (1970). Allotransplantation of joints. *J. Bone Jt. Surg.*, **52B**, 49
65. Graham, W.C. (1954). Transplantation of joints to replace diseased or damaged articulations in the hands. *Am. J. Surg.*, **88**, 136
66. Berg, E.M. and Trevaskis, A.E. (1967). Metacarpal transplant and joint reconstruction following a power mower injury. *Plast. Reconstr. Surg.*, **39**, 287
67. Buncke, H.J. *et al.* (1967). The fate of autogenous whole joints transplanted by microvascular anastomoses. *Plast. Reconstr. Surg.*, **39**, 333

CHAPTER 26

External Fixation

This is a method of immobilizing fractures by means of pins passed through the skin to transfix the fragments and firmly connected to an external rod or bar. It is generally attributed to Malgaigne[1], the Parisian surgeon, at around 1840, but, as we have seen (p. 37), the essential principle was recognized by Hippocrates, who did the best he could with the means available to him.

In 1840, Jean-François Malgaigne described the use of a spike introduced into the upper fragment of a fractured tibia, held by an encircling strap, and intended to hold the fragment down against the unbalanced pull of the quadriceps. This deforming force has long been recognized and has been dealt with, by E A Nicoll in England, among others, by incorporating a Steinmann pin in the plaster cast. In 1843, Malgaigne devised a more elaborate apparatus with four prongs, two above and two below, with a connector adjustable by a screw mechanism, which he used mainly for fractures of the olecranon. He recognized that the method was uncomfortable, and often very painful for the patient; in many cases it was vitiated by sepsis, so he does not seem to have persevered.

In 1850, Rigaud of Strasbourg treated olecranon fractures simply with two screws tied together[2]. His countrymen, Amédée Bonnet and Béranger-Feraud improved on this by connecting the screws with wooden or metal bars[3]. In 1886, at the 15th Surgical Congress in Germany, Langenbeck reported a series of long bone fractures treated with two screws remote from the fracture site and connected by an external rod. One assumes that most cases suppurated; Malgaigne had admitted as much.

In 1894, Clayton Parkhill, a surgeon in Denver and professor of surgery at the University of Colorado, a Philadelphia graduate of 1883, wrote, 'We believe that the time has come when a more accurate fixation of the bones, both after resection for cases of pseudarthrosis and for malunion, and also for fractures with a tendency to displacement, particularly if they be compound, should be used.' For this, he devised a steel clamp incorporating

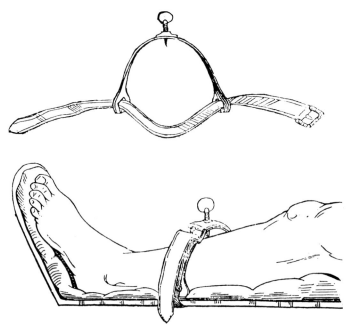

Figure 231   Malgaigne's spike to fix a fractured tibia, 1840

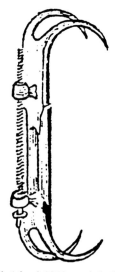

Figure 232   Malgaigne's 'claw' 1843, mainly for olecranon fractures

four one-cortex screws, the clamp consisting of two halves clamped together once reduction has been secured, and in 1897 he reported 14 cases so treated, all successfully[4,5].

At very much the same time, though his publication was a little later, in

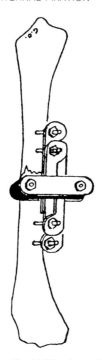

Figure 233 Parkhill's clamp (1897)

1902, Albin Lambotte, in Belgium (see Figure 234) was using an essentially similar apparatus for fractures of the femur, tibia, forearm, humerus, clavicle and metacarpals, which he argued had very considerable advantages: it was simple and rigid, and wounds were accessible for observation and dressing, union could be assessed before removing the device (which, when done, left no residual foreign material), and it might sometimes obviate the need for amputation[6].

In 1934, Henri Judet, in France, was the first to transfix both cortices and wrote on instrumentation for osteosynthesis by external fixator[7]. It is gratifying to note that his more famous sons, the Parisian orthopaedic surgeons, Robert and Jean Judet, were contributing to the same technique a quarter of a century later[8]. Obviously, this principle could be applied either after securing reduction of the fracture, or by initial transfixation and using the pins and plate to guide the fragments together, a form of secondary correction for which the term 'osteotaxis' was coined by Hoffmann in Switzerland in 1938[9].

However, the name probably most often associated with external fixation is that of Roger Anderson[10], in the USA, who had started by incorporating pins in a plaster cast but then used pins only, attached to adjustable metal yokes. Some American military surgeons tried to use the method during the Second World War, but there were problems, including sepsis and muscle adhesion at the transfixion sites, and it was officially forbidden and the

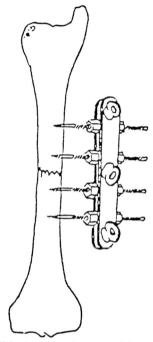

Figure 234 Lambotte's external fixator (1902)

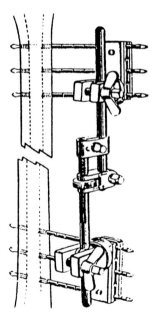

Figure 235 Hoffman external fixator (1938)

apparatus even confiscated!

One may, perhaps, surmise that the Harrington method[11,12] of instrumentation for correction of scoliosis was merely an adaptation of this same principle; though used within the body, it was still 'external' to the structures concerned.

In modern methods of internal fixation of fractures, the external bar is very light and infinitely adjustable and bony union can be assessed by electrical methods without having to remove it. For those interested in the philosophy of orthopaedic surgery, external fixation may be regarded as the opposite pole to Küntscher's intramedullary fixation.

REFERENCES

1. Malgaigne, J.-F. (1847). *Traité des fractures et des luxations.* (Paris)
2. Cucel, L.R. and Rigaud, R. (1850). Des vis metalliques enfoncées dans le tissu des os pour le traitement de certaines fractures. *Rev. Méd. Chir.*, **8**, 113
3. Béranger-Feraud, L.J.B. (1870). *Traité de l'immobilisation directe dans les fractures.* (Paris, Delahaye)
4. Parkhill, C. (1897). A new apparatus for the fixation of bones after resection and in fractures with a tendency to displacement. *Trans. Am. Surg. Assoc.*, **15**, 251
5. Parkhill, C. (1898). Further observations regarding the use of the bone clamp in ununited fractures, fractures with malunion, and recent fractures with a tendency to displacement. *Ann. Surg.*, **27**, 553
6. Lambotte, A. (1913). *Chirurgie opératoire des fractures.* (Paris, Masson)
7. Judet, H. (1932). Instrumentation pour ostéosynthèse à fixateur externe. *Soc. Chir. Paris*, **24**, 400
8. Judet, R. and Judet, J. (1958). Remarques à propos des fixateurs externes dans le traitement des fractures ouvertes de la jambe. *Mém. Acad. Chir.*, **84**, 288
9. Hoffmann, R. (1938). Rotules à os pour la réduction dirigée non-sanglante des fractures (ostéotaxis). *Helv. Med. Acta.*, **5**, 844
10. Anderson, R. (1934). An automatic method of treatment for fractures of the tibia and fibula. *Surg. Gynaecol. Obstet.*, **58**, 639
11. Harrington, P.R. (1973). The history and development of Harrington instrumentation. *Clin. Orthop.*, **93**, 110
12. Harrington, P.R. (1962). The treatment of scoliosis. *J. Bone Jt. Surg.*, **44A**, 591

CHAPTER 27

Nerves*

Joseph Swan (1791–1874) was an early English investigator of nerve degeneration and regeneration. Originally an assistant in his father's general practice in Lincoln, he moved to London at the age of 40, having won the Jacksonian Prize of the Royal College of Surgeons of England in 1819 for his essay, *The Treatment of Local Morbid Affections of the Nerves*, republished in 1834 as *A Treatise on the Diseases and Injuries of Nerves*. This was based on section of the sciatic nerve in rabbits, where the ends were joined by new tissue and some imperfect function returned after a few months, whereas excision leaving a half-inch gap gave little or no recovery.

His contemporary, Marie Jean Pierre Flourens[1], who graduated at Montpellier and went to Paris, divided the two nerves supplying the flexors and extensors of the cock's wing and did a crossover suture so that new paths had to be used for old movements – a very early use of nerve suture. Recovery ensued. (Nerve suture had been suggested by Avicenna, and actually practised by Salicet in the 13th century.)

A little earlier, in 1795, Cumberland Cruikshank[2], assistant to John Hunter, had also experimented on nerves and found that regeneration was possible after their division, fibres sprouting from the proximal towards the distal stump. But suture was something that surgeons refrained from in clinical practice, fearing convulsions, and contenting themselves with coaptation of the adjacent soft tissues. As to the natural method of repair, Augustus Waller[1], of Kent in England (though a Paris graduate of 1840) gave his name to the pulpy degeneration he noted in the distal stumps after dividing the nerves to the frog's tongue, whether motor or sensory. He noted that regeneration was by new fibres growing distally, very slowly over months, and not by immediate union, faster in young frogs and in warm weather and *vice versa*. Türck noted a similar degeneration in the pyramidal

---

*Much material on the lesions of nerves in peace and war is given elsewhere, for example at pp. 263, 627, 651 and 672.

tract after cerebral haemorrhage in papers published in 1851[3] and 1853[4].

It is interesting that Sir James Paget, in his 1853 *Lectures on Surgical Pathology*, distinguished between secondary healing, similar to that of divided tendons, with recovery – if any – in not less than 12 months, and primary healing due to immediate union after end-to-end apposition, with restoration of conduction within two weeks! This because of ignorance about the effects of territorial overlap and ingrowth and of the difference between epicritic and protopathic sensation.

In 1873, Carl Hueter, in his *Allgemeine Chirurgie*, described suture by epineural stitches, and this remained the method of choice for a hundred years, and is still largely employed, though there is a marked trend to fascicular suture.* However, even with improved suture material and the use of a lens, there were only some 50 per cent good results until recent decades[10]. There was also a vogue in the 1960s for ensheathing the suture-line in microfilter (millipore) material[11,12], absorbent collagen membranes[13,14] and silastic sheaths[15,16], but not with notably improved results. Those interested may consult McKibbin's review of the subject[17].

Victor Horsley, the pioneer London neurosurgeon at University College Hospital, did successful suture of the muscular branch of the median nerve and neurolysis of the sciatic in the 1880s and 90s. In 1882, while still a registrar, he assisted Christopher Heath in removing a tumour behind the knee, leaving a six-inch gap in the peroneal nerve; Horsley suggested splitting the tibial nerve and suturing one half to the lower end of the peroneal, and this was done with a fair outcome.

In London, in 1895, Charles Ballance[18] sutured the accessory nerve to the distal stump of the divided facial nerve and got some recovery. At the London Hospital, in 1903, the neurologist Henry Head divided some cutaneous nerves in his own arm, noting that deep sensibility of muscles, tendons, joints and bones was never lost, that protopathic sensation for pain, heat and cold returned not less than six weeks after suture, but that restoration of sensation for light and discriminatory touch (epicritic) could take up to two years. Evidently, this last was supplied only by the divided nerve in its own territory, protopathic sensation partly by its neighbours, and deep sensation by the motor branches of the nerve itself proximal to section and of other intact nerves.

Jules Tinel (1879–1942), of Rouen, wrote in 1917 an excellent book[19] on the nerve injuries of World War I (which barely refers to suture), and described his sign of 'formication', evoked by percussion over the injured trunk, indicative of the process of regeneration. Distal migration of the sensitive site with time was evidence of progressive regeneration, while its persistent location at the site of injury confirmed complete interruption and the impossibility of spontaneous regeneration.

---

* This actually dates back at least to 1917, when Langley and Hashimoto[5] reported on suture of separate nerve bundles in a nerve trunk, and further papers on 'funicular suture' or microsurgery were published by Sunderland[6] in 1953, Michon and Masse[7] in 1964, Millesi[8] in 1967 and Smith[9] in 1964.

Rang[20] has written interestingly on the history of the Lasègue straight-leg raising sign in sciatica. It was *not* described by Lasègue himself, but by his pupil Forst[21] in Paris, who had learnt it from the master. However, it had been reported the previous year by the Yugoslav, Lazarevic, who had also shown that it could be elicited by getting the patient to try to sit up in bed with his legs extended, useful with malingerers. Forst had thought that the sign must be due to sciatic compression by the tautened hamstrings, but a little later de Beurmann[22] showed in cadaver experiments, where the nerve was replaced by rubber tubing, that straight-leg raising caused an elongation of several centimetres.

Nerve grafting is referred to elsewhere (p. 674). We need only refer here to an early experience of Foerster in 1916[23], and repeat that while suture gives better results than grafting when suture is practicable, the reverse may be true if suture is possible only under tension. This was the case with the older technique of epineural suture and applies even more to interfascicular grafting. Keith says that Eduard Albert (1841–1900), of Vienna, had tried to fill a gap in the median nerve with a graft from the tibial nerve of an amputated leg as far back as 1876, and that Mayo Robson did likewise in England in 1888, but gives no references.

The work of Armand Duchenne (1806–1875) on birth palsies, the concept that movement is to be conceived as due to the action of groups of muscles rather than individual muscles, the effects of loss of proprioception in tabes, and the various muscular atrophies and palsies, are dealt with elsewhere.

REFERENCES

1. Keith, A. (1919). *Menders of the Maimed*. (London)
2. Cruikshank, C. (1795). Experiments on the nerves, particularly on their repro-duction, and on the spinal marrow of living animals. *Philos. Trans.*, **85**, 1777
3. Türck, L. (1851). Über sekundäre Erkrankung einzeln Rückensmarkstränger und ihre Fortsetzung zum Gehirne. *Akad. Wissensch. Wien.*, **6**, 288
4. Türck, L. (1853). Über sekundäre Erkrankung einzeln Rückensmarkstränger und ihre Fortsetzung zum Gehirne. *Akad. Wissensch. Wien.*, **11**, 93
5. Langley, J.N. and Hashimoto, M. (1917). On suture of separate nerve bundles in a nerve trunk. *J. Physiol. Lond.*, **51**, 318
6. Sunderland, S. (1953). Funicular suture and funicular exclusion in the repair of severed nerves. *Brit. J. Surg.*, **40**, 580
7. Michon, J. and Masse, P. (1964). Le moment optimum de la suture nerveuse dans les plaies du membre supérieur. *Rev. Chir. et Orthop.*, **2**, 205
8. Millesi, H. *et al.* (1967). Erfahrungen mit der Mikrochirurgie der peripheren Nerven. *Chir. Plastica*, **3**, 47
9. Smith, J.W. (1964). Microsurgery of peripheral nerves. *Plast. Reconstr. Surg.*, **33**, 317
10. Björkesten, G. (1947). Suture of war injuries to peripheral nerves: a clinical study of results. *Acta Chir. Scand.*, **95**, 119
11. Campbell, J.B. *et al.* (1961). Microfilter sheathing in peripheral nerve surgery. *J. Trauma*, **1**, 139
12. Böhler, J. (1962). Nervennaht und homoioplastische Nerven transplantation mit Milliporeumscheidung. *Langenbachs Arch. f. Chir.*, **301**, 900

13. Braun, R.M. (1964). Experimental peripheral nerve repair. *Surgical Forum*, **15**, 452
14. Kline, D.G. and Hayes, E.C. (1964). The use of resorbable wrapper for peripheral nerve repair. *J. Neurosurg.*, **21**, 737
15. Ducker, T.B. and Hayes, G. (1968). Experimental improvement in the use of Silastic cuff for peripheral nerve repair. *J. Neurosurg.*, **28**, 6, 582
16. Midgley, R. and Woodhouse, F. (1968). Silicone rubber sheathing as an adjunct to neural anastomosis. *Canad. Med. J.*, **98**, 550
17. McKibbin, B. (ed.) (1983). *Recent Advances in Orthopaedics*. (Edinburgh and London, Churchill Livingstone)
18. Ballance, C.A. and Stewart, P. (1901). *The Healing of Nerves*. (London)
19. Tinel, J. (1917). *Nerve wounds* (trans. F. Rothwell). (London, Baillière)
20. Rang, M. (1968). *Anthology of Orthopaedics*. (Edinburgh and London, Livingstone)
21. Forst, J.J. (1881). Contribution a l'étude clinique de la sciatique. *Medical thesis*, Paris, No 33
22. de Beurmann, L. (1884). *Arch. Physiol. Norm. Path.*, **16**, 375
23. Foerster, O. (1916). *Münch. Med. Wschr.*, **63**, 283

CHAPTER 28

Plaster

At various places elsewhere we have referred to methods of external fracture fixation; the grave splints of ancient Egypt, the resinated dough of Hippocrates, the bark splints of the Susruta era in India, Cheselden's egg-white and flour (which he had learned from a bonesetter). The *ambulances volantes* of Larrey in the Napoleonic Wars introduced from Spain a bandage impregnated with wine, lead acetate, camphorated spirits and egg-white, so hard and heavy as to be suitable only for the treatment of leg fractures in bed. We discuss under Belgium (p. 313) the starched bandage of Baron Seutin, the *appareil amovo-inamovible*, but this did not harden for 2–3 days and even when Velpeau (1795–1867) in Paris used dextrin instead of starch, it still took six hours to set, so that in both cases there was a period when it was necessary to continue with traction.

In 970, in his book on pharmacology, the Persian Abu Mansur Muwaffak advised that for fractures and other bony injuries the limb should be coated with plaster. The Arabs had used plaster-of-Paris in the 10th century, had discovered the miracle by which the addition of water to a soft powder of anhydrous calcium sulphate produced the hard hydrated crystalline form. William Eton, former British consul in Basra, wrote to a Petersburg doctor in 1798 about such treatment for an Arab soldier who had broken his leg falling from a cannon[1]. This consisted of pouring liquid plaster on the limb in a trough or box, the casts (upper and lower) being made separately. Eton's letter was copied in some European journals but the first new publications were in Russian, by von Huebenthal in 1816. The first Westerner to use plaster seems to have been a Professor Pieter Hendriks (1779–1841) in Groningen in Holland in 1814[2]. Dieffenbach (1792–1847) used the method frequently in Berlin and wrote a monograph about the virtues of liquid plaster in fracture treatment in 1831[3]; it was adopted in England and France. Lafargue, of Montpellier, in 1839, used layers of linen with warm starch paste mixed with plaster powder between the layers. All this was cumbersome and was replaced by Seutin's method after 1840.

The inventor of the plaster bandage in something approaching its modern form was a Dutch army surgeon, Antonius Mathysen (1805–1878), Dutch because, although he was born in Budel in 1805 when Belgium and the Netherlands were not separate countries, Belgian independence in 1830 left Budel in Holland. Moreover, his famous book on the plaster bandage was published in 1852 in Haarlem[4], and he is described on the title-page as medical officer (first class) to the Haarlem garrison and the bandage is described as a contribution to military surgery.

Mathysen rejected Seutin's bandage because it was slow to harden, could shrink, and was easily contaminated by pus and urine. The ideal bandage, he wrote, must be easily applicable, rapidly setting, giving easy access to the injured part and moulding to the limb; it should be unaffected by suppuration or moisture and not too heavy or extensive. Of plaster-of-Paris he wrote:

> 'Although it is widely known that this material was already used in earlier centuries ... its use, however, by no means found general application and it is not even spoken of any more. I believe that this is not due to the material but must be ascribed to the inappropriate manner of its application up to now. Improvement of the method can therefore perhaps form the means of returning to this material again.'

Of course, he must have been aware of the use of plaster by another Dutchman in nearby Groningen earlier in the century, for that had been a matter of interest to the Army Health Inspectorate. And what happened now, in 1852, was that as early as April a Dutch military commission had

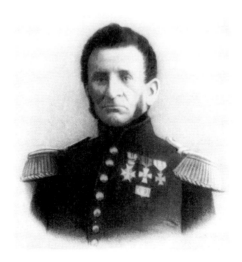

Figure 236   Antonius Mathysen (1805–1878): Dutch inventor of the plaster bandage

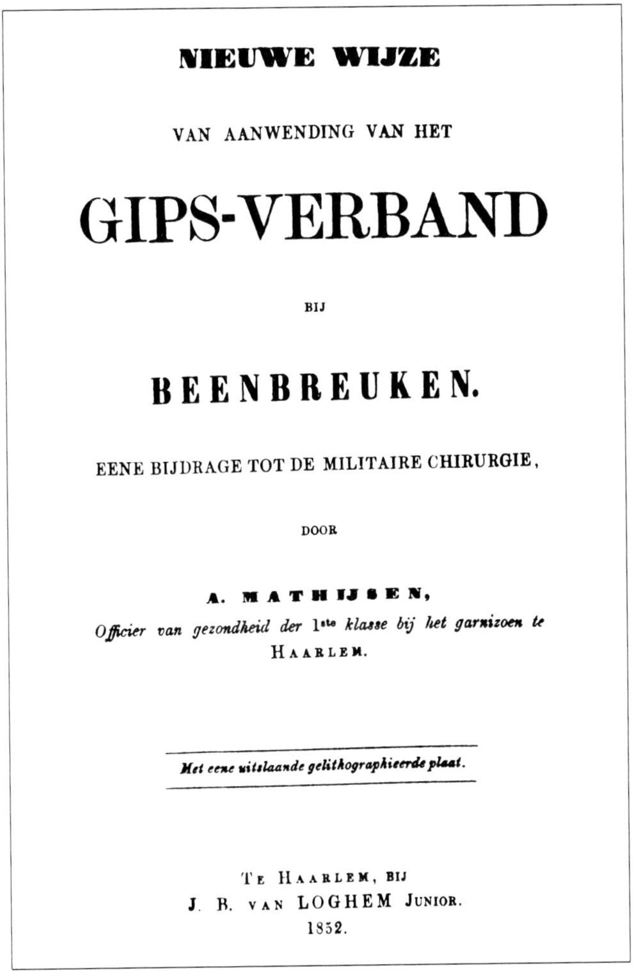

NIEUWE WIJZE

VAN AANWENDING VAN HET

GIPS-VERBAND

BIJ

BEENBREUKEN.

EENE BIJDRAGE TOT DE MILITAIRE CHIRURGIE,

DOOR

A. MATHIJSEN,

Officier van gezondheid der 1ste klasse bij het garnizoen te
HAARLEM.

Met eene uitslaande gelithographieerde plaat.

TE HAARLEM, BIJ
J. B. VAN LOGHEM JUNIOR.
1852.

Figure 237   Title page: Mathysen's book on the plaster bandage (1852)

called the new method 'a real benefit for mankind in general, while in
particular it promises to be of the utmost importance in military practice,
especially on the battlefield ... we venture to forecast that from now on the
transport of the severely wounded will be able to take place much more
easily and safely, and thus the limbs and lives of hundreds and thousands
in wartime will be preserved. Humanity and the Treasury would both benefit
thereby at the same time.' Only a civil servant could have penned the last
sentence.

The method was not widely known until Mathysen was posted to Venlo
at the end of that year and met a local physician, Johannes Petrus Huseritus
van de Loo (1812–1883), who became a great propagandist and showed it
in Brussels (where they had been using starched linen, to which plaster

adheres poorly) and then triumphantly in Paris and other European cities, immersing the bandage in water where Mathysen had wetted it with a sponge. Mathysen had initially tried layers of plaster powder between compresses, a sort of poultice; the limb was laid on the bandage, which was moistened and folded around the part. Next, he sprinkled and spread the powder with a spatula on an already applied bandage. The final version was to impregnate a cotton bandage before it was applied, so that, when setting, the newly-formed crystals intertwined in the bandage mesh.*

Mathysen asserted that his bandage set at once, was easy to apply, porous to fluid and needed no other appliance (though he did later have to invent plaster shears). Dieffenbach had previously used the plaster cast for the treatment of club-foot and demonstrated this in Paris in 1834. Now, another Dutchman, one Blumenkamp, used the new bandage for the same purpose in 1853[5]. This was obviously not the present-day bandage, for Mathysen says it could be easily removed by wetting and unrolling like an ordinary cotton bandage; and he suggested its use in veterinary practice.

Roughly speaking, the new plaster treatment found favour in continental Europe and disfavour in England and America. Hugh Owen Thomas and Robert Jones thought it risky, a method of adventure that constricted and embarrassed the local circulation, shutting out light and air and the surgeon's enquiring eye. Jones only held this opinion initially, but for long enough to remark: 'Nothing so barbarous as plaster-of-Paris is used any longer' and he continued to use tin splints for Colles' fractures to the end of his life. In New York, James Knight (1810–1887), almost an exact contemporary of Mathysen, an apostle of the brace and buckle and director of the Hospital for the Ruptured and Crippled, wrote, 'The discoveries, inventions and mechanical appliances in accordance with physiological laws and surgical science we make available, but we carefully avoid compression of the respiratory organs by encasing them in plaster-of-Paris, or impeding the arterial circulation by compressing bands of the limbs. All such adventurous treatment is avoided in this hospital.' For Knight and his conservative colleagues, Sayre's suspension plaster jacket of 1877 was therefore anathema, as odious as Ridlon's use of the Thomas splint in 1888, after visiting Liverpool, was to be to Shaffer at St Luke's (p. 402). Knight was a self-styled 'surgico-mechanic' who regarded any innovations and all operations as undesirable; it may be that Sayre's demonstration tour of Europe in 1877 – where he complained that the dampness of the British Isles interfered with the setting of his bandages – was due to the fact that he was without honour in his own country. Under these circumstances, the foreign tour followed by a triumphant return is a standard way of gaining kudos.

However, plaster gained universal popularity because in many cases of leg fractures it kept ambulant patients who would otherwise have been bedridden, an enormous contribution to rehabilitation. It also proved of great value in the 'closed plaster' management of war wounds, popularized, but not

---

*The writer recalls that, as a medical student, one of his chores was to prepare plaster bandages in just this way.

invented, by Trueta (p. 661); there is evidence that it had been used earlier by Pirogoff in the Russian wars of the mid-century. At the 2nd Congress of the German Orthopaedic Association in Berlin in 1903, Hoffa said that 'the plaster bandage will remain the essence of orthopaedics for all time'. And in 1928, on the 50th anniversary of Mathysen's death, Putti wrote, 'He deserves great credit ... for the effectiveness of this simple bandage, which gives miraculous rest and immobility to the painful organ, the broken bone and the diseased joint and gives unsurpassed help in the fight against the forces of deformity[6].

REFERENCES

1. Monro, J.K. (1935). History of plaster of Paris in the treatment of fractures. *Brit. J. Surg.*, **23**, 257
2. Hendriks, P. (1838–9). Editorial. *Netherlands Lancet*, **1**, 357
3. Dieffenbach, J.F. (1831). *De cruribua fractis gypso-liquefacto curando.* (Berlin)
4. Mathijsen, A. (1852). *Nieuwe Wijze van Aanwending van het Gips-Verband bij Beenbreuken.* (Haarlem, J.B. van Loghem)
5. Blumenkamp, C. (1853). Eenige waarnemingen van behandelnde beenbreuken met het gipsverband. *Geneesk. Courant.*, **18**
6. Putti, V. (1938). Antonius Mathijsen. *Chir. Org. Muov.*, **24**, 1

CHAPTER 29

Arthroscopy of the Knee

Endoscopy of certain parts of the interior of the body – the ear, larynx and optic fundus – became a practical possibility in the first half of the 19th century. Gastroscopy and cystoscopy followed at around 1880, the invention of the carbon filament light bulb by Edison accelerated developments, cystoscopy was routine at the turn of the century, and a little later Jacobaeus designed the laparoscope. This was the instrument used by the Swiss surgeon, Eugen Bircher, in a series of experimental endoscopies of cadaver knee joints in 1919–20. In 1920–1 he published his famous paper – in the *Zentralblatt für Chirurgie*[1] – of its use in 18 patients. This was the first ever publication on clinical arthroscopy, and in 13 cases he was able to make a diagnosis confirmed by subsequent operation. The procedure was carried out under general anaesthesia in nearly every case, in joints filled with oxygen and nitrogen.

In 1922, Bircher reported on meniscus injuries in 20 knees so examined, successfully diagnosing eight out of nine meniscus injuries[2]. 'Arthroscopy,' he wrote, 'is superior to all other methods of investigation and, like endoscopy of the bladder, can be used to define certain indications for surgery. It will meet with resistance, as did cystoscopy, but, like the latter procedure, will gain in popularity and develop to the point at which it becomes indispensable.'

Arthroscopy must have been 'in the air', since Takanagi in Japan had experimented with a cystoscope within the knee in 1918 and had developed a special device for the joint in 1920[3]. Its calibre, at 7.3 mm, was too great and it was not until 1931 that he produced a 3.5 mm instrument, filling the knee with saline[4]. The first western report was by Philip H Kreuscher[5], of Chicago, in 1925. Work was also done at the New York Hospital for Joint Diseases in the early 1930s by Burman and others[6,7], using local anaesthesia and irrigation with Ringer's solution. Shortly before World War II, the method was tried by both surgeons[8] and rheumatologists in Germany; Vaupel[9] was one of the latter and in 1937 reported serial arthroscopy to study the changes in the synovial membrane in the course of disease. He also tried – without great success – to obtain photographic records. There was an excellent review of the subject by Wilcke[10] in 1939, but it was pessimistic, 'Its value is not such that it could be recommended for routine use in living patients.' The main thrust next came after the second world war, in Japan, where Watanabe, Sato and Kawashima reported to the Japanese Orthopedic Association in 1953, and where the first *Atlas of Arthroscopy* was published in 1957[11].

Arthroscopic surgery also began in Japan, where, on 5th April 1962, Watanabe did the first partial meniscectomy. The method was popularized in the West by a regrettably short-lived American surgeon, Richard L O'Connor (1933–1980), who trained in arthroscopy with Watanabe in Tokyo and introduced arthroscopic surgery in California, developing new instruments for meniscectomy. He was rather a lone pioneer, a founding member of the International Arthroscopy Association and wrote a textbook in 1977. The method was then taken up by European surgeons, such as Dandy in England[12]. The first US course in arthroscopic surgery was in Maine in 1977 and the first European course at Nijmegen in 1978.

Arthroscopy of the knee has now become a common procedure, but, one sometimes suspects, used by many surgeons 'to keep up with the Joneses'; there are many excellent surgeons who prefer to manage without it, and operative arthroscopy is not without its hazards. Arthroscopy has also been extended to the shoulder and other joints, and even to the spine, where it has been used for disc operations. One is bound to wonder if such ingenuity is not sometimes self-defeating.

REFERENCES

1. Bircher, E. (1921). Die Arthroendoskopie. *Zbl. f. Chir.*, **48**, 1460
2. Bircher, E. (1922). *Bruns' Beitr. z. klin. Chir.*, **127**, 329
3. Watanabe, M. (1954). The development and present status of the arthroscope. *J. Jap. Med. Inst.*, **25**, 11
4. Takagi, K. (1933). Practical experience using Takagi's arthroscope. *J. Jap. Orthop. Ass.*, **8**, 132
5. Kreuscher, P.K. (1925). Semilunar cartilage disease, a plea for early recognition by means of the arthroscope and early treatment of this condition. *Ill. Med. J.*, **47**, 290
6. Burman, M.S. (1931). Arthroscopy, or the direct visualization of joints. An experimental cadaver study. *J. Bone Jt. Surg.*, **13**, 669
7. Burman, M.S., Finkelstein, H. and Mayer, L. (1934). Arthroscopy of the knee joint. *J. Bone Jt. Surg.*, **16**, 255
8. Sommer, R.L. (1937). Die Endoskopie des Kniegelenks. *Zbl. Chir.*, **64**, 1692
9. Vaupel, E. (1938). Die Endoskopie des Kniegelenks. *Z. Rheum.*, **1**, 210
10. Wilcke, K.H. (1939). Endoskopie des Kniegelenks an der Leiche. *Bruns' Beitr. klin. Chir.*, **169**, 75
11. Watanabe, M., Takeda, S. and Ikeuchi, H. (1969). *Atlas of Arthroscopy*, 2nd edn. (Tokyo)
12. Dandy, D.J. (1981). *Arthroscopic surgery of the knee*. (Edinburgh and London, Churchill Livingstone)

CHAPTER 30

Tendon Transplantation

Probably the best historical review of tendon transplantation is that by J Hilton Waterman in the *Medical News* of July 12th, 1902, and reproduced in full by Mercer Rang in his *Anthology of Orthopaedics*, although attention had previously been directed to it by Bick.

The earliest known case is that of Missa, reported in the *Gazette Salutaire* of 1770, when, for a severed middle finger extensor tendon, both ends were implanted into the ring extensor. What Waterman does not tell us is that both Velpeau (1829)[1] and Malgaigne (1862)[2] in their textbooks recommended that cut tendons be grafted into adjacent intact tendons. In the 1870s, several French surgeons – Tillaux, Duplay, Polaillon – reported cases of divided finger extensors in which the peripheral ends only were so implanted. Such procedures are properly described as tendon anastomoses rather than true transplants, and they were done because retraction of the proximal ends made direct suture impossible, even though tendon suture had evidently long been commonplace.

However, a quite new step was taken when Nicoladoni, in Vienna in 1881[3], used the tendons of active muscles to activate that of a paralysed muscle when he transferred the proximal ends of the divided peroneal tendons into the Achilles tendon of a calf paralysed by poliomyelitis and responsible for calcaneus deformity in a boy of 16. There was some benefit, but it did not last; Nicoladoni moved away and did not follow the case and the union separated. One wonders whether, at the time, his mind reverted to that first tendon operation described by Homer in the Iliad, when Achilles barbarously slit the heel cords of the slain Hector and inserted leather straps so as to be able to drag his corpse behind his horses. A few colleagues – Helferich[4], Hacker[5], Maydl[6] – repeated the procedure, again for calcaneus, but with disappointing results, and abandoned it before the end of the 1980s.

In 1892, Parrish in New York[7], who maintained that his procedure was original, operated on a child aged nearly four years with paralytic valgus dating from the first year of life. Assisted by Lewis Sayre and Sayre's son,

Reginald, he sewed the extensor hallucis longus tendon to that of the tibialis anterior with the foot held in inversion. Neither tendon was actually cut; they were laid alongside, 'coapted', and the foot held in plaster for a month. It was not the brilliant success Parrish had hoped for and he did not pursue it, though he did claim to have established the important principle of having a live muscle do the work of a dead one. If the tendons had actually been divided and resutured end-to-end, the outcome might have been different; as it was, the action of the donor muscle was embarrassed and not effectively transferred to the recipient tendon. Also in New York, Milliken reported 'A new operation for deformities' in the New York Medical Record for 26th October 1895.

However, in 1896 a Pole, one Drobnik, writing in a German journal[8], reported sustained trials in a series of 16 cases, some with outstanding results. In some cases he split the donor tendon to preserve some of its original function. He repeated Parrish's procedure but divided the extensor hallucis completely to give its belly a direct pull. In the upper limb – the first such procedure for poliomyelitis of the upper extremity – he transplanted the radial wrist extensors into the finger and thumb extensors with benefit. In some instances the transferred tendon was attached subperiosteally. These were modern procedures.

In 1894–6, Goldthwait[9] began tendon transfer in Boston, initially believing his method to be original and only later learning of the work of Nicoladoni and Parrish; but he went further and transplanted the lower end of the muscle belly of the sartorius to the rectus femoris tendon for quadriceps paralysis. This proved less satisfactory than Lange's 1898 method[10] of transplanting the biceps tendon into the patella, confirmed by Krause[11] and introduced into the USA by Painter in 1902[12]. In 1897, Bradford[13], also in Boston, reported 27 transplants (which he called 'tenoplastic operations') and in 1898 Vulpius, of Heidelberg, who was to acquire a great reputation in this field, published 30 cases[14–16].

By the turn of the century, and until 1914, tendon transplantation became fashionable and was thought by some to offer the ultimate solution to various outstanding problems (see p. 626). Schanz, of Dresden, told the Second Congress of the German Orthopaedic Association in 1903, 'If I had to sum up my experience ... in a sentence, I would say that I regard the new method as the greatest advance that orthopaedic treatment has to show in recent years.'

The trouble lay in regarding the method as a panacea in itself and not as part of a balanced programme including arthrodeses or bone-block operations. There was a common concept that transplantation, performed early enough in young children, would provide a permanent solution to paralyses, but this was usually disproved as the child aged and the foot grew heavier.

Another important figure at that time was Alessandro Codivilla (1861–1912), director of the Rizzoli Institute at Bologna. In 1899, in an important early paper[17] (see also at p. 287), he laid down the principles of first eliminating any contractures and then redistributing the available muscle forces to restore equilibrium. He acknowledged the difficulty of gauging the function of the muscles before transfer and at their new site of attachment.

He favoured Drobnik's total donor section and end-to-end suture, transferred the tibialis posterior forward through the interosseous membrane, and devised an opponens transplant for the thumb using the superficial flexor of the little finger. In another paper[18] he recognized the importance of preserving the glide mechanism by passing the transferred tendon through the emptied sheath of the replaced tendon. He also saw that arthrodesis might be better in some cases but does not seem to have regarded the two methods as complementary.

Fritz Lange's work on transplantation, in particular his use of silk strands to prolong the line of a short transplant, is mentioned at p. 202; it did not gain wide acceptance and was superseded by the autogenous fascial strips used by Codivilla, Payr[19] and others. The cooperative studies of Leo Mayer and Biesalski relevant to both the gliding mechanism and fascial prolongation are discussed elsewhere.

In 1939, Willis Campbell wrote, 'Nicoladoni, Velpeau, Helferich, Salvia, Lange, Vulpius and Codivilla, and in this country (the USA) Parrish, Goldthwait and Milliken, were responsible for making tendon transference practicable. Hundreds of varieties of the pioneer procedures have since been described'[20]. This remark, as all the foregoing material, was based mainly on transfer for imbalance due to poliomyelitis, and that mainly in the foot; attempts to apply the method to paralyses around the shoulder were less successful, for here there were no sufficiently-long, readily-accessible tendons. The problem of deltoid paralysis was never really solved, but certain transfers in the upper limb, such as of part of the pectoralis major for loss of elbow flexion, could give brilliant results. In some cases it seemed better to move muscle origins *en bloc*, as in Steindler's procedure to restore elbow flexion by proximal transfer of the common flexor origin[21,22].

Soon, tendon or muscle transfer was applied to spastic paralysis, and later to the paralyses of spina bifida, but the indications were less clear-cut and the outcome less predictable. Only its employment in peripheral nerve lesions, including congenital or traumatic brachial plexus palsies, approached the purity of the original concept. It has to be said that the results in spastic paralysis were far less satisfactory than in poliomyelitis, and for obvious reasons. The patients were often mentally retarded and emotionally disturbed; the transferred spastic muscle had never been truly under voluntary control; there was a possibility of overcorrection, as when hamstring transfer to the patella led to genu recurvatum; it was difficult to distinguish between the effects of simple release from the deforming pull and those of a genuinely functioning transplant; but, most of all, operation was useless without reeducation and was often shown to be unnecessary if individual attention to retraining were thorough. It was – and is – common to perform elaborate procedures which gave anatomically impressive results but failed to improve original function, or even worsened it, especially in the case of transfers around the hip, and it came to be seen that operation should be confined to special centres where expertise could be concentrated along with sufficient ancillary staff.

Also, in certain situations, there were alternatives, such as the partial peripheral neurectomies of Stöffel (p. 201). Overall, cerebral palsy remains a field in which surgical enthusiasm has been tempered by experience. It is worth repeating Little's remarks of 1862, 'I have had many of these cases under observation from one to twenty years, and may mention as an encouragement to other practitioners that treatment based upon physiology and rational therapeutics effects an amelioration surprising to those who have not watched such cases ... even cases which exhibit impaired intellect may be benefited in mind and body to an unexpected extent[23].' This is entirely consistent with the attitude of Phelps, as set out on p. 442.

Somewhat similar considerations apply to surgery for muscle imbalance in spina bifida. Here, one of the greatest problems is to prevent the relatively overacting hip flexors and adductors from dislocating the hip. Transference of the iliopsoas through a hole in the ilium into the great trochanter has often proved beneficial, more in prophylaxis than in treatment; and yet in many cases the transplant is not actively working and the improvement is due to removal of the deforming force.

For peripheral nerve palsies the situation is entirely different and tendon transfer remains efficient, though sometimes as a supplement to arthrodesis. Thus, the fully developed transplant for radial palsy, which we owe to Robert Jones, has proved outstandingly successful over the years, as has Sterling Bunnell's procedure for loss of thenar opposition[24,25]. Transfers to restore function in the hand paralysed by the peripheral neuritis of leprosy are particularly associated with the work of Paul Brand, in Vellore, India, and have proved of value when applied for nerve injuries in the West.

REFERENCES

1. Velpeau, A.A. (1839). *Nouveaux éléments de médecine opératoire.* 2nd edn. (Paris)
2. Malgaigne, J.-F. (1862). *Leçons d'Orthopédie.* (Paris)
3. Nicoladoni, K. (1882). Nachtrag zur Pes Calcaneus und zur Transplantation der Peroneal Sehnen. *Arch. f. klin. Chir.,* **27**, 660
4. Helferich, H. (1882). Über Muskeltransplantation beim Menschen. *Verh. d. dtsch. Ges. f. Chir.*
5. von Hacker (1886). Behandlung des Pes Calcaneus mittels Transposition der Peroneus und Achillessehnen. *Wien. med. Presse,* **26–27**, 882
6. Maydl (1886). Behandlung des Pes Calcaneus mittels Transposition der Peroneus und Achillessehnen. *Wien. med. Presse,* **26–27**, 882
7. Parrish, B.F. (1892). A new operation for paralytic talipes. *N.Y. Med. J.,* **56**, 402
8. Drobnik (1896). Über die Behandlung der Kinderlähmung mit Funktionsteilung und Funktionsübertragung der Muskeln. *Dtsch. Ztschr. f. Chir.,* **43**, 473
9. Goldthwait, J.E. (1895). Tendon transplantation in the treatment of deformities resulting from infantile paralysis. *Boston Med. Surg. J.,* **133**, 477
10. Lange, F. (1900). Über periostale Sehnenverpflanzung bei Lähmungen. *Münch. med. Wchschr.,* **47**, 486
11. Krause, F. (1902). Ersatz des gelähmten Quadriceps femoris durch die Flexoren des Unterschenkels. *Dtsch. med. Wchschr.,* **28**, 118
12. Painter, C.F. (1902). A case of transplantation of the biceps femoris tendon. *Boston Med. Surg. J.,* **147**, 381
13. Bradford, E.H. (1879). Tenoplastic surgery. *Ann. Surg.,* **26**, 153

14. Vulpius, O. (1897). Zur Kasuistik der Sehnentransplantation. *Münch. med. Wchschr.*, **16**
15. Vulpius, O. (1898). *Trans. Am. Assoc. Orthop. Surg.*, **11**, 439
16. Vulpius, O. (1910). *Behandlung der spinale Kinderlähmung.* (Leipzig)
17. Codivilla, A. (1899). Sur trapianti tendinei nella practica orthopaedica. *Arch. di Ortop.*, **16**, 225
18. Codivilla, A. (1900). Il trattamento chirurgio moderni della paralysi infantile spinale. *Policlinico*, **7**, 110
19. Payr, E. (1914). *Arch. f. klin. Chir.*, **106**, 235
20. Campbell, W. (1939). *Operative Orthopaedics.* (St Louis, Mosby)
21. Steindler, A. (1919). Operative treatment of paralytic conditions of the upper extremity. *J. Orthop. Surg.*, **1**, 187
22. Steindler, A. (1923). *Reconstructive Surgery of the Upper Extremity.* (New York)
23. Little, W.J. (1862). On the influence of abnormal parturition, difficult labour, premature birth and asphyxia neonatorum on the mental and physical condition of the child, especially in relation to deformities. *Trans. Obstet. Soc. London*, **3**, 283
24. Bunnell, S. (1927). Surgery of the nerves of the hand. *Surg. Gynaecol. Obst.*, **44**, 145
25. Bunnell, S. (1938). Opposition of the thumb. *J. Bone Jt. Surg.*, **20**, 269

CHAPTER 31

Electricity in Osteogenesis and Fracture Treatment

Current interest in the use of electricity to promote the union of sluggish fractures has obscured the fact that this has quite a long history. Indeed, it can be traced back as far as Galvani in 1791, via Benjamin Franklin and the somewhat uncritical use of electrical machines in the London hospitals of the early 19th century.

The first reports of the use of 'electrical fields' passed by 'acupuncturation' to induce the union of tardy fractures relate to the practice of a Mr Birch of St Thomas's Hospital in London in 1812. As Leonard F Peltier[1], the distinguished orthopaedic historian, has pointed out, when Alexander H Stevens, Professor of Surgery at the Medical Institution of New York, translated Alexis Boyer's surgical treatise[2] in 1816 he added this footnote:

> 'The late Mr Birch, one of the surgeons of St Thomas's Hospital, London
> ... informed me that he had succeeded in procuring a firm osseous
> union in several cases of ligamentous connexion of bones after fracture,
> by means of electricity. He stated that, in his hands, that remedy had
> never failed of success ... One of these patients, whom I often visited
> during his illness, entered St Thomas's Hospital in the month of January
> 1812 with an unconsolidated fracture of the tibia below the middle of
> thirteen months' standing. The leg below the fracture could be easily
> moved in any direction and without exciting much pain. Shocks of
> electric fluid were daily passed through the space between the ends of
> the bones, both in the direction of the length of the limb and that of its
> thickness ... After the limb was electrized, the ordinary apparatus for
> fractures of the leg was applied. At the expiration of two weeks the limb
> had evidently become less flexible in the situation of the fracture; and
> after a continuation of the same treatment for six weeks, the man was
> able to walk and left the hospital cured.'

This seems to be the first report of the method, and it stimulated another

New York surgeon, Valentine Mott, to try it; he was able to report two cases of ununited fracture successfully treated by this method in 1820[3]. In 1841, Hartshorne[4] wrote on the electrical treatment of pseudarthrosis in the *American Journal of Medical Science*, and the method must have continued in vogue since Lente published three 'successful' cases in the *New York Journal of Medicine* in 1850[5]. Only one of these is convincing, that of a recalcitrant negro woman of 25 with a midshaft fracture of the femur totally ununited after six months on the inclined plane and 'starch applications'. 'Directed the limb to be secured to the double inclined plane, so as to have that portion of the thigh adjacent to the seat of fracture exposed. Ordered electricity by means of Pike's galvanic apparatus three times a week, with acupuncture, the needle being passed to the periosteum on either side of the fracture.' Union was firm after eight weeks and the patient discharged after a further seven weeks.

The second case was a woman of 35, with a fracture of the tibia and fibula ununited at ten weeks despite treatment in the 'fracture box' and with the starch apparatus, 'Electricity with acupuncture to be applied every other day, the limb, in the interval, to be kept in the immovable apparatus.' Treatment was for ten minutes at a session, union was firm after four weeks and the patient discharged. The third case was another fracture of the tibia and fibula, unconsolidated at nine weeks, treated by electricity with daily acupuncture, the limb kept in the 'immovable apparatus'. It was firm after three weeks and the patient given a starch bandage and crutches and discharged seven weeks later, cured.

These two cases were early fractures that might well have joined anyway in the box; and it may be that the acupuncture itself stimulated osteogenesis. Lente refers to treatment by rubbing the bone-ends together and by passing a seton between them, the 'American method' used by Physick, which the latter had probably acquired from John Hunter. But electricity, wrote Lente, 'to be at all efficient, must be applied in connection with acupuncturation. It appears to have little or no effect when the poles of the battery are applied merely to the soft parts on either side of the fracture, as the current does not appear to reach the bone.' He added, 'We have also had several cases [of nonunion] during the same period treated by other means, by the starch apparatus, by seton, and by sawing off and wiring together the ends of the bones.'

In 1853, the *US Medical Times and Gazette* reported that a Mr Hall, house surgeon at York County Hospital, cured an ununited fracture of over a year's duration. 'He introduced a needle from each side of the limb into the interspace between the bones, and then passed a continuous current through. The operation was repeated every day for about a fortnight and a cure ultimately resulted[6].'

In 1861, Garratt wrote a book on electrotherapeutics, published in Boston, and described the insertion of needles into femoral fractures[7].

Whatever the genuineness of the central phenomenon, it must soon have become surrounded by quackery, as mesmerism had earlier, and have attracted similar condemnation. As the great German surgeon, Dieffenbach, who was noted for his caustic wit, said in a public lecture in 1840, '... no matter how peverse an idea may be in science, once it is thought of someone or other will actually put it into practice ... I need only remind you of how such a one has claimed to restore a sluggish fracture by applying one galvanic plate in the mouth and the opposite one in the anus ...[8].' Possibly the method was overtaken by Listerism and the resulting enthusiasm for operation, for the literature is silent for nearly a century. We note only von Baeyer's tantalizing observation in 1908–9[9,10] that when copper and zinc were implanted in animals, the connective tissue cells aligned themselves axially along the path of the corrosion current.

The modern interest stems from Japan. In 1953, Yasuda published two important papers. One, on the piezoelectric effect[11], showed that when a bone is stressed or deformed, a potential difference is created and current passes. The other, dealing with fractures, showed that small amounts of current applied to bone stimulated osteogenesis at the cathode or negative electrode[12]. In 1957, Fukada and Yasuda[13] confirmed that an electrical charge separation (i.e. a voltage) is produced when a bone is mechanically stressed as one aspect of the piezoelectric phenomenon, and this was later confirmed by American workers and considered to be the physical mediator of Wolff's Law (p. 190). The work was originally published in rather obscure Japanese journals, and we owe its later development and practical application almost entirely to Bassett and his colleagues in New York at the College of Physicians and Surgeons of Columbia University. This had to overcome an initial scepticism which has not, in some quarters, entirely subsided.

It is not possible to list Bassett's researches in detail. His fundamental work in the 1960s on the piezoelectric effect[14], on the effects of electric currents on bone *in vivo*[15] and on the behaviour of fibroblasts *in vitro*[16] led naturally to the concept that such currents might be used in the treatment of delayed union and nonunion in fractures. The early trials confirmed the Japanese finding that the best results were obtained with the cathode actually implanted in the fracture gap, a semi-invasive method which was perhaps an historical echo[17,18]. This was followed by totally invasive methods which consisted of implanting a small power pack with a trailing wire cathode which was inserted between the fracture ends or at the site of an attempted arthrodesis of the spine[19] or of large joints[20]. In the usual case of slow tibial union, the pack was implanted just below the knee under the skin or muscle. The more invasive method allowed accurate positioning and a precise current flow, but required two operations, one for insertion and one for removal (unless a pull-out method was used leaving a small permanently indwelling component) and it was inapplicable to infected fractures. Unidirectional direct or bidirectional alternating currents seemed equally effective, and current levels of 5–20 microamperes the most efficacious. Both the invasive and semi-invasive methods found wide application despite scepticism.

However, Bassett came down in favour of stimulating bone repair by means of pulsed electromagnetic fields (PEMF)[21–23] induced at a time-varying current by two coils mounted on the skin or plaster cast, and so usable with outpatients, which generated weak currents at the fracture. These fields were found to promote the synthesis of fibroblasts *in vitro* and to augment bone repair. According to Bassett, PEMF increases the calcium ion content of the chondrocytes at the discontinuity and triggers calcification of the fibrocartilage blocking union to allow normal terminal ossification. It is not effective if there is a fibrous bridge or pseudarthrosis, unless mechanical stresses are eliminated by immobilization and non-weight bearing; then the fibrous tissue may become fibrocartilage, which will respond; but it is essential to eliminate tension and torque[24]. Union occurs with little external callus, and metal fixation devices are not a contraindication to treatment.

This is an entirely noninvasive method, the current differs from that of implanted electrodes, and careful calibration is required to generate a voltage in the narrow therapeutic range of 1.0–1.5 mv/cm at the fracture site. Acceptance of the validity of the method was grudging. Most of the fractures treated are tibial, and since PEMF requires continued plaster fixation and non-weightbearing it is difficult to assess the effects of electrical treatment as such as distinct from those of the continued immobilization. What is impressive is that PEMF can give up to 100 per cent success in fractures ununited despite efficient *internal* fixation, though when that fixation is loose the success rate falls to only around 60 per cent. Nonmagnetic metals seem not to be corroded by PEMF and the rate of healing is unaffected by their presence.

Nevertheless, even such an enthusiast as Sharrard[25], who has even said that this method can dry up sinuses and lead to absorption of sequestra in infected cases, could not demonstrate an advantage over conventionally treated cases in a controlled series. A fairly general opinion might be that, while the treatment may not increase the proportion of tibial fractures that unite, it markedly speeds the process. Until recently, it has been used as a last resort after the failure of other conservative and operative measures; but if it is really effective it might be logical to use it earlier, i.e. for the fractured tibia not united at three of four months which might otherwise be managed by bone-grafting[26]. Such early treatment is compatible with the continued plaster fixation that is in any case required; the disadvantages are that the apparatus is costly to buy or rent, somewhat tedious to use, and has to be rationed in a busy fracture department.

Despite lack of general acceptance, there are certain conditions in which spontaneous bony union is so rare, and union so difficult to achieve by operation, that the success of electrical treatment under the most daunting circumstances is striking. These include established nonunion of the scaphoid[27], failed arthrodesis for Charcot joints, and – particularly impressive – congenital pseudarthrosis of the tibia[28]. Here, the success of the treatment seems undeniable. Bassett's claims that it also acts against infection and bone necrosis are more debatable.

It is unfortunate that, historically, electrotherapy has always attracted quacks, and perhaps the unfair association lingers on. It is unlikely to become routine until its application becomes simpler and cheaper. And, as the history of effective osteogenesis is a matter of barely 30 years, little more should be added at this stage. It is clear, however, that the implications for the future biological managment of fracture healing, and possibly much more besides, are very considerable.

REFERENCES

1. Peltier, L.F. (1981). A brief historical note on the use of electricity in the treatment of fractures. *Clin. Orthop.*, **161**, 4

2. Boyer, A. (1816). *Traité des maladies chirurgicales.* Translated by Stevens, A.H. as *A Treatise in surgical diseases and the operations suited to them.* (New York)

3. Mott, V. (1820). Two cases of ununited fractures successfully treated by seton. *Med. Surg. Register*, **1**, (Part 2) 375

4. Hartshorne, E. (1841). On the causes and treatment of pseudarthrosis and especially of that form of it sometimes called supernumerary joint. *Am. J. Med. Soc.*, **121**, 143

5. Lente, F.D. (1850). Cases of ununited fractures treated by electricity. *N.Y.J. Med.*, **5**, 317

6. Stillings, D. (1974). Electrically stimulated bone growth in animals and man. *Clin. Orthop.*, **8**, 259

7. Garratt, A.C. (1861). *Electro-Physiology and Electro-Therapeutics.* (Boston, Ticknor and Fields)

8. Valentin, B. (1961). *Die Geschichte der Orthopädie.* (Stüttgart, Thieme)

9. von Baeyer, H. (1909). *Munch. med. Wschr.*, **56**, 2416

10. von Baeyer, H. (1908). *Beitr. klin. Chir.*, **58**, 1

11. Yasuda, I. (1953). Piezoelectricity of living bone. *J. Kyoto Pref. Univ. Med.*, **53**, 325

12. Yasuda, I. (1953). Fundamental aspects of fracture treatment: electrical callus. *J. Kyoto Med. Soc.*, **4**, 395

13. Fukada, E. and Yasuda, I. (1957). On the piezoelectric effect of bone. *J. Physiol. Soc. Japan*, **12**, 1158

14. Bassett, C.A.L. and Becker, R.O. (1962). Generation of electric potentials by bone in response to mechanical stress. *Science*, **137**, 1063

15. Bassett, C.A.L., Pawluk, R.J. and Becker, R.O. (1964). Effects of electric currents on bone *in vivo*. *Nature*, **204**, 652

16. Bassett, C.A.L. and Herman, I. (1968). The effect of electrostatic fields on macromolecular synthesis of fibroblasts *in vitro*. *J. Cell Biol.*, **39**, 9a

17. Friedenberg, Z.B. and Kohanim, J. (1968). The effect of direct current on bone. *Surg. Gynaecol. Obstet.*, **127**, 97

18. Friedenberg, Z.B., Harlow, M.C. and Brighton, C.T. (1971). Healing of nonunion of the medial malleolus by means of direct current. A case report. *J. Trauma*, **2**, 883

19. Dwyer, A.F. and Wickham, G.G. (1974). Direct current stimulation in spinal fusion. *Med. J. Austral.*, **1**, 73

20. Bigliani, L.U. *et al.* (1983). The use of pulsing electromagnetic fields to achieve arthrodesis of the knee following failed total knee arthroplasty. A preliminary report. *J. Bone Jt. Surg.*, **65A**, 480

21. Bassett, C.A.L. (1978). Pulsing electromagnetic fields: a new approach to surgical problems. In Buchwald, H. and Varco, R.L. (eds.) *Metabolic Surgery.* (New York, Grune and Stratton)

22. Bassett, C.A.L., Mitchell, S.N. and Gaston, S.R. (1981). Treatment of ununited tibial diaphyseal fractures with pulsing electromagnetic fields. *Clin. Orthop.*, **154**, 136

23. Bassett, C.A.L., Mitchell, S.N. and Schink, M.M. (1982). Treatment of therapeutically resistant nonunion with bone grafts and pulsing electromagnetic fields. *J. Bone Jt. Surg.*, **64A**, 1214

24. Bassett, C.A.L. (1984). The development and application of pulsed electromagnetic fields (PEMF) for ununited fractures and arthrodeses. *Orthop. Clin. N. Am.*, **15**, 61

25. Sharrard, W.J.W. *et al.* (1982). The treatment of fibrous non-union of fractures by pulsing electromagnetic stimulation. *J. Bone Jt. Surg.*, **64B**, 189
26. Compere, C.L. (1982). Electromagnetic fields and bone. *J. Am. Med. Assoc.*, **247**, 669
27. Bora, F.W., Osterman, A.L. and Brighton, C.T. (1981). The electrical treatment of scaphoid nonunion. *Clin. Orthop.*, **161**, 33
28. Kort, J.K. *et al.* (1982). Congenital pseudarthrosis of the tibia: treatment with pulsing electromagnetic fields. *Clin. Orthop.*, **165**, 124

CHAPTER 32

Implants in Orthopaedic Surgery

As Sir Thomas Browne wrote of the song the Sirens sang, though the date at which an orthopaedic implant was first used cannot be ascertained with any certainty, yet it is not beyond all conjecture. Leaving aside such cosmetic devices as Tycho Brahe's silver nose, we are concerned initially with the use of metal or other sutures to control the position of fractures. This must have been a nagging temptation to surgeons aware of both what needed to be done and the hazards of intervention, of which infection was the least. We know that the Etruscans and Greeks wired teeth for fractured jaws. In the 17th century, a Neapolitan surgeon, one Severino (1580–1656) was perhaps the first to counsel suture for fracture of the patella. We have no details, but anthropologists have reported that for a very long time the South African tribes sutured fractures with catgut-like material obtained from the dorsal spinal ligament of camels. Moreover, Jacques Croissant de Garengeot (1668–1759), in his *Traité des Instruments les Plus Utiles* of 1725, refers to the 'ancient' classification of operations into *synthesis, diaeresis, exeresis* and *prosthesis*; and one wonders about the last. In 1775, the *Journal Français de Chirurgie* contained a report by Icart of two Toulouse surgeons, Lapoyde and Sicre, on the use of brass wire for fracture suture, which excited fierce opposition.

It was probably first seriously attempted in the late 18th or early 19th century and what we may assume with virtual certainty is that these attempts, before anaesthesia, antisepsis, asepsis and antibiotics, were uniformly disastrous. It meant creating an open fracture; and right up to the second half of the 19th century an open fracture spelled death or amputation for the majority of patients[1].

For as late as 1883, when Listerian principles were at least partly accepted in Europe, and when Lister had wired his first patella in 1877, Beauregard[2], reviewing 49 cases of patellar fracture wired with silver, steel or platinum or sutured with silk in various European countries, did not find it especially remarkable that these endeavours resulted in one amputation and four

587

deaths. In earlier days, then, the deliberate opening of a simple fracture was to tempt Fate, an act of surgical *hubris* which rarely went unpunished.

At any given period, the status of orthopaedic implants has to be considered in the light of the contemporary technology and of the status of orthopaedics itself. Metallurgy reached its peak in the latter half of the 19th century when it transformed the western world[3], but orthopaedics did not become a separate discipline until the turn of the century or even later; and even then, as was pointed out at the first congress of the German Association for Orthopaedic Surgery, the wish to associate was tempered by the fear that separation from general surgery would reduce them once more to the status of mere 'bandagists'[4]. Even in the first decades of the 20th century, when implants were very much in vogue, and later still with the expansion in plastics at the midcentury, tissue reactions to materials were still not fully understood and there was still no adequate science of biomechanics.

One of the problems was the well-known tendency of metal implants in living tissue to corrosion, of varying intensity and pace and with varying damage to the tissues, sometimes with rapid disintegration of the implant, sometimes – as with the 'noble' metals – with negligible change. That metals were not physiologically inactive in the body had been known since Galvani's discovery in 1779[5], but the physical basis of corrosion as an electrochemical process was first elucidated by Sir Humphrey Davy in the 1820s[6], followed by Michael Faraday[7], and the theory was refined by many other later workers.

In 1804, Bell of New York was using steel-tipped silver pins for wound closure and noted the galvanic corrosion that occurred[8] and in 1829 another American, Levert, experimented with gold, silver, lead and platinum implants in dogs and found platinum the least irritant buried wire sutures[9]. The surgeon's quandary was well exemplified by Malgaigne, in France. He wanted to fix unstable fractures but believed that metal implants caused hospital gangrene, so in 1837 he designed the first external fixator, an apparatus of clamps with screws attached to percutaneous hooks into the bone that permitted compression. This was successful in six tibial fractures in 1840[10] and four successes with patellar fractures were published in 1847[11]. He was surprised at his own success, for 'such innocuousness ... is still, to my thinking, one of the most surprising things that one can mention in surgical pathology.' (See p. 557)*.

It was therefore possible to have the right idea at the wrong time, to develop a concept of treatment which could not be supported by the current technology. Thus Langenbeck, in Germany, had attempted fixation of femoral neck fractures in the 1870s[12] but his metals were unsatisfactory and X-rays had yet to be invented. It is fascinating that total replacement of the hip joint for osteoarthritis was attempted as long ago as 1890 by one Themistocles Gluck[13–15] using an ivory ball and socket fixed to the upper femur with nickel-plated steel screws, with a primitive 'cement' of pumice powder, plaster and glue. (Carnochan, in New York, had tried implantation of a piece of

---

* It was not totally innocuous; there was a good deal of sepsis.

wood after excision of an ankylosed temporomandibular joint as far back as 1840[16].) It must have been galling to be so premature. Lister developed antisepsis during the years 1860–70, but, even before its general acceptance, Gurlt in 1862 was describing techniques of nailing, screwing and wiring for fresh, particularly juxtarticular, fractures[17]. Even before this, subcutaneous fractures such as those of the patella and olecranon had been wired[18] and when Wahl reported a patellar suture with silver wire and catgut in 1883 it was evidently a commonplace and gave good union and function despite minor sequestration[19]. But with the advent of Listerism, metallic internal fixation really began to take off.

An early pioneer was Hansmann in 1886[20], who fixed fractures with strips of unhardened nickel-plated sheet steel and nickel-plated screws, one end of the plate being bent at a right angle to protrude through the skin and facilitate removal after 6–8 weeks. This he reported to the 15th Surgical Congress in Germany, and two visitors were impressed: Halsted (p. 411) took some plates back to Johns Hopkins in the USA and Lambotte, of Belgium saw this as the ideal future treatment of fractures (p. 316). Until the end of the century open reduction, with or without internal fixation, was generally only used when conservative treatment had long failed; and the use of plates and screws was rare until the advent of X-rays in 1895 when, as Delbet wrote[10], 'we know more of what we have to do, of what we are doing, and of what has been done'. (Though one may wonder if this was an unmixed blessing and whether strenuous efforts to obtain demonstrable anatomic reduction, pleasing to the eye and to the law courts, often at the expense of function, are always justified when a policy of 'watchful neglect' and early rehabilitation may yield better results without the risk of iatrogenic disability.)

In 1905, Fritz Koenig, of Altona in Germany used wires (including hemicirclage wiring), ivory pegs and bone inserts in order to avoid postoperative fixation and favour mobilisation[21]. In 1891, Berthold Ernst Hadra (1842–1903), a German who had emigrated to Texas, was able to ask, 'Since we fix other fractures by clamps, nails, wires, sutures and so on, why not do so for spinal fractures?'[22], and proceeded to do so by wiring the spinous and even the transverse processes to safeguard the cord, later extending this technique to Pott's disease of the vertebral column. At much the same time, in 1894, Jules Emile Péan (1830–1898), of the Hôpital St Louis in Paris, refers to fixing fractures with aluminium plates and screws or silver wire[23]. He also used platinum replacements for syphilitic nasal bones and inserted an aluminium plate after resecting a tuberculous orbit. He records the insertion of a large rubber and platinum prosthesis to replace the upper end of a humerus excised for tuberculosis and offers this principle as an alternative to disarticulation after resection of major parts of the skeleton. As we shall see, the offer was taken up.

But it is Sir William Arbuthnot Lane (1856–1938), in London, who must be regarded as the great precursor in internal fixation[24]. After an early trial of silver wire, he began early in the 1890s to fix oblique tibial fractures with ordinary steel screws, on the grounds that this secured better alignment of ankle joint fractures and promoted rehabilitation[25]. This was with his new 'no touch' technique, and since, in his hands, infection was rare, it became possible to distinguish the failures due to corrosion. In 1905 he proceeded to the use of plates and though not the originator of the method was the first to apply it safely and systematically[26]. These screws and plates were made of plain high-carbon steel and were intended 'to bring together and maintain the opposing surfaces of the bone into the most accurate and forcible apposition', an aim that must have resounded in the compression enthusiasts of the 20th century. In Lane's plates the transition from the curve round the screw hole to the shank of the shaft was an abrupt one and it was here that mechanical failure occurred. In 1912, Sherman reported the treatment of 55 femoral shaft fractures with Lane's plates, three of which broke at this junction[27]. He considered that the plate should be sufficiently ductile and elastic to bend rather than break, introduced a high-carbon steel containing vanadium, and redesigned the plate to reduce the 'necking' between holes. Sherman's plates served in good stead and were recommended by the US Bureau of Standards and the Committee on Fractures of the American College of Surgeons in 1932 and again in 1947[11] and are still to be found in some parts of the world. Still, even in the 1920s, Sherman's plates, though usually mechanically sound, often loosened or caused local iron staining[28], and it is fair to say that up to 1920, despite experiments with many materials, some rather dubious, nothing totally reliable had been found and implants were generally removed once union was achieved. Such modifications as the rectangular Venable plate were an improvement. It is interesting that a contemporary of Sherman's, F J Cotton, in 1912, thought that, 'no matter how good a rigid plate is, it necessarily exposes the patient to the danger of pulling out screws. It seems to me that much is in favour of a slightly flexible elastic plate, one which can be fitted to the case in hand,' the actual metal used being unimportant[29]. The point was a good one, better perhaps than Cotton realised, and will be returned to.

Much credit is due to the brothers Lambotte, in Belgium. Elie Lambotte

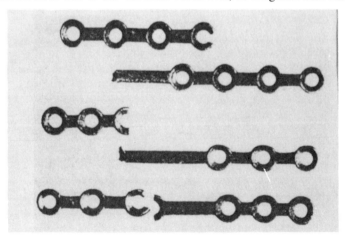

Figure 238   Lane's plates, illustrating their general form and the type of mechanical failure that often occurred

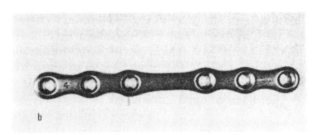

Figure 239   The Sherman plate

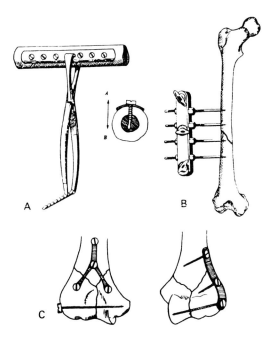

Figure 240   Forceps, bone plates and external fixator, after Lambotte

had used wires and screws for oblique tibial fractures in the 1890s with good results[30] but was discouraged by criticism. His brother Albin was made of sterner stuff and used plates and screws, transfixion pins, external fixators, curved or Y-shaped plates for condylar fractures at the lower ends of the humerus or femur, and thin guided nails for the scaphoid[31,32]. His 1909 paper had dealt with the fate in the bone of alloys such as brass and also of aluminium, silver, copper and magnesium, all of which proved malleable and corrodable, so that he settled on soft steel plated with gold or nickel. Some contemporary work by von Baeyer[33,34], on cellular reactions to implants, anticipating much later work on piezoelectricity, noted that if copper and zinc were implanted close together the connective tissue cells aligned themselves axially along the path of the corrosion current.

Thus, as Mears has well said, for fifty years after the introduction of asepsis, though internal fixation was propounded by the few who saw its potential, the metals and alloys then available were mechanically unsound and not inert to the tissues. Sherman was the first to grasp the metallurgical and mechanical requirements of the situation and to act to meet them.

Another pioneer in the field was Ernest William Hey-Groves (1872–1944), a village general practitioner in England who became a surgeon in Bristol and rapidly developed an innovative enthusiasm for orthopaedics, doing much animal experimental research on methods of fracture fixation[35]. Like Cotton, he anticipated that really rigid fixation, if it could be achieved, might delay union. On tissue tolerance he noted that magnesium rapidly disintegrated and dissolved but that nickel-plated steel was inert; also that continued minor movement between metal and bone led to irritation, bone

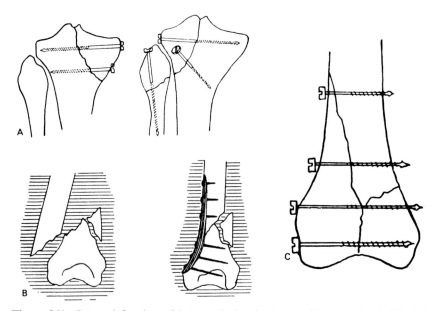

Figure 241   Internal fixation of intra-articular fractures of the proximal tibia (A) and the femur (B and C), after Lambotte

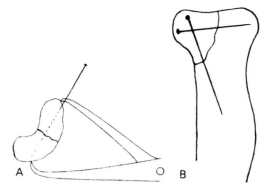

Figure 242 Method of immobilizing a scaphoid fracture (A), and a fracture of the radial styloid (B), after Lambotte

resorption, sepsis and sinuses.

In 1924, Zierold studied metal corrosion extensively in dogs[36], noting that iron and high and low carbon steels rapidly dissolved, their erosion affecting the bone. Inserts of copper, nickel, zinc and aluminium alloy all discoloured bone, but there was no reaction to gold, silver, lead (though this was systemically toxic), or pure aluminium – materials too soft for plates though useful for wires or plating other metals. Stellite, a cobalt alloy, was very well tolerated but, strangely, not further studied at this time. 1926 saw the introduction of 'stainless' steel, with 18 per cent chromium and 8 per cent nickel, more resistant than vanadium steel but still liable to disintegrate[37–39]. This was followed by the austenitic 18-8-SMo steel with 2–4 per cent molybdenum which was very corrosion-resistant, though it did not gain early acceptance when first patented[40].

In 1929 a nonferrous alloy of cobalt with chromium and molybdenum, similar to Zierold's stellite and labelled vitallium, began to be used in dentistry and its complete inertness and suitability for orthopaedic implants were noted by Venable and Stuck in 1936[11]. Similar inertness to tantalum was noted at this time[11], but its poor mechanical properties made it fitter for neurosurgeons and plastic surgeons. Titanium and its alloys appeared around 1947 and trial implants of the pure metal proved it very inert and corrosion-resistant. Specifications for the various metals and alloys were laid down by the American Committee on Fractures in 1947[41] and after 1950 there were few new developments.

Corresponding with these three decades of the study of plates between 1920 and 1950, there developed a theory of the microstructure of metals and how this was altered by mechanical deformation or alloying; this has been well summarized by Cottrell[42,43]. We may add here that, much later, experience with total hip replacement revealed, in a minority of cases, the existence of a tissue sensitivity to metals of an allergic rather than an electrolytic nature, one which can be detected by patch testing before operation[44].

Plates for fracture fixation have developed with great variety in recent decades and need not be described in detail. It became increasingly recognised that, because a fracture of a long bone normally heals with minimal absorption at the bone ends and slight shortening and collapse, a very rigid plate might prevent such collapse and even delay healing indefinitely unless the patient was lucky enough to have the plate break. One way of dealing with this was to use a slotted plate in which the screws could move axially, but the really important advance was recognition of the role of compression.

This was far from a new idea but it was not developed systematically until after World War II. In 1947, Robert Danis (1880–1962) of Brussels, dissatisfied with current fixation techniques, wrote a famous book[45] in which he stated that, with really rigid aseptic internal fixation, so little callus forms that it is not even visible ... the process seems to take place without the participation of the surrounding tissues ... the periosteum does not play a very important part.'

Danis poohpoohed the notion that callus is essential to fracture healing. 'It should be regarded as a pathological structure whose formation can usually be prevented by internal fixation, which should produce and maintain interfragmentary pressure ... mainly directed along their axes.' This was what he called *soudure autogène* or primary cortical healing. As Cave wrote in 1958, '... the more accurately a fracture is aligned, the less demand there will be for callus'[46]. Danis therefore, in 1947, introduced a compression plate, especially for forearm fractures, to bring about such healing, which differs essentially from normal biological healing with ensheathing callus, incidentally popularising the existing European term 'osteosynthesis'.

Although the importance of compression had been recognised at least as far back as Lambotte, and by Key in securing arthrodesis[47], Danis's work started a revolution in fracture treatment. In the early 1950s three Swiss workers – M E Müller, M Allgöwer and H Willenegger – began to study compression systems in a converted watchspring factory and in 1958 founded the now famous *Arbeitsgemeinschaft für Osteosynthesefragen* or Working Party on Problems of Internal Fixation, generally known as AO[48]. They developed lag screws, compression plates and tension band wires and powered equipment and special tools for their insertion. They preferred ductile coaptable material to unyielding devices, and studied their effects on bone healing. This is a technique obviously related to Charnley's work on compression arthrodesis[49] and since it acts by cortical approximation and dispenses with external callus it can be employed immediately, whereas with conventional plate fixation a delay of 7–10 days is advisable to allow the fracture haematoma to begin organising and so reduce the risk of delayed union. Further, the compression system had advantages in the presence of infection. Earlier, the emphasis had been on removing foreign material from infected fractures, but maintaining rigid compression fixation of such fractures gave better union than other treatment and without the proliferative callus usually seen in sepsis[50].

The AO system is now so widely used that any criticism may seem carping. Nevertheless, one thinks of Hugh Owen Thomas's dictum that 'screws, if there be any strain on them, do not long maintain their hold on living matter', and his condemnation of surgeons who treated the human body 'as if it were a watch, with no automatic self-repairing quality of its own' and imposed their own solutions, willy-nilly[51]. Compression, it is true, must ultimately act by biological processes but end-to-end cortical union is not the natural method of repair, it is often achieved only by the introduction of a great mass of metal, it calls for an expertise often denied to the contemplative surgeon who prefers to do the minimum and leave the rest to the tissues, it is expensive, and worse, it is basically contemptuous of the normal method of fracture healing. This it supplants, rather than supplements, surely an error in historical perspective.

On the other hand, compression theory was valuable in stressing the importance of axial forces in long bone healing. As Bassett has pointed out[52], tensile and torque forces at a fracture are deleterious and tend to produce a bridge of fibroblasts rather than chondrocytes. This had been recognised by Gerhard Küntscher (1900–1972) in Germany at the beginning of World War II, but his solution, stimulated by the recent successes of hip nailing, had been to pass a long stout nail down the medullary cavity to secure fixation and convert all stresses into axial ones[53,54]. The concept was not entirely novel, for Hey-Groves had used the identical principle in 1916, inserting a bone-peg retrograde at the fracture site, driving it out through the great trochanter and hammering it back into the lower fragment[55]. Also, a similar technique had been employed by Müller-Meernach in 1933, using an open method in which the nails were not removed[56], while a little later Lambrinudi was fixing forearm fractures with intramedullary Kirschner wires[57].

However, it was Küntscher who made medullary nailing an accepted technique, using it widely during the war before it became known in Britain and America. The nail was initially V-shaped in section but was soon altered to clover-leaf shape so as to impinge everywhere on the walls of the canal and channel stresses longitudinally. It was moderately flexible and introduced blindly from above over a guide under X-ray screening. Open exposure of the fracture and retrograde insertion were employed only if closed reduction was impossible or, in malunion, an osteotomy necessary. Küntscher stressed the value of his method for early mobilisation under wartime conditions, favoured it – with qualifications – for compound and pathological fractures, and adapted it with a slotted-in 'signal arm' to trochanteric fractures and extended it to the ankle for arthrodesis of the knee[58].

Medullary nailing, extended to the tibia and forearm bones and humerus, has long been a standard procedure. Most surgeons now prefer open insertion, though closed nailing of femoral fractures has its adherents[59,60]. Reaming of the shaft to allow insertion of the widest possible nail was added by Maatz in 1942[61] and the general principle became the basis of the Rush system[62] and of systems of multiple medullary wires or pins developed by Hackenthal – 'stacked nailing'[63,64] and by Ender for trochanteric fractures[65]. The method obviously competes with plating in the treatment of fresh transverse or short oblique shaft fractures, it is generally simpler in suitable cases and can be performed alone or in combination with cancellous bone grafting for delayed or non-union.

To bring internal fixation up-to-date, we should refer to the introduction of carbon fibre, a very strong material which, reinforced with epoxy resin, has been used as plates fixed with conventional screws. Because these plates have some elasticity, they avoid the stress osteopenia due to rigid metal plates[66]. Carbon fibre threads are also used to substitute tendons and ligaments, particularly the cruciate and collateral ligaments of the knee and seem to have few disadvantages[67]. Very recently, biodegradable fixation systems[68] and systems allowing tissue ingrowth have been tried[201] but it is too soon to assess the results.

HIP FRACTURES

Langenbeck's attempts at nailing these in the mid-19th century were sporadically imitated but with general lack of success because the nails were inaccurately inserted without X-rays available, open reduction was dangerous, the metals were not inert and a nail could not control rotational stresses.

In 1898, Boeckmann and Gillette in the US made a lateral approach, divided the trochanter, and placed an ivory peg in the neck and another to reattach the trochanter[69], and in 1900 Davis opened old ununited fractures, freshened them, and fixed them with steel pins or ivory pegs[70]. At about this time, Sayre in New York was using a gimlet and nuts and the great J B Murphy in Chicago also tried his hand with nailing from 1902 on[71]. Hey-Groves used bone and ivory pegs in 1913[35] and in those prewar years Delbet, Lambotte and others devised screws and guides for their insertion[72]. Hey-Groves thought that bone pegs might give a better hold than the screw 'which is still used by many surgeons' (1926)[73], because pegs would become incorporated in the new bone. He also took out a loose head and bolted it back with an ivory peg or replaced it with an ivory prosthesis, whereas Robert Jones resigned himself to wrapping the stump of the neck in gold foil.

Soon after the end of World War II a renewed attack on the problem was made in many quarters. In 1922, Martin and King in New Orleans performed closed nailing under X-ray control[74] and in 1925 Smith-Petersen in Boston inserted a triflanged nail under direct vision in 24 patients, though he did not report this until 1931[75]. This nail was sharply pointed and its strength and shape enabled it to withstand, as no previous implant had done, the bending (shear) and rotational stresses in the femoral neck. It was made first in stainless steel and then in vitallium. In 1932, independently, Johansson in Sweden[76] and Westcott in Virginia[77] cannulated the nail so that it could be inserted blindly over a guide under X-ray control after manipulative reduction. When Smith-Petersen reassessed the position in 1937[78] he acknowledged that though he had considered accurate reduction without soft part interposition impossible without open exposure, he now admitted that he had been proved wrong, and he stressed the value of Leadbetter's manoeuvre in reduction to produce slight valgus[79] and of the lateral X-ray view.* Along this line of progress only details remained to be added, such as Hillebrand's advocacy of carrying the fixation on into the pelvis[80], Thornton's addition of a small plate on the outside of the femur to prevent extrusion[81], Garden's replacement of a single nail with two compression screws[82] and other modifications.

With the recognition that cervical nails could not be expected to control trochanteric fractures on their own, and although such fractures nearly, but not quite always unite, and in order to reduce hospital stay and morbidity, a spate of angled nail-plates or blade-plates appeared, as one- or two-piece systems[83], followed inevitably by similar systems incorporating compression[84]. Such systems, with or without compression, rapidly became popular for internal fixation of the intertrochanteric osteotomy introduced by McMurray for hip arthrosis and fractures[85], thus avoiding long incarceration in plaster.

Perhaps, before passing to further and deeper aspects of hip surgery we should, for completeness, refer to the principle of the external fixator for fractures since this does involve metal implants in the form of transfixion pins, albeit temporary. This continues to be reinvented from time to time, but we have seen that Malgaigne had devised a primitive version as far back as 1837 and doubtless others in that century improved on it. Lambotte found it useful for infected fractures and nonunions, since it allowed easy inspection. Nevertheless, its assembly and stability and the incidence of pintrack infection were a nuisance. Shortly before World War II, Roger Anderson produced a much more reliable version[86] and this was modified in 1954 as a three-plane system by Hoffmann in Switzerland[87] and by Adrey at Montpellier[88] and others. It is mainly for shaft fractures but is also applicable to comminuted fractures of the lower radius[89] and to control arthrodeses and massive bone resections. As with every other complicated technique, though valuable in the hands of those who like and understand it, external fixation is 'caviar' to the general fracture surgeon, who will tend to prefer less exacting methods. (See also p. 557.)

We should also refer, with unfair brevity, to internal fixation for unstable fracture-dislocations of the thoracolumbar and cervical spine. The massive internal spinal instrumentation devised by Harrington, of Texas, for the correction of scoliosis, in which a metal rod anchored to the spine by fixation hooks is distracted[90,91], a method adapted by Dwyer, in Australia, to act on the anterior spinal elements[92], is discussed elsewhere (p. 543).

HEMIARTHROPLASTY OF THE HIP

Since high subcapital fractures of the femoral neck are so often followed by necrosis and collapse of the head due to loss of blood-supply, and this despite the most meticulous reduction and fixation, it was a logical step, at any rate in older patients, to remove the head and replace it with a metal prosthesis

---

*Guy Whitman Leadbetter was Professor at George Washington Medical School. His 1933 paper described a manoeuvre of reduction which has never been surpassed, though he followed it with a hip spica cast from nipple to toes, using Whitman's method (see p. 436).

as the primary treatment. In 1942, Austin T Moore (1899–1963) reported in a South Carolina journal[93] and later in a more august medium[94] the case of a very heavy negro with a recurrent osteoclastoma of the upper end of the femur in whom he replaced – for the first time – the entire upper portion of the bone with a vitallium prosthesis a foot long, with a round head, loops for muscle attachments, and a lower end slipping over the cut shaft and bolted to it. The patient died 20 months later from other causes, after good function. This led to the development of the wellknown self-locking fenestrated femoral head prosthesis, which was initially employed as a hemiarthroplasty in arthrosis of the hip, leaving the acetabulum untouched[95]. At about this time a basically similar device was introduced by Thompson[96,97].

Although these possessed the essential factor of intramedullary anchorage of the stem in the femur, the results in arthrosis were not outstanding, largely because of lack of congruity of the head in the socket. When, however, it was realised that these prostheses could provide an immediate and satisfactory solution to the subcapital fracture[98], they at once gained and retained popularity. They are best reserved for the elderly as, if the patient lives long enough, the metal head will always sink into the pelvis, and it became common to fix them in the femur with cement once that had been developed. Because of the risk of dislocation, the Monk or similar modifications, in which the head is contained within a mobile metal or plastic shell fitting in the acetabulum, may have some advantages[99]. Some authors now advocate primary total hip replacement for selected hip fractures[100].

One way or another, it is fair to say that what Kellogg Speed (1879–1955), who organised the first fracture service at Cook County Hospital, Chicago, called 'the unsolved fracture' in 1935[101] has long been solved, as a technical problem, in one way or another, though not by bony union in more than half the cases, and that the real problems now are logistic – early operation and ambulation and intensive rehabilitation. Where these are not available, too many orthopaedic hospital beds are blocked by these patients even when their fractures themselves have been competently dealt with.

TOTAL REPLACEMENT OF THE HIP JOINT

We shall consider this subject in considerable detail, because it embodies all the problems inherent in the use of massive permanent endoprostheses and because it is a very striking success story based largely on the continuing exertions of two British surgeons. But first, we must go back quite a long way.

The idea of arthroplasty arose early in the 19th century, or even before, because of the many joints stiffened by pyogenic or tuberculous infection or by severe injury. Excisional arthroplasty in one form or another has never been entirely abandoned and is still used, especially in the Third World. It is discussed elsewhere. We refer here only to the two important aspects of *excision* of diseased joint surfaces and *interposition* of natural or synthetic materials.

We noted that, as far back as 1890, Gluck[13,14] replaced the hip joint (and also the knee) with ivory, a good idea woefully ahead of its time. Delbet replaced the femoral head in 1903[102] and Hey-Groves substituted an ivory ball and stem in 1922[103,104]. As to interposita, Hoffa in 1906[105], Hübscher[106] and others used silver, magnesium and zinc; and ivory had quite a vogue[107]. Others used celluloid and gutta percha, which caused irritation and reankylosis. Much of this work derived from the observation that even careful reshaping of the head and acetabulum by itself, which had been very thoroughly worked out by J B Murphy early in the century using male and female reamers, and by European surgeons for old unreduced congenital dislocation of the hip[108,109], was not often followed by good results and that even the good results did not last, so much so that some returned to the simple resection of the previous century[110]. Inorganic interposita were not successful in Murphy's hands. The use of free or flap grafts of autogenous tissue, which did give considerable success and persisted well into the 20th century, is referred to elsewhere.

During the second and third decades of this century, Smith-Petersen in Boston pursued the famous series of interposition studies which led to the evolution of mould arthroplasty of the arthritic hip joint[111]. Essentially, these essays consisted of removing the articular surface of the head and reshaping it with a reamer and covering it with a cup of synthetic material; the acetabulum was also reamed. In 1923 he used glass, in 1925 viscaloid, which proved a severe irritant, in 1933 pyrex glass and in 1937 bakelite, not arriving at the vitallium mould until 1938. All of these stages were faithfully recorded, but it was not until his experience with vitallium that he felt able to write definitively of 'Arthroplasty of the hip: a new method'[112].

What Smith-Petersen had originally intended was that, as the cup moved over the head and also within the acetubulum – for it was not intended to be firmly fixed – the underlying bone would undergo metaplasia into a new smooth fibrocartilage and that it would eventually be possible to remove the cup and leave a smooth gliding joint. Fibrocartilage could and did develop, sometimes impressively so, but somehow removal of the cup often proved impracticable or unnecessary and it was usually left in place. At special centres, in skilled hands and in younger patients, good results were obtainable[113,114]. But it was a costly method as prolonged hospitalisation and physiotherapy were required; in average hands periarticular fibrosis was severe, and even the substitution of materials such as plexiglass[115] or fixing the cup firmly to the femoral head[116] did little to help, especially as no type of cup could prevent necrosis and absorption of the neck if its blood-supply were compromised.

Some workers began to see the need to give the acetabulum its own prosthesis[117] but in general the mould arthroplasty as elaborated by Smith-Petersen and the reshaping with fascial interposition often successful in the hands of Willis Campbell[118] seemed to have reached their limits; and, in orthopaedics, operations that cannot be expected to succeed routinely in the hands of the average surgeon are not the answer to common and disabling diseases.

The solution had been anticipated even before the Second World War. In the 1930s, at the Middlesex Hospital in London, Philip Wiles performed six total hip replacements for the effects of Still's disease, using all-metal components – a cup screwed to the acetabulum and a femoral head connected by a stem in the neck to a plate bolted to the outer side of the shaft. Wiles was a surgeon of great courage

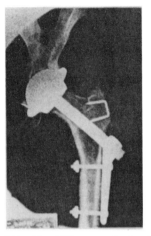

Figure 243   The Wiles prosthesis of 1938

and one wonders how much he was influenced by his chief, A S Blundell Bankart, the man who elucidated the pathology and repair of recurrent dislocation of the shoulder and did not hesitate to excise the acetabulum for tuberculosis of the hip joint. Wiles's pioneer procedure was halted by the war but later he was able to report considerable longterm success[119]. One of his bilateral cases had excellent function after 13 years.

In the third and fourth decades of the century, then, interposition arthroplasty began to yield to true replacement of the head or socket, or both. If Wiles's principle of total replacement was not immediately developed – though, as we shall see, there were those engaged in it – this was because of a dazzling new arrival. This took the form of the 'resection–reconstruction' for hip arthrosis introduced in 1946 by Robert and Jean Judet, in Paris, in which the femoral head was replaced by a knob of polymethylmethacrylate (PMMA) incorporating a plastic stem

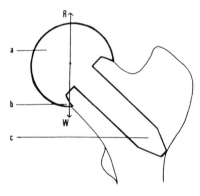

Figure 244   Judet prosthesis: (a) acrylic femoral head, (b) rim of head, (c) acrylic stem with metal core

passing axially down the neck[120]. This was a hemiarthroplasty, the acetabulum untouched, it was an easy operation, little or no special instrumentation was required, and the immediate results were stunningly successful; a new era seemed to have opened.

However, disappointment followed in a very few years, or even months. Pain and instability returned, and when these hips were reexplored it was found that the plastic surface had crazed or fissured, the stem broken or the entire assembly loosened. Although the Judets themselves had better results than most – because of better selection and attention to detail, and because the quality of the implants deteriorated with mass production, as happened with Sherman's plates – most surgeons had to remove the prostheses and effect the best possible salvage.

The reason for this failure was failure to conceive the relevant biomechanics. The plastic had previously only been used for dental implants in the 1930s and, briefly, for one form of cup arthroplasty[121]. The stresses it would have to withstand at the hip had not been properly analysed and the alignment in the bone not understood. There was an unwarranted trust in the mechanical properties of PMMA, but these were impaired by heat sterilisation and cooling while formaldehyde sterilisation gave rise to sinuses[122]. Attempts were made to remedy this by giving the stem a steel core and by a bewildering range of variations[123-127].

Without a consensus on the right step to take next, there was a temporary sense of bafflement. Nevertheless, as Scales pointed out later[128], the Judet operation had been a milestone in orthopaedic surgery and good results of replacement operations were to be expected eventually if the necessary preliminary research was made in animals and man into the relevant mechanical, chemical and biologic factors with accelerated wear tests. One good outcome was the acceptance of the intramedullary shaft. At first this retained the PMMA head[129-131] but the definitive solution tended to be a one-piece vitallium insert[95,96,123,132,133]. Some of these prostheses were very elaborate[134]. By 1954, the American Committee for the Supervision of Construction of Femoral Head Endoprostheses reported on nearly 40 different types. The metals were vitallium and various steels. The plastics included acrylic, polyethylene, nylon and polyamid. The metals behaved well in the tissues but the new plastics tended to be troublesome[135]. The Judets issued revised versions of their model[136].

Throughout this period, the two Englishmen – McKee in Norwich and Charnley in Manchester – had been reflecting on the problems of materials, construction and fixation. McKee had produced a prototype as far back as 1940[137] and continued entirely in metal. Charnley settled on a metal femoral component and a plastic acetabular replacement. But which plastic, and how were the components to be held in place?

To consider the first the matter of fixation, a wide range of tissue adhesives were already available (see p. 606). Of these PMMA had been in use as a self-curing acrylic cement in dentistry in the USA from the 1930s. Charnley had met this on a visit to California and it seemed ideal for anchoring the femoral stem. (The cup was originally *not* cemented, but fixed in the acetabulum by a spigot in hole mechanism.) There is some question whether it is a true adhesive or rather a grouting agent locking into the interstices of the spongiosa[138], but Charnley found it effectively eliminated slip between prosthesis and femur[139] and later wrote about it at length[140].

By good fortune, Charnley had engineering interests. He saw more clearly than most the need to understand the mechanical properties of the tissue to be replaced and the stresses imposed, the planes of movement, the properties and limitations of the implant, and the mechanisms of lubrication. He also saw that a method successful in a common disorder must allow for early discharge from hospital on grounds of cost.

Much discussion went on between Charnley, mechanical engineers and students of the new science of biomechanics[128,141,142]. McKee published his early trials of an all-metal system as early as 1951[143] but Charnley waited another decade before announcing 'Arthroplasty of the hip – a new operation'[144], an echo of Smith-Petersen. He would, in hindsight, have been entitled to say 'a new era', but the delay was due to his perfectionism in reaching a final form and even then he would not speak of longterm results for another decade[145]. At one stage he had tried simple reshaping of the femoral head and surfacing it with a polytetra-fluorethylene shell, but though the early results were good the head often necrosed and loosened so that total replacement proved essential. The original metal head was as large as that of a Moore's prosthesis ($1\frac{5}{8}''$ diameter) and was only later changed to the present small sphere which enabled him to use the much thicker cup that is steadier against rotation strains.

He also decided on an anterolateral approach with temporary resection of the great trochanter, wired back afterwards, the site of reattachment being variable to increase the moment of the abductors. Initially he used a plaster splint after operation and forbade weightbearing for some weeks, but these cautions were abandoned as it became clear that very early ambulation was possible and little or no aftertreatment required. The problem of the shape and composition of the femoral component having been early settled, there remained the matter of lubrication. He disparaged the lubricating properties of synovial fluid; they might even be the consequence rather than the cause of movement. Even if it did lubricate a normal joint, it would not necessarily lubricate a prosthesis. If friction between head and socket were too high, this could only loosen the hold of the stem in the shaft (which was what had happened in some of the Judet prostheses); surface-to-surface characteristics were all-important. Therefore he sought an ideal plastic for the cup of his 'low friction arthroplasty' and thought to have found it in teflon, until several years of wear proved to give rise to irritative particles and tissue fibrosis. He then changed to the thick polyethylene we now know.

Little need be said more about the low friction arthroplasty as such. Though it has been modified in innumerable ways, surgeons throughout the world continue to perform the operation exactly as Charnley postulated, though not always using the 'greenhouse' or 'theatre within the theatre' and operator's diving equipment he devised to reduce the risk of infection. Infection, which may occur during operation, or arise endogenously at any time thereafter, though uncommon, is the great hazard. By itself, as does loosening or fracture of one or other component, it may call for revision and replacement, always difficult, and sometimes the only solution is permanent removal of implanted material to leave a Girdlestone type of pseudarthrosis. Incorporation of antibiotics in the cement at the primary operation is thought helpful by some[146-148].

The operation can be done through other incisions and without removing the trochanter and with a variety of prostheses, but the essential principle is constant.

It remains the first really successful and widely applicable method of joint replacement and has conferred untold benefit.

We must add that the McKee metal-to-metal system, though equally effective, has not proved so popular. Also that, working on somewhat different lines and without cement, Ring devised a system in which the acetabulum was not reamed but a metal or later plastic cup fixed by a screw into the ilium[149]. Because the details of recent developments will be familiar, little more need be said on these. There has been a revival of interest in hip resurfacing[150-152], using eccentric shells with a metal cup cemented over a reshaped head and a polyethylene socket, but the problem of necrosis and collapse of the head will not go away.

The success of total hip replacement of course led to its application to the knee, ankle and other joints. Of knee replacement, recent and still in evolution, we need say only that the difficulties with a bulky implant so close to the skin make it a much less reliable procedure than hip replacement, as the multiplicity of methods implies. The biomechanical problems are difficult and the early designs had a five-year failure rate of 10–25 per cent. Despite great success at special centres, failure – usually due to sepsis – is still too common and may lead to amputation; the best outcome in such circumstances is arthrodesis, with severe shortening, but even this is often difficult to achieve[153]. Total ankle replacement is feasible enough[154] but the consensus is that, if the tarsal joints are mobile, little is to be gained from this surgical *tour de force*.

Of the metal replacement arthroplasties, though they exist for the shoulder (Neer)[155] and elbow[156], perhaps the most useful were the hinged finger joints for the rheumatoid hand devised by Flatt and others[157,158], but their stems were not fixed in the bone and they did not allow for the lateral and rotary movements of fine use, and they were expensive. Earlier essays at finger prostheses had been made, in 1959[159], but the best results so far have been with the flexible implants of Swanson[160,161] made of silicone rubber (see below).

We should add, in connection with hip and other endoprostheses, that ceramic materials have been used[162] and also porous or porous coated metal implants designed to further incorporation[163] though recent opinion is not wholly favourable[164].

It remains to be said, on the subject of joint replacement, that many of the problems cannot be predicted before operation and may not become apparent until the implant has been long in place. These include problems of stability, wear and tissue reaction. Wear products may prove irritant and a stable implant may become unstable if the bone stock undergoes resorption. More important, fundamentally, is that the massive implant is never really accepted or incorporated in the body; it is, at best, tolerated. Therefore there has been reluctance to do hip replacements in young patients for fear of longterm complications; nevertheless, brilliant results have been obtained by Arden and coworkers in older children and adolescents crippled by Still's disease[165,166]. Moreover, we are to consider, as Dr Johnson would have put it, that expectations change and that well within the professional lifetimes of many living orthopaedic surgeons, even in the West, arthrosis of the hip and similar ailments used to be suffered resignedly as a part of life, without a thought of cure. Even such a one as the late Sir George Pickering, Regius Professor of Medicine at Oxford, having undergone hip replacement and pleased to be relieved of his torment, nevertheless regretted it as an old friend and useful ally against life's demands.

Taking a long view, one may wonder whether joint replacement, though a brilliant tactical success, represents the true path of progress in orthopaedics or whether it represents a very specialised but temporary makeshift. Without decrying the enormous achievement of Charnley and his followers, this writer opines for the latter view and risks saying that a more fundamental knowledge of the biology of the cartilage cell, as discussed by Mankin[167], may lead to presently unconceived methods of preventing and treating chronic arthritis that will leave joint replacement as dead as the dinosaur.

MASSIVE ENDOPROSTHETIC REPLACEMENT AFTER LOCAL RESECTION OF BONY OR OSTEOARTICULAR SEGMENTS

We must now turn to the use of massive replacements of metal or plastic or both after extensive but local skeletal resections. As already noted, Péan in 1894 had written an essay on prosthetic measures intended to secure repair of the bony parts and suggested this as an alternative to disarticulation after major skeletal excisions. Pending the development of suitable material and techniques, little came of this until after World War II. The tendency was rather to seek repair in such cases by bony or osteoarticular grafts or heroic homogenous transplants (see p. 200). However, the matter could not remain in abeyance, for certainly in the case of locally extensive but nonmalignant lesions such as fibrous dysplasia of a long bone amputation was to be regretted if an alternative offered, and this was to be extended to tumours of low malignancy such as chondrosarcoma without evidence of metastasis. Some would go even further, 'There is no proven evidence that ablative surgery is superior to radical local surgery of bone tumors in the process of survival. When locally radical bone tumor resection is anatomically possible, such a procedure is advantageous ... For replacement of large defects, custom-made endoprostheses serve a useful purpose regarding limb function'[168].

Certainly, such prosthetic replacement of the upper arm after resection of a lesion of the scapula or humerus has the enormous advantage of saving function of the hand. Allografts (a convenient term for synthetic inserts) can also replace all or part of the end of a long bone, including the joint surface, after tumour excision[169] and can be combined, as can an intramedullary rod, with local bone grafts[170]. The same principle can be applied to local resection of malignancies at the hip or pelvis[171], tailoring the device to the individual patient, as did Austin Moore in 1942 after resection of an osteoclastoma of the upper femur[93,94].

To typify these endeavours, we may refer to the long programme at the Royal National Orthopaedic Hospital associated with the names of the late Jackson Burrows[172] and of J T Scales, a pioneer in biomechanics[173,174]. A fairly recent article reviews this work in terms of the proximal femur and acetabulum, which began with a polythene replacement of the upper two thirds of the femur in 1949[175,176]. Although the early implants of plastic remained satisfactory for many years, a change was soon made to metal – vitallium, pure titanium or, best, titanium alloy. These were initially attached to the lower femur by ensheathing plates and bolts but a move was soon made to an intramedullary stem plus cement[177], and a cup was placed in the acetabulum. The hazards included early dislocation or infection and late fracture or loosening, but the survival rate in terms of the prosthesis was much the same as for standard total hip replacement while patient survival in osteoclastoma or chondrosarcoma was as good as with alternative treatment, including amputation, and the limb was spared.

The method has been adapted to many parts of the skeleton – for benign and malignant tumours, for metastases and after failed joint replacements. The results are often brilliant but we must enter the same caveat as for hip replacement; the inserts are at best tolerated, and when we have learned to control malignancy by biologic means such heroic feats will be seen to have merely held the line.

PLASTICS

We have seen that rubber, ivory, inorganic materials and certain synthetics were already in use in orthopaedics in the 19th century and that Smith-Petersen tried various plastics in developing the mould arthroplasty. But the plastic revolution which began in the early 1900s with celluloid and bakelite did not take off until the 1930s with the synthesis of acetylene and ethylene polymers, while the urethanes and silicones emerged in the 50s.

Polymethylmethacrylate was an early polymer-based compound and was followed by polyethylene, polyethylene terephthalate, polytetrafluoroethylene, polyacrylonitrile, the polyamides, polyvinyl alcohol, polypropylene, the epoxy resins, polyurethanes, polyalkycyanoacrylates and many others. After a time it began to be possible to predict the requirements of a plastic implant and to synthesize the molecule accordingly, avoiding waste on unlikely starters[178].

The *silicones* are organic radicles attached to a silicon atom and then polymerised. The simplest polymer, dimethylpolysiloxane, is an oily liquid; this and its fellows can be gelled, and oxidation of the gels gives rubbers known as silastics. Liquids and gels are very stable, slippery and inert; the oils hold oxygen and the rubbers withstand bending indefinitely without fatigue fracture. The original enthusiasm has abated. Silicone oil is little used now for facial and breast contouring and its injection to lubricate arthritic joints also seems to have been abandoned, as has injection into the sole under callosities. Silastic sheet has been used to sheath sutured nerves and tendons to prevent adhesions[179], solid silicone as a pad over the bone-end in an amputation stump[180] and silastic rods have been inserted as temporary fillers after resecting damaged finger flexor tendons to create smooth tunnels for later tendon grafts.

However, current usage is largely restricted to:

(1) Swanson's flexible double-stemmed finger joint implants (see above),
(2) Replacement of excised carpal bones, especially the scaphoid and lunate[181], and
(3) As a 'spacer' after resection of the radial head or of the base of the proximal phalanx in hallux rigidus.

Silicone oil, as a nonwetting oxygen-rich medium, is sometimes used as a bath for dirty wounds or exercising injured hands[182].

Useful as they are in these limited fields, it would be difficult now to agree with

Helal, in 1969, that their clinical applications would provide answers to many previously insoluble problems[183].

ADHESIVES IN ORTHOPAEDIC SURGERY

This topic was well reviewed by Weber and Chapman in 1984[184] and by Mueller earlier[185]. The idea of an adhesive that would instantly glue tissues together and bond fractures without need of metal fixation has always been attractive. We recall Gluck, in 1890, hopefully using a 'cement' of pumice powder, plaster and glue to anchor his ivory hip and bone replacements. A practical bone-bonding, and preferably biodegradable, agent could fix small osteoarticular fragments and hold comminuted fractures in good position; and, in fact, PMMA has proved useful in trochanteric fractures[186] and pathologic fractures[187], but as an adjunct to metal osteosynthesis.

In 1931, Hedri's 'ossocol' – a mix of heterogeneous collagen and connective tissue proteins – proved too allergogenic[188]. In the 50s and after, epoxy resins were generally inadequate, incompatible, unabsorbed and impaired healing[189–192]. 'Ostamer', a polyurethane foam, was also nondegradable and gave rise to problems of infection, wound healing and nonunion[193]. In the late 60s and the 70s, the cyanoacrylates, which bond strongly to wet tissues, found favour with the Russians, who were enthusiastic over the early results[194,195]. This was used in the West as 'Biobond', but its breakdown products were toxic, at least one malignancy resulted, fracture nonunion was common and good reports rare.

Homogeneous human fibrin adhesives were used with moderate success at Oxford as far back as 1940 for the repair of peripheral nerves[196]. Its first experimental use in osteosynthesis was reported by Passl et al. 1976[197], using what was known in Germany as FKS (Fibrinklebesystem) composed of fibrin, thrombin, calcium and Factor XIII. It was tried clinically[198] but adhesion was poor and there was a risk of hepatitis, so it was used mainly to stick back small osteochondral fragments. The role of PMMA has been reviewed in the context of total hip replacement. It need only be added here that its use as the sole agent for bone fragment fixation is unsatisfactory, the rate of nonunion being too high[199]. However, it has proved valuable at many sites as an adjunct to other treatment and can, for instance, be employed as a filler after removal of a cervical intervertebral disc or around the cervical spinous processes after wire fixation[200].

REFERENCES

1. Billroth, T. (1866). *Die allgemeine chirurgische Pathologie und Therapie.* (Berlin, Georg Reimer)
2. Beauregard (1883). De la suture osseuse dans les fractures transversales de la rotule avec écartement. *Bull. et Mém. Soc. Chir. Paris,* **9**, 804
3. Mears, D.C. (1979). *Materials and Orthopaedic Surgery.* (Baltimore, Williams and Wilkins)
4. Hoeftman (1902). In *Verhandlungen der deutschen Gesellschaft für orthopädische Chirurgie.* (Stuttgart)
5. Galvani, A.L. (1791). De Viribus Electricitatis in Motu Musculari Commentarius.

Bonon. Sci. Art. Inst. Acad. Comm. Bologna, **7**, 363
6. Davy, H. (1824). *Phil. Trans. Roy. Soc.*, **114**, 151
7. Singer, C., Holmyard, E.J. and Hall, A.R. (eds.) (1954). *A History of Technology*, p. 375. (London, Oxford University Press)
8. Bell, B.A. (1804). *A System of Surgery*, p. 22. (New York, Penniman)
9. Levert, H.S. (1829). *Am. J. Med. Sci.*, **4**, 17
10. Chigot, P.L. and Moinet, P.H. (1972). The background of orthopaedics in France. *Clin. Orthop.*, **82**, 268
11. Venable, C.S. and Stuck, W.G. (1947). *The Internal Fixation of Fractures*, p. 5. (Springfield, Illinois, Charles C. Thomas)
12. Langenbeck, B. (1878). *Verh. d. dtsch. Ges. f. Chir.* (7th Congress), **1**, 92
13. Gluck, T. (1890). Die Invaginationsmethode der Osteo- und Arthroplastik. *Berl. klin. Wschr.*, **19**, 732
14. Gluck, T. (1891). *Arch. klin. Chir.*, **41**, 186 and 234
15. Zippel, J. and Meyer-Ralfs, M. (1975). Themistocles Gluck (1853–1942), Wegbereiter der endoprosthetik. *Z. Orthop.*, **113**, 134
16. Carnochan, J.M. (1860). *Arch. de Méd.*, 284
17. Gurlt, E. (1862). *Handbuch der Lehre von den Knochenbruchen*, p. 119. (Berlin)
18. Lente, F.D. (1850). Cases of ununited fractures treated by electricity. *N.Y. Med. J.*, **5**, 317
19. Wahl, M. (1883). Naht einer Patellefraktur. *Dtsch. med. Wschr.*, 18
20. Hansmann, H. (1886). *Verein Dtsch. Ges. f. Chir.*, **15**, 134
21. Koenig, F. (1907). *Langenbeck's Arch. klin. Chir.*, **76**, 23
22. Hadra, B.E. (1891). *Med. Times Register*, **22**, 423
23. Péan, J.E. (1894). Des moyens prosthétiques destinés à obtenir la réparation des parties osseuses. *Gaz. Hôp.* (*Paris*), **67**, 291
24. Lane, W.A. (1893). On the advantage of the steel screw in the treatment of ununited fractures. *Lancet*, **i**, 1500
25. Lane, W.A. (1894). *Trans. Clin. Soc. London*, **27**, 167
26. Lane, W.A. (1914). *The Operative Treatment of Fractures.* (London)
27. Sherman, W.D. (1912). *Surg. Gynaecol. Obstet.*, **14**, 629
28. Bechtol, C.H., Ferguson, A.B. and Laing, P.G. (1959). *Metals and Engineering in Bone and Joint Surgery.* (London, Baillière Tindall)
29. Cotton, F.J. (1912). *J. Am. Med. Assoc.*, **49**, 354
30. Lambotte, E. (1890). *Presse méd. Belge.*
31. Lambotte, A. (1909). *Presse méd. Belge.*, **17**, 321
32. Lambotte, A. (1913). *Chirurgie Opératoire des Fractures.* (Paris, Masson)
33. von Baeyer, H. (1909). *München. med. Wschr.*, **56**, 2416
34. von Baeyer, H. (1908). *Beitr. klin. Chir.*, **58**, 1
35. Hey-Groves, E.W. (1913). An experimental study of the operative treatment of fractures. *Brit. J. Surg.*, **1**, 438
36. Zierold, A.A. (1924). *Arch. Surg.*, **9**, 365
37. Speed, K. (1935). The unsolved fracture. *Surg. Gynaecol. Obstet.*, **60**, 341
38. Harris, R.I. (1938). Experiences with internal fixation in fresh fractures of the neck of the femur. *J. Bone Jt. Surg.*, **20**, 144
39. Paagaard, O. (1939). Some comments on complications occasioned by a rustless surgical nail. *Acta Chir. Scand.*, **82**, 475
40. Large, M. (1926). Krupp steel wire as a bone suture material. *Z. orthop. Chir.*, **47**, 250
41. Williams, D.F. and Roaf, R. (1973). *Implants in Surgery*, p. 10. (London, W.P. Saunders)
42. Cottrell, A.H. (1949). *Prog. Met. Phys.*, **1**, 77
43. Cottrell, A.H. (1953). *Prog. Met. Phys.*, **4**, 205

44. Rooker, G.D. and Wilkinson, J.D. (1980). Metal sensitivity in patients undergoing hip replacement. *J. Bone Jt. Surg.*, **62B**, 502
45. Danis, R. (1947). Théorie et Pratique de l'Ostéosynthèse. (Paris, Masson)
46. Cave, E.F. (1958). *Fractures and other injuries.* (Chicago Year Book Publications)
47. Key, J. (1932). Positive pressure in arthrodesis for tuberculosis of the knee joint. *South. Med. J.*, **25**, 909
48. Müller, M.E., Allgöwer, M. and Willenegger, H. (1965). *Techniques of Internal Fixation.* (Berlin, Springer-Verlag)
49. Charnley, J. (1953). *Compression Arthrodesis.* (Edinburgh, Livingstone)
50. Pittmann, W.W. and Perren, S.M. (1974). *Cortical Bone Healing After Internal Fixation and Infection.* (Berlin, Springer-Verlag)
51. Le Vay, D. (1957). *The Life of Hugh Owen Thomas*, p. 88. (Edinburgh, Livingstone)
52. Bassett, C.A.L. (1982). The development and application of pulsed electromagnetic fields (PEMF) for ununited fractures and arthrodeses. *Orthop. Clinics N. Am.*, **15**, 61
53. Küntscher, G. (1940). Die Marknägelung von Knochenbruchen. *Arch. klin. Chir.*, **200**, 443
54. Küntscher, G. (1967). *The Practice of Intramedullary Nailing.* (Springerfield, Illinois, Charles C. Thomas)
55. Hey-Groves, E.W. (1916). *On Modern Methods of Treating Fractures.* (Bristol)
56. Müller-Meernach (1933). *Zbl. Chir.*, **60**, 29
57. Lambrinudi, C. (1940). Intramedullary Kirschner Wires in the treatment of fractures. *Proc. Roy. Soc. Med.*, **33**, 153
58. Le Vay, D. (1950). *J. Bone Jt. Surg.*, **32B**, 694
59. Gross, H.P. and Glebink, R.R. (1967). Blind nailing of the femur. *J. Trauma*, **7**, 591
60. Rothwell, A.G. (1982). Closed Küntscher nailing for comminuted femoral shaft fractures. *J. Bone Jt. Surg.*, **64B**, 12
61. Maatz, R. (1944). Erfahrungen der Kieler Klinik bei der Marknagelung von Knochenbruchen. *Bruns. Beitr. Z. Klin. Chir.*, **1**, 175
62. Rush, L.V. (1955). *Atlas of Rush Pin Techniques.* (Meridian, Miss., Berivan)
63. Hackethal, K.H. (1961). *Die Bundel-Nagelung.* (Berlin, Springer-Verlag)
64. Durbin, R.A., Gottesman, M.D. and Saunders, K.C. (1983). Hackethal stacked nailing of humeral shaft fractures. *Clin. Orthop.*, **179**, 168
65. Ender, J. and Simon-Weidner, R. (1970). Die Fixierung der trochantären Brüche mit runden elastischen Condylennägeln. *Acta. Chir. Austriaca*, **2**, 40
66. McKibbin, B. (1883). New materials in orthopaedics: carbon fibre. In: McKibbin, B. (ed.) *Recent Advances in Orthopaedics.* (Edinburgh and London, Churchill Livingstone)
67. Jenkins, D.H.R. and McKibbin, B. (1980). The role of flexible carbon fibre implants as tendon and ligament substitutes in clinical practice. *J. Bone Jt. Surg.*, **62B**, 497
68. Klawitter, J.J. *et al.* (1976). Tissue ingrowth and mechanical locking for anchorage of prostheses in the locomotor system. In *Artificial Hip and Knee Joint Technology.* (Berlin, Springer)
69. Boeckmann, E. and Gillette, A. (1898). *Trans. Am. Orth. Assoc.*, **11**, 241
70. Davis, G.G. (1900). *Trans. Am. Orth. Assoc.*, **13**, 134
71. Murphy, J.B. (1913). Old ununited fractures of anatomic neck of femur. *Southern. Med. J.*, **6**, 387
72. Preston, M.E. (1914). New appliances for the internal fixation of fractures of the femoral neck. *Surg. Gynaecol. Obstet.*, **18**, 260
73. Hey-Groves, E.W. (1926). Some contributions to the reconstructive surgery of the hip. *Brit. J. Surg.*, **14**, 486

74. Martin, E.D. and King, A.C. (1922). Preliminary report of a new method of treating fractures of the neck of the femur. *N. Orleans Med. Surg. J.*, **75**, 710
75. Smith-Petersen, M.N., Cave, E. and Vangorder, G.W. (1931). *Arch. Surg.*, **23**, 715
76. Johansson, S. (1932). *Acta Chir. Scand.*, **3**, 262
77. Westcott, H.H. (1932). Preliminary report of a method of internal fixation of transcervical fractures of the neck of the femur in the aged. *Virginia Med. Monthly*, **59**, 197
78. Smith-Petersen, M.N. (1937). Treatment of fractures of the neck of the femur by internal fixation. *Surg. Gynaecol. Obstet.*, **64**, 287
79. Leadbetter, G.W. (1933). Treatment for fracture of the neck of the femur. *J. Bone Jt. Surg.*, **15**, 931
80. Hillebrand, H. (1933). Treatment of fractures of neck of femur by the Hotz femoropelvic screwing method. *Beitr. klin. Chir.*, **157**, 266
81. Thornton, L. (1937). The treatment of trochanteric fractures: two new methods. *Piedmont Hosp. Bull.*, **10**, 21
82. Garden, R.S. (1961). Low angle fixation in fractures of the femoral neck. *J. Bone Jt. Surg.*, **43B**, 647
83. Evans, E.M. (1949). The treatment of trochanteric fractures of the femur. *J. Bone Jt. Surg.*, **31B**, 190
84. Massie, M.E. (1958). Functional fixation of femoral neck fractures: telescoping nail technic. *Clin. Orthop.*, **12**, 230
85. McMurray, T.P. (1939). Osteoarthritis of the hip. *J. Bone Jt. Surg.*, **21**, 1
86. Anderson, R. (1934). An automatic method of treatment for fractures of the tibia and fibula. *Surg. Gynaecol. Obstet.*, **58**, 639
87. Hoffmann, R. (1954). Osteotaxis. *Acta Chir. Scand.*, **107**, 72
88. Adrey, J. (1970). *Le Fixateur Externe d'Hoffmann.* (Paris)
89. Anderson, R. and O'Neil, G. (1944). *Clin. Orthop.*, **78**, 434
90. Harrington, P.R. (1962). The treatment of scoliosis. *J. Bone Jt. Surg.*, **44A**, 591
91. Hirsch, C. (1971). Harrington rods in scoliosis. In: Proceedings of the *Symposium on Operative Treatment of Scoliosis*, Amsterdam
92. Dwyer, A.F. (1969). *Clin. Orthop.*, **62**, 192
93. Moore, A.T. (1942). *Recorder of Columbia Med. Soc. (S. Carolina)*, **6**, 12
94. Moore, A.T. and Bohlman, H.R. (1943). Metal hip joint: a case report. *J. Bone Jt. Surg.*, **25**, 688
95. Moore, A.T. (1957). The self-locking metal hip prosthesis. *J. Bone Jt. Surg.*, **39A**, 811
96. Thompson, F.R. (1952). Vitallium intramedullary hip prosthesis; preliminary report. *N.Y. J. Med.*, **52**, 3011
97. Thompson, F.R. (1954). Two and a half years' experience with a vitallium intramedullary hip prosthesis. *J. Bone Jt. Surg.*, **36A**, 489
98. Chapchal, G. (1950). *Z. Orthop.*, **79**, 417
99. Long, J.W. and Knight, W. (1980). Bateman UPF prosthesis in fractures of the femoral neck. *Clin. Orthop.*, **152**, 198
100. Campbell (1987). *Operative Orthopaedics*, Vol. 3, p. 1770 (7th edn.). (St. Louis, CV Mosby)
101. Speed, K. (1935). The unsolved fracture. *Surg. Gynaecol. Obstet.*, **60**, 341
102. Delbet, P. (1903). *Bull. Soc. Nat. Chir.*, **24**, 1172
103. Hey-Groves, E.W. (1923). Arthroplasty. *Brit. J. Surg.*, **11**, 234
104. Hey-Groves, E.W. (1927). Some contributions to the reconstructive surgery of the hip. *Brit. J. Surg.*, **14**, 486
105. Hoffa, A. (1925). *Lehrbuch der Orthopädischen Chirurgie*, 7th edn. (Stuttgart, Enke)

106. MacAusland, R.W. (1924). Arthroplasty of the hip. In *6th Congress Society of International Chirurgerie,* Vol. 1, Brussels
107. König, F. (1913). Über die Implantation von Elfenbein zum Ersatz von Knochen und Gelenkenden. *Bruns' Beitr. klin. Chir.,* **85**, 613
108. Ewens, J. (1897. *Trans. Brit. Orth. Soc.,* **2**, 16
109. Margary, F. (1884). Cura operativa della lussazione congenita dell'anca. *Archiv. Ortop.,* **1**, 381
110. Allison, M. and Brooks, B. (1913). The mobilisation of ankylosed joints. *Surg. Gynaecol. Obstet.,* **17**, 645
111. Smith-Petersen, M.N. (1948). Evolution of the mould arthroplasty of the hip joint. *J. Bone Jt. Surg.,* **30B**, 59
112. Smith-Petersen, M.N. (1939). Arthroplasty of the hip. A new method. *J. Bone Jt. Surg.,* **21**, 269
113. Aufranc, C.E. (1957). Constructive hip surgery with the vitallium mould. A report of 1000 cases. *J. Bone Jt. Surg.,* **39**, 237
114. Law, L.A. (1962). *J. Bone Jt. Surg.,* **44A**, 1497
115. Lange, M. (1951). *Orthopädische und Chirurgische Operationslehre.* (Münich)
116. Adams, J.C. (1953). A reconsideration of cup arthroplasty of the hip. *J. Bone Jt. Surg.,* **35B**, 199
117. Urist, M.R. (1957). The principles of the hip-socket arthroplasty. *J. Bone Jt. Surg.,* **39A**, 786
118. Campbell, W.C. (1939). *Operative Orthopaedics.* (St. Louis, C.V. Mosby)
119. Wiles, P. (1958). The surgery of the osteoarthritic hip. *Brit. J. Surg.,* **45**, 488
120. Judet, J. and Judet, R. (1952). *Résection-reconstruction de la hanche: arthroplastie par prothèse acrylique.* (Paris, Expansion Scientifique Française)
121. Harmon, P.H. (1943). Arthroplasty of the hip joint for osteoarthritis using foreign body cups of plastic. *Surg. Gynaecol. Obstet.,* **76**, 347
122. Scales, J.T. and Zarek, J.M. (1954). Biomechanical problems of the original Judet prosthesis. *Br. Med. J.,* **1**, 1007
123. Timmermans, L. (1956). Experimenti di artroplastica dell'anca con trapanto articolare mettalico totale. *Clin. Orthop.,* **8**, 252
124. Anderson, R. (1952). Femoral head. (Seattle, Tower Company Bulletin)
125. Marino-Zuco, C. (1956). Les prothèses acryliques dans la chirurgie de la hanche. *Rev. Chir. Orthop.,* **42**, 314
126. Movin, R. (1954). Judet's arthroplastic hip operation (Comparative pressure tests with a new angled prosthesis). *Dan. Med. Bull.,* **1**, 55
127. Valls, J. (1952). A new prosthesis for arthroplasty of the hip. *J. Bone Jt. Surg.,* **34B**, 308
128. Scales, J.T. (1967). Arthroplasty of the hip using foreign materials: a history. In *Lubrication and wear in living and artificial human joints, paper No. 13, Proceedings of the Institute of Mechanical Engineers,* London
129. Gosset, J. (1950). Arthroplastie de la hanche par plastic acrylique cervico-capitale. *Sem. Hop. Paris,* **26**, 4494
130. Rettig, H. (1952). Die Hüft arthroplastik mit Spezialprothese. *Z. Orthop.,* **82**, 290
131. D'Aubigné, R.M. (1966). *10th Congress SICOT,* Paris
132. De Palma, A.F. (1951). An improved type of arthroplasty of the hip joint. *J. Bone Jt. Surg.,* **33A**, 437
133. Güntz, E. (1952). Die Behandlung der Hüftgelenksarthrose. Zugleich ein Beitrag zur Verwendung von Metallprothesen beim Kopf-Hals-Schwind. *Z. Orthop.,* **82**, 28
134. Lippmann, R.K. (1957). The transfixion hip prosthesis. *J. Bone Jt. Surg.,* **39A**, 759

135. Contzen, H. (1966). Der alloplastische Ersatz von Geweben und Organteiles mit Kunststofformen. *Arbeitsmed. Sozialmed. Arbeitshyg.*, **1**, 126
136. Judet, J. (1962). Nouvelles prothèses fémorales brevetées. Paris. Drapier
137. McKee, G.R. (1970). *Clin. Orthop.*, **72**, 85
138. Wiltse, L.L. *et al.* (1957). *J. Bone Jt. Surg.*, **39A**, 961
139. Charnley, J. and Kettlewell, J. (1965). The elimination of slip between prosthesis and femur. *J. Bone Jt. Surg.*, **47B**, 56
140. Charnley, J. (1970). *Acrylic Cement in Orthopaedic Surgery.* (London, Livingstone)
141. Scales, J.T., Duff-Barclay, I. and Burrows, H.J. (1964). In *Biomechanics and Related Bioengineering Topics*, Proceedings of a Symposium held at Glasgow in September, p. 205
142. Charnley, J. (1967). Factors in the design of an artificial hip joint. In Lubrication and wear in living and artificial human joints, *Proceedings of the Institute of Mechanical Engineers*, London, pp. 104–11
143. McKee, G.R. (1951). Artificial hip joint. *J. Bone Jt. Surg.*, **33B**, 465
144. Charnley, J. (1961). Arthroplasty of the hip – a new operation. *Lancet*, **ii**, 1129
145. Charnley, J. (1972). The long term results of low-friction arthroplasty of the hip performed as a primary intervention. *J. Bone Jt. Surg.*, **54B**, 61
146. Buchholz, H.W. and Engelbrecht, H. (1970). Uber die Depotwirkung einiger Antibiotica bei Vermischung mit den Kunstharz Palacos. *Chirurg.*, **41**, 511
147. Buchholz, H.W. and Gartman, H.D. (1972). Infektionsprophylaxe und operative Behandlung der schleichender tiefen Infektion bei der totale Endoprothese. *Chirurg.*, **43**, 446
148. Hughes, S., Field, C.A., Kennedy, M.R.K. and Dasg, C.H. (1979). Cephalosporins in bone cement. *J. Bone Jt. Surg.*, **61B**, 96
149. Ring, P.A. (1978). Five to 14 year interim results of uncemented total hip arthroplasty. *Clin. Orthop.*, **137**, 87
150. Amstutz, H.C. *et al.* (1981). Surface replacement of the hip with the THARIES system. *J. Bone Jt. Surg.*, **63A**, 1069
151. Freeman, M.A.R. *et al.* (1978). Cemented double cup arthroplasty of the hip. *Clin. Orthop.*, **134**, 45
152. Head, V.C. (1981). Wagner surface replacement arthroplasty of the hip. *J. Bone Jt. Surg.*, **63A**, 420
153. Knutson, K., Hovelius, L., Lundstrand, A. and Lidgren, L. (1984). Arthrodesis after failed knee arthroplasty. *Clin. Orthop.*, **191**, 202
154. Newton, S.E. (1975). Total ankle replacement: an alternative to ankle fusion. *J. Bone Jt. Surg.*, **57A**, 1033
155. Neer, C.S. *et al.* (1977). Total shoulder replacement: a preliminary report (abstract). *Orthop. Trans.*, **1**, 244
156. Dee, R. (1972). Total replacement of elbow joint in rheumatoid arthritis. *J. Bone Jt. Surgery*, **54B**, 88
157. Flatt, A.E. (1961). Restoration of rheumatoid finger joint function. *J. Bone Jt. Surg.*, **43A**, 753
158. Flatt, A.E. (1974). *The Care of the Rheumatoid Hand.* (St Louis, C V Mosby)
159. Brannon, E.W. and Klein, G. (1959). Experience with a finger joint prosthesis. *J. Bone Jt. Surg.*, **41A**, 87
160. Swanson, A.B. (1968). Silicone rubber implants for replacement of arthritic or destroyed joints in the hand. *Surg. Clinics N. Am.*, **48**, 1133
161. Swanson, A.B. (1973). *Flexible Implant Resection Arthroplasty in the Hand and Extremities.* (St Louis, C V Mosby)
162. Hulbert, S.F. *et al.* (1970). Potential of ceramic materials as permanently implantable skeletal prostheses. *J. Biomed. Mater. Research*, **4**, 433

163. Hahn, H. and Palich, W. (1970). Preliminary evaluation of porous metal surfaced tantalum for orthopaedic implants. *J. Biomed. Mater. Res.*, **4**, 571
164. Haddad, R.J., Cook, S.D. and Thomas, K.A. (1987). *J. Bone Jt. Surgery*, **69A**, 1459
165. Arden, G.P., Harrison, S.H. and Ansell, B.M. (1970). *Brit. Med. J.*, **4**, 604
166. Arden, G.P., Taylor, A.R. and Ansell, B.M. (1970). *Ann. Rheum. Dis.*, **29**, 1
167. Mankin, H.J. (1983). Orthopaedics in 2013: A prospection. *J. Bone Jt. Surgery*, **65A**, 1190
168. Nilsonne, V. (1984). Limb-preserving radical surgery for malignant bone tumors. *Clin. Orthop.*, **191**, 21
169. Parrish, F.F. (1973). Allograft replacement of all or part of the end of a long bone following excision of a tumor. *J. Bone Jt. Surg.*, **55A**, 1
170. Enneking, W.F. and Shirley, P.D. (1977). Resection–arthrodesis for malignant and potentially malignant lesions about the knee using an intramedullary rod and local bone grafts. *J. Bone Jt. Surg.*, **59A**, 223
171. Enneking, W.F. (1966). Local resection of malignant lesions of the hip and pelvis. *J. Bone Jt. Surg.*, **48A**, 991
172. Burrows, H.J. (1968). Major prosthetic replacement of bone: lessons learned in 17 years. *J. Bone Jt. Surg.*, **50B**, 225
173. Scales, J.T. (1979). Aspects of major bone and joint replacement and its cost effectiveness. In Kenedi, R.M., Paul, J.P. and Hughes, J. (eds.) *Disability*. (London, Macmillan)
174. Scales, J.T. (1979). *30 years' experience of major bone and joint replacement*. Report to the Department of Health and Social Security. London, July
175. Dobbs, H.S., Scales, J.T., Wilson, J.N., Kemp, H.B.S., Burrows, H.J. and Sneath, R.S. (1981). Endoprosthetic replacement of the proximal femur and acetabulum. *J. Bone Jt. Surg.*, **53B**, 219.
176. Wilson, P.D. and Lance, E.M. (1973). Surgical reconstruction of the skeleton following segmental resection for bone tumours. *Instruction Course lectures, Amer. Acad. Orth. Surg.*, Vol. XVIII 1962–69. p. 45. (St. Louis, C.V. Mosby)
177. Seddon, H.J. and Scales, J.T. (1949). A polythene substitute for the upper two thirds of the shaft of the femur. *Lancet*, **ii**, 795
178. Kranzberg, M. and Purcell, W. (eds.) (1967). *Technology in Western Civilisation*, p. 183. (London, Oxford University Press)
179. Ashley, F. *et al.* (1967). *Plastic Reconstr. Surg.*, **39**, 411
180. Swanson, A.B. (1966). Interclinic Information Bull., **5**, 1
181. Stork, H.H., Zornel, N.P. and Ashworth, C.R. (1981). Use of a hand-carved silicone-rubber spacer for advanced Kienböck's disease. *J. Bone Jt. Surgery*, **63A**, 359
182. Helal, B., Chapman, R., Ellis, M. and Gifford, D. (1982). The use of silicone oil for mobilisation of the hand. *J. Bone Jt. Surg.*, **64B**, 67
183. Helal, B. (1969). In Apley, A.G. (ed.) *Recent Advances in Orthopaedics*. (London, Churchill)
184. Weber, S.C. and Chapman, M.W. (1984). Adhesives in orthopaedic surgery. *Clin. Orthop.*, **191**, 249
185. Mueller, M.E. (1962). Die Verwendung von Kunstharzen in der Knochenchirurgie. *Arch. Orthop. Unfall.-Chir.*, **64**, 513
186. Muhr, C., Tscherne, H. and Thomas, R. (1979). Comminuted trochanteric femoral fractures in geriatric patients: The results of 231 cases treated with internal fixation and acrylic cement. *Clin. Orthop.*, **138**, 41
187. Sim, F.H., Daugherty, T.W. and Ivins, J.C. (1974). The adjunctive use of methylmetacrylate in fixation of pathological fractures. *J. Bone Jt. Surg.*, **56A**, 40
188. Hedri, W. (1931). Ein neues Prinzip der Osteosynthese. *Arch. Klin. Chir.*, **167**,

145

189. Golovin, G.V. (1956). Frakturfixierung mit Kunststoff. *Vestb. Khir.*, **77**, 125
190. Block, B. (1958). Bonding of fractures by plastic adhesives. *J. Bone Jt. Surg.*, **40A**, 804
191. Rietz, K.A. (1964). Polymer osteosynthesis. *Acta Chir. Scand.*, **128**, 387
192. Meyer, G. *et al.* (1979). Bone-bonding through bioadhesives, recent status. *Biomater. Med. Devices Artif. Organs*, **7**, 55
193. Mandarino, M.P. and Salvatore, J.E. (1959). Polyurethane polymer: its use in fractures and diseased bone. *Am. J. Surg.*, **97**, 442
194. Tkachenko, S.S. and Rurski, V.V. (1969). Osteosynthesis with methylmethacrylate and cyanoacrylate adhesives. *Vestn. Khir.*, **103**, 135
195. Movshovich, I.A. *et al.* (1976). Experimental union of bony tissue with cyacrin. *Eksp. Khir. Anestezol.*, **6**, 61
196. Young, J.Z. and Medawar, P.B. (1940). Fibrin suture of peripheral nerves. *Lancet*, **ii**, 126
197. Passl, R. *et al.* (1976). Die Homologe Reine Gelenkknorpeltransplantation im Tierexperiment. *Arch. Ortho-Unfall. Chir.*, **86**, 243
198. Bosch, P. (1981). Die Fibrinspongiosaplastik. *Wien. klin. Wschr.* (Suppl.) **93**, 1
199. Enis, J.E., McCollough, N.C. and Cooper, J.S. (1974). Effects of methylmethacrylate in osteosynthesis. *Clin. Orthop.*, **105**, 283
200. Kristaps, J.K., Southwick, W.O. and Keller, J.K. (1976). Stabilization of the spine using methylmethacrylate. *J. Bone Jt. Surg.*, **58A**, 738
201. Böstrom, O. *et al.* (1987). Biodegradable internal fixation for malleolar fractures. *J. Bone Jt. Surg.*, **69B**, 615.

Much of the material used in this survey has been derived from the following: Williams, D.F. and Roaf, R., *Implants in Surgery.*, W.B. Saunders 1973. Mears, D.C., *Materials and Orthopaedic Surgery*, Williams and Wilkins, Baltimore 1979

Section 4

The Turn of the Century

CHAPTER 33

1900: The Turn of the Century

A conspectus of activities in the orthopaedic world and around the commencement of the 20th century shows how much had already been achieved (a quite surprising amount for those who may think these were days of darkness), whither endeavour (sometimes misconceived) was striving, and the historical links with past and modern practice.

The onlooker is struck by the *repetitiveness* of orthopaedic history, how the same problems recur and resist the boldest of attacks until the necessary materials and techniques arrive on the scene. He will also see surgeons making the same mistakes until led into new paths, swept by often misguided enthusiasms, loquacious, itinerant, exhibitionist, often cantankerous. But he cannot fail to be impressed by the quite extraordinary drive manifested in Europe and America to solve the great problems of the day, whether these were of hip surgery or paralysis or lesions of tendons and nerves, a drive that may well have been fuelled in many cases by egoism or ambition, but also by disinterested devotion (one thinks of Putti and Robert Jones) and which constituted an often confused but generally forward movement in the struggle against crippling disease.

In 1900, the 14th session of the American Orthopedic Association convened in Washington. The Association was the first nationally affiliated group of orthopaedic surgeons in any country. It had been founded in 1887, with P Gibney as its first President. He had been succeeded by, among others, Newton M Shaffer, E H Bradford, De Forest Willard, John Ridlon, Royal Whitman, R W Lovett and, at this 14th session, Arthur G Gillette. Ridlon was the Secretary (and power behind the scenes), Lovett and Joel Goldthwait were nominees on the executive committee from the Congress of American Physicians and Surgeons, and 51 members were listed. The Honorary Members included William Adams of the Royal National Orthopaedic Hospital in London, O Lannelongue of the *Hôpital Trousseau* in Paris, William Macewen, Professor of Surgery in Glasgow, Leopold Ollier of Lyon and Lewis A Sayre, Professor of Orthopaedic Surgery at Bellevue Hospital Medical College in New York.

Five Honorary Members had died; they included William Detmold, C Fayette Taylor and the great William John Little of London, who had been elected in 1889.

The list of Corresponding Members is a roll-call of the great orthopaedic surgeons of Europe. They included M Bilhaut, editor of the *Annales d'Orthopédie et de Chirurgie Pratique* of Paris, Bernard Brodhurst, Senior Surgeon of the Royal Orthopaedic Hospital in London, Julius Dollinger, professor of orthopaedics at Buda-Pest, A Hoffa, Privatdozent in surgery at Würzburg University, Robert Jones of the Royal Southern Hospital, Liverpool, E Kirmisson, surgeon at the *Hôpital des Enfants Assistés*, Paris, Sigfried Levy, surgeon to the Society for the Relief of Crippled and Mutilated Children, Copenhagen, Ernest Muirhead Little of the Royal National Orthopaedic Hospital, Adolf Lorenz of Vienna, Howard Marsh, assistant surgeon at St Bartholomew's Hospital in London and surgeon to the Hospital for Sick Children, Pietro Panzeri, director of the *Istituto dei Rachitici*, Milan, Alfred H Tubby of the Westminster and National Orthopaedic Hospitals in London, Oscar Vulpius, lecturer in orthopaedic surgery and director of the *Orthopädische Heilanstalt* at Heidelberg, and Noble Smith, senior surgeon at London's City Orthopaedic Hospital.

Two Corresponding Members had died, both from the (then) British Isles; Hugh Owen Thomas, of Liverpool, elected in 1890, a year before his death, and Nicholas Grattan of Cork. Of Thomas we speak at length elsewhere. Of Grattan, the 1897 President of the AOA, Samuel Ketch, said that 'as far as we know, he is the only surgeon in Ireland who has made a specialty of orthopaedic surgery'. (The Irish–American link antedated the foundation of the Association. Sayre had demonstrated his suspension plaster jacket in Cork in 1877 – the plaster had not set very well, which Sayre blamed on the dampness of the climate, 'which prevents the plaster from setting so soon as with us', and Grattan had adopted it, though acknowledging the risks when he sometimes first extended his children with Pott's disease over chairs, and preferring not to continue with the jacket too long for nontuberculous lateral curvature[1].)

At Washington in 1900 the incoming President was Harry M Sherman of San Francisco. In his address[2], he pointed out that, of the 76 medical colleges in the USA, only 38 were teaching orthopaedic surgery as such, i.e. only half the American medical schools thought orthopaedic teaching worthy of mention in their prospectuses (the only less regarded speciality was genitourinary surgery, the highest was gynaecology) 'It must be because the general surgeon still considers that genitourinary surgery is his own, just as, in many instances, he thinks that orthopedic surgery is his own, and continues to practice each specialty as a part of general practice.'

However, the picture had vastly improved. Before 1887, only six schools had taught orthopaedics: Bellevue in New York (Sayre), Detroit, Illinois, Western Pennsylvania, St Louis (Bauer) and Iowa. Rush Medical College and the University of California had had orthopaedic professors but the chairs were now vacant. Between 1887 and 1900, 17 institutions initiated or resumed teaching and newly-founded institutions seem to have done so from the start. Of the Association's 51 active members in 1900, 26 were into teaching and were responsible for 60 per cent of all orthopaedic instruction in the country. Teaching, said Sherman, was important in relation to the child, 'because the acts committed on him when he is helpless and young reach out and affect him when he is neither ... the child has to be contented or discontented for all his life with the result of the orthopaedist's work.'

At this meeting, Abel Mix Phelps[3] advocated operation for all joint abscesses, tuberculous or not, 'No surgeon of any reputation would ever think of trusting a case of osteomyelitis or tubercular abscess to nature.' Joel Goldthwait, reporting 38 operations for non-tuberculous conditions of the knee-joint[4], said his object was 'to remove a dread which many surgeons seem to have of opening the knee-joint.' Surgeons were more fearful of opening a joint than the skull or abdomen, but arthrotomy and biopsy were often essential to diagnosis, and to prevent rheumatoid disease from being treated as tuberculosis. Nine of his cases were medial meniscus tears. Two were stitched back, but in the others the injured portion was removed, 'I am sure this is the best operation.' 'Synovial fringes' were often regarded as a clinical entity, but sound more like arthrosis. (They have, possibly, been revalidated since by arthroscopy.)

John Ridlon reported 35 cases of forcible correction of spinal deformity in Pott's disease (see Calot, p. 266), also in 'rheumatic disease' and rickets, using manual traction at the head and heels and often as much force on the gibbus as he could exert with both hands[5]. 'There was almost always some crunching of the bones, which was startling at first.' There was no immediate mortality, and no paraplegia; in fact, he did it *for* paraplegia, and with benefit, subsequently using a frame or plaster. (Earlier, Bradford and others had done this even when the spine was ankylosed. The method was, in fact, as old as Hippocrates, but never really became popular except in France.) Goldthwait advised against plaster jackets in hyperextension because, of its nature, the correction of tuberculous destruction could not be maintained. The general opinion was against Ridlon.

Shortening of the limb with a tuberculous hip was recognized as due to retardation of the epiphyseal growth and to reflex trophic factors. Bradford[6] advocated open operation for congenital dislocation of the hip because of capsular obstruction and noted that, in most cases, anteversion 'a twist of the neck in the femur' required subsequent osteotomy at the middle or lower third of the shaft. All of his own cases had relapsed after the 'bloodless' method of reduction.

Gwilym G Davis was using open operation for old ununited intracapsular femoral neck fractures[7], freshening the bone ends and fixing them with steel pins or ivory pegs. He referred to a paper by Boeckmann and Gillette, who made a lateral approach, sectioning the trochanter, and used an ivory peg for the neck and another to reattach the trochanter. Sayre had used a gimlet and nuts. There were lengthy papers by Phelps and others on the mechanism and treatment of scoliosis, as much a plague of orthopaedic surgeons in the late 19th century as it has been till more recent times. And tendon transplantations were now coming into vogue[8].

We may now look a little further back. Foundation of the Association had initially been discussed at Shaeffer's house in New York on 29th January

1887. Gibney and Shaffer had independently planned such an organization but agreed to merge, with Gibney as the original Chairman and Lovett as Secretary, and the first Annual Meeting was in New York on 15–16th June of the same year, its *Transactions* appearing as Volume I in 1889 in a private edition of 500 copies printed by L P Kellogg and Son, of 15 Milk Street, Boston.

The 35 initial Members included Buckminster Brown and E H Bradford (Boston), Virgil P Gibney (New York), Benjamin Lee (Philadelphia), R W Lovett (Boston), John Ridlon (New York), Lewis Sayre (New York), Newton M Shaffer (New York), C Fayette Taylor (New York) and De Forest Willard (Philadelphia). Of the 35, 19 were from New York or its environs, four from Boston and five from Philadelphia. There was only one Corresponding Member; Bernard Roth, of London.

At the 1887 meeting, Sayre reported excision of the femoral head in a boy of ten for what seems to have been suppurative arthritis[9], and the discussion referred to the difficulty of eradicating the acetabular component of the disease. (It is possible that this had been achieved by Schede and Volkmann; it was certainly being done for tuberculosis by Blundell Bankart at the Middlesex Hospital in London in the 1930s.)

The Second Annual Meeting was in Washington in 1888. Gibney[10] was treating club-feet with Thomas's wrench, but he was also operating, 'I think there is not a single member of this Association ... that is afraid to divide the tendo Achillis in a case of congenital club-foot and get the greatest possible amount of extension and separation of the ends of the tendon ... The foot, you know, is wonderfully subservient to the surgeon.' In a long and thoughtful paper, Bradford reported on the treatment of 101 cases of congenital equinovarus[11]. He stressed the primacy of mechanical treatment by splintage, whether operation was done or not, 'Tenotomy without the aid of a thorough mechanical treatment is evidently irrational and useless.' Deliberate overcorrection led to efficient retention ('half-cures are no cures'), and though he was conservative with young children, tenotomy and bone operations saved time in older patients, though tarsal resection or osteotomy of the talus was reserved for the severest cases where other methods had not achieved full success. 'In no branch of surgery can a cure be more confidently predicted than in the treatment of club-foot, and in few surgical undertakings do half-measures occasion greater annoyance.' T G Morton[12] was using vigorous correction by manipulation under ether, with the application of the 'tarsoclast', using a strong footplate with a lateral arm that was an evolutionary successor of Venel's splint and a predecessor of Denis Browne's, but much more forcible. For adult deformity, he excised the cuboid or did a wedge tarsectomy.

There was a paper on excision of the knee-joint, by A J Steele[13], for either tuberculosis or vicious ankylosis, the bone-ends sometimes being transfixed with bone-pegs or removable steel nails. 'The results of excision of the knee in this country have been better than in England. Probably our material is better, less constitutional taint and closer antiseptic precautions.'

George W Ryan, of Ohio, gave what may have been the first clinical account of spasmodic flat-foot[14], a case of 'reflex valgus' with severe peroneal spasm in a boy of ten. He thought it a neurosis, though nothing in the child's nature pointed to hysteria, 'The neuroses of joints must have ... a peculiar fascination for every orthopaedic surgeon'. Other surgeons had seen cases and had divided the peroneal tendons, but with questionable benefit.

Scoliosis was a perennial problem; what caused it, why was it commoner in girls, why did puberty seem to produce it? It was a condition that continued to baffle clinicians for many years, for which operative treatment had not yet been envisaged (save for the ill-advised and contentious multiple tenotomies and myotomies carried out by Guérin[15] in Paris in the early 19th century), and was managed by corsets or Sayre's plaster jacket, sometimes in suspension[16], coupled with vigorous 'remedial' exercises[17].

Osteotomy for lower limb deformities was now well established in 1888, under Listerian safeguards, and advised by Willard[18] if manual fracture or osteoclasis was inadequate. He used careful skin preparation by shaving, soap and water, towels soaked in 1:2000 mercuric chloride, ether anaesthesia, the instruments placed in boiling water (no time stated) and then in 1:20 carbolic. A simple linear osteotomy, without a wedge, was adequate if the angulation was less than 90°; no tourniquet was used because the haemorrhage had the desirable effect of preventing air entry, the wound was irrigated with mercuric chloride, no drainage, plaster in overcorrection. But for a wedge osteotomy in more severe deformities an Esmarch bandage helped visualization, asepsis was particularly important, the fibula was divided first and the wound drained, (one thinks of Macewen, 'I have never ventured beyond six osteotomies at one time, but as high as ten have been performed[19].')

Vance, of Louisville, spoke of femoral osteotomy for the correction of fixed flexion-adduction deformity resulting from hip-joint disease, inserting a chisel through a small incision; he also did supracondylar section for fixed knee flexion[20]. Phelps insisted that the surgeon undertaking osteotomy must practise antiseptic surgery, 'When germ life produces suppuration and septicaemia ... it has been introduced into the wound either by the chisel or by the hands of the operator or his assistants[21].' He himself reported no instance of suppuration or nonunion in 200 osteotomies, a record one might be proud of today, but he also used the Rizzoli osteoclast for angulations if they were remote from joints; if they were juxtarticular, there was a risk of epiphyseal damage.

Charles N Dixon Jones, of Brooklyn, speaking on 'The Etiology and Pathology of Rhachitic Deformity'[22], while reporting 158 consecutive osteotomies without suppuration, speculated admirably on the nature of the disease, 'It is primarily a diet disease ... caused by a rhachitic diet just as certainly as scurvy by a scorbutic diet, and which can be cured as certainly by an antirhachitic diet. (Ironically, Kassowitz, in a paper entitled *Die Phosphorbehandlung der Rachitis* in the *Berliner Klinische Wochenschrift* in 1884, had already reported the cure of rickets with phosphates; ironically because these were given suspended in cod-liver oil, regarded as an inert base!). Jones incriminated a lack of animal fat and poor environmental conditions and gave an excellent account of the disturbed histology of epiphyseal ossification. He reviewed the history of the first osteotomy, for hip ankylosis in malposition, by Rhea Barton in 1826 (see p. 381), followed by Langenbeck in 1852 (subcutaneous osteotomy with a narrow saw, also for hip ankylosis), Volkmann in 1875 (two cases of knee ankylosis, using antisepsis and a small skin incision) and then Macewen, also in 1875. 'These two influences, the introduction of Listerism and the subcutaneous method of Langenbeck, have made osteotomy one of the safest operations in surgery ... the honour of introducing antisepsis into osteotomy is due to the distinguished Volkmann, of Halle.' Osteotomy could be performed with 'trephines, bone perforators, gimlets, chain-saws, round saws, trocar saws and electro-saws ... but the last and best of all is the chisel.' Of this last, there were two types: the carpenter's chisel and the double-tapering instrument that Macewen called his 'osteotome' (though we note elsewhere – at p. 183 – that this name had been applied very much earlier by Bernhard Heine, of Würzburg, to an instrument he had devised on a very difficult principle). 'Macewen,' said Dixon Jones, 'should be canonized as the ideal scientific corrector of bone deformities', but he considered the osteoclast 'an instrument of tremendous and brutal power, which I hope will never be generally adopted by American surgeons.' He practised a linear or cuneiform bone section, using an Esmarch bandage and plenty of 1:1000 mercuric chloride, and sometimes drained the wound with horsehair or catgut, or even by a counterincision at the apex of the bony wedge, followed by plaster.

To round out our survey of American orthopaedics at the end of the century, let us refer to Volume 10 of the AOA's *Transactions*, of 1897. This includes a number of passable X-rays and a rather wistful contribution by Noble Smith, of London, on 'An Englishman's View of Orthopaedic Surgery as Practised in America'[23]. Americans, said Smith, had advanced far more in orthopaedic surgery than in any other field of surgery and had done far more than Britain. This was because Americans were practical men and orthopaedic surgery was a practical discipline; because they were untrammelled by the prejudices of the old country, so that any surgeon with the necessary mechanical aptitude could turn to orthopaedic surgery unafraid of tradition; and because they devised their appliances themselves and were not dependent on instrument-makers, as in Britain. (There had never really been a self-perpetuating class of 'mechanicians' in the USA.) The plaster jacket had emanated from America.

An admirable paper by Gibney on 'Operative Procedures in Orthopaedic Surgery'[24] laid down some unexceptionable principles. The orthopaedic surgeon must be prepared to conduct a case from start to finish, to operate if apparatus failed, and to operate 'as well as any general surgeon can do it'. It is evident from his remarks that some orthopaedists relied on appliances alone, or mainly so, and others on operations alone, but an orthopaedic surgeon had to be able to meet any emergency that might arise. Here Gibney was able to draw on an enormous experience at the Hospital for the Ruptured and Crippled, where, in the previous ten years, there had been 828 operations on 515 cases of hip disease, including 99 subtrochanteric osteotomies for deformity and 119 excisions; 69 operations for Pott's disease, mostly for abscesses and sinuses but with 'removal of the focus' attempted, albeit unsatisfactorily, in a few cases; 356 operations for tuberculosis of the knee, ranging from aspiration through excision to amputation; 471 operations for club-foot, the most favoured procedure being tenotomy, followed by manipulation under anaesthesia, with a few wedge tarsectomies and supra-malleolar osteotomies; and 78 operations for poliomyelitis and hemiplegia – tenotomy (usually subcutaneous), myotomy and tendon transplanation.

So much for American orthopaedics at the beginning of the 20th century. We see it best, perhaps, as the Englishman Noble Smith saw it: surgical adventurism in the best sense of the word, a willingness to undertake new and unexampled responsibilities coupled with a devotion to detail and an analysis of results that were to become the hallmark of orthopaedics in the USA as the century advanced.

Let us now turn to Britain. On 3rd August 1894, 'it having been felt for some years by Surgeons interested in Orthopaedic practice that the opportunities afforded for meeting together and exchanging opinions on subjects associated with this important branch of Surgical practice were inadequate, an informal meeting was held during the Annual Meeting of the British Medical Association at University College, Bristol on August 3rd, 1894, at which were present Messrs Ewens, Robert Jones, Murray, Noble Smith, D'Arcy Power, Freer and Keetley.' It was resolved to form the British Orthopaedic Society and Noble Smith was voted Chairman. The Council were; W J Walshmann, E Muirhead Little, D'Arcy Power, Noble Smith, C T Holland, H A Reeves, S Sunderland, J Ewens, Robert Jones and Grattan of Cork. The Secretaries were E Luke Freer of Birmingham and A H Tubby of London. There were 31 members[25].

The new Society did not last long, and only four volumes of its *Transactions* were published, for the years 1894–1900. The First General Meeting, on 3rd November 1894, was at the Holborn Restaurant, London; we have no details of its proceedings, or even of the menu. At the Second Meeting, on 31st January 1895, at the Royal Medical and Chirurgical Society's rooms in Hanover Square, clinical cases were shown, including examples of wedge tarsectomy (of talus and os calcis) for 'inveterate talipes equinovarus' by E M Little[26], an operation practised, as we have noted, by Bradford in Boston and evidently common at this time. At the Third Meeting, in Liverpool on 24th May 1895, Robert Jones said, of intractable talipes equinovarus, that 'the foot is not cured until the patient can voluntarily place it in the position of valgus ... in other words, until the act of walking becomes a beneficial factor in the correction of the deformity[27].'

The current treatment included manual correction, wrenching, subcutane-ous section of ligaments and tendons, tarsoclasis, osteotomy, tarsectomy, and removal of the cuboid or astragalus (the latter done by Lund with good results). Jones himself had done astragalectomy six times and tarsectomy 13 times, but the feet were stiff and he had abandoned operation in favour of the Thomas wrench and Achilles tenotomy, with an occasional osteoclasis for internal rotation of the tibia as a final step. (Of course, bone operations for congenital talipes were already *vieux jeu*. Richard Davy, of the Westminster Hospital, in a paper in the *British Medical Journal* in 1883[28], said that he had advocated such procedures for intractable club-foot for ten years, the main difficulty being the reluctance of some of the adults afflicted, e.g. crossing-sweepers, to relinquish a lucrative deformity, a reluctance that had been commented on much earlier by Dieffenbach. Davy either excised the cuboid or took out a midtarsal wedge, using a saw rather than a chisel and a gum and chalk bandage or an unpadded plaster cast, not to be wriggled out of. His youngest patient was aged 16 months! There was one death, from septicaemia.)

The Fourth Meeting, on 30 July 1895, was at the National Orthopaedic Hospital* at 234 Great Portland Street, London. Noble Smith[29] reported successful laminectomy for late onset Pott's paraplegia. Muirhead Little[30] stated that Dr V Ménard, of Berck-sur-Mer, had recently reported the treatment of such paraplegia by division of a rib, removal of the corresponding transverse process, and seeking the abscess, possibly the earliest instance of costotransversectomy. The operation was repeated by Little and Tubby. There was disagreement on the management of chronic abscesses in Pott's disease; most members were conservative, but evidently some radical operations were being done. The British Medical Journal of 1883, 1, 812, contained a report 'On the relief of Pott's paraplegia by trephining' by Charles Atkins, about an operation by Mr Arthur Jackson at the Sheffield General Infirmary in 1882 on a girl of 12 with spastic paraplegia of 6 months' duration. The spine and laminae of T9 were removed: 'No pus was found, but the spinal cord rose to the opening made in the bone'. She regained bladder control in a week, sensation and slight voluntary power returned, and the spasms disappeared. No late result is given.

The First Annual Meeting was on 18th December 1895, at the Royal Orthopaedic Hospital in Oxford Street. Keetley[31] described a case of increasing hip deformity in a child which he thought was not congenital dislocation but 'varus of the neck'. Evidently, the two conditions were easily confused before the arrival of the X-ray. For the 1896 Session there were 34 members. William Thomas[32] reported a case of 'Severe acquired lateral curvature of the spine', which his description clearly shows to have been a sciatic scoliosis (and known as such, though the recognition of the prolapsed disc still lay in the future). On congenital dislocation of the hip, Noble Smith[33] considered that 'surgical opinion at the present day is adverse to heroic operations for making acetabula'; some children died and the best results were far from perfect. Tubby felt that 'the whole question of the general treatment of CDH was so far absolutely chaotic'[34]. Some German surgeons were making claims they believed to be true, but patients coming to London after operation in Germany or Vienna were still waddling or lordosed, and some were ankylosed. (A contemporary surgeon remarked that, before operation, Hoffa's patients walked like ducks, and after operation like operated ducks!) The bugbear seems to have been the difficulty and danger of trying to enlarge the acetabulum: Kirmisson in Paris had had three deaths, but these risks were not stopping surgeons from trying. Keetley referred to Ogston's removal of a piece of bone involving the entire thickness of the acetabulum, while Ewens[35] claimed that *he* was refashioning the acetabulum successfully.

---

*The nomenclature of the various London orthopaedic hospitals before their final amalgamation into the Royal National Orthopaedic Hospital in Great Portland Street is confusing and is dealt with at p. 125. There is an excellent history by Cholmeley.

At the Second Annual Meeting at the City Orthopaedic Hospital in Hatton Garden, Noble Smith referred to Calot's forcible reduction of Pott's kyphosis at Berck (see also p. 619)[36]. Manual pressure was applied under chloroform anaesthesia, followed by a plaster jacket for 5–6 months, leading to 'cure'. (Calot, at the *Académie de Médecine*, Paris, December 1896, reported on 37 cases; 35 were cured, two required laminectomy. The British visitors were sceptical.) At this meeting, Keetley[37] described open reduction for congenital dislocation of the hip in a girl of 13, in whom he had gouged out the acetabulum and lined it with a musculo-periosteal flap to cover the head of the femur, an anticipation of Hey Groves and Colonna.

However, the 1897 Session returned, as if fascinated, to Calot's method, which had infected even Robert Jones[38], who had been to see it and demonstrated it with slides. Now, under chloroform, with bandage traction to the head and four assistants pulling on the limbs, forcible reduction of the kyphosis was obtained with a crack and a plaster jacket applied in suspension. The procedure was repeated little and often; Jones had done it himself. The entire episode is rather extraordinary when we recall that Pott himself, in 1779, had recognized the dangers of violent correction, that to draw the carious bones asunder must interfere with the natural mode of healing by coalescence of the diseased segments. A much sounder opinion had been expressed by Edmund Owen, of St Mary's Hospital in London, in the *British Medical Journal* for 1882, *1*, 690, 'Let us all recognise ... that we are simply treating the diseased vertebrae ... by securing for them the nearest approach to that absolute physiological rest of which our Hilton was the High Priest. And let us stretch our hand across the Atlantic ... to give our fraternal greetings to Professor Sayre, who has systematised and brought to us a practical means of helping those countless children whom we had almost begun to regard as surgical outcasts.' This was a reference to the plaster jacket; but Owen combined it with bed-rest and stated that Sayre did not consider suspension essential.

Also at this meeting, Jones[39] reported some 60 arthrodeses (ankle excisions) for poliomyelitic paralysis. Jackson Clarke[40] reflected the growing interest in coxa vara in children, thought to be rachitic. As to fractures, Keetley[41] was doing open reduction and wiring for fractures of the lateral condyle and capitellum of the humerus, 'There was no doubt that the introduction of the Röntgen rays had given them a means whereby they might often come to a very easy decision of what they ought to do.' And Noble Smith, 'There was no doubt a great deal might be done by cutting down on fractures. It seemed to him that in all fractures in the neighbourhood of the joints ... it would become the practice to cut down on the fracture, clear out the clots, put the bones as neatly as possible together and close the wound[42].' There were fractures in which the bones separated so far that instead of there being an excess of callus, there might be no callus at all; this was frequent in Pott's fracture with fracture of the medial malleolus, 'and in all such fractures they ought to cut down and suture the separated fragments.' (Open reduction was very far from new. Beauregard[43], in 1883, had collected 49 cases of patellar suture from various European countries, in which silver wire was most often used but also steel, platinum and silk; four of these patients died and one was amputated. Septic complications seem to have been taken for granted[44].

Keetley, on rheumatoid arthritis, 'The primary difficulty is due to our not knowing what rheumatoid arthritis is. Not many years ago we were in the same difficulty with regard to tubercle. Bacteriology has put us in a better position in respect of that disease. But the far-seeing and acute had a shrewd guess at the nature of tubercle long before the bacillus was demonstrated[45].' It is clear that operations for non-tuberculous arthritis were by now commonplace: removal of osteophytes and lavage.

Tubby and Robert Jones[46] had treated a girl of 12 with congenital dislocation of the hip by an operation 'aimed at fibrous ankylosis' by denuding the head and socket plus cervical osteotomy for anteversion. Reeves riposted that, even without operation, these children could run and get about, so that reposition operations were 'simple madness'. There was much dispute as to whether there was ever a useful acetabulum afterwards to make operating worthwhile, but some agreement on pulling down the limb by traction for a time before attempting manipulative or open reduction.

T H Openshaw made an important contribution on 'tendon implantation'[47]. He referred to the pioneering operation by Nicoladoni[48] in 1881. This was for a girl of 16, left with paralytic calcaneovalgus after poliomyelitis at the age of two. He had transferred the peronei into the Achilles tendon and, though the wound sloughed, it was healed at seven weeks and the child walked and regained active plantarflexion three months after operation. In 1893, Pochas, of Lille, had treated paralytic valgus in a child of four by buttonholing the distal divided tibialis anterior through the extensor pollicis longus (the rationale is obscure). In 1893, Milliken had reported in the New York Medical Record 'a new operation for deformities following infantile paralysis'; for paralysis of the tibialis anterior only with valgus, he split and dovetailed the tibialis anterior and extensor pollicis longus below the annular ligament with plaster immobilization, getting a perfect result. Goldthwait had reported three cases. In 1897, Mr Eve, of the London Hospital, reported four cases of tendon transplantation in the foot; but Openshaw's comment was that three of these had had equinus, that the Achilles tendon was divided as part of the procedure, and that this might be responsible for the improvement, a perennially sobering thought in tendon transplantation.

Openshaw himself reported six successful cases of peroneal transfer to the paralysed tibialis posterior and laid down these postulates: (1) All fixed contractures must be cured by tenotomy or other means as a preliminary, (2) strict asepsis was to be observed, (3) the tendons were to be disturbed as little as possible and kept warm during operation, (4) the tendon sheaths were to be opened widely, (5) tendons were to be united firmly, (6) there was to be postoperative immobilization for 2–3 weeks, (7) the donor muscle must be healthy and, if the joint were flail, arthrodesis was preferable (8) the best results were with limited pareses (9) the donor muscle must be one whose action was close to that of the paralysed muscle, but (10) it might be good to take an antagonist because it weakened the one side while strengthening the other, though care was required not to produce an opposite deformity. Evidently, sloughing, suppuration and stitch abscesses were common and troublesome; of the various suture materials, catgut was safest.

Openshaw quoted Goldthwait in the American *Transactions* in 1897 on three cases of sartorius transplant for quadriceps paralysis, a method that seemed likely to gain wide future use (see also p. 576). During the 1899–1900 Session, W E Bennett[49], of Birmingham, referred to a case of ulnar nerve injury at the elbow treated by a $1\frac{1}{2}$ inch graft of rabbit sciatic nerve with success. (Nerve suture, immediate or delayed, had been carried out with varying success since at least the 1880s. Paget, in his *Lectures on Surgical Pathology* (London 1853)[50] had thought that cleanly divided nerves 'might coalesce by immediate union ... We may ... always endeavour to bring into contact and immediately unite the ends of divided nerves, and we need not in all such cases anticipate a long-continued suspension of the sensation and other functions of the part the nerves supplied.' Paget thought that divided nerves healed like divided tendons, even if functional restoration of conduction took a few weeks; and this was because he was ignorant of overlap of nerve territories and the distinction between protopathic and epicritic sensation established by Henry Head of the London Hospital in 1903 after experimental section of his own nerves. Page[51], of St Mary's Hospital in London, claimed a success in 1881 after immediate suture of the median nerve two inches above the elbow; at ten months the only motor residue was loss of flexion of the terminal interphalangeal joint of the index, but with some persistent anaesthesia. 'For all practical purposes, the function of the median nerve has been restored', which is manifestly untrue for the reasons against Paget's optimism. He used catgut neurilemmal sutures, though silk and even silver wire had been tried; but suppuration tended to vitiate the results. 'If the mode of dressing which is known by Mr Lister's name can with certainty ensure that wounds shall heal without suppuration ... then it will play an essential part in the restoration of nerve continuity.' Secondary suture had been thought useless by many, including Létiévant in 1873 in his *Traité des Sections Nerveuses*[52] and Tillaux in *Affections chirurgicales des Nerfs*; both Hulke and von Langenbeck had reported successes in 1880[53,54]. Nerve *grafting* had been tried by Albert in 1876, using the tibial nerve of an amputated leg to fill a gap in the median, also by Mayo Robson in England; but of course, if Seddon was right in World War II, ideally the graft should not be intact but predegenerated.)

To resume our session, there was a reference to Phelps on radical operation for severe equinovarus, in which he cut all the contracted medial and plantar structures, osteotomized the neck of the talus and resected a wedge of cuboid if necessary[55]; but Robert Jones[56] preferred Lund's operation of astragalectomy to all other procedures, for it had yielded the most satisfactory results, though in all these operations the aftertreatment was the most important part.

Keetley*[57], on coxa vara, described the adolescent type as 'rachitic', even

---

* Charles Bell Keetley (1848–1909)[95] was always a general surgeon interested in orthopaedics, whose career was at the West London Hospital from 1878 until his death. He was overshadowed by his exact contemporary. Macewen, and by Lane, Robert Jones and Tubby. He was one of the founders of the *Annals of Surgery* and anticipated Capener's anterolateral decompression for Pott's paraplegia by 40 years, essentially describing the operation in 1890. He performed subtrochanteric osteotomy for slipped epiphysis in 1888.

if there were no other features of rickets (but his 'rachitic deformity of the upper epiphyseal region of the femur 'was evidently slipped epiphysis'). These adolescent cases were rare, and interest had been aroused by Keetley's article (not modest) in the *Illustrated Medical News* of September 29, 1888. Kocher had excised all four joints in two bilateral cases! Keetley favoured osteotomy and time.

Robert Jones[58] described a case of 'multiple enchondromata', which is clearly one of congenital myositis ossificans affecting the spine and other regions; he recognized that it was rather like myositis, but that it differed in various respects, and this may have been the first such observation. He also said, in a discussion on the treatment of spastic paralysis, that 'exercise and reeducation ... were not of the slightest use in the absence of surgical measures ... his practice had been to adopt treatment by tenotomy, no matter how early the case and no matter how slight the deformity[59].' He also operated from above downwards. Subcutaneous adductor tenotomy was 'worse than useless' and he excised a 'lump' of the muscles and often divided the Achilles tendon and the hamstrings. All this was quite contrary to his usual care and conservatism. Though the discussion revealed much disagreement on the place of operations and the usefulness of appliances, it was generally accepted that the physicians were wrong in condemning surgery, and that 'a good deal of the discredit that had fallen upon orthopaedic measures in these cases was due to idiotic children having been operated upon' (Tubby).

On hip ankylosis, Jones[60] advocated traction for 'unsound' fibrous lesions and oblique transtrochanteric abduction osteotomy for bony fusion with shortening; he treated bilateral bony ankylosis by excisional pseudarthrosis and had ideas about capping the bone-ends with photographic film or aluminium foil to prevent refusion, still at that time a rather novel and aggressive approach to late deformity in tuberculous and suppurative arthritis.

Jones seems to have dominated this session. On hallux valgus, he stressed the sinister role of the extensor hallucis longus tendon, to be divided or excised. Then if necessary, he removed (a lot of) the head of the metatarsal, 'There is a big chunk of bone obviously in the wrong place and the course is simply to remove it.' Osteotomies were a complete failure.

Still at this same 1899–1900 session, Jackson Clarke[61] showed photographs and sciagrams of a 'fracture' of the neck of the femur in a girl of 14, evidently an acute on chronic slipped epiphysis. 'Should they call it coxa vara or not? The patient had no obvious signs of rickets and ... he thought it more likley to be an actual fracture of the neck, but whether a separation of the epiphysis or not he could not be quite sure.'

However, 1900, far from marking a resurgence of the British Orthopaedic Society, saw its end. No further meetings were held, and the British Orthopaedic Association as we now know it was not founded until after the First World War. Why the Society failed is obscure; it seems to have collapsed quite suddenly.

In France, the *Revue d'Orthopédie* was a bimonthly edited by Kirmisson, Professor of the Clinical Surgery of Childhood in the Paris Faculty of

Medicine, surgeon to the *Hôpital des Enfants Malades* and corresponding member of the American Orthopedic Association. It is evident from the journal's Second Series, Volume 9, of 1908, that the subject was still not detached from paediatric surgery in general, for the contents, though mainly orthopaedic, contained items of general surgery affecting children.

Kirmisson himself wrote on the dislocations following osteomyelitis of the hip[62]. Reduction was virtually impossible and treatment therefore usually palliative, for severe adduction deformity could be treated by subtrochanteric osteotomy but he himself had not done it. We are still not much further forwards in this matter of loss of the femoral head in neglected suppurative arthritis. By now, X-rays were revealing hitherto unsuspected lesions, such as nonunion of fractures of the lateral humeral condyle, subluxations of the radial head accompanying ulnar fractures, etc.

E H Burckhardt[63], of Bâle, reported two cases of open reduction for compound supracondylar humeral fractures and he noted, and Kirmisson confirmed, that passive mobilization was resented and self-defeating, while the elbow left to itself recovered more rapidly, a fact noted long before by Verneuil. This view was reinforced by Vignard and Barlatier of Lyons in a paper: *De l'intervention sanglante dans les fractures récentes du coude*[64]. Admittedly, remodelling could occur without intervention, but some cases seemed to demand operation and they reported six cases with excellent clinical and radiological results. The concept of remodelling ought to be abandoned in favour of reduction at all costs; otherwise 'it would be better to leave them to the bonesetters for imperfect immobilization and massage.'

This volume carries a report of the Proceedings of the Section of Paediatric Orthopaedics at the French Congress of Surgery in Paris in 1907, which includes an important discussion on tendon, muscle and nerve transplants in the treatment of paralyses. Gaudier[65], of Lille, described suture or 'anastomosis' of tendon to tendon, either side-to-side or end-to-side, total or partial (splitting) transplants, and periosteal suture to bone, either direct or by prolongation with silk sutures. Kirmisson found it difficult to assess the results of tendon transplantation when so many were done in conjunction with tenodesis, tendon shortening, arthrodesis, etc., and when some surgeons were proponents of transplantation as an entire system of treatment while others used it as an adjunct to operations on bones and joints. *He* relied primarily on correction of deformity, with transplantation as a second stage; and for severe deformities, arthrodesis was the method of choice. There was no future for tendon transplantation in Little's disease.

It seems that transplant techniques differed from those used today. There was a common use of the term 'total descending transplantation', which seems to have meant what Hoffa described as insertion of the lower end of the entire tendon of an active muscle into the tendon of a paralysed fellow[66]. One could also transect a paralysed tendon and insert the peripheral end into the substance of an active tendon; or the active tendon could be split lengthwise and one half transferred into an inactive one (this last technique is still useful as a two-tailed procedure with the tibialis anterior.) (There was also tendon *shortening*. Keetley[67] had described in 1884 six cases of partial resection of the quadriceps tendon for poliomyelitis, while Walsham[68], in the same year and journal, had reported four cases of paralytic calcaneus treated by segmental excision of the Achilles tendon.)

Robert Jones, taking part in this congress, referred to 253 transplants: to reinforce a weak group or replace a nil group; to weaken an overstrong (unbalanced) group; to shift a malaligned group (as with lateral transfer of the Achilles tendon) or to supplement an arthrodesis. Suture to bone or periosteum was best. He sometimes excised an oval of skin on the weak side, so that the scarring aided correction, a procedure practised by the Japanese in the early 19th century for the repair of club-foot and probably of European origin. Jones operated only on children after the age of five, and not less than two and a half years after the paralysis. He obtained maximal preoperative correction, excised the skin flap, moved the tendons in a straight line, sutured them firmly to bone or periosteum, and kept the part overcorrected in plaster until voluntary contraction was visible in the transplant, weight not to be taken on the limb while waiting. For paralytic calcaneus he moved the peroneus longus or flexor hallucis longus to the Achilles tendon; for equinovarus he took the tibialis anterior to the outer side of the foot; for Little's disease he transferred the hamstrings into the patella.

The Germans, who were largely responsible for this transplant furore, were represented at this French congress by Lange, of Munich, and Oscar Vulpius, of Heidelberg.* Lange advised transfer of the tendon together with its sheath and fatty paratendon, with suture in the foot rather than the leg for fear of adhesions. He liked prolonging a short tendon to its desired insertion with silk strands. Vulpius waited a year after the paralysis, advised the total transfer of powerful muscles (preferring the antagonists), and saw no need for silk prolongation – it was always possible to use the distal end of the paralysed tendon. Better results were obtained for peripheral nerve injuries than for the paralysis of poliomyelitis; failure was often due to poor follow-up in poor patients.

Not all agreed with this. Williams, of Ghent, found the great majority of his transplants for paralytic feet total failures. A Broca, of Paris, doubted that antagonists could take over function, and felt that the early successes of transplantation were usually late failures; he preferred tenotomy plus an appliance for minor cases and arthrodesis for severe ones.

The debate on congenital disloction of the hip shows that pseudoreduction, i.e. anterior transposition of the femoral head, was still a method of treatment. Le Damany, of Rouen, who made great contributions to the subject (see p. 268), advocated a retentive appliance that allowed movement and so promoted deepening of the acetabulum[70,71]. Judet, of Paris, father of Robert and Jean Judet, thought that about half the early cases ended in anterior transposition after manipulative 'reduction', but that most of the later cases did achieve anatomic position.

---

* Vulpius was a very active and innovative figure. Thus, in 1907 he successfully arthrodesed the shoulder for poliomyelitis, using silver wire, with good results, an operation only attempted previously[69].

For Italy, it is worthwhile to go back as far as Volume I of the *Archivio di Ortopedia*, of 1884, because the editorial introduction indicates the problems facing orthopaedics in its struggle for existence as a discipline separate from the general body of surgery. The editors did not believe that they would incur 'Malthusian condemnation' in producing this new journal, since the subject was topical and expanding and urgent, especially in the operative field; and it would raise its voice to support the 'splendid concept' of the foundation of special institutes and of departments in general hospitals.

The first article in this first issue is by a leading figure in Italian orthopaedics for many years, F Margary[72], on the operative management of resistant club-foot. This starts with a valuable historical review. Cuboidectomy had been done by Little in 1854 and by Solly in 1857, astragalectomy in 1872 by Lund. Tarsal osteotomy or wedge resection was reported by Hueter (1877), Weber (1866), Davies-Colley (1877) and Rupprecht (1882). Astragalectomy was favourably regarded by Boeckel in Paris in 1885: it was a rival to tarsectomy, results were improved by resection of the lateral malleolus, it could be combined with resection. Supramalleolar osteotomy for residual equinus and internal rotation was practised by Hahn in 1881 (and is still useful to overcome the severe valgus sometimes found with spina bifida).

This is a long and thoughtful essay, covering all aspects of manipulation, splintage (he used various stiff impregnated bandages, mentioning potassium silicate but not plaster-of-Paris), tenotomy (of the Achilles tendon, tibialis anterior and posterior) and bone operations (five astragalectomies, various resections). Margary stressed that treatment must start early and that operation was but a part of continued supervision. All the tarsal bones, especially the talus, were deformed, he thought, in congenital talipes.

In the 1880s, osteotomy was now in full swing, and there is a typical report by Novaro[73] on subtrochanteric section for ankylosis in flexion-adduction, an operation intended by some to create a pseudarthrosis, as Barton had done in 1826 (p. 381). This issue contains the report of an 'electro-osteotome', a new instrument for the performance of osteotomy, in the *Medical Record* of New York, 27th October 1883. It was battery-driven by 10 zinc-carbon elements at 6000 revolutions a minute. 'It divides rapidly, easily and safely the smallest and the largest bones, the softest and the hardest, in any direction and depth without damage to the soft parts and with transverse, longitudinal, simple or cuneiform resection.'

Margary himself[74] discussed the operative treatment of congenital dislocation of the hip, which was beginning to make slow headway in Europe against the orthodoxy of Lorenz's 'bloodless reduction', i.e. manipulation. Margary reserved operation for older pubertal children, enlarging the socket with a chisel and making a new capsule that included an iliac periosteal flap. His first case, in 1882, a patient of 15, died of 'catgut sepsis' on the 11th day and so he moved on to 'decapitation' – resection of the head and neck, followed by traction for two months. In seven cases a 'neoarthrosis' formed and corrected the lordosis, limp, flexion and trochanteric prominence. This procedure was practised by other European surgeons of the period; it evidently resulted in fair function, and was probably a historical encouragement to Girdlestone, of Oxford, when he introduced his pseudarthrosis, initially for tuberculosis with severe secondary sepsis.

Panzeri[75], of the University of Pavia, in a lecture course on orthopaedics – described as a novelty – pointed out the great contribution of the Italian school to the development of a morbid anatomy of deformity and of scientific indications for treatment. It is worth pursuing his review because of its insight into early 19th century developments.

Palletta, in 1788, had made a study of congenital limp and of the kyphosis of Pott's disease. The great Scarpa, in his classic *Sui Piedi Torti* of 1803[76], had founded rational concepts of treatment on a study of structure which was to have a marked influence on Delpech at Montpellier. Cittadini in 1820 and Du Camin in 1839 had already operated for pseudarthrosis, while Portal and Gherardi had done osteotomy for nonunion. Bruni in Naples and Carbonai in Florence had established orthopaedic institutes (see p. 284) which published their own journals and attracted official recognition of the speciality. Rizzoli made deliberate use of a femoral fracture to compensate for preexisting shortening of the other leg, and this led him to the concept of deliberate osteoclasis for deformity and the invention of his *macchinetta ossifraga*. This he used to correct malunited fractures and the flexed ankylosed knee, and to fracture the healthy femur in old dislocations of the opposite hip and other luxations to obtain equal leg-length. (Deliberate osteoclasis, manual or mechanical, had been around since the late 18th century, but it was Rizzoli's machine of 1849 that popularized the method, which, though it fought a losing battle against an osteotomy made safer by antisepsis, was still in vogue up to 1900 and beyond[77].

Moving to Volume 17 of the *Archivio* and the year 1900, the first article, by Ferrando[78] of Genoa, may well have been the first ever on the substitution of the fibula for a tibia lost from osteomyelitis and has an excellent X-ray. (If not the first, it is rivalled by Poirier[79] in 1895 and 1896, with reports of two similar cases with good results. Here again, it took the brilliance of Girdlestone to develop this concept fully.)

Bajardi[80], of Florence, reported open reduction of an anterior hip dislocation in a girl of five, where the labrum was found to be the obstructive factor. He quoted Dessault[81], in Paris in 1830, as having either conceived or actually performed open reduction for dislocation of the talus. Volkmann had done or tried to open hip reduction in 1874, without success, and the first satisfactory operation may have been done by Polaillon in France in 1883. Guidelines for operation in traumatic dislocation had been laid down by Giovanni Fiorani of Milan in 1872 and 1887[82,83], but he seems not to have done the operation himself. Various surgeons then tried. Some were successful in repositioning the femoral head, but there is a long list of others who admitted failure and had to compromise by decapitation, neck resection or osteotomy[84,85]. All these were very late operations by our standards. The difficulties were due to this late diagnosis, with fibrous filling of the acetabulum, shortening of the flexors and adductors, and calcification of the soft tissues. Ollier[86] had pointed out in 1891 that reflection of the trochanter made access much easier. There had also been successes; though some reductions suppurated and some died, the turning-point towards operative success seems to have been the late 1880s.

Italian orthopaedics, like orthopaedics everywhere, was much occupied with problems of rickets and skeletal tuberculosis. The third quarter of the century was marked by a conflict between those, like Syme, who operated for joint tuberculosis (by excision) and those like Thomas, who condemned this utterly and relied on conservatism. In 1900 the pendulum was swinging towards intervention, and Filipello[87], of the Turin *Istituto dei Rachitici*, reported 97 cases of tuberculosis of the knee in which only 12 were treated purely conservatively, 13 by initial conservatism and eventual operation, and 72 by immediate operation. Conservatism consisted of ambulation with a brace under good inpatient conditions, sometimes with intraarticular iodoform or systemic iodine. Over half the operations consisted of partial or complete resection, but some were amputated and one case was disarticulated at the hip. There were many recurrences; the best results were with ankylosis in extension.

An interesting example of an idea whose fruition had to await the right techniques and the right time was Vanghetti's complex but well-reasoned theoretical proposal[88] to utilize the tendons of amputated limbs as motors for appliances, a proposal motivated by the amputation of the hands of Italian soldiers by Abyssinian tribesmen in the colonial war of that period, but not practised on any scale until the First World War.

At the time when patients with congenital hip dislocation from all over Europe were visiting Lorenz in Vienna for treatment by 'bloodless' reduction and plaster splintage, with 'brilliant' results, Codivilla[89] made a forward stride by stressing the pathology of the condition. Anteversion, attributed to intrauterine pressure, was important, and another cause of redisplacement after manipulative reduction was adhesion of the capsule to the ilium above the acetabulum, to be treated by extirpation of the sac. Other factors were torsion, coxa valga and shallow acetabula, and all these might need to be dealt with operatively. Between March 1899 and October 1900, Codivilla 'operated' on 76 cases (this included the bloodless method, which was successful in 66, but the rest were truly operated).

Codivilla, referred to elsewhere at p. 287, was a notable figure in contemporary European orthopaedics. In 1903 he introduced skeletal traction via an os calcis pin; not for fractures, but for coxa vara, femoral curvatures or old femoral fractures with shortening, after osteotomy. The subject was reviewed by Almerini in the *Archivio* in 1906. Codivilla also wrote on congenital pseudarthrosis of the tibia, noting the absolute failure of all previous procedures, stressing the abnormal bone structure at the apex of the angulation as shown in X-rays and postulating a vascular cause. He resected the pseudarthrosis, osteotomized the fibula, and packed osteoperiosteal chips from the healthy tibia around the lesion and reported two successes.

Putti's name is not as prominent in the early years of the 20th century as it was to become, but he appears in the *Archivio* for 1906, **23**, 4, describing interscapular arthrodesis for a case of progressive muscular atrophy, a procedure first suggested by von Eiselberg.

In Germany, the First Congress of the *Deutschen Gesellschaft für orthopädische Chirurgie* was held in Berlin in April 1902. It met under the shadow of the death of Julius Wolff a few weeks earlier. Wolff's Berlin doctoral thesis had been an experimental study; *De artificiale ossium productione*. He went on to study the structural and developmental conditions for ossification under normal and pathological states and collaborated with engineers to elaborate his famous Laws governing the laying down of bone[90]. (See p. 190).

The German association had arisen partly due to the efforts of Florian Beely, also of Berlin, who died a few weeks after its first meeting, Beely had been impressed by the success of the young American Orthopedic Association. He was more interested in appliances than operating, thought it more important to establish orthopaedic workshops in liaison with surgeons, and never hesitated to call in a general surgeon when necessary.

On the very first page of the transactions, Hoeftman[91] contrasted the *wish* of orthopaedic surgeons to associate with the *fear* that separation from general surgery would reduce them to mere 'bandagists' (i.e. truss-makers). However, the expansion of surgery was now too great for anyone to comprehend entire: hence the need for orthopaedic specialization, both clinical and academic. The point had been reached when it took great audacity to demonstrate an appliance at a general surgical meeting; but orthopaedists were useless without appliances, and the most useful appliances were now American in origin; Taylor's hip splint and kyphosis apparatus, Sayre's plaster corset and Buck's traction. The unqualified bandagists, said Hoeftman, need not worry if the doctors assumed the responsibility for orthopaedic treatment; there would always be work for them, and the success of the American orthopaedists showed the advantages of a German association. Separation would help both parties; orthopaedists would become independent and offer such help to general surgeons as to enable the latter to dispense with the knife in many cases. After all, it was German surgeons – Stromeyer, Dieffenbach, Langenbeck – who had given orthopaedics its great impetus. It is a quite fascinating glimpse of a situation, reproduced in other countries, where the demands of an energetic and growing and increasingly operative discipline were driving orthopaedists into an autonomy they rightly recognized as essential to further progress, but which they also feared might entail initial 'loss of face' because it might, for a time, link them too closely, in the minds of the public and their general surgical colleagues, with the mechanicians whose ancestry led back to the quacks and charlatans of the Middle Ages.

At this meeting, Albert Hoffa[92] (p. 192) spoke of neurogenic scoliosis. Paralytic scoliosis, after poliomyelitis, had first been described by Bernhard Heine in 1840, followed by Laborde, Monserrat, Messner, Kirmisson, Sainton and Mirailler. Hoffa had seen 320 scolioses in 1889–1900, 34 of which were due to poliomyelitis; 29 of the latter were static, due to leg shortening or contracture, while 5 were truly paralytic, i.e. muscular. It also occurred in progressive muscular atrophy, polyneuritis, hemiplegia and, especially, in Friedreich's ataxia, where it existed in not less than half the cases. It was rare in tabes, common in syringomyelia. There was also hysterical scoliosis, mainly a postural curve in pubertal girls, first widely described by the French, and finally there was sciatic scoliosis. On this last he quoted Nicoladoni, who had said, presciently, that the nerve roots were swollen on the affected side and that the scoliosis was aimed at relief by widening the foramina.

Adolf Lorenz[93] was still pontificating on the avoidance of bloody procedures on defective hips by the use of 'relatively harmless bloodless methods'.

Vulpius[94] dealt with the longterm results of the immediate correction of 'spondylitic' (i.e. tuberculous) gibbus. This was Calot's *redressement brusque*, already mentioned elsewhere (pp. 266, 625). Calot's results had originally been very impressive but experience showed disadvantages, including paralyses; however, with care, its value was not to be underestimated. (We have noted, with some surprise, Robert Jones's advocacy of the method, and it is convenient here to refer to a paper given by Jones and Tubby at a meeting of the New York Academy of Medicine, section of orthopaedic surgery, on 19th January 1900, on *The reduction of deformity in spinal caries*, the essence of which was that (1) it was not, in itself, a great threat to life, (2) nor was it necessarily a cause of paraplegia, (3) many curves could be greatly reduced, even cured, and (4) though some paraplegias may have been due to redressment, if correction was made in small stages at monthly intervals, 'far from causing paraplegia, the operation is in fact a curative measure' without risk of spreading the disease. This met with general approval and the decision to set up a commission of investigation; rarely an aid to clarification.

Codivilla was Director of the *Istituto Ortopedica Rizzoli*, and no doubt influenced by Rizzoli's use of osteoclasis, described the forcible correction of genu valgum, with subsequent plaster fixation. Osteoclasis for this condition had continued in vogue throughout the 1880s and 90s, but it was not competing with the osteotomy made safer by Listerian principles, while the newly-discovered X-rays were showing that forcible correction was often at the expense of the epiphyses and might even partially separate the lower femoral epiphysis.

Hoffa opened the Second Congress, at Berlin on 2nd June 1903, by stating that simple methods could obtain just as satisfactory results as operation, and that the plaster bandage would remain the 'soul' of orthopaedics for all time.

We have referred elsewhere to the contemporary enthusiasm for tendon transplantation. Schanz, of Dresden, now said, 'If I had to sum up my experience with our new operative methods in a sentence, I would say that I regard the new method as the greatest advance that orthopaedic treatment has to show in recent years', while Vulpius, quoted by Spitzy, affirmed that 'orthopaedics stands under the sign of tenoplasty' and wrote a book on the subject.

At this meeting, Codivilla reported on 250 tendon operations during 1899–1903, 202 of which were tenoplasties or transplants of various kinds, and only 10 of which were combined with arthrodesis. He was an enthusiast, even claiming the cure of paralytic hip subluxation by a Nicola type of transplant of the ligamentum teres through a tunnel in the femoral neck; there were plenty of other enthusiasts. The enthusiasm spread to include nerves. Spitzy reported on his experimental animal work on the reinnervation of paralysed muscles. (By 1908, he had extended his method to clinical practice, inserting nerve transplants into muscles paralysed from poliomyelitis; this proved useless in the leg but 'of immense value' in the upper limb, with 70 per cent of partial or total cures. What were these 'cures'? Was it just a matter of ordinary recovery or trick movements? It is not clear.)

Finally, we refer to the 7th Congress in Berlin on 25 April 1908, when Schulthess, of Zürich, said of Esmarch, *L'invention d'Esmarch (bande d'Esmarch) fut le don de joyeux avènement de l'empire allemand reconstitué a l'humanité.*

The most impressive paper was by Förster, of Breslau, on section of the posterior spinal roots, usually at L3-5, for spastic paralysis; this abolished the reflexes causing spasm and led to a proper gait. However, three of the five cases died (the operations were done by Förster's chief assistant, Tietze).

Ludloff described a medial (adductor) approach for congenital dislocation of the hip; and Lorenz, still steering clear of operative measures, advised deliberate anterior transposition for old dislocations. Hoffa was treating late cases by resection of the femoral head and implantation of the neck stump into the acetabulum; a similar procedure especially after nonunion of fractures, sometimes placing the actual trochanter, covered by a vitallium cup, into the socket, lingered on until far into the 20th century (and was certainly done by the present writer).

This cross-section of orthopaedic activity at and around the turn of the century is as dazzling and as confusing as a flower-shop; but it must be remembered that a cross-section is, by definition, an artefact. More important is to see this period in the context of the whole body of orthopaedics, in its evolution, spread out in space and time. We may regard our ancestors with some amusement, but it must be affectionate amusement. We certainly cannot afford to laugh at them, struggling against imperfections of knowledge and technique, because we are in exactly the same condition ourselves. What is important is the rate and direction of change, what is retained and developed, and what is discarded. We may be sure that, in fifty years' time, if not sooner, when our crude attempts at surgical solutions will have been obviated by a better understanding of the biology of bone and cartilage cells, much of our present practice and much of what we are now most proud of will be pityingly regarded as prehistoric.

REFERENCES

1. Grattan, N. (1882). *Br. Med. J.*, **1**, 693
2. Sherman, H.M. (1901). *Trans. Am. Orthop. Assoc.*, **13**
3. Phelps, A.M. (1901). *Trans. Am. Orthop. Assoc.*, **13**, 13
4. Goldthwait, J.E. (1901). *Trans. Am. Orthop. Assoc.*, **13**, 25
5. Ridlon, J. (1901). *Trans. Am. Orthop. Assoc.*, **13**, 38
6. Bradford, E.H. (1901). *Trans. Am. Orthop. Assoc.*, **13**, 124
7. Davis, G.G. (1901). *Trans. Am. Orthop. Assoc.*, **13**, 134
8. Townsend, W.R. (1901). Tendon transplantation in the treatment of deformities of the hand. *Trans. Am. Orthop. Assoc.*, **13**, 192
9. Sayre, L.H. (1889). *Trans. Am. Orthop. Assoc.*, **1**
10. Gibney, V.P. (1889). *Trans. Am. Orthop. Assoc.*, **1**, 75
11. Bradford, E.H. (1889). *Trans. Am. Orthop. Assoc.*, **1**, 89
12. Morton, T.G. (1889). *Trans. Am. Orthop. Assoc.*, **1**, 31
13. Steele, A.J. (1889). *Trans. Am. Orthop. Assoc.*, **1**, 180

14. Ryan, G.W. (1889). *Trans. Am. Orthop. Assoc.*, **1**, 116
15. Guérin, J. (1839). Traité des déviations latérales de l'épine par myotomie rachidienne. *Gaz. Méd. Paris*
16. Roth, B. (1882). The treatment of lateral curvatures of the spine. *Br. Med. J.*, **1**, 691
17. Stöffel, A. (1884). Die orthopädische Gymnastik als Grundlage der Therapie der Scoliose. *Zbl. f. Chir.*, **10**
18. Willard De, F. (1889). *Trans. Am. Orthop. Assoc.*, **1**, 138
19. Macewen, W.S. (1884). *Transactions of the 8th International Medical Congress*, Copenhagen
20. Vance, M. (1889). *Trans. Am. Orthop. Assoc.*, **1**, 149
21. Phelps, A.M. (1889). *Trans. Am. Orthop. Assoc.*, **1**, 163
22. Jones, C.N.D. (1889). *Trans. Am. Orthop. Assoc.*, **1**, 242
23. Smith, N. (1897). *Trans. Am. Orthop. Assoc.*, **10**
24. Gibney, V.P. (1897). *Trans. Am. Orthop. Assoc.*, **10**, 210
25. (1896). *Trans. Brit. Orthop. Soc.*, **1**
26. Little, E.M. (1896). *Trans. Brit. Orthop. Soc.*, **1**, 3
27. Jones, R. (1896). *Trans. Brit. Orthop. Soc.*, **1**, 20
28. Davy, R. (1833). *Br. Med. J.*, **1**, 899
29. Smith, N. (1896). *Trans. Brit. Orthop. Soc.*, **1**
30. Little, E.M. (1896). *Trans. Brit. Orthop. Soc.*, **1**
31. Keetley, C.R.B. (1896). *Trans. Brit. Orthop. Soc.*, **1**, 49
32. Thomas, W. (1897). *Trans. Brit. Orthop. Soc.*, **2**
33. Smith, N. (1897). *Trans. Brit. Orthop. Soc.*, **2**, 10
34. Tubby, A.H. (1897). *Trans. Brit. Orthop. Soc.*, **2**
35. Ewens (1897). *Trans. Brit. Orthop. Soc.*, **2**, 16
36. Smith, N. (1897). *Trans. Brit. Orthop. Soc.*, **2**, 46
37. Keetley, C.R.B. (1897). *Trans. Brit. Orthop. Soc.*, **2**, 50
38. Jones, R. (1899). *Trans. Brit. Orthop. Soc.*, **3**, 2
39. Jones, R. (1899). *Trans. Brit. Orthop. Soc.*, **3**, 7
40. Clarke, J.J. (1899). *Trans. Brit. Orthop. Soc.*, **3**, 17
41. Keetley, C.R.B. (1899). *Trans. Brit. Orthop. Soc.*, **3**, 25
42. Smith, N. (1899). *Trans. Brit. Orthop. Soc.*, **3**, 26
43. Beauregard (1883). De la suture osseuse dans les fractures transversales de la rotule avec écartement. *Bull. et Mém. Soc. Chir. Paris*, Nov. 7
44. Wahl, M. (1883). Naht einer Patellafraktur. *Dtsch. med. Wschr.*, 18
45. Keetley,C.R.B. (1899). *Trans. Brit. Orthop. Assoc.*, **4**, 59
46. Jones, R. and Tubby, A.H. (1899). *Trans. Brit. Orthop. Assoc.*, **3**, 68
47. Openshaw, T.H. (1899). *Trans. Brit. Orthop. Assoc.*, **3**, 78
48. Nicoladoni, C. (1881). *Arch. f. klin. Chir.*, **27**, Sect. 3, 660
49. Bennett, W.E. (1901). *Trans. Brit. Orthop. Soc.*, **4**
50. Paget, S. (1853). *Lectures on Surgical Pathology.* (London)
51. Page, H.W. (1881). Immediate suture of divided nerves. *Br. Med. J.*, **1**, 717
52. Létiévant, J.J.E. (1873). *Traité des sections nerveuses.* (Paris)
53. Hulke, J.W. (1880). *Lancet*, **i**, 288
54. von Langenbeck, B. (1880). *Berl. klin. Wschr.*, **8**
55. Phelps, A.M. (1897). *Trans. Med. Soc. N.Y.*, 414
56. Jones, R. (1901). *Trans. Brit. Orthop. Soc.*, **4**
57. Keetley, C.R.B. (1901). *Trans. Brit. Orthop. Soc.*, **4**, 21
58. Jones, R. (1901). *Trans. Brit. Orthop. Soc.*, **4**, 25
59. Jones, R. (1901). *Trans. Brit. Orthop. Soc.*, **4**, 38
60. Jones, R. (1901). *Trans. Brit. Orthop. Soc.*, **4**, 56
61. Clarke, J.J. (1901). *Trans. Brit. Orthop. Soc.*, **4**, 99

62. Kirmisson, E. (1908). *Rev. d'Orthop.*, **9**, 31
63. Burckhardt, E.H. (1908). *Rev. d'Orthop.*, **9**, 97
64. Vignard, P. and Barlatier, R. (1908). De l'intervention sanglante dans les fractures récentes du coude. *Rev. d'Orthop.*, **9**, 207
65. Gaudier (1908). *Rev. d'Orthop.*, **9**, 163
66. Hoffa, A. (1899). *Berl. klin. Wschr.*, **30**
67. Keetley, C.R.B. (1884). Resection of muscles in infantile paralysis. *Br. Med. J.*, **1**, 1058
68. Walsham (1884). *Br. Med. J.*, **1**, 147
69. Vulpius, O. (1907). *Z. f. orth. Chir.*, **19**, 130
70. Le Damany, P. (1908). *Z. orthop. Chir.*, **21**, 129
71. Le Damany, P. and Sauget, J. (1910). *Rev. Chir. (Paris)*, **45**, 572
72. Margary, F. (1884). *Archivio di Ortop.*, **1**, 3
73. Novaro, G.F. (1884). *Archivio di Ortop.*, **1**, 49
74. Margary, F. (1884). *Archivio di Ortop.*, **1**, 381
75. Panzeri, P. (1884). *Archivio di Ortop.*, **1**, 424
76. Scarpa, A. (1803). *Memoria chirurgia sui piedi torti congenita dei fanciulli e sulla maniera di corregere questa deformita.* (Pavia)
77. Valentin, B. (1958). Die Geschichte der Osteoklasie. *Arch. orthop. Unfall. Chir.*, **49**, 467
78. Ferrando, I. (1901). *Arch. di Ortop.*, **17**, 1
79. Poirier (1896). Remplacement de la diaphyse tibiale par la diaphyse péroneale. *Rev. de Chir.*, **1**, 918
80. Bajardi, D. (1901). *Arch. di Ortop.*, **17**, 145
81. Dessault, P. (1830). *Oeuvres chirurgicales*, Vol. 1, p. 436. (Paris)
82. Fiorani, G. (1872). *La meccanica delle lussazioni recenti del femore a della loro riduzione.* (Lodi)
83. Fiorani, G. and Vecelli (1887). Riduzione cruenta della lussazioni del femore. *Gazz. Med. Ital.*, **28**
84. Jones, S. (1884). *Lancet*, **ii**, 870
85. Bloch, O. (1889). *Jahresbericht der gesamten Medizin*, **2**, 449
86. Ollier, L. (1891). *Traité des Résections et des Opérations Conservatrices.* (Paris)
87. Filipello, G.B. (1901). *Arch. di Ortop.*, **17**, 176
88. Vanghetti, G. (1901). *Arch. di Ortop.*, **17**, 305
89. Codivilla, A. (1901). *Arch. di. Ortop.*, **17**, 428
90. Wolff, J. (1892). *Das Gesetz der Transformation der Knochen.* (Berlin)
91. Hoeftman (1902). *Verh. d. dtsch. Ges. f. orthop. Chir.*, **1**, 1
92. Hoffa, A. (1902). *Verh. d. dtsch. Ges. f. orthop. Chir.*, **1**, 4
93. Lorenz, A. (1902). *Verh. d. dtsch. Ges. f. orthop. Chir.*, **1**, 92
94. Vulpius, O. (1902). *Verh. d. dtsch. Ges. f. orthop. Chir.*, **1**, 115
95. Harrold, A.J. (1957). Charles Bell Keetley. *J. Bone Jt Surg.*, **39B**, 572

Section 5

The Effects of War on Orthopaedic Surgery

CHAPTER 34

World War I

Omne quod contusum, necesse est ut putrescat, et in pus vertetur
Everything that is contused necessarily putrefies and is converted into
pus.*

Hippocrates

Those who forget the past are condemned to repeat it.

Santayana

The ancients were well acquainted with the wounds of war and how to deal
with them. The Iliad, as we have pointed out, is a useful handbook of military
surgery, for Homer was an acute observer of (mainly transfixion) wounds,
and the Homeric poems show that surgical procedures were often practised
by the heroes themselves. It was they who withdrew the arrows and
spearheads and dressed and bandaged the wounds; surgery had become
laicized. Nevertheless, a good regimental surgeon, like Machaon, was himself
'worth a regiment of men'.

Celsus wrote an excellent book dealing *inter alia* with principles that are
still valid – the removal of foreign bodies, debridement, counter-drainage.
The advent of gunpowder changed all this. It also abolished the function of
the armourer, who often now turned to the manufacture of orthopaedic
appliances. Methods that had sufficed for the treatment of injuries made by
arrows or cold steel were no longer adequate for those caused by guns and
bombs and military surgeons had no guide to the management of gunshot
wounds that could be borrowed from the ancients or from the Arabs; they
had to improvise.

Their first – and lasting – idea was that these wounds were *poisoned*:

'It is not gratifying enough for the Devil that, through wicked persons'

---

* Quoted by Sergeant–Chirurgeon Richard Wiseman, attendant to Charles II in exile
in the 17th century.

help, this gun, previously unheard of and so deadly for the human race, was ever invented. For he still proceeds daily with new inventions to accumulate such evil engines, and ... some accursed persons apply dangerous deadly poison to the bullets, so much so that even the least wounds therefrom prove fatal[1].'

Everything pointed to this – the blackish wounds, the stupor, the serious complications. It was because of this belief that the Strasbourg surgeon, Braunschweig, at the end of the 15th century, embedded lard in the wound to absorb the poison and drew setons through the wound to bring it out, or gave theriac internally to expel it[2]. It was because of this that Jean de Vigo recommended the red-hot iron or boiling oil[3]. Unfortunately, the idea was false; and as false ideas always lead to falsity in practice, it became routine to apply heated iron or oil or other caustics, thus uselessly augmenting the suffering and danger of the wounded. The reform initiated by Paré was an accident. After an engagement with numerous wounded, he lacked oil to boil and passed the night in cruel anxiety, fearing that the morning would find the wounds worse and his patients dead or dying; but he was agreeably surprised to find them in better condition than those who had been submitted to the conventional treatment. It was obvious that the 'poison' was imaginary, and that gunshot wounds had to be managed by quite other principles.

On the whole, British and American civilian surgeons had little or no experience of war wounds during the 19th century, certain episodes (the Crimean War, the American Civil War) apart; and even these were mostly left to the professionals, the military surgeons who tended to decry the authority and expertise of their civil counterparts in the field. They were still in the condition of the 18th century, when surgeons debated endlessly whether a gunshot wound with a comminuted fracture should or should not be amputated forthwith and, if not, how to avert grave complications. The general conclusion was for amputation; perhaps it was often performed unnecessarily, but this was far outweighed by the inevitable dangers of not amputating and, of course, immediate amputation was far more practicable on the battlefield, where transport, even when available, could only exacerbate the pain and danger of fractures.

This did not always apply in continental Europe, where commotions tended to occur under one's drawing-room window. In France, for instance, in 1814, 1830 and 1848, not to mention the *Commune*, the civilians did have firsthand experience.* Baron Dupuytren, of the *Hôtel-Dieu* in Paris, was one of these and had much to say in a series of lectures[4]. Without going into detail, we may stress the importance of those of Dupuytren's conclusions retailed to us by Littré[5].

From the most general aspect, it was clear that the main task of the surgeon was to arrange the parts so that Nature could effect the cure. Art

---

* On one such occasion, Talleyrand, surveying the scene from above, remarked, 'I see we are winning.' 'Yes, Minister,' said one of his retinue, 'but who are "we"?' 'I will tell you that tomorrow,' replied Talleyrand prudently.

without Nature was *always* impotent, but the latter, without the aid of Art, was often incapable of repairing the disordered parts. If the wound margins were not approximated, scarring would not take place; but the actual scarring was the work of the organism. If the ends of a fractured bone were not held in proper position, union either did not occur or occurred slowly and irregularly; callus formation was an organic process.

WORLD WAR I

This is what a great British authority wrote retrospectively, in 1922, of the history of the surgical services of the First World War:

'The outbreak of war in August 1914 found surgical opinion in a fairly settled state regarding the main principles governing the treatment of wounds. These principles were based on experience gained in the practice of the surgery of civilian life and that of the South African War, substantially consolidated by succeeding campaigns, notably the Russo-Japanese. Surgeons, therefore, entered upon the work of the war with small anticipation that views cherished and implicitly relied on were destined to be rudely shaken, or that experience gained during half a century of continuous progress was shortly to be tested by a repetition of nearly every step which had progressively led up to the position of surgical security which it was assumed had been reached[6].'

This was because few surgeons in 1914 were familiar with the course and treatment of grossly infected wounds in the pre-Listerian epoch. Listerism had shielded them from this; but the confidence Lister had given them in the enormous expansion of planned civilian surgery in peace-time was of no avail under military conditions in north-west Europe. The bullet wounds of the Boer War, inflicted under sunny, dry semi-desert conditions, always did well; with shell wounds on the heavily manured soil of France, and if evacuation were delayed, things were quite otherwise.

At the commencement of the war, most surgeons inclined to the belief that a prompt application of a solution of iodine in spirit would suffice for the primary disinfection of a wound of moderate size, for this was the common practice prior to planned surgical procedures. Also freely used were hydrogen peroxide, mercuric chloride, formalin, carbolic 1:20, lysol, camphor, etc.* Moreover, the archetypal idea of an implanted 'poison' had evidently lingered in the surgical unconscious, so much so that leading authorities in London aimed at the equivalent of the *therapia sterilisans magna* that Ehrlich had achieved with 606 for syphilis, that is, they advised the immediate treatment of wounds with phenol, either pure or in strong solutions. In November, 1914, a War Office memorandum, ascribed to Sir Rickman Godlee, once a

---

* Lucas-Championnière, who gave a first account in France of antiseptic surgery after a visit to Glasgow in 1868[7], wanted to use carbolic acid at the front in the Franco-Prussian War but was forbidden to do so by his superiors.

junior to Lister, proposed that recent wounds be swabbed out with pure carbolic acid! 'Carbolic acid, by preference pure, for the first purification of a wound which is possibly infected with the organisms of tetanus or spreading gangrene. Victor Horsley protested against this in the British Medical Journal of 14th November 1914 and a correspondence followed in which the surgical adviser to the British Expeditionary Force, Colonel (later Sir) G H Makins, author of the quotation at the head of this section, reassured Horsley. However, other voices were raised in favour and a comparative trial was in fact made of pure phenol vs 2 per cent iodine in 100 cases, bacteriologically supervised by Almroth Wright and others. The iodine cases were not greatly harmed, but the wounds treated with phenol were heavily scabbed with eschar and extensively infected.

Phenol was therefore abandoned, but not the idea of chemical antisepsis. Other early methods included painting with iodine and dressing with cyanide gauze in the field ambulance, a pre-war policy that was liable to cause blistering but had no effect on sepsis. In February 1915, Sir Watson Cheyne's 'borsal' powder of salicylic and boric acids combined in pastes of varying composition with phenol or cresol which were squeezed into the wound, often after irrigation with hydrogen peroxide or 1 : 20 carbolic, was thought to be so effective that the only additional treatment likely to be required would be drainage at the base hospital for signs of sepsis. This was based on Lister's idea of an 'antiseptic reservoir' pending proper inspection and drainage, which had never been intended as a definitive treatment. The wounds became blocked with an evil mess of powder, paste and clot with choked-up spreading infection. The reservoir system proved powerless to inhibit infection and introduced new dangers of its own.

Still, in the early months, forward medical officers were so confident in the effectiveness of primary antisepsis that they sutured less extensive wounds and amputations; most of these cases, and the unsutured, arrived at the base hospital in a terrible state, with sepsis, gangrene or tetanus. 'All cases, except those of the simplest types of bullet wounds, were infected at the time of reception into the base hospital. Less than five per cent of primarily sutured amputations healed primarily; the vast majority had extensive suppuration and had to be reopened.'

The function of the base hospital was thus very largely the management of wounds and compound fractures that were already grossly infected. Before we come to this, we must chronicle a vitally important change of attitude summed up in a paper by Milligan* in 1915, on *The early treatment of projectile wounds by excision of the damaged tissues*[8]. He pointed out that the ingrained infective material was inseparably attached to the devitalized tissue, which acted as a culture medium, and that cleaning by antiseptics could not be effective. Therefore, it was necessary to 'boldly cut out' the skin

---

* Edward Thomas Campbell Milligan (1886–1972) was an Australian who graduated at Melbourne in 1910, served in the Australian Expeditionary Force in France in 1914–18, and then settled in practice in London, where he was a senior colleague of the writer at the Woolwich Memorial Hospital.

wound completely, also the superficial and deep fascia and damaged muscle, and to enlarge the incision so as to provide ample exposure and drainage, removing foreign bodies and dead matter. A wide-open wound without drainage-tubes was better than a deep narrow wound with tubes. 'It is not wise to impair the resisting and offensive powers of the artificially obtained healthy tissue surfaces by the use of strong or injurious antiseptics'; in this way healing might be obtained without suppuration in superficial wounds, though not in many compound fractures. Thus, though Milligan did not use the actual words, wound excision amounted to sterilization by mechanical means (in recent, if not in old, wounds, a practice not absolutely new since something like it had been advocated by Dessault in Paris at the early part of the 19th century. The war was, in fact, a practical exercise, on a very large scale, in the bacteriological management of wounds.

Although Milligan seems to have been entirely unaware of it, the *idea* of wound excision was not, in fact, new. Larrey in the Napoleonic Wars, had emphasized early excision. Mathysen, the Dutch military surgeon who invented the plaster-of-Paris bandage, described excision and closed plaster treatment. In 1897, a German surgeon, P L Friedrich, demonstrated experimentally the crucial importance of excision of dead tissue in open wounds and advocated their clinical excision as if they were neoplasms[9]. These workers and others[11-15] are quoted by Trueta in his *Principles and Practice of War Surgery*, of 1943, based on his experience in the Spanish Civil War (see p. 661). The earlier authors also emphasized the importance of *debridement* in its proper sense of *unbridling*, i.e. of incising the deep fascia to relieve tension, and it is a great pity that the word has been debased by confusion to indicate the removal of extraneous matter.

Early excision thus became the forward alternative to the previous simple incision and drainage after 1915 at casualty clearing stations in quiet periods, but was not adopted at the front on a large scale until the First Battle of the Somme in 1916, when it became regular practice and was also found to be best way of preventing gas gangrene. Even then, it was found to be most important not to excise any skin, although free incisions to get at the deeper parts were required. It had been established that it was futile to try to obtain definitive primary sterilization of wounds with antiseptics, that it was futile and positively harmful to attempt primary wound closure, and that all wounds were infected by the time they came to be definitively dealt with. 'The one positive advantage gained from the use of antiseptics ... was the safety ensured by decreasing the liability on the part of the surgeon to carry infection from patient to patient.'

To return to the infected wound at the base hospital, the establishment of granulation tissue was the vital first line of defence; later, this tissue could become chronically infected, a 'pyogenic membrane', yet interference with this barrier could set up a dreaded flare of infection. In the early days, a fresh wound was treated by drainage, or incision and drainage, but its walls were not touched; later there was excision and closure (in some cases); but chronically infected granulation tissue could not be so dealt with, and the whole point of antiseptic treatment, if it had a point, was to allow secondary closure as soon as possible and before the inevitable complications.

It may be added that treatment was always affected by logistic considerations, more favourable on the Western than the Eastern Front. Early in
the war, it was possible for a wounded French soldier to arrive in hospital
in Paris on the same day as a battle, and for his British comrade to be home
again within 24 hours. At first, the wounds were sloughing, infected, held
foreign bodies and bone fragments, and were full of anaerobes. Later, they
arrived having been incised and drained, though not yet excised; later still,
after the adoption of excision, drainage and splintage, especially with the
Thomas splint, they were often in excellent state, and the anaerobes had
been replaced by cocci. Transport always upset a wound, and so had less
effect on an excised and sutured and *properly splinted* wound. At the
beginning of the war, virtually all patients with gunshot fractures of the
femur died. It was not until 1915 that it became clearly recognized how
much the subsequent satisfactory progress of any case of gunshot fracture
depended on efficient splintage prior to transport. Early on, fractured femurs
were 'fixed' with the long lateral splint that went back to Liston. 'After the
general introduction of the Thomas splint for the treatment of this fracture,
the improvement in results was too great not to attract attention.' (We recall
that Thomas offered his splint to the French Army in the Franco-Prussian
War, and that the offer was rejected.)

At the base hospital, the wounds were opened up freely and treated locally
with fomentations or weak carbolic or iodine irrigation. Some improved
rapidly, suppurated and granulated; but there was a marked tendency to
induration and indolence so that healing progressed slowly. Others died
from the spread of suppuration and toxaemia. 'During the whole of this
period a host of efforts were made to try to arrest the spread of infection by
the local application of antiseptics, although the conviction was steadily
strengthening that the only effective means at the disposal of the surgeon
were mechanical in nature and consisted in the judicious use of the knife
and scissors.' It was therefore laid down that cleansing and drainage were
primary, suturing proscribed, and that the wound was to be exposed as far
as possible.

This was all very well, but did not deter the interventionists, the least
harmful of whom was probably Almroth Wright with his method of irrigation
with hypertonic saline 'to draw out the bad lymph' and replace it with good –
the 'physiological method'. It was abandoned after 1915. Then came the era
of hypochlorite irrigation, associated with the names of Carrel in France
and Dakin in England. Hypochlorous acid and hypochlorites, or Eusol (for
Edinburgh University solution), had been popular even before Lister as the
lotio sodio chlorinati, a nontoxic germicide which was actively proteolytic
and dissolved organic debris. Something of the same nature was used by the
Union forces in the American Civil War. In 1893 Dr Henry G Davis of
Massachusetts[16] reported on 50 years' experience with evacuating joint
abscesses, 'washing out with blood-warm water and injecting a French
preparation of chlorine', i.e. a procedure which antedated the Carrel–Dakin
method by 70 years. (The solution was even given intravenously, in doses of
60–100 ml, for septicaemia!) The method was revived, without great success,
for the treatment of burns, by a dental surgeon in Britain, John Bunyan, in

World War II, using a closed 'envelope'[17]. It was difficult or impossible to apply this to compound fractures because of difficulties with splintage.

The results of well-managed hypochlorite irrigation were a great improvement on those general before; it was a solvent rather than an antiseptic which degraded into nontoxic products by interaction with pus and tissues. This illustrated the paradox that, though the supporters of antisepsis seemed to have gained an initial success over those opposed to them, their success really depended on the skill of the surgical means used to deploy that system, for the importance of prior drainage had first to be learned and never was drainage more thoroughly accomplished than as a preliminary to the Carrel–Dakin procedure. (Later, when the primary excision had been thorough, further drainage at the base could be largely dispensed with.)

Carrel made a regular 'bacterial count' of his wounds, taking a particular low threshold value as an index of the safety of secondary suture. This was a rival to the surgeon's clinical impression of suitability for closure and was eventually abandoned, but only after valuable service and after having established the principle of systematic bacteriologic investigation of wounds; and the common and successful use of secondary suture was certainly due to the introduction of the Carrel–Dakin method, and even brought into remote view the ideal of primary suture. And yet, 'even enthusiastic supporters of the antiseptic system discovered that in a wound treated by exposure to the sun, the same mathematical estimate of the length of time necessary for its closure could be made as with the Carrel–Dakin system, and that the period necessary was practically the same in both cases.' Secondary suture was not always technically easy; it sometimes called for reexcision, or relieving incisions and/or skin-grafting, and was sometimes combined with BIPP impregnation (see below).

Another approach arose from the observation that wounds treated in the forward area with saline tablets and a gauze pack and nothing more – a no-dressing method analogous to the closed-plaster treatment of Trueta in the Spanish Civil War – in many cases arrived at base in good condition despite a stink and mild fever. Cognate with this was the use of BIPP – bismuth-iodoform-paraffin paste – by Rutherford Morison in 1916. Gauze impregnated with this was packed into every wound crevice and the dressings changed only infrequently, a system often valuable in old deep wounds and compound fractures that could also be used as an aid to the staged closure of a septic wound. (The mastisol sealing of wounds had been tried in the Russo-Japanese War, and 'closed' treatment with infrequent dressings seems to have been used, of necessity, by Pirogoff in the Crimean War.) However, BIPP could cause poisoning, more from the bismuth than from the iodoform. In 1917 there was considerable popularity for the flavine dyes and brilliant green; but, though these certainly cleaned the wound, they were found to impair the healing process, with fine pale granulations and an indurated wound margin retarding epithelialization. Other agents that sustained the never altogether abandoned hope of a panacea included iodine, alcohol, picric acid, ether, hydrogen peroxide, potassium permanganate, salicyclic acid, boric acid, urea, camphor, saturated magnesium sulphate, petrol, liquid paraffin, boric acid and urea.

Makins' rather cynical opinion was that the only outcome of the strenuous efforts of an army of pathologists and surgeons over a continuous period of four years was a return to the fundamental edict of Hunter: 'the injury done has in all cases a tendency to produce the disposition and the means of cure. The stimulus of imperfection taking place immediately calls forth the action of restoration.'

We now revert to the dazzling prospect of successful primary closure of war wounds that haunted military surgeons everywhere. We have seen that such closure, in the early months, was always disastrous and had to be officially forbidden. Secondary suture was the rule (if possible), or, at best and not very often, delayed primary suture. Nevertheless, at an Inter-Allied Surgical Conference in Paris in March 1917, it was laid down that 'when the wound had been properly prepared by excision and removal of foreign bodies, etc., primary suture may give good results, especially in the case of wounds of the joints. Primary suture is not to be undertaken unless the wound is only of some hours' standing (at the most eight hours) *and only when the surgeon can retain the patient under his own observation for 15 days*' (author's italics). It should be added that no clear distinction had been laid down between delayed primary and secondary suture. To the extent that primary or delayed primary suture succeeded, it was dependent on the availability of good medical services in close proximity to the fighting and on a stationary front.

Looking back after the War, Makins wrote, 'The surgeon of the future ... has not, however, an easy task before him in attainment of the ideal of "primary closure". The mechanical elimination of the infection-bearing tissue in a gunshot injury needs experience and meticulous precaution far beyond that required to ensure success in many of the greatest operations of surgery in civil practice.' The general impression, therefore, left by the experience of World War I was that primary suture, however desirable, was too risky ever to be attempted except in occasional cases. So lasting was this impression that, to leap ahead to World War II, there was a brief period in that conflict when the wounds of American Air Force personnel, stationed in England but injured in the air over Europe, were treated very tentatively but with considerable success by primary suture, but with the comment that, if these wounds had been sustained on the European soil below, no such treatment could have been contemplated.

It is the more surprising, therefore, and a fact that does not appear to be widely known, that deliberate primary suture for troops on the ground in northern France *was* tried out on a large scale, and with great success, and is well documented. The official history of the British service states that, because sutured wounds did so badly in the early days, suture was not tried again until 1917, when 'under good aseptic conditions and after the excision of damaged tissues and the removal of all foreign bodies, it was soon found that very good results could be obtained ... experience in all areas showed that the great majority of wounds could be safely sutured if the patients were treated within about 24 hours, and if no virulent streptococci were present.'

Thus at No. 22 General Hospial, in August/September 1918, out of 5539 arrivals with wounds 48 hours old, there had been 741 primary sutures with

88 per cent successes, despite the involvement of bones or joints in a quarter of the cases, while 192 had delayed primary suture with 81 per cent successes; there were similar statistics from other areas. These striking results seem to have been buried with the armistice and, like other lessons of the war, had to be learned all over again. The abiding impression, up to and well after World War II, was that primary suture was an adventure not to be attempted.

Yet, in contradistinction to Makins' rather gloomy attitude, Sir A A Bowlby, Major–General and Advisory Casualty Surgeon to the British Expeditionary Force in France, wrote, 'It may therefore be concluded that excision and suture were regarded at the end of the war as the ideal method of treatment for most gunshot wounds.' It had the very great advantage of speed of convalescence and the avoidance of secondary infection, especially by streptococci from carriers on the staffs of hospitals. Extensive or oozing wounds were lightly packed with gauze with delayed primary suture at the first dressing one to five days later, provided that the part was fully immobilized and the patient kept recumbent for several days under continued supervision. Although various antiseptics were still used in sutured wounds, the general feeling favoured thorough surgery and no antisepsis. 'As experience of suture increased, it was found safe to operate upon and suture many wounds which had been left untreated for as long as 48 hours or more.'

The treatment of severe war wounds in hospitals at home in the United Kingdom lagged behind that in the base hospitals in France, and had to be painfully learned by civilian surgeons quite unfamiliar with extensive infected wounds. Radiological, pathological and physiotherapy services were either absent or woefully rudimentary at the outset, and there was not usually any system or staff for the manufacture of appliances such as calipers, so that there was much unnecessary bedrest and disuse atrophy. (This applied in varying degree to all the warring nations.) The importance of the preventive factor was not at first appreciated in orthopaedic work; but later in Britain, with Robert Jones as director, preventive as well as curative teamwork developed. The civilian doctors often worked in isolation, without exchange of information, to a degree worse even than the army doctors in France, and the classification and segregation of like cases, whether orthopaedic, genitourinary, spinal or other came only slowly.

Eventually, special hospitals were devoted to orthopaedic cases and similar wounds, as femoral fractures, were even grouped in the same wards. 'The essential requirement was to get medical officers to understand that the efficient surgical treatment of the vast proportion of all wounds really involved the observance of orthopaedic principles,' wrote Jones, 'and to get them to realise that it was often possible by rectifying disabling influences such as joint stiffness early in the case to preclude the need for many of those remedial opeations and restorative exercises which formed such a considerable part of the daily work of the orthopaedic institutions.' This was especially true for compound fractures of the femur and for nerve and tendon injuries.

It is this truth, this realization that the prompt and proper treatment of wounds is a major exercise in prophylactic orthopaedics, that justifies – if justification were needed – the inclusion of a lengthy section on military surgery in any history of our subject.

NOTES ON CERTAIN SPECIAL ASPECTS

The value of the Thomas splint was immensely increased by the invention, in 1915, in the British First Army of the 'stretcher suspension bar'. The splint was in general use by the end of 1915 at casualty clearing stations and base hospitals, and at the end of 1916 in field ambulances. The anatomic reduction of the fracture was left to later; it was early traction that was important. The splint was adapted for fractures of the humerus as an angled elbow splint.

Spine fractures were managed by rapid evacuation, without any fixation except the stretcher itself, with great care to prevent sores by padding and, initially, by regular catheterization; but as this invariably led to cystitis, the forward policy was to allow distension with overflow.

As for blood transfusions, despite a history of centuries of misguided endeavour, including transfusion of animal blood, it was only definitively established in therapy by the Americans. It was used in England by Moynihan from 1908, but it took the first world war to popularize it. The British initially used the direct arm-to-arm method, while the Canadians and Americans in 1916–17 used the indirect method with preserved blood.

Gas gangrene was comparatively rare before 1914. 'In no previous campaign had the disease figured to any great extent, but ... it quickly assumed a position of tragic importance, more especially on the Western Front.' Even at that time, however, the important distinction was made between relatively harmless 'gaseous cellulitis' and 'massive' or muscular gangrene[18], and the role of muscle ischaemia was recognized and the primary importance of death of tissue. Also there emerged the difference between gas gangrene of a single muscle or muscle group and massive 'segmental' gangrene distal to a complete arterial lesion. Treatment had to be early; by resection of muscle, amputation, serum. The British were unenthusiastic about serum because there was no adequate supply of any one particular type, the opinions of those who used it conflicted and the collection of observations was difficult. It was more favoured by the French and Germans.

Though practice differed as regards amputations in different countries, in the West the ordinary circular amputation was not a guillotine, but a division of tissues at successively higher levels from without inwards, plus skin traction on the stump; this worked well in infected cases, especially when secondary suture became possible. At this time the length of bone left was the maximum, and there were no sites of election as in World War II, while the transcondylar or Gritti–Stokes and Syme's amputations were favoured. Through-knee amputations proved unsatisfactory, too bulky for limb-fitting and generally reamputated; and, in general, many of the long and bulky stumps gave difficulty and required refashioning or shortening. By the end of the war, definite ideas on ideal sites of election had emerged, e.g. seven inches for the ideal below-knee amputation, with a two-inch minimum if an artificial knee-joint were to be fitted; and for below-knee amputees it was found that weight-bearing at the tibial tuberosity caused pressure-sores and was replaced by ischial bearing.

During the Napoleonic Wars, Larrey wrote in his diary, after a night in which he had performed over 200 amputations, that it ought to be possible to utilize the healthy muscles remaining in the stump for practical purposes. Sauerbruch remembered this in World War I on the German side and devised methods of creating skin-lined tunnels through the muscles in which inserted pegs could be activated. The Italians had foreseen this possibility before the war (see p. 484) and seized the opportunity to apply it. In the end this seemed more an ingenious trick, rather than a genuinely useful method; moreover, it was aesthetically repellent to the average amputee in the West. Even more repellent was the Krukenberg operation of splitting the forarm of a hand amputee longitudinally and skin-grafting the cleft to create a crude 'forceps' limb; if these were ever used much, it was in private; few cared to be seen in public except with a decent artificial limb or an empty sleeve.

As for arterial injuries, these were generally treated by ligation, with the corresponding risks of amputation to follow. Repair by suture was rare: Makins could collect only 39 cases, with good results in half, about equal to those of ligation[19]. In general, there was neither the time nor the technique to try harder, though Tuffier, in France, did attempt the maintenance of continuity with glass or metal (silver) tubes to bridge gaps, sometimes lined by vein-grafts, as far back as 1915[20]. In ordinary ligation, there was a heated debate as to whether the accompanying main vein should be tied simultaneously. Makins argued that this was necessary to minimize the risk of gangrene, others that it must be left intact; the matter was never settled. As we shall see, the surgery of arterial wounds remained almost entirely in the field of ligature during both world wars and then entered rapidly into the sphere of repair (see p. 679). At all times, the damaged popliteal artery bore a sinister reputation; rarely did the victim escape amputation.

During the first world war, little was known about the appropriate treatment of injuries of peripheral nerves; these were never fully documented or followed up and the subject was virtually closed in 1918, so that a fresh start had to be made in 1939. Platt and Bristow, of England, reporting to the International Society of Surgery in 1923, found end-to-end suture best and autogenous grafting to be inadvisable, or only for unbridgeable gaps (the French thought better of it).

The French experience in World War I was similar to that of the British, with whom there was fairly close collaboration. They seem to have similarly favoured regular wound excision, used large tubes for dependent drainage and plaster-of-Paris splints that were retained for weeks. Their essential role in the Carrel–Dakin treatment has been noted.

In general, the surgeons of the American Expeditionary Force followed Anglo-French practice for gunshot wounds of the limbs. By the end of the war, Colonel Eugene Pool and Colonel Joseph A Blake were recommending delayed primary suture as usually possible without risk, and resisted the free removal of bony fragments. Wounds of the knee joint were debrided, the capsule closed and the superficial wound dealt with by delayed suture. With these methods, in the days before chemotherapy or antibiotics, there were over 80 per cent of satisfactory results. Pool's methods were never in general use in the American Army in that war because of the independent American involvement; their orthopaedic experience was brief and these methods were limited to a few top-ranking officers and not relayed to the forward hospitals. The war was over before the information appeared in the medical literature. When a military manual entitled *Orthopaedic Subjects* was issued in 1942 under the auspices of the Committee of Surgery of the Division of Medical Sciences of the National Research Council, and though this was edited by outstanding orthopaedic surgeons who had served in World War I, it was mainly a compendium of reconstructive procedures suitably only for fixed base hospitals and was almost devoid of specific directives for the primary care of injuries in forward zones. Thus, wounds of joints are dismissed in half a page, 'Splints can be improvised at the scene of the accident if they are needed.' The text was defective because it was written from the standpoint of civilian practice, and the material that would have avoided the trial and error method by which the management of bone and joint injuries was finally evolved in World War II remained buried and forgotten in the British and American official histories of the first world war. American surgeons therefore entered World War II with no clear-cut concepts of the optimum procedure for the management of these casualties (see p. 675, ff)[21].

I have dealt with the surgical history of World War I mainly from the British point of view because this is the one most easily accessible to me. It was marked by the development of a 'surgery of the front' based on the casualty clearing station staffed by specialist surgeons which had not existed in any previous war in which Britain was involved. These were intermediate between field ambulances and base hospitals, they were largely predicted on a virtually stationary front-line, and they were indispensable. We may note that initially there were no X-ray facilities at all, and that even by January 1915 there was only one mobile X-ray vehicle available for the whole First Army and another for Second Army; by 1917 many clearing stations had their own lorry-powered units, for X-rays were far more important at the front than at the base.

Finally, an important advance was the routine dissemination of information as to methods and techniques among medical officers at all levels; by the end of 1916 discussion meetings had become a commonplace. In the official medical British history of the Second War, Ogilvie wrote, 'There are many reasons why a war should initiate a phase of surgical advance, but underlying them all is the fundamental fact that war brings surgeons back to a study of the basis of their craft, the reactions of the human body to injury and infection.' In peace, surgeons work independently, often in the ignorance of the efforts of others, advance and fall back haphazardly; there is a survival of the fittest. Despite the vast expansion of journals and informational exchanges, there is still far too little operational research – the presentation of what individual surgeons are actually *doing* in day-to-day practice. In World War I – eventually – all efforts were pooled and analyzed, everyone was notified of successes and drawbacks, new techniques were made available, young men seconded for instruction and experienced surgeons visited and encouraged at the fronts. The war *accelerated* progress. As in most wars, in surgery as in battle, Britain had largely forgotten the lessons of the past, or remembered them too well, and had to relearn them the hard way; but ended superbly equipped and successful.

REFERENCES

1. Hildanus, G.F. (1646). *Opera observationum et curationum*, p. 1228. (Frankfort)
2. Braunschweig, H. (1497). *Buch der Chirurgia*. (Strasburg)
3. Vigo, J. (1514). *Practica copiosa in arte chirurgica*. (Rome)
4. Dupuytren, G. (1834). *Traité theorique et pratique des blessures par armes de guerre, rédigé d'après les leçons cliniques de M. le Baron Dupuytren, par MM. A. Paillard et Marx*. (Paris)
5. Littré, E. (1872). *Médecine et Médecins*. (Paris, Didier)
6. Makins, G.H. (1922). Medical Services: Surgery of the War. In *History of the Great War*, Vol. I, p. 248. (London, HMSO)
7. Lucas-Championnière, J. (1876). *Chirurgie Antiseptique*. (Paris, Baillière)
8. Milligan, E.T.C. (1915). The early treatment of projectile wounds by excision of the damaged tissues. *Br. Med. J.*, **1**, 1081
9. Friedrich, P.L. (1897). *Arch. f. klin. Chir.*, **57**, 288
10. Trueta, J. (1943). *Principles and Practice of War Surgery*. (St. Louis, Mosby)
11. Duval, P. (1916). Wound excision in Flanders. *Bull. et mém. Soc. Chir. Paris*, **42**, 2229
12. Duval, P. (1917). Wound excision in Flanders. *Bull. et mém. Soc. Chir. Paris*, **43**, 1739
13. Duval, P. (1919). *Surg. Gynaecol. Obstet.*, **45**, 222
14. Gaudier and Hamart (1916). *Rev. Gén. de Clin. et de Thérapie*, **30**, 95
15. Borchard, A. and Schmieden, V. (1920). *Die deutsche Chirurgie im Weltkrieg 1914–18*. (Leipzig)
16. Davis, H.G. (1893). Treatment of abscesses. *Trans. Amer. Orth. Assoc.*, **6**, 150
17. Bunyan, J. (1940). Envelope method of treating burns. *Proc. Roy. Soc. Med.*, **34**, 65
18. Qvist, G. (1941). Anaerobic cellulitis and gas gangrene. *Br. Med. J.*, **2**, 217
19. Makins, G.H. (1919). *Gunshot injuries to the blood vessels*. (Bristol, John Wright)
20. Tuffier (1915). De l'intubation dans les plaies des grosses artères. *Bull. Acad. Méd. Paris*, **74**, 455
21. Cleveland, M. (1956). Introduction to Surgery in World War II. In *Surgery in World War II, Medical Department of the US Army: Orthopaedic Surgery in the European Theater of Operations*. (Washington, Office of the Surgeon General)

CHAPTER 35

Between the Wars

We can now see that the First and Second World Wars were essentially the same conflict: what Rowse has called 'the two maniacal German bids for power that have devastated the twentieth century'. This was not apparent in 1928, when the 70th birthday of Sir Robert Jones, whose life and achievements are dealt with elsewhere (p. 137), was celebrated by the production of *The Robert Jones Birthday Volume*, edited by H A T Fairbank, W Rowley Bristow and Harry Platt, which included contributions from a galaxy of international orthopaedic figures and gives an excellent picture of the state of the art *entre deux guerres*[1]. Such a celebration or *Festschrift* is uncommon in England; but we should recall that Jones did an enormous amount to foster collaboration between British orthopaedic surgeons and their European and American counterparts, that he could do so because he was lovable as well as able, and that the textbook he wrote jointly with Lovett, of Boston, continued the earlier tradition of Lovett and Bradford.

The first scientific paper was by Robert B Osgood, professor of orthopaedic surgery at Harvard, on 'The frequent association of intestinal stasis with spinal and sacroiliac arthritis'. This was not connected with the very genuine association now recognized between ulcerative colitis, chronic dysentery and arthritis, with its HLA-B27 antigenic context, but stemmed from Arbuthnot Lane's bogus theories of colonic stasis and related ideas about septic foci[2]. The treatment extended to ileo-sigmoidostomy and even right hemi-colectomy for 'ileocaecal stasis causing arthritis[3]' and its only virtue is that it may help us at the present time to see how past enthusiasms look in perspective.

Vittorio Putti, then professor of orthopaedic surgery at the University of Bologna, wrote on the segmental resection of tumours at the knee, using massive bone-grafts to bridge the defect. He stressed the errors in radiologic diagnosis and the importance of biopsy, bearing in mind that accurate histologic diagnosis must depend on examination of the *whole* tumour.

Ernest W Hey Groves, professor of orthopaedic surgery at Bristol, England, dealt with the treatment of congenital dislocation of the hip, with special reference to open operative reduction. It was, he wrote, a disease 'mysterious in its origin, insidious in its course and relentless in its final crippling results', and one regarded as incurable until about the beginning of the 20th century. At the time of Groves' paper, 60 years ago, recognition was still rare before walking, was often missed in infancy, sometimes not even achieved before school age; but there were, of course, good descriptions of the morbid anatomy of advanced untreated cases, with their late hour-glass constriction of the capsule. Manipulation was always to be tried first, after preliminary traction in abduction; even if successful, a rotation osteotomy of the neck or shaft might be needed for anteversion. Open reduction was often necessary, and could be combined with capsulorrhaphy, correction of anteversion, deepening of the socket (risking stiffness) or a shelf operation. In particular, Groves described an open reduction with capsular arthroplasty by interposition after deepening of the acetabulum which seems to have foreshadowed the Colonna operation.

Nathanial Allison, professor at Harvard and chief of orthopaedic services at the Massachusetts General Hospital, gave a long historical review of the treatment of congenital dislocation and concluded that the place of manipulative reduction was limited by age, that few experienced surgeons were satisfied with the results of manipulative treatment, and that it was also dangerous. There could be no complacency about the end-results because of the risk of late degeneration of the femoral epiphysis and of atrophy of bone and muscle from long plaster fixation. So much so that he favoured preliminary skeletal traction before gentle efforts at reduction, open replacement for resistant cases and early function. Operation comprised simple capsular division and restoration of the head in younger children, capsulotomy and acetabular clearance in older cases, sometimes rotation osteotomy. Adults required a shelf operation or a Lorenz bifurcation osteotomy, though the latter was of dubious value. The whole emphasis was on early diagnosis to allow gentle manipulative reduction, and operation without waiting for cases to become resistant.

R C Elmslie, of St Bartholomew's Hospital and the Royal National Orthopaedic Hospital in London, gave a good clinical description of osteitis fibrosa cystica and its differential diagnosis, referring to the finding of a parathyroid tumour at post mortem in such a case by Dawson and Stanley in 1923[4], and to the then recent parathyroid extract developed by Collip[5]. It is strange that he did not take the logical next step of exploring the parathyroids, merely advising curettage of the cysts, splintage and corrective osteotomy in the later stages of deformity. He did, however, comment that further investigation of excessive parathyroid activity was certainly indicated, so that, historically, we are here at the very brink of the solution of the problem.

Elmslie, incidentally, seems to have been the first, or one of the first, to have described infantile or cervical coxa vara as an individual entity[6-8], though there were several other contributions on the subject just after the turn of the century[9-11]. Of course, the separated triangular fragment at the base of the femoral neck had not been recognized until the advent of X-rays in 1895. In the *Birthday Volume*, H A T Fairbank of the Great Ormond Street Hospital for Sick Children in London gave an excellent account of the condition.

Clarence L Starr, professor of surgery at the University of Toronto, remarked, of acute osteomyelitis, that early diagnosis was essential but that X-rays were useless in the acute stage.

On lateral curvature of the spine, McCrae Aitken, of the Shropshire Orthopaedic Hospital and St Vincent's Orthopaedic Hospital in England, remarked that the aetiology of scoliosis was still very vague (as it still is), and that it was possibly due to 'a disturbance of reflex coordination of postural muscles'. One wonders whether we are much further forward. He stated that, in the early part of the 20th century, under Robert Jones in Liverpool, the only gymnastic treatment was that devised by those trained in the Swedish system. Treatment by plaster jackets, even when applied with suspension and lateral pressure, had been unsatisfactory until Hoke of Atlanta, in 1903–5, pointed out the rotary element in the deformity and used plasters that compressed the prominence of the chest with windows over flattened areas[12]. Abbott had stressed the importance of flexing the spine when applying the plaster jacket[13,14] and Aitken applied his plasters with the patient supine in a frame, with side-slings for lateral pressure and spine hyperflexed at 90°. His clinical photographs in this volume leave no doubt as to the very considerable degree of improvement, even in severe curvatures, obtained in this way.

There were three papers on knee-joint surgery in the volume. T P McMurray, of Liverpool, discussed the diagnosis of internal derangements, referring to Hey's classical descriptions (p. 94) and warning against using exploration for diagnostic purposes. He stressed the vaguer clinical picture of posterior and lateral meniscal lesions, mentioned the characteristic clunk produced by the latter, and described his wellknown method of examination (the McMurray sign) and the importance of removing the entire meniscus for cysts. This last point was also made by Rowley Bristow, of St Thomas's Hospital, London, who quoted earlier descriptions of cystic changes in the menisci[15,16].

The transitional stage of management of internal derangements of the knee was indicated by Alwyn Smith, of the Shropshire Orthopaedic Hospital and the Welsh National School of Medicine, in a paper on *Sidelights on Knee Joint Surgery*. He indicated that the subject was moving from the hands of lay practitioners (still not insignificant in Wales in numbers and influence) into those of surgeons, and that this was a recent development. He discussed osteochondritis dissecans, first described by König in 1888. The torn medial meniscus was to be removed entirely, making an additional posterior incision if necessary. Smith had done much work on repair of the anterior cruciate and lateral ligaments[17], originally by silk repair and later using the fascial strips advocated by Hey Groves, but he also mentioned the work of Edwards with tendons retaining their muscle attachment[18].

That modest but courageous and innovative orthopaedic surgeon, A S Blundell Bankart, of the Middlesex and Royal National Orthopaedic Hospitals, London (see p. 155), wrote on shoulder dislocations. He considered that there was little tendency to redisplacement after reduction of an ordinary subcoracoid displacement, so that movements could be resumed early. Recurrent dislocation was entirely different in nature and produced by a different mechanism, i.e. not by a fall on the outstretched hand but by a thrust on the humeral head from behind forwards, shearing off the capsular labrum from the glenoid rim, an injury typical of athletes and epileptics and one that should be repaired.

There was an interesting contribution by Jacques Calvé, of the well-known French orthopaedic long-stay institute on the coast at Berck-Plage, near Boulogne, dealing with 'infantile vertebral osteochondritis' or vertebra plana. Calvé's original description of 1924 had been of a localized affection of the spine suggesting osteochondritis of a vertebral body within the clinical aspects (angular kyphosis and pain) of Pott's disease. The vertebral body became flattened, but the adjacent discs were never involved and regeneration always occurred. He thought it due to a combination of trauma and vascular changes causing transient localized osteomalacia analogous to Perthes' disease, though it is now usually ascribed to a local manifestation of eosinophil granuloma[19].

Sir William Ireland De Courcy Wheeler, of Dublin, wrote on bone-grafting as part of the *conservative* treatment of advanced cases of Pott's disease, indicating that it should be regarded as conservative in that it most favoured rapid recovery and rehabilitation. Spinal disease at that time was the commonest form of skeletal tuberculosis and Wheeler built on the work of Albee, an enthusiast, Girdlestone and others. He considered operation only an incident in treatment, though strongly indicated in paraplegia[20,21].

Gathorne Robert Girdlestone, of the Wingfield-Morris Orthopaedic Hospital (later to become the Nuffield Orthopaedic Centre), a brilliant, courageous and compassionate but not entirely unassuming man, known to the writer and considered by him as easily the outstanding orthopaedic surgeon of his time, contributed a paper on arthrodesis and other operations for tuberculosis of the hip. He warned that recurrence and deformity could occur after a good initial response, that sound healing was rare in adults, and that essentially the end-result should be either a freely mobile joint or one soundly ankylosed. In children, arthrodesis could be achieved by extra-articular fusion alone; but adults required radical excision, plus fusion, sometimes combined with osteotomy to correct deformity. He described the technical requirements of grafting, and how to operate with the patient on a frame. There was also a place for deliberate creation of a pseudarthrosis for severe secondary sepsis by wide excision of the femoral head and neck, with the wound left wide open (and this was also the basis of the famous Girdlestone pseudarthrosis for osteoarthritis of the hip.) Sometimes, only disarticulation could save the patient. All the same, Girdlestone revealed his underlying modesty, related to his profound religious beliefs, in his very last line, 'Arthrodesis is the achievement of osteoblasts.'

At this period, foot deformities due to poliomyelitis were very common and so were operations to correct them. Here, Naughton Dunn gave a masterly account of his triple arthrodesis. Dunn, a former pupil of Robert Jones, did his main work at Birmingham, England, and in 1919 had described an operation he had used for some years for calcaneocavus, supplementing fusion with transfer of the peroneal and tibialis posterior tendons to the Achilles tendon. In 1921 he reported its application to other types of paralytic deformity. He resected the midtarsal and subtaloid joint surfaces and, and this is important, displaced the foot backwards. He had done 535 such operations during 1918–27, most of these were for paralysis; a very few for congenital talipes equinovarus. The patients walked in plaster after a month and remained in plaster for six months. This is a masterly statement of an essentially unchanged procedure.

A final paper, by E Laming Evans of the Royal National Orthopaedic Hospital, dealt with astragalectomy, with a fascinating historical review. This is considered in conjunction with other historical material in the section on club foot (p. 503).

REFERENCES

1. Fairbank, H.A.T., Bristow, W.R. and Platt, H. (1928). *The Robert Jones Birthday Volume*. (London, Oxford University Press)
2. Lane, W.A. (1915). *Operative Treatment and Intestinal Stasis*. (London)
3. Smith, R. (1922). *Ann. Surg.*, **6** (4), 515; *J. Bone Jt. Surg.*, 1928, **10**, 62
4. Dawson, J.W. and Stanley, F.W. (1923). *Edinb. Med. J.*, **39**, 421
5. Collip, J.B. (1925). Extraction of a parathyroid hormone which will prevent or control parathyroid tetany and which regulates the level of the blood calcium. *J. Biol. Chem.*, **63**, 395
6. Elmslie, R.C. (1905). *Jacksonian Prize Essay*. (Royal College of Surgeons of England, London)
7. Elmslie, R.C. (1907). *Lancet*, **i**, 410
8. Elmslie, R.C. (1913). *Coxa Vara*. (London, Henry Frowde)
9. Whitman, R. (1902). *Ann. Surg.*, **36**, 746
10. Hoffa, A. (1905). *Dtsch. med. Wschr.*, **31**, 1257
11. Openshaw, T.H. (1906). *Clin. Soc. Trans. London*, **39**, 241
12. Hoke, M. (1903). A study of a case of lateral curvature of the spine: a report on an operation for the deformity. *Am. J. Orth. Surg.*, **1**, 2
13. Abbott, E.G. (1912). Correction of lateral curvature of the spine. *N.Y. Med. J.*, **95**, 833
14. Abbott, E.G. (1917). Principles of treatment of scoliosis. *Am. J. Orth. Surg.*, **3**, 4
15. Ebner, A. (1904). *Münch. med. Wschr.*, **51**, 1737
16. Ollerenshaw, R. (1921). *Brit. J. Surg.*, **8**, 409
17. Smith, S.A. (1918). The diagnosis and treatment of injuries to the crucial ligaments. *Brit. J. Surg.*, **22**, 176
18. Edwards, H.A. (1920). Operative procedure suggested for repair of collateral ligaments of knee joint. *Brit. J. Surg.*, **8**, 266
19. Calvé, J. (1925). Sur une affection particulière de la colonne vertébrale chez l'enfant simulante le mal de Pott. Ostéochondrite vertébrale infantile? *J. Radiol. Electrol.* **9**, 22
20. Girdlestone, G.R. (1923). *Brit. J. Surg.*, **10** (39), 372
21. Girdlestone, G.R. (1931). The place of operation for spinal fixation in the treatment of Pott's disease. *Brit. J. Surg.*, **19**, 121

CHAPTER 36

The Spanish Civil War (1936–1939): Trueta and the Closed Plaster Method

Advances in the treatment of compound fractures have always been due to experience in war, and the essential is the treatment of the wound; that of the fracture is ancillary. By a lucky historical accident, Josep Trueta, of Barcelona, was brought to England shortly before the outbreak of World War II and there published his *Treatment of War Wounds and Fractures*[1] which was to have a great influence on the larger conflict.

Trueta was generous to his predecessors; rightly so, since the idea was not original. The principle of enlarging wounds to release exudate, remove foreign bodies and provide drainage goes back at least as far as Celsus, and is described by Paré. It was confirmed in the Napoleonic Wars by Larrey[2] and others, but dressings then were frequent and each redressing tore the fresh granulations and introduced secondary infection. In the Crimean War, Pirogoff used sealed dressings which were changed infrequently and in the Franco-Prussian War Ollier, of Lyon, also employed an 'occlusive' treatment[3]. Winnett Orr, of Nebraska, noted in 1918–19 that the wounds of American soldiers shipped home undisturbed in plaster were in surprisingly good condition and he made use of this observation in the treatment of chronic osteomyelitis. In civil life, Orr also treated many infected fractures and settled his indecision about whether to treat the fracture or the infection by using a plaster cast including the adjacent joints and covering the wound, noting the importance of rest for the soft tissues as well as for the bones; and he always insisted on the importance of securing free drainage before enclosing the wound. However, insofar as his principle was accepted, it was mainly in relation to chronic osteomyelitis and it did not much affect the general run of fracture management[4–9].

Plaster (as 'poured' plaster) had been used for compound fractures as far back as around 1000 AD by the Arabs in the Persian Gulf; and the idea of putting an injured limb into a 'fracture box' or 'bran box' and leaving it alone was not unknown in the remote rural parts of the United States in the 19th century. Some German surgeons, such as Schede[10], used casts in World War I, but these were windowed casts. Even Hippocrates had castigated the practice of exposing splinted wounds in compound fractures, rather than covering and mildly compressing them (p. 36), but the lesson always seems to have to be relearnt. When the present writer worked in a Zimbabwe hospital during the civil war in 1980, he found scores of compound fractures of the tibia (mainly in civilians injured by land-mines) being treated in windowed casts, their wounds stubbornly refusing to heal until the windows were closed and the patients sent home for a few weeks.

Surgeons had to *see* the results of closed treatment to believe them. Trueta refers to the British Sir Joseph Gamgee, who wrote a book in 1853 *On the Advantages of the Starched Apparatus in the Treatment of Fractures and Diseases of the Joints*, which must have been influenced by the work of Baron Seutin in Belgium (p. 313). Gamgee mentions the case of a French soldier wounded in Russia in the *Grande Armée* of 1812 who arrived back in France with the original splintage and dressing undisturbed and the wound healthy and healing. He stressed the importance of immobilization and *pressure* on the soft parts (the pressure one would apply to a lady's hand)[11,12]. But even though the importance of immobilization was stressed by Robert Jones and others in World War I, the wound was usually exposed and given frequent antiseptic dressings.

Trueta's results showed that, both in soldiers and civilians, oedema and stagnation were caused by windows, that the rest and pressure of an unwindowed cast inhibited infection and encouraged granulation – Nature's first line of defence – and that patients could be mobilized even in a hip spica and discharged from hospital. This was very useful in a modern war for both soldiers and civilians, especially when circumstances demanded their transfer. For the shoulder and humerus he used a thoracobrachial cast, sometimes combined with traction, for hip and femoral fractures a spica applied in traction.

The closed plaster method had a great impact on British practice in World War II, especially where, as in the Desert campaigns, the injured had to be transported over long distances. But, as time passed, and logistics allowed, many or most of the cases that would have been so treated or had been initially so treated were managed by delayed suture or skin-grafting, so saving much time and rehabilitation. Nevertheless, one might – and still may – always have to fall back on the closed method, which has one supreme advantage, that it is *safe*.

REFERENCES

1. Trueta, J. (1939). *The Treatment of War Wounds and Fractures*. (London, Hamish Hamilton).
2. Larrey, D. (1812) *Mémoires de chirurgie militaire et campagnes d'Amérique, d'Italie, d'Espagne et de Russie*. (Paris)
3. Ollier, L. (1872). *Congrès Médical de France*, p. 192
4. Orr, H.W. (1919). *Surg. Gynaecol. Obstet.*, **55**, 222
5. Orr, H.W. (1920). *J. Orthop. Surg.*, **2**, 196
6. Orr, H.W. (1927). *Am. J. Surg.*, **35**, 146
7. Orr, H.W. (1922). *J. Am. Med. Assoc.*, **79**, 255
8. Orr, H.W. (1925). *Lancet*, **i**, 515

 9. Orr, H.W. (1928). *J. Bone Jt. Surg.*, **10**, 605
10. Schede, F. (1915). *Dtsch. Z. f. Chir.*, **133**, 617
11. Gamgee, J. (1871). *On the Treatment of Fractures of the Limbs.* (London)
12. Gamgee, J. (1878). *On the Treatment of Wounds.* (London)

CHAPTER 37

World War II

'At the beginning of the Second World War, Great Britain was in the fortunate position of still having available the orthopaedic surgeons who had laid the foundation of the work during the previous World War. They not only had vast experience over these cases but had been able to watch and evaluate their results over the years. It was possible, therefore, to lay down early in the war detailed information concerning diagnosis and treatment for the information of the younger generation.'

These remarks, taken from the official New Zealand History of the Second World War[1], have an obvious and general truth. But they were over-sanguine, since many of the lessons had been forgotten, or only half-learned, the conditions of the war were very different, weapons far more destructive and entirely new forms of treatment available. And they do not allow for the fact that, in certain fields – and it is ironic that nerve injury, to which this quotation actually refers, was one of these – the first world war had constituted an experiment that was still unsolved by the Armistice, and that the second world war was to take a stage nearer solution. They ignore the changes necessitated when a war of movement replaced a war of position. What treatment was used between 1939 and 1945 depended largely on circumstances: whether or not the front was stationary, the nature of the terrain, the ease of transport.

It is also ironic that, after primary suture had at least begun to be established on the British Front in the later stages of World War I, the official British history of the second world war[2] states that, while the newer generation of surgeons had to relearn the folly of antiseptics, they often had to relearn the folly of primary suture, ignoring the remarkable contributions of transfusion, anaesthesia and chemotherapy; but the remark has this justification, that once a wound was closed it was essential for the same surgeon to be able to watch his patient for the next 7–10 days, and troop movements and transport problems very often made this impossible.

Wound treatment was widely influenced by the Trueta closed plaster method; but this was by no means universally known or its principles understood, and its incorrect use could and did lead to disasters. These were invited by applying an unsplit and unpadded plaster over an unexcised wound; but the advantages of plaster in splintage and transport made it very attractive and, properly used, it could be followed by delayed suture or skin-grafting at the base. The more so since it became apparent, as the war advanced, that far quicker recovery could be obtained by early closure than by persisting with closed plaster as the definitive treatment throughout, as Trueta had done, or had had to do. It was often used with topical sulphonamides, though these were more valuable systemically. Ultimately, with the advent of pencillin, chemotherapy became so dramatically effective that it became necessary to remind surgeons that antibiotics did not and could not replace excision of damaged tissue. The heyday of the sulphonamides in the British Army was in the Middle East, especially for systemic infection; its use with a field dressing was more a matter of morale. Penicillin was nontoxic and had a wider spectrum of action, but was not then available in oral form.

In general (this is written mainly from the Anglo-American viewpoint), the rules for primary closure had become rather puritan: not later than 6–8 hours after wounding, less if muscle damage were severe, an extension allowed for facial wounds. Whether simple bullet wounds should be excised or just sutured was a question with various answers, and still is, though the havoc wrought by new high velocity weapons favours exploration. A new factor was the phosphorus contamination of incendiary or tracer bullet wounds, requiring wide exposure and irrigation with sodium bicarbonate and 1 per cent copper sulphate. The crucial factors were the intervals between wounding and primary surgery and between primary and secondary surgery, though replacement of lost fluid, protein and electrolytes with blood, plasma or aminoacid transfusion, even at the front itself, tended to allow greater licence. One problem was the greater destructive power of missiles since 1918. Blast, often fatal, was common; it had been noticed, but not understood, in World War I. There was the crush syndrome, especially in civilian air-raid casualties. Vehicles, both on land and in the air, were much faster and more lethal, and, like parachuting, caused multiple injuries rather than a single impact lesion.

The main features of first aid were speed, splintage, warm covering under as well as over the body, fluid, morphine; tourniquets were discouraged. The primary surgery involved cleaning skin and wound with a mild agent like cetyl-tetra-ammonium bromide (CTAB), excision (minimal for the skin), haemostasis with minimal catgut (which had been recognised as promoting tissue oedema and sometimes turning the scale to sepsis), preservation of even loose bone fragments as the scaffolding for future repair, and no (or not much) internal fixation of fractures. Drainage was by a light dry gauze pack and immobilization by closed plaster, with rest and elevation for a week or ten days. It was found that joints resisted infection longer than compound fractures, and that excision and closure were practicable after longer delays, or at any rate closure of the capsule, even if severe damage to the articular surfaces eventually required arthrodesis or arthroplasty. It was also noted that extensive muscle damage could liberate materials causing severe shock, and sometimes made early amputation essential.

For infected wounds of over 24 hours' duration, it was accepted that incision, not excision, was proper; but it may be noted here that more recent military experience, in Cyprus, the Middle East and Vietnam, has suggested that the wound seen late should be treated by exactly the same excision as a fresh wound.

Plaster casts for forearm or lower leg injuries enclosing the joints above and below the wound caused few problems, provided only that they were padded and immediately split; otherwise, gangrene was always a potential tragedy. A classical shoulder abduction spica for upper arm injuries was too obtrusive when space was limited and was replaced by a thoraco-brachial cast with the limb at the side. A full hip spica was similarly impracticable; there was often not enough water or plaster or a traction table and, if applied, the patients suffered agonies in transport; so the Australian 'Tobruk' splint was widely used – skin traction in a Thomas splint encased in a plaster cylinder. By the end of the war, the usual practice of the British was closed plasters for major soft tissue wounds, with or without fractures; but in the American Army the directive was to treat fractures of the long bones by skeletal traction, so that many of these cases could not easily be in plaster.

The overall treatment objective at this time, as far as Britain and American were concerned, was delayed primary or early secondary suture; and, although penicillin proved a great help[3], this could be achieved simply by prompt and efficient surgery. Indeed, penicillin, like the Carrel–Dakin irrigation of the first war, may have been given credit unduly for the results of improved surgery.

As regards rehabilitation, this was now right in the forefront and there was a rapid expansion of all aspects of orthopaedic surgery. The principle of segregation, mainly at the base, was observed, notably in the Royal Air Force, where there were teams of orthopaedic specialists and their assistants, secretaries, radiographers, plaster technicians, remedial gymnasts, occupational therapists, photographers, orthopaedic theatre nurses, combined with early discharge to energetic specialized rehabilitation centres, a system that has endured in postwar civilian life.

The mass of large chronically infected wounds with compound fractures that had so often characterized the base hospitals of the first world war was not seen in the west in World War II, though they were still common in Russia and the guerilla campaigns of eastern Europe and in the far east. They were handled gently, not injured further with antiseptics, the closed plaster method was common and, if skeletal traction were used, it was often incorporated. It was recognized that distraction led to nonunion and must be avoided. Sequestrectomy was done early, except for whole-shaft sequestra of the femur or tibia, where the development of an involucrum was awaited. Established joint infection was managed by incision, drainage, immobilization and chemotherapy, not by the wide articular excision still sometimes practised in Europe and Russia.

Gas gangrene was now less common, and its mortality reduced to around 10 per cent. It was not reliably to be diagnosed from air felt in the tissues, or seen in the X-rays, or from the odour, and some limbs were removed unnecessarily for what was only anaerobic cellulitis of subcutaneous areolar tissue. The typical features were severe toxaemia with peripheral vascular collapse within 48 hours of wounding, i.e. the diagnosis was to be made on clinical and not bacteriological grounds, from examination of the whole patient and the pulse-chart, even without opening up a plaster to inspect the wound. Tetanus was also rare by now and so was secondary haemorrhage. But wounds were complicated by burns far more than in World War I and fat embolism seems to have been commoner, though it may simply have often been missed in the earlier conflict – it was not a matter of much discussion even shortly before 1941[4].

Amputations[5] were done far less often than in the first world war, and usually only for gangrene, severe muscle toxaemia and loss of blood supply; irremediable devascularization, not bone or soft tissue damage, however extensive, was the only absolute indication. It was not inevitable for gas gangrene, except for the massive spreading form; but it might be required for less severe injuries when transport to the base was unreliable. Prostheses were now far better. The work of the British Ministry of Pensions in and after World War I had stabilized the mode and site of amputations. Long end-bearing stumps were now abandoned for a standard five and a half inch below-knee stump, a thigh stump eleven inches from the tip of the trochanter, a seven inch forearm stump and an eight inch upper arm stump (measured from the tip of the acromion) wherever possible. There was still a place for Syme's amputation, and it was sometimes desirable to conserve part of the foot, provided it remained plantigrade or could be made so.

However, British Army Medical Directorate orders were to conserve all possible tissue in cases treated in the front line and advanced clearing stations, and to leave definitive amputations to the base hospitals; if amputation had to be done forward to save life, it must be at the lowest possible level and not at the optimal sites listed above, and this allowed revision if necessary. This was for fear of sepsis ruining an unwise definitive amputation; so low-level ablation with flaps left open was done forward by the British, or a guillotine by the Americans. The flaps were transverse and included the fascia but no muscle, the nerves simply sharply divided without crushing or injection; under these conditions, drainage was unnecessary; definitive secondary closure, not necessarily requiring further removal of bone, was done under more relaxed conditions. However, with chemotherapy, these provisional stumps often healed well and were then too long, so that it was advised they be done not less than three inches above the joint. Later still, the forward primary amputation was often deliberately done at the site of election and there was no provisional amputation at all. In any definitive amputation, haemostasis was very important, for haemorrhage could ruin a procedure and lose a knee-joint.

The problem of the painful stump was little better than in World War I. The Americans tried embedding the neuromata in bone and there was some (unreliable) help from sympathectomy. Painful phantoms were commoner in arm than in leg amputations.

The initial British assumptions were that the life of an end-bearing stump was limited, that the best artificial limbs required observance of the optimal sites of election listed above, and that nonseptic stumps were better than septic. Only this last point is beyond debate. Thus, for end-bearing, the

British experience in the first war was against the Syme and Gritti–Stokes stumps, while the Americans and Canadians favoured both. By the end of World War II, it became widely accepted that the Syme was better than a below-knee stump, especially for bilateral amputees, in the hands of a good surgeon and if sound primary healing were ensured. The argument for short stumps was that they were easier to fit, provided they remained in the socket of the prosthesis and retained the insertions of the controlling muscles; shortly before his death, Watson-Jones was urging that even an inch of tibia was worth preserving. The only major change in British practice was a trend to through-wrist in place of forearm amputation, retaining rotation.

In limb-fitting, the important factors were preparatory psychological and physical rehabilitation, stump exercises and amputation at the sites of election. In the thigh, it was initially felt that ischial bearing remained essential, and, in the arm, stump control from the shoulder. Shoulder control fell from 53 per cent in World War I to 15.5 per cent in World War II, with a move to suction sockets without any shoulder suspension at all. In the lower limb, through-knee amputations could be accommodated, but without room for a knee-joint mechanism. With the below-knee stump, weight-bearing was partly tibial, partly at the thigh; ischial bearing was used only if there was a risk of breakdown. Even very short stumps of one to one and three-quarter inches could be fitted with polycentric joints, and the kneeling position of the past abandoned. Even very short thigh stumps could be given an above-knee type of limb, much better than a tilting-table limb. Thigh sockets without pelvic bands or much or any ischial bearing began to appear. The modern fitting for the Syme was with most or all of the weight-bearing at the tibial condyles, however.

The cineplastic procedures originally envisaged by Vanghetti in Italy before the first war and adopted in that conflict still remained popular in Germany and, to a limited extent, in the USA[6], but not in Britain or France. The Krukenberg forearm procedure was done quite often in Germany and Russia in the second world war, possibly because of the lack of prostheses[7].

The various services tended to suffer different types of injury. Thus, air crashes gave rise to multiple injuries, often associated with burns. Pilots could sustain fractures of the talus, due to forcible dorsiflexion of the ankle, often compound, with the bone rotated or extruded, later often necrotic. If the bone were totally lost, the best results were from tibio-calcaneal fusion.

Parachuting injuries[8–10] occurred mainly on landing and were mainly ankle injuries and concussion, also knee and shoulder injuries. Fractures formed only 8.5 per cent of all parachute injuries in the UK, where landing was with the feet together; in the USA, where landing was with the feet apart, there fractures were 19 per cent of injuries until the British method was adopted.

Spinal fractures in airforce personnel could be limited by reducing flexion strains with a harness for the shoulders and upper spine as well as the waist, and by seating passengers facing backwards. They were reduced by hyperextension and held in plaster jackets, and early and energetic rehabilitation sometimes even led to men returning to flying duties wearing plaster jackets. Cord injuries were transferred to special centres. The prolapsed intervertebral disc, recognized by Mixter and Barr in Boston in 1934, was now related to wartime injuries; but diagnosis by air or lipiodol myelography, and treatment, whether operative or conservative, returned only 50 per cent of such cases to duty.

Ankylosing spondylitis was surprisingly common in the services and only irradiation, now frowned upon, enabled many to resume duty. Of course, many servicemen sustained ordinary types of orthopaedic disability and there was a definite place for elective orthopaedic surgery in service hospitals, provided such treatment gave a reasonable prospect of return to duty (and, very often, even if no such hope existed). Thus, recurrent dislocation of the shoulder was common, and best managed by the Putti-Platt or Bankart procedures. For the fractured scaphoid, operation was avoided except to excise a dead proximal fragment or to fuse the wrist. Tendon surgery and treatment for fracture-dislocation of the hip gave excellent functional results, compatible in many cases with some form of duty. Internal derangement of the knee, and consequent meniscectomy, was very common and treated on civilian lines but with more emphasis on rehabilitation.

Such intensive rehabilitation was extended to orthopaedic patients in civilian hospitals in the wartime Emergency Medical Service in Britain, with instructors and group exercises, often in the open air, resisted and assisted gymnasium exercises and occupational therapy.

Certain service injuries had a poor prognosis: os calcis fractures in navy personnel due to upthrust from the deck when torpedoed, or in foot-soldiers injured by land-mines; tibial fractures, very common in despatch-riders; and femoral fractures more often than not led to invaliding.

Some interesting notes on the German military medical establishment were published in Washington in 1965[11], based on American findings. What the Americans found – bearing in mind that they were advancing against a defeated and retreating enemy in the closing stages of the war – was a flexible system of hospitalization favouring the lightly wounded at the expense of more serious cases. (Penetrating abdominal injuries were liable to be treated as *Spritzefälle* – syringe cases – with lethal or near-lethal injections of morphine.) There was little care for asepsis, cross-infection in ward rounds and dressings was common and wound infection taken for granted. Formal excision of fresh wounds was rarely done, merely decompression incision, drainage, dressing and splintage, perhaps because of the enormous numbers of casualties and the very rapid advances and retreats.

Transfusion services were very poor compared with those of the US or UK, there were no blood-banks, and the blood that was given rarely exceeded 200–300 ml and never more than a litre. No blood, plasma or blood substitutes, apart from Periston, were available at field hospitals, and no penicillin, though sulphonamides were used. Also, the medical officers were of poor quality, with little liaison or continuity; but it was a medical organization predicated on a successful blitzkrieg, not on a long drawn out war. The policy was not to operate at all for apparently clean through-and-through wounds. Compound fractures of the femur were treated in field and general hospitals with Kirschner wire skeletal traction, possibly incorporated in plaster or a wire frame. Some simple and compound femoral fractures were managed in a walking hip spica, *à la* Trueta, but only at a late stage. There was a vogue for the new Küntscher medullary nailing in the hands of a few surgeons (though it was not encouraged from above), mainly for mid-femoral fractures, but with some osteomyelitis and some deaths from shock or fat embolism (see p. 208).

Another American source states, 'When the 217th (US) General Hospital took over the *Hôpital de la Pitié* in Paris in late August—September 1944, it was filled to capacity with German wounded. The incoming staff were impressed with the lack of cleanliness, paper bandages, Kramer wire and metal trough splints instead of traction, the over-generous use of morphine and the high incidence of osteomyelitis and amputees[12]. But, as we have said, these Allied encounters were with the medical services of a defeated army.

SPINAL CORD INJURIES

The history of these injuries in World War I had been depressing, with an early mortality of over 50 per cent and a three-year death-rate of 80 per cent, while those who had not been lucky enough to die were left as institutional wrecks. In England, in World War II, the decision was to segregate these patients in special hospitals, of which Stoke Mandeville, now world-famous, was the earliest and largest.

In primary care, careful movement from the site of injury was important, the patient turned on his back as a unit (though some advocated the prone position); there must be no flexion or extension, risking turning a partial into a complete cord lesion. The stress was on transfusion, rapid evacuation, if possible by air, maintenance of nutritional status, by intravenous methods if necessary, less early operative interference, chemotherapy, suprapubic cystotomy if required. On this basis, the overall death-rate in 351 cord injuries fell to around 7 per cent if we exclude unrelated conditions, and this vast improvement was paralleled elsewhere in the West. Thus, the Canadian figure was 7.8 per cent[13], and the Americans gave even lower figures of under 4 per cent.[14]. It should be noted, however, that all statistics are dubious. The main causes of death were urinary infection, bedsores, or both. It was not noted that, in aviators, the pilot's harness had transferred the site of injury from the dorsolumbar junction to the upper dorsal or cervical region.

The director of Stoke Mandeville, Ludwig Guttmann, a refugee from Nazi Germany, later knighted, stressed a conservative approach. Even cautious manipulation could produce or exacerbate the cord damage, while the open reduction advocated by some[15,16] in the early stages of the war found no place. Better was the nonoperative reduction of dorsolumbar spinal injuries by gradual hyperextension and of cervical displacements by skull traction[17]. Certainly, immediate operation was indicated for compound injuries: debridement, dural closure and antibiotics; also, possibly, for cauda equina injuries, to free and straighten the roots, but there seem to be no data on successful root suture at this level. The British view was that there was no place at all for operation in closed lesions with complete paraplegia, and not in partial paraplegia unless a progressive subdural haematoma was worsening the picture, or if the X-ray was normal but there was a manometric block.

As for late operations, laminectomy was useless in complete lesions and of dubious value for incomplete ones[18]; but it was, or might be, indicated for incomplete lesions where the neurologic status was deteriorating due to adhesions, callus, chronic meningitis or osteomyelitis.

It was found that plaster beds or jackets were detrimental and produced renal stasis and infection, sores, fixed deformities and muscle wasting. Very careful, regular, frequent turning was the answer, so a high staff/patient ratio was essential. Spasms were best treated by preventing distension of the bladder and rectum, resting the limbs in the correct position and passive movements. The intrathecal injection of prostigmine and other drugs was of doubtful value. Useful procedures included obturator neurectomy and achilles tendon elongation, possibly tenotomy of the tibialis posterior and long toe flexors or inner hamstrings. Anterior or posterior root section proved unsuccessful, weakened the back and impaired sexual activity. But there did seem to be a place for intrathecal alcohol[19,20]. The best treatment for *pain* was to reduce or abolish drugs by early mobilization and rehabilitation.

For the bladder, no intervention was advised for the first 24 hours, after which manual expression or possibly suprapubic aspiration were used. After 24–48 hours a sterile catheter was inserted, at first intermittently, later indwelling, and then intermittently again as automaticity developed. A suprapubic cystotomy always led to ascending urinary tract infection, and therefore Guttmann denied that this was the method of choice as advocated by some[21,22]. If it were done, it should be by high open operation or with a trocar and cannula; stones were to be prevented by irrigation, antibiotics and postural change.

Bedsores were to be at all costs prevented by the turning regime, great care of bed surfaces, maintenance of protein nutrition, judicious use of the prone position. If they did develop, early slough excision and plastic repair were called for.

In general, it was necesary to prevent contractures by physiotherapy, to stimulate the muscles electrically, to over-develop the shoulder girdle and upper limb muscles by exercises and sports such as archery, to encourage walking in long light calipers (even though the majority of patients eventually settled for a wheelchair) and to provide interesting and remunerative work.

PERIPHERAL NERVE INJURIES

This, with spinal cord injuries, was the problem still awaiting a solution at the end of the first world war[23], and in the UK there were plans for a special organization for treatment and research in the new conflict, plans associated particularly with the name of Herbert Seddon (p. 154). Little was really learned about their management in the first war; they had never been properly documented or followed up.

Some half-dozen centres were set up in Britain, with records systematized on a basis agreed with the Medical Research Council. The newer techniques now available included regular electrical stimulation of paralysed muscles during the period of denervation, electrical testing of nerve function, electromyography, sweat tests and fibrinogen cement for suture. It was generally felt that the best treatment was by the earliest possible secondary suture, at 3–4 weeks at soonest, with preliminary healing of wounds and fractures; primary suture was rarely indicated. End-to-end suture remained the ideal, but if gaps were above a certain critical size, specific for each nerve, such that they could be closed only by acute flexion of adjacent joints, this meant that later extension led to traction damage precluding useful recovery[24,25]. End suture could often be secured by various devices: really lengthy exposure and nerve freeing and stripping of branches, transposition, bone shortening (in the arm). Results were better with distal unmixed nerves, and with the radial rather than the median. Recovery of the intrinsic muscle power and discriminatory sensation in the hand was usually poor. The sciatic nerve as such recovered poorly, and the tibial branch gave better results than the peroneal.

No operations were of any use for future guidance unless their results were carefully assessed numerically as far as possible. There had to be uniform charting of motor power, sensation and electrical reactions, with a minimum of five years' follow-up. The Medical Research Council grading of muscle power from 0 to 5 was invaluable (0 = total paralysis; 1 = a flicker; 2 = movement with gravity eliminated; 3 = movement against gravity; 4 = movement against gravity + resistance; 5 = full normal power) and was later used for poliomyelitis worldwide. Sensory examination was made better with von Frey hairs than cottonwool, with compasses for two-point sensation and with a needle for pain. The alizarin sweat-test was described by Guttmann and Guttmann. Electrical tests stressed the importance of strength-duration curves rather than simple galvanic and faradic testing. The electromyogram was developed by Weddell and others at Oxford. All these, taken together, gave a precise estimate of the state of the injured nerve.

Seddon made a classification of nerve injuries which was and remains fundamental: neurotmesis (anatomic division of the whole nerve), axonotmesis (the fibres damaged within an intact sheath) and neurapraxia (the 'stunned' nerve, a benign and mainly motor lesion).

Maintenance of joint mobility and prevention of oedema during the waiting period before operation were vital, especially if there were delays in transit to the centre. There must be a full passive range of movement at least once daily, as even a paralysed muscle can contract; splintage need not be in the fully relaxed position but near the neutral; the muscles should be galvanized regularly, especially those of the hand.

Even when there was a clean incised wound, early secondary repair was thought better than primary, where the nerve suture would end tied up in the general scar; it was best to tack the ends together with an identifiable suture and close the wound and repair the nerve after a few weeks, when the extent of intraneural fibrosis would have become visible (or palpable), the epineurium thickened enough to hold sutures safely, and wide mobilization safe from risk of sepsis would be possible. The official policy was to explore every case with complete conductivity loss, even though, in half of all war nerve injuries, the nerve was not divided, for as there was an even chance that repair would be required the best prospect for complete paralysis was to look and see rather than wait and see. The main problem in *judgment* was what to do if the nerve were found in continuity. It might be only an axonotmesis, which would recover spontaneously. If there were a fusiform indurated neuroma, trial incision of the damaged segment usually revealed that the damage was worse than expected; and if the scar exceeded half an inch, it was best to resect and suture. The great *technical* problem was closure of gaps. The critical lengths of gaps, above which closure by flexion of adjacent joints inevitably led to later traction damage were established by Highet and others: about seven cm for the median and radial, six cm for the ulnar, and so on. Alternatively, if suture required joint flexion exceeding 90–100°, failure was almost certain. In such cases, cable grafts were very useful; they had to be autogenous and were needed in some 8–9 per cent of cases and the results were as good as those of suture in about 38 per cent of cases. For larger and longer grafts, a nerve pedicle ensured a better blood supply, but closure of really large gaps was the greatest problem, and often insoluble. Allogenous grafting was a total failure. New suture materials were devised – human hair, fibrin plasma clot. I find no records of use of the operating microscope or of bundle suture during World War II (see p. 564).

The follow-up showed that low repairs were better than higher; gave the critical gaps as stated; and laid down the period of critical delay, after which little or no recovery was to be expected even from a good operation: nine months for motor power in intermediate and high median lesions.

Seddon summed up, 'Provided the interval between injury and operation does not exceed a year, and that end-to-end suture is not employed where the gap in a nerve is more than seven cm, a worthwhile result is obtained in most cases of radial, median and internal popliteal nerve injury.' Repair of the lateral popliteal or of the ulnar proximal to the elbow was hardly worth attempting. Work by J Z Young showed that a nerve's intrinsic circulation was adequate even with extensive longitudinal mobilization; but regional ischaemia, as with Volkmann's contracture, produced very severe vascular impairment. He confirmed that allografts were a total failure, while heterografts fixed in alcohol or formaldehyde produced violent reactions; they had been used by the French in World War I with poor results and were therefore not used by the Allies in the second war.

The *New Zealand* official medical history of World War II[1] relates largely to the campaigns in the Western Desert and Italy. The basic lines of primary wound treatment was as for the British and, after Alamein, had to be predicated on rapid movement of the front line. Closed plaster, or plaster plus a Thomas splint or Kramer wire splint, with sulphonamides locally and systematically until the advent of penicillin in 1943 were routine. If plasters were not split before transfer to the rear, blood supply could be endangered and, in any case, wounds so treated stank and there was long healing, wasting and loss of function, often a secondary (pyocaneus) infection. Therefore, delayed primary or at least early secondary suture was desirable. There was also some diphtheria infection of desert wounds, with severe toxaemia.

The New Zealanders found ward cross-infection a problem; the only real safeguard was closure, but after delay skin-grafting tended to replace secondary closure. Primary suture, and primary amputation at the site of election, were attempted but were unsatisfactory under conditions of mobile warfare; but there was some success when these were repeated in the later stages of the war, when done forward with little delay and not much pressure of work, provided the patients were retained for observation. It was always possible to do an immediate amputation at the site of election, using flaps left open for delayed primary suture.

The *Australian* history[26] states that, at the onset of the second world war, military surgery was little advanced beyond that of 1918. Essentially, the army surgeon of 1939 was situated much like his predecessor of 1918 as regards wound treatment: by excision, as advocated in the Napoleonic Wars and by Milligan – against opposition – in World War I, with delayed primary suture the best outcome, secondary closure the least satisfactory, initial primary suture more an unattainable ideal.

The outcome was, that although advocated by some, primary suture was officially and strictly forbidden in the field, except for injuries of the skull, chest, abdomen, large superficial joints, face and jaw. Treatment was by gauze pack and plaster, if it was possible to keep the patient for 24 hours to check for constriction and bleeding; or a plaster could be used for purposes of transport only, and the wound then inspected, fractures reduced and a new cast applied. Sulphonamides were given systemically with a large loading dose, using fluids and alkalis to safeguard the kidneys and watching the blood-count. In severe wounds, it was necessary to combat protein loss and vitamin deficiency.

American experience is set out in great detail in the official surveys of the Medical Department of the United States Army under the direction of the Surgeon General[11]. Of the 381 350 men wounded in action in Europe, two thirds had injuries of the limbs. These were efficiently managed because:

(1) There was careful assignment of the relatively few orthopaedic surgeons.
(2) Many medical officers and technicians were trained in basic military orthopaedic surgery in overseas posts.
(3) There was prompt publication and distribution of uniform combat-tested methods, not always identical with those of civilian life (contrasted with an almost total lack of dissemination of information in the first world war).
(4) There was continuous supervision, not only of patients, but also of those treating them and, most important, specialization.
(5) Orthopaedic surgery was a recognized speciality with an overall European Theater consultant to supervise training and visit hospitals and other installations, some of which had no trained orthopaedic staff, and to disseminate directives and promote clinical investigations in the field. Not all individual field armies in Europe had their own orthopaedic consultants; where these existed, as in North Army, they were concentrated in the evacuation hospitals with a striking improvement in management. Finally,

(6) There was segregation of cases.

243 fully or partly trained orthopaedic surgeons and other medical officers trained in orthopaedic work in post cared for a maximum troop strength of 3 065 505 men and treated about 250 000 hospitalized patients plus prisoners of war and outpatients between 1st February 1942 and 8th May 1945. An orthopaedic surgeon was not normally regarded as necessary in a field hospital, and qualified orthopaedists were not so used in the European Theater. Wound excision forward was done by trained general (and even ENT) surgeons; an orthopaedic surgeon was most usefully assigned to an evacuation hospital to supervise other surgeons' work, and most were assigned to general and base hospitals.

It was not the responsibility of forward units to obtain anatomic reduction of fractures, but to secure early evacuation in comfort and safety. No internal fixation of any kind was allowed; the aim was to treat most long bone fractures by skeletal traction. External fixators of the Roger Anderson type were rarely used; they were in fact forbidden and the appliances confiscated! Steinmann pins incorporated in casts were also frowned on. All plasters had to be padded, all circular casts split; except for transport, closed plaster as definitive treatment was abandoned in favour of adequate early excision and delayed primary suture or grafting. However, as stated earlier, in special circumstances, as in Army Air Force personnel stationed in England, living in clean conditions and wounded at high altitudes, excision and immediate closure gave uninfected primary healing in 90 per cent of cases, whether supplementary chemotherapy or antibiotics were given or not. These results were *not* considered applicable to troops on the ground.

However, delayed primary closure was not smoothly and universally accepted. Many surgeons in Europe clung to repeated changes of closed plaster with healing by granulation until the facts told. Poor initial excision forward meant repeat debridement or drainage at the base. Paradoxically, therefore, the most radical forward excision was really the most conservative treatment: debridement by a longitudinal incision through the wound (if possible), excision to bleeding tissue, wide opening of the fascia, removal of foreign bodies, conservation of skin and bone, haemostasis, one wire stitch to approximate a nerve, the wound irrigated and drained, if necessary, by a separate stab (especially in the thigh and buttock), followed by a fine-mesh gauze pack without vaseline, a pressure dressing and a split padded plaster cast for transport only without concern for anatomic reduction and penicillin when available. In the European Theater there was a very definite preference for the hip spica over the Tobruk splint. At the base, the essence of treatment for compound fractures was skeletal traction.

Amputation was indicated for:

(1) Irretrievable shattering.
(2) Destruction of the main artery (vascular repair was very time-consuming and endangered the treatment of other wounded and rarely worked; there were repeated reports of total lack of success after repair of the popliteal artery, exactly echoing the experience of World War I).

(3) Gas gangrene if spreading and toxaemic, but not for the localized or segmental variety.

Originally, both the guillotine and circular methods were authorized; but by 1945, the guillotine was discarded and the circular method mandatory, without primary closure and with skin traction.

REFERENCES

1. Duncan, T. and Stout, M. (1954). *Official History of New Zealand in the Second World War 1939–45 War Surgery and Medicine*. (Department of Internal Affairs, Wellington, New Zealand)
2. Cope, Z. (1953). *History of the Second World War: United Kingdom Medical Series: Surgery*. (London, HMSO)
3. Bentley, F.H. (1944). The treatment of flesh wounds by early secondary suture and penicillin. *Brit. J. Surg.*, **32**, 132
4. Aberle, V. (1907). Über Fettembolie nach orthopädischen Operationen. *Z. f. orth. Chir.*, **19**, 89
5. Kelham, R.D.L. and Perkins, G. (1942). *Amputations and Artificial Limbs*. (London, Oxford University Press)
6. Rank, B.K. and Henderson, G.D. (1946). Cineplastic forearm amputations and prostheses. *Surg. Gynaecol. Obstet.*, **83**, 373
7. Eyre-Brook, A.L. (1947). *Postgrad. Med. J.*, **23**, 263
8. Tobin, W.J., Cohen, L.J. and Dover, J.T. (1941). Parachute injuries. *J. Am. Med. Assoc.*, **117**, 1318
9. Lord, C.D. and Coutts, J.W. (1944). Typical parachute injuries. *J. Am. Med. Assoc.*, **125**, 1182
10. Essex-Lopresti, P. (1946). The hazards of parachuting. *Brit. J. Surg.*, **34**, 1
11. Wiltke, C.M. (1965). The Medical Department: Medical Service in the Mediterranean and Minor Theatres. Appendix D, p. 601 in *United States Army in World War II: the Technical Services*. (Washington)
12. Wiltke, C.M. (1965). Orthopaedic Surgery in the European Theatre of Operations. In *United States Army in World War II: the Technical Services*. (Washington)
13. Botterall, E.H., Jousse, A.T., Aberhart, C. and Cluff, J.W. (1948). Treatment Services. *Bull. Dept. Veter. Aff., Ottawa*, **3**, 11
14. Prather, G. (1947). *J. Urol.*, **57**, 15
15. Albee, F. (1940). *Bone Graft Surgery*. (New York and London)
16. Taylor, J. (1941). *Proc. Roy. Soc. Med.*, **34**, 447
17. Watson-Jones, R. (1941). *Proc. Roy. Soc. Med.*, **34**, 454
18. Cutler, C.W. (1945). *J. Am. Med. Assoc.*, **129**, 153
19. Guttmann, L. (1947). *Proc. Roy. Soc. Med.*, **40**, 219
20. Sheldon, C. and Borg, E. (1948). *J. Neurosurg.*, **5**, 385
21. Ward, O. (1944). *Surgery of Modern Warfare*. (Edinburgh, Hamilton Bailey)
22. Riches, E.W. (1944). *Proc. Roy. Soc. Med.*, **37**, 77
23. Platt, H. and Bristow, W.R. (1924). More results of operation for injuries of the peripheral nerves. *Brit. J. Surg.*, **2**, 535
24. Highet, W.B. and Holmes, W. (1943). *Brit. J. Surg.*, **30**, 212
25. Highet, W.B. and Sanders, F.K. (1943). *Brit. J. Surg.*, **30**, 355
26. Walker, A.S. (1952). *Australia in the War of 1939–1945*. Series Five: Medical Vol. I: Clinical Problems of War. (Canberra)

CHAPTER 38

Some Subsequent Conflicts

KOREA

Delayed primary wound closure remained the preferred wound treatment[1]. However, there was a great leap forward in the treatment of arterial injuries. Competent authorities in World War II had found that simple ligature gave an amputation rate of 48.9 per cent, but that this was reduced to 35.8 per cent by arterial suture[2]. Ligature in Korea gave a very similar amputation rate of 48.9 per cent, but in this theatre the figure now fell to 13 per cent with repair by suture[2]. Reconstruction therefore became the treatment of choice for arterial injuries and these ceased to be a major indication for amputation. Although repair was sometimes possible by lateral suture, patch arterioplasty or (less commonly) end-to-end suture, it was effected mostly by vein-grafting. It was clear that repair gave far better results than ligature.

This lesson was applied to the *Yom Kippur War* of 1973 by the Israelis[3]. Here, it was found important also to repair the major veins, as impaired venous return could vitiate a successful arterial repair. (This had been advocated even in World War I by some and keenly disputed by those, like Makins, who believed that the prognosis for the limb was improved by tying the veins.) It was also found that extensive fasciotomy and hyperbaric oxygen were valuable adjuncts.

VIETNAM

By this time, it could be stated in a semi-official report 'the repair of vascular injuries is now routine'[4]. And this was due to technical surgical advances, more and better-trained surgeons, rapid casualty evacuation to properly equipped bases, and new instruments and antibiotics. The vessel wound itself had to be debrided (very conservatively) and irrigated, then managed by suture, resection and anastomosis or vein graft, with insertion of a plastic prosthesis as the last resort, with delayed primary closure of the main wound. The amputation rate after repair now fell to 8.3 per cent, and this was so impressive that arterial injuries tended to become an indication for internal fixation of fractures for stabilization. The amputation rate fell correspondingly. 'Since the Korean War,' wrote King in 1969, 'primary arterial suture has become standard practice in army medical services and as the patients are usually young, the results are good[5].

The nature of the wounds was changing. Landmine injury of the foot was now common; and the Armalite rifle wound caused so much more internal destruction than the old rifle bullet that even the smallest wound had to be explored thoroughly. However, the basic principles remained; adequate longitudinal skin and fascial incision, removal of dead and damaged bone and foreign bodies, delayed primary or secondary suture or split-skin grafting. There was now a trend to cleaning and replacing even quite loose bone fragments, for they would be needed. In joint injuries the synovium, but not the skin, was closed primarily, after debridement and copious irrigation. (Irrigation, always a feature of elective orthopaedic surgery in the USA, is even more important in the management of war wounds.) Bivalved casts were frequently used.

Early in the war, there was considerable reluctance to use internal fixation for compound fractures. Later, it came to be seen, especially by Australian surgeons, that fixation offered great advantages. It was felt that the wound could be closed by primary suture if not severely contaminated and there was no undue tension and that, if internal fixation were required for stability, it could be done at the time of the primary excision, even for late contaminated cases (though these could not be sutured immediately.) McNeur had a very high success rate – 1 infection in 31 cases of fixation[6].

This marked a reversal of the traditional view that metal insertion promoted osteomyelitis; rather, it seemed that the immobilization minimized this risk, also that (in civil life) severe osteomyelitis in compound fractures was three times greater in patients treated conservatively than when primary osteosynthesis was used[7]. McNeur stated unequivocally that internal fixation reduced infection, and that an infected stable fracture was much better than an infected unstable one, the same justification that Küntscher had advanced for his medullary nailing of borderline cases in World War II.

The only indications for amputation in the field in Vietnam were massive uncontrollable gas gangrene, to save life, overwhelming infection, vascular gangrene and severe mangling. It was performed as low as possible and left open. Laminectomy was routine for penetrating spinal wounds with neurological deficit, and for closed injuries with a deficit that was not improving.

Vietnam expanded the rapid direct air evacuation first practised on a large scale in Korea, from an advanced aid station, or even the battlefield, to a base hospital. It was now possible for a casualty to have definitive surgery less than an hour from wounding, and also to be directed to the appropriate facility. It was an immense change from a semi-official stricture of 1966: 'In the surgery of war wounds, primary closure must never be done[8].'

REFERENCES

1. Fisher, D. (1953). Delayed primary closure of Korean War wounds. *Surg. Gynaecol. Obstet.*, **96**, 696

2. DeBakey, M.E. and Simeone, F.A. (1958). Battle injuries of the arteries in World War II. *Ann. Surg.*, **123**, 534

3. Schramek, A. and Hashmonai, M. (1977). Vascular injuries in the extremities in battle casualties. *Brit. J. Surg.*, **64**, 644

4. Elton, R.C. (1971). Orthopaedic war surgery, 85th Evacuation Hospital, Viet Nam 1968. *J. Bone Jt. Surg.* (abstract) **53A**, 1231

5. King, K.F. (1969). Orthopaedic aspects of war wounds in South Vietnam. *J. Bone Jt. Surg.*, **51B**, 112

6. McNeur, J.C. (1970). The management of open skeletal trauma with particular reference to internal fixation. *J. Bone Jt. Surg.*, **52B**, 54

7. Holstad, H.A. (1962). Primary osteosynthesis versus conservative treatment of compound fractures of long tubular bones. *J. Oslo City Hosp.*, **12**, 225

8. Heaton, L.D. *et al.* (1966). Military Surgical Practices of the United States Army in Viet Nam. In *Current Problems in Surgery*. (Chicago Year Book Medical Publishers)

Index